Jennie Longbottom
MSc BSc MCSP MBAcC
Alied Tutor

Clinical Mastery
in the Treatment
of Myofascial Pain

Senior Acquisitions
Development Edi
Senior Marketin
Project Editor:
Artwork: Kir
Composit
Printer:

Co

Clinical M
in the Treatment
of Myofascial Pain

Lucy Whyte Ferguson, DC
Robert Gerwin, MD
With Contributors

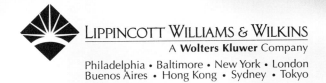

LIPPINCOTT WILLIAMS & WILKINS
A **Wolters Kluwer** Company

Philadelphia • Baltimore • New York • London
Buenos Aires • Hong Kong • Sydney • Tokyo

Editor: *Pete Darcy*
ors: *David Payne, Betsy Dilernia*
g Manager: *Christen DeMarco*
Christina Remsberg
Battista
r: *Maryland Composition*
ourier-Kendallville

Printed in the United States of America

Library of Congress Cataloging-in-Publication Data

Clinical mastery in the treatment of myofascial pain [edited by] Lucy
    Whyte-Ferguson, Robert Gerwin.
        p.; cm.
    Includes bibliographical references and index.
    ISBN 0-683-30620-0
    1. Myofascial pain syndromes. I. Whyte-Ferguson, Lucy. II. Gerwin, Robert, 1938–
    [DNLM: 1. Myofascial Pain Syndromes—rehabilitation. 2. Exercise Therapy.
    3. Myofascial Pain Syndromes—diagnosis. 4. Pain—rehabilitation. 5. Self Care, WE 500
    C6415 2005]
    RC927.3.C557 2005
    616.7′4–dc22

                                                                                2004048593

The publishers have made every effort to trace the copyright holders for borrowed material. If they have inadvertently overlooked any, they will be pleased to make the necessary arrangements at the first opportunity.

To purchase additional copies of this book, call our customer service department at **(800) 638-3030** or fax orders to **(301) 824-7390.** For other book services, including chapter reprints and large quantity sales, ask for the Special Sales department.

For all other calls originating outside of the United States, please call **(301)714-2324.**

Visit Lippincott Williams & Wilkins on the Internet: http://www.lww.com. Lippincott Williams & Wilkins customer service representatives are available from 8:30 am to 6:00 pm, EST, Monday through Friday, for telephone access.

04 05 06 07 08 09
1 2 3 4 5 6 7 8 9 1

DEDICATION

We dedicate this book to Dr. Janet G. Travell,
in memorium, and to Dr. David G. Simons, our mentors,
our inspiration, our guides, and our friends.
Their dedication to myofascial pain medicine opened
a path that we and others have followed.
Without their enormous dedication, little of what we are doing would be possible.
We also dedicate this book to our spouses, Allen Ferguson and Brenda I. Gerwin.

Contributors

Gregory M. Berkoff, DC
Private Practice
La Jolla Village Family Medical Group
La Jolla, California

Jan Dommerholt, PT, MPS, FAAPM
Director of Rehabilitation Services
Pain and Rehabilitation Medicine
Janet G. Travell MD Seminar
International Myopain Academy
Bethesda, Maryland

James Fricton, DDSs, MS
Professor
Division of TMD and Orofacial Pain
University of Minnesota School of Dentistry
Minneapolis, Minnesota

Robert Gerwin, MD
Private Practice
Pain and Rehabilitation Medicine
Bethesda, Maryland

Shannon P. Goossen, AP, LMT, CMTPT
Comprehensive Myofascial Therapy Associates
Jacksonville, Florida

Christian Gröbli, PT
Schmerzmedizin und Rehabilitation
Winterthur, Switzerland

Rhonda Kotarinos, MS, PT
Private Practice
Oakbrook Terrace, Illinois

Richard M. Kushner, DPM
American Board of Disability Analysts
Private Practice
New York, New York

Mary L. Maloney, PT
Team Rehab
Danbury, Connecticut

Lewis E. Mock, DC
Private Practice
Colorado Springs, Colorado

Jill Maloney Newman, P.T.
Team Rehab
Danbury, Connecticut

Margaret W. Royson, DO, MSW
Diplomate, American Board of Family Practice
Private Practice
Albuquerque, New Mexico

Michael Schneider, DC, PhD (candidate)
Private Practice
Pittsburgh, Pennsylvania

Roberta F. Shapiro, DO, FAAPMR
Albert Einstein College of Medicine
Private Practice
New York, New York

Nancy L. Shaw, CMTPT, CMTPT, MS
Director
Myofascial Pain Treatment Center
Springfield, Virginia

Arnold Graham Smith, MD, FRCS, FACS
Private Practice
Jacksonville, Florida

Tasso G. Spanos, BS, CMTPT
Center for Pain Management
Pittsburgh, Pennsylvania
Pittsburgh School of Pain Management
Pittsburgh, Pennsylvania

Lucy Whyte Ferguson, DC
Private Practice
Taos/El Prado, New Mexico

Foreword

The opportunity to contribute this foreword is a special pleasure for me because it marks a major step ahead in the maturation of the field of myofascial trigger points. Lucy Whyte Ferguson and Robert Gerwin have collaborated beautifully to sandwich between these two covers a stellar assembly of outstanding pioneers in the clinical practice of myofascial trigger points, almost all of whom I know personally. They represent the cream of the crop. We are beginning to assume the proportions of a critical mass for sustained progress in this field. In these days of *increasingly* rapid progress and explosion of knowledge, one must run fast just to stand still.

Lucy's specific role, to elucidate the relationship between myofascial and articular dysfunction, helped them reach a goal toward which we have been striving for many years: to describe the effective integration of articular dysfunctions and myofascial trigger points in the management of musculoskeletal problems. The 1983 edition of Volume 1 of *Myofascial Pain and Dysfunction: The Trigger Point Manual* bypassed the integration of articular dysfunctions and myofascial trigger points except in the area of temporomandibular dysfunction. The 1992 edition of Volume 2 noted articular dysfunction as a related condition to be considered. The 1999 (second) edition of Volume 1 tried to call specific attention to the importance of articular dysfunction in relation to myofascial trigger points in many muscles. In this new book, for example, Chapter 3: "Neck Pain and Restriction Following Whiplash," masterfully integrates identification and treatment of both articular dysfunctions and myofascial trigger points.

A survey of the current conventional literature on patients with whiplash injury makes it clear that there is serious distress and perplexity concerning the lack of understanding as to what is causing the prolongation of pain and dysfunction, that there is distress over the poor therapeutic results generally obtained in many of these patients with whiplash injury, and that there is almost a total lack of competent recognition of the combined effects of myofascial trigger points and articular dysfunctions in patients with whiplash injury. The last point can be made regarding pain in many other regions of the body that are covered in this book, including headache and low back pain. This volume fills these voids remarkably well. We hope that more medical training programs and research investigators will get and promote the message of this book. Of the three chapters that I reviewed in detail, all integrated myofascial trigger points and articular dysfunction issues so seamlessly and completely that one wonders whether the title of the book should not include the integration of these two medical disciplines.

Do not overlook the Preface. The rest of the book tells you what to do. The preface tells you why and how to do it. Lucy first encountered Janet Travell at a dental seminar in Bethesda, Maryland, in 1983, where Janet presented and demonstrated the treatment of myofascial trigger points. Janet was a master clinician with a genius mind and a flair for fascinating clinical demonstrations. She was inspired by her father, who was a pioneering physician and an accomplished amateur magician. Lucy was literally stunned by the realization that myofascial pain was really a missing piece of the puzzle of pain that explained a lot of what she had been seeing in her patients. I had experienced a quite similar revelation with my first exposure to a Janet Travell presentation/demonstration some 20 years earlier. That experience changed the course of my life as well.

Bob Gerwin came under the spell of Dr. Travell when he agreed to help her write a clinical paper on myofascial trigger points, which led him to become one of the early outstanding and dedicated pioneers in this field. This intense advanced course from her on meticulous attention to detail and insistence on statements that are clear and unambiguous has stood him in good stead through the years. Janet and Bob were soon exchanging consultations based on Bob's expertise as a neurologist. As early as 1991, he published a trail-blazing paper in a pain journal on the present and future role of myofascial trigger points in pain management from the perspective of a specialist in myofascial pain. The chapters in this book have benefited greatly from his mature judgment and dedication that is based on his early inspiration and training from the master.

Lucy attended more Travell presentations, began to integrate myofascial trigger point concepts into her clinical practice, and began to exchange difficult-patient referrals with Janet and with Bob Gerwin—a fruitful learning experience for all. By the late 1980s, Lucy was being invited to present at myofascial trigger point seminars. Soon both Bob and Lucy were involved in hands-on training seminars. Nothing stimulates learning a subject more than the teaching of it. Bob continued to be a leader in the field, with an additional biennial series of international seminars, FOCUS ON PAIN, that emphasized the role of myofascial trigger points.

At one point, Lucy canceled an entire week of patients to attend (and it turned out, participate in) the recording of videotapes of Dr. Travell demonstrating the diagnosis and treatment of myofascial trigger points in muscles throughout the body. Janet loved to teach, and Lucy was an eager sponge. I providentially had a comparable experience with Janet in the early 1970s, some 20 years earlier, that permanently changed my concept of the practice of medicine.

The Preface clearly warns of something that the clinical achievements of the other authors of this volume have demonstrated so eloquently: it takes many years of dedicated learning and practice to become truly proficient in the complexities of this subject. The preface also promises that each chapter is a 5-course meal: conventional treatments, contribution of the myofascial (integrated with an articular) approach, case histories, discussion of this approach (with understanding of basic mechanisms and serious consideration of the cause of the pain), and finally, a summary treat-

ment protocol (but fortunately NOT a cookbook approach). When I first encountered this outline, the thought struck me, "What a lofty goal!" It made me curious to see how well it was fulfilled. To my delight, the chapters that I reviewed in detail exceeded my hopes, and the commitment had been fulfilled masterfully. Clinician readers are encouraged to enjoy and digest the many gourmet meals offered in this volume. When well digested and applied, they can nurture your practice and greatly benefit your patients.

David G. Simons, MD
Coauthor of
Travell & Simons' Myofascial Pain and Dysfunction:
The Trigger Point Manual

ORIGIN

This text grows out of the contagious enthusiasm and dedication of Janet Travell, MD, and David Simons, MD, who devoted so much of their lives to research, writing, and teaching about myofascial pain and dysfunction. Many of the contributors to this text have been extremely fortunate to have had the experience of learning from them. We saw how our practices were literally revolutionized by what we learned. We attained a better and more precise understanding of the origins of pain experienced by our patients, and we increased our skills in relieving that pain many-fold. It took years to become proficient in integrating the concepts of myofascial pain management into our examination and treatment procedures and to develop reliable treatment protocols. As our skills increased, we were able to help more patients, with ever more complex pain conditions, and more efficiently. Nevertheless, each time we felt more competent, we were challenged by a patient with a new complex pain problem. The gratitude we felt for being taught by Drs. Travell and Simons and by our challenging patients then translated into an understanding that we had a similar responsibility to pass on to others what we had learned. We realized that although we could each help a certain number of individuals through direct examination and care, we could help many more by sharing our learning with other health practitioners.

This book does not replace the seminal texts <u>Myofascial Pain and Dysfunction: The Trigger Point Manual</u>, (Volume 1, 2nd edition, and Volume 2). Those volumes are the building blocks on which our treatment approaches are predicated. We encourage all practitioners interested in myofascial pain to have them in their clinics. They are an invaluable resource for the clinician. Despite our years of training and clinical experience, we find ourselves referring to them quite regularly.

GOALS

This book developed out of three distinct ideas. First, we wanted to pass on what we and our colleagues have learned, to assist a larger number of pain practitioners in the development of effective rehabilitation strategies. Second, we wanted to save other practitioners the lengthy and arduous process of discovering by trial and error how to apply the techniques of Drs. Travell and Simons in the management of specific pain problems. Third, in recognition of the limitations of our own experience and skills, we have drawn on the knowledge and skills of our colleagues, who have unique talents and who have applied the concepts of myofascial

medicine to their specific areas of expertise. Because we, the editors, have already been able to improve our own clinical skills in treating a variety of conditions by learning from our colleagues (including the contributors to this book), we are excited about presenting this information to our readers and are confident of its usefulness.

A fourth goal took shape as the book developed. By providing a working definition of a comprehensive myofascial and articular approach to a particular pain problem, we hope to promote research that will accurately assess the effectiveness of this care. The concept of referred pain is key to accurate diagnosis and treatment of myofascial pain and also is key to accurately focusing research on efficacy. For example, patients often fail to experience lasting relief from trigger point injections that are performed only on the tender spots in the area of referred pain, rather than on the trigger points in muscles that are the source of that pain and are often located elsewhere. This is a diagnostic failure and precludes effective treatment. Likewise, studies of the effectiveness of trigger point injections in treatment of low back pain will produce misleading results if the areas examined and treated are restricted to the low back. Low back pain frequently is referred pain from trigger points in muscles located elsewhere. Joint dysfunction is also a frequent source of low back pain and is a perpetuating factor for myofascial pain. Assessment and treatment of joint dysfunction is, therefore, included in our treatment protocol for low back pain. It should be a consideration in research projects that study the effectiveness of the combined myofascial and articular approach. We hope that this text also serves as a resource for clinical researchers, and we encourage efforts to assess the efficacy of these approaches.

COMPREHENSIVE ASSESSMENT FOCUS

In the tradition of Janet Travell's commitment to thorough and detailed evaluation of patients, we intend with this book to provide practitioners with tools to aid in careful patient assessment. As therapists and practitioners, we may not be able to spend an hour or two talking with the patient on the first visit, as Dr. Travell was known to do. Nevertheless, we need to allow enough time to truly listen and assist them in exploring factors that may lead to more effective diagnosis and treatment. In this age of time-limited managed health care, we are asked to develop a short-cut thought process analogous to a digitized computer process or to the algorithms that are developed for clinical decision-making. The patient either has this or that, yes or no, and thus the course of care is dictated. Although algorithms are useful in clinical decision-making, it is important to have a broad and inclusive thought process, to see the big picture, because elements that constitute the big picture may provide precisely the critical information needed to discover why previous care has not been fully effective.

An example of Dr. Travell's comprehensive approach is her examination of a runner with chronic neck and upper back pain and a history of numerous failed treatment interventions. Not only did she identify trigger points in the scalene muscles that reproduced his neck and upper back pain, she also observed that the runner did not use his diaphragm properly in breathing. He was therefore overloading the scalene muscles, which are accessory muscles of respiration. She could focus the treatment process to both alleviate the source of the pain and treat a critically important perpetuating factor, because she did a comprehensive evaluation.

Moreover, to get the big picture, we need to perform more than a regional examination. An everyday occurrence in our practices is finding that problems in the back or pelvis have an impact on problems in the head, neck, and shoulder. The book is organized around specific pain problems such as headache, pelvic pain, or heel pain. The skilled clinician needs to understand how these problems interrelate. For example, it may be difficult to strengthen a knee when there is a hip problem that causes weakness of hip and knee flexor muscles. It may be difficult to address chronic neck pain when a myofascial disorder pulls the shoulder forward, putting excessive stress on the neck. As we learn to integrate the myofascial and articular aspects of dysfunction into our approach, our ability to help the patient with each of these pain conditions will be enhanced. We will also be able to more easily develop successful treatment approaches.

THE IMPORTANCE OF PATIENT RAPPORT

Technical proficiency and taking a broad and inclusive approach with our patients is not sufficient. We also have to become part of the healing process for our patients. There was something more to Dr. Travell's evaluations than taking a history. She was willing to travel to the terrain inhabited by the patient with his or her pain. She was willing to sit as a witness to patients' suffering, to listen to how they experience pain and how it affects their lives. Touch was also very important for Dr. Travell. When her knowledgeable fingers found tender trigger points and reproduced the pain complaint, patients were both surprised and relieved that someone finally understood their pain. Trust and hope were established in this first encounter. Her touch in examining the patient initiated the healing process.

When we work at our best, we can recognize the same rapport that develops between ourselves and our patients. We have to be willing to "go there," and the rewards are well worth the effort. An example from Dr. Whyte Ferguson's practice:

A patient suffered from highly debilitating pain and anxiety, and his back or neck frequently "went out" not long after treatment. Besides receiving treatment of his neck and back muscle and joint dysfunction, he was taught stretching techniques, proper body mechanics, and better breathing and relaxation approaches, but his condition remained volatile. One day he came for treatment in a very agitated state. I felt certain that, no matter what I did in treatment, he would feel the same within half an hour after he left the office as he did when he entered. I told him I was "giving up." I asked him to help me to look further into his situation to discover clues that might help us. When asked to describe how he was feeling at that moment, he said that he felt very agitated and out of control of his life and very distressed by this. When asked whether he could remember any other time or the first time that he had felt this way, he thought and then replied that he had felt just this same way one summer when he was picked up and brought home from summer camp because his father had died and was told, "Now you are the man of the family." This revelation became the key to the patient's healing. He sought counseling and was slowly able to reclaim his life. He told me later how grateful he was that I "gave up" that day. I could have remained more removed from his situation and could simply have said that his emotional state was interfering with his response to treatment. It made a difference that I was willing to "go there" with him and clearly wanted to help.

We do not suggest that the clinician must identify strongly with the patient's problems and pain, but that the most effective clinicians are those who listen well to their patients. If we can work together to discover the sources of the patient's pain and the factors that have been perpetuating that pain, our efforts are likely to be more beneficial and more cost-effective. We can avoid the pitfall of blaming our difficult patients when they fail to respond to our care. Our listening and problem-solving skills are essential and often can help individuals with chronic disabilities to reclaim their lives. This is a central aspect of the legacy derived from the work of Janet Travell and David Simons.

COLLABORATIVE APPROACH

Comprehensive management of chronic pain requires an understanding of how to work with other health care professionals as a team, whether under one roof or in separate offices. In a sense, this text is the outgrowth of just such collaboration. Those of us who worked in the greater Washington, D.C. area and had received training in diagnosis and management of myofascial pain syndromes from Dr. Janet Travell often sent our most challenging patients to each other for assistance in evaluation and treatment. We learned a tremendous amount by seeing what other health professionals discovered about our patients, and by seeing the effectiveness of their treatments. As a chiropractor, Lucy Whyte Ferguson learned how much trigger point injections could help with treatment of muscles that had not released with manual techniques. Bob Gerwin, a neurologist, developed a keen interest in the understanding of joint dysfunction because he saw how this affected his patients. We both saw the usefulness of working with trained physical therapists, certified trigger point myotherapists or neuromuscular therapists, dentists, psychologists, and others in the medical community. Despite our very different backgrounds, as we delved into the myofascial pain problems of our patients, we found that our approaches overlapped more and more. We adapted and came to speak a common language, so that the protocols developed by each one of us made sense to all of us. This book therefore attempts to communicate in this common language. We define those terms that are particular to each profession so that they can be understood by all. The interdisciplinary nature of this book reflects the developing interdisciplinary field of myofascial pain management.

REDEFINING THE PROBLEM

A myofascial approach dramatically changes the way we diagnose and treat most common pain conditions. In fact, this change is often so significant that it alters how we define the problem that we are treating. For example, the fact that myofascial pain can serve as a trigger in some kinds of migraine headache alters how we define and classify headaches. The fact that myofascial treatment can alter the course of care when treating both tendonitis of the elbow and plantar fasciitis raises the possibility that the tenderness may arise primarily as a referral phenomenon from trigger points rather than arising from true tissue inflammation. Similarly, the fact that treating abnormal joint mechanics and shortened muscles can improve a "frozen shoulder" raises doubts that adhesions or a tightened joint capsule are the critical pathologic entities in this disorder. Most of the chapters in this text explore the important issue of redefining the painful presenting condition.

COMPREHENSIVE TREATMENT PROTOCOLS

Treatment of myofascial pain that is based on only a partial understanding of the factors behind trigger points is ineffective; therefore, we stress the importance of developing and refining treatment protocols that are comprehensive, and that consider the multiple factors that can be involved in the initiation and perpetuation of the patient's pain. This text is a step toward developing these comprehensive protocols, for the purposes of both providing a wide range of practitioners with treatment techniques that we have found successful and, as mentioned, to encourage studies that can evaluate their effectiveness. Although the treatment protocols at the end of each chapter attempt to distill the approach suggested in the chapter, they should not be used as a "cookbook" approach to treatment. Rather, the reader should recognize that pain is often a complex problem and presents unexpected challenges for which no formulaic approach will suffice.

ORGANIZATION AND FEATURES

This book addresses the most common pain problems that we see in our own practices. It is structured so that each chapter addresses a particular pain problem in a particular region of the body, beginning with the head and progressing downward. Thus, the book opens with a chapter on headache and ends with a chapter on heel pain. Each chapter begins by considering the conventional treatment approaches for the particular type of pain problem, and discusses the ways in which a myofascial medicine approach may differ from or enhance current conventional care. Case histories are presented to illustrate this approach. Each chapter then thoroughly discusses this approach. Listed below are the key chapter features:

- Chapter outline—provides a quick overview of the contents of each chapter

- Case history—relates real-life patient cases and the treatment provided by the therapist

- Technique box—presents information on specific techniques to treat myofascial pain

- Treatment protocol—provides step-by-step guidelines on treating a particular condition

- Focus on manual myofascial release techniques—each chapter includes extensive discussion of how to integrate manual myofascial release techniques into the treatment of myofascial pain, either in the body of the chapter or in a special Manual Myofascial Release Technique section at the end of the chapter.

FINAL NOTE

The usefulness of myofascial concepts in diagnosis and treatment is confirmed in our practices on a daily basis. When we elicit the patient's pain during the examination, we can usually develop an effective treatment plan. Even if we cannot elicit the pain, we can treat the muscles most likely to be the sources of that pain, based on the patient's history and the pain pattern. Therefore, in each treatment session, we test a clinical hypothesis and we confirm the usefulness of the myofascial/articular approach. It is our hope that the reader will find this text useful in a similar way, to help better focus the diagnostic process, suggest effective treatment, and identify important perpetuating factors. We hope that clinicians will find that these treatment approaches prove to be useful on a daily basis with their own patients. We encourage others to build on our efforts and further the development of this remarkable field of health care.

Editor's Note on the Nature of the Trigger Point

Robert Gerwin, MD

Myofascial pain syndrome (MPS) is a myalgic condition characterized by local and referred pain that originates in a myofascial trigger point. The term *myofascial trigger point* was coined to describe a hardened band within the muscle on which there is a zone of intense pain. The trigger point has two clinical attributes that must be explained for there to be a more complete understanding of the nature of myofascial pain. One attribute is a motor dysfunction of the muscle that is characterized by a constant, discrete hardness within the muscle. It is usually palpable as a taut band or as a nodule within the muscle. The other attribute is a sensory abnormality that is characterized primarily by pain. The pain can be both local to the site of the muscular abnormality and referred to another part of the body. The hardness within the muscle or the taut band is a constant feature of the trigger point and can be present in the absence of pain. The taut band appears to be a primary muscle response to some kind of stress, whether metabolic or physical. Ischemia may be an important factor in the development of the taut band, if not a dominant factor.

The taut band and pain are both dynamic features of the muscle trigger point, in that they vary in their presence and activity from being spontaneously painful to being quiescent, or painful only when stimulated mechanically or metabolically. The taut band itself has unique characteristics not found in normal muscle. For example, it is persistently hard. It is considered to be a contracted band of muscle. It also has the additional property of contracting sharply when mechanically stimulated, for example, by plucking it manually or by putting a needle into it.

The mechanism that underlies development of the taut band is not known, but altered activity of the motor endplate, or neuromuscular junction, is best supported by the literature. Increase in acetylcholine (ACh) release, upregulation of acetylcholine receptor (AChR) activity and of the number of receptors, and depression of acetylcholinesterase (AChE) activity are consistent with known mechanisms of end plate function, and well explain the changes in end plate activity that occur in the myofascial trigger point. Pain develops after muscle hardening, and occurs because of the release of substances, such as bradykinin and K^+, from the trigger point, and from the presence in the extracellular fluid around the trigger point of protons from the acidic milieu that occurs in ischemia and in exercise. These substances activate peripheral nociceptors and also induce the release of calcitonin gene-related peptide (CGRP) from the motor nerve terminal, which in turn increases end plate activity and enhances sensory nerve activation.

Certain features of the myofascial trigger point relevant to the problem of how it develops and is maintained are well established. Likewise, certain pathophysiologic changes in exercised muscle are known that are relevant to the development of muscle pain and myofascial pain syndromes. Finally, additional aspects of neurophysiology that are well established are relevant to an understanding of the trigger point, particularly to aspects of sympathetic nerve function and of nociceptive sensory receptor activation and modulation.

1. At a clinical level, a taut muscle band may be present without tenderness. However, tenderness is always associated with the taut band. Treatment of the tender, taut band by injection of local anesthetic, dry needling without anesthetic, or by manual compression and stretching of the tender area on the taut band without use of any anesthetic results in clinically evident softening of the taut band and an increase in the pressure pain threshold (PPT) not seen in a control, nontender muscle.

2. A marked increase in the frequency of miniature end plate potential activity is found at the point of maximum tenderness in the taut band in the human and in the neuromuscular junction end plate zone of the taut band in the rabbit model.

3. Areas of intense focal sarcomere contraction have been described in the muscles of animals with naturally occurring trigger points, and in animals in which AChE activity has been pharmacologically blocked or inhibited. In studies in which AChE was blocked or inhibited, supercontraction of sarcomeres occurred at the neuromuscular junction.

4. Studies by Jay Shah and associates at the National Institutes of Health indicate that a number of biochemical alterations are found by microdialysis sampling techniques at the active trigger point site. Among the changes found are elevated calcitonin gene-related peptide (CGRP) levels, and lowered pH when compared with inactive (asymptomatic) trigger points and normal controls.

5. Exercise under ischemic conditions and eccentric muscle exercise result in muscle pain. Delayed-onset muscle soreness occurs after ischemic exercise. Muscle that is maximally eccentrically contracted shows evidence of muscle fiber destruction similar to changes seen in exercised ischemic muscle. Unaccustomed eccentric exercise (forced lengthening of a contracting muscle) causes immediate damage to muscle and delayed muscle soreness in the succeeding days. Muscle soreness is

the result of local muscle damage, inflammatory changes, and nociceptor sensitization. Metabolic disorders that impair energy production in muscle are associated with exercise-induced muscle pain.

6. Tendon organs (sensory receptors located at the muscle–tendon junction in skeletal muscle) are responsive to active tension generated by contractions of groups of motor units. They are particularly sensitive to active muscle force but also respond to muscle stretch.

7. Intramuscular hypoperfusion occurs in fibromyalgia and myofascial pain patients.

8. Hypoxia (extremely low pO_2) is associated with the trigger point, compatible with the concept of hypoperfusion, which results in hypoxia.

9. Persons with work-related trapezius myalgia have a deficit of cytochrome C oxidase, suggestive of an energy crisis within the muscle, perhaps associated with mitochondrial dysfunction. This correlates with reports of low levels of adenosine triphosphate (ATP) and adenosine diphosphate (ADP) in persons with trapezius myalgia. A high degree of mitochondrial disorganization also was seen in the muscles of these persons. Moreover, there was a decrease in the number of capillaries per fiber area in these subjects. These data support the concept of an ischemia-induced energy crisis in the development of exercise-induced muscle pain.

10. Alpha-adrenergic agonists that inhibit sympathetic nerve activation reduce abnormal miniature end plate activity by approximately 60%.

These points, taken together, suggest that a possible initiating event in myofascial pain syndrome is exercise under conditions that limit the availability of an energy supply, possibly by the development of high pressures within the contracting muscles that result in vascular constriction or closure and the subsequent development of muscular ischemia. The increase in CGRP that can arise as a result of ischemia-induced muscle injury could result in an apparent increase in acetylcholine receptor activity and an inhibition of acetylcholinesterase activity, resulting in the development of the taut bands seen in myofascial pain syndrome. The mechanism whereby the sympathetic nervous system (SNS) modulates end plate noise may be explained as adrenergic activity–modulated release of ACh from the motor nerve terminal. The SNS could produce some degree of vasoconstriction that is focally superimposed on other factors that predispose to focal hypoperfusion, and thereby turn a marginal state of ischemia into a pathologic state.

In summary, current literature supports the hypothesis that the initial event in trigger point formation is an acute or repeated muscle overload such as eccentric or maximal contraction, with contractile forces distributed irregularly through a hypoperfused muscle. Focal areas of muscle injury and ischemia develop, causing low tissue pH and hypoxia. Initial motor nerve–induced release of ACh and CGRP increases AChR function. CGRP and low pH both inhibit AChE activity, increasing the synaptic concentration of ACh. CGRP also causes upregulation of AChR. Moreover, sympathetic activation of alpha-adrenoreceptors on the motor nerve synaptic terminal can increase ACh release. Increased ACh concentration, and more and widespread AChR, produce abnormal end plate noise (increased miniature end plate potential frequency), and cause intense, focal sarcomere compression under the end plate, which becomes self-sustaining. Such compression further constricts local capillaries, increasing hypoperfusion and ischemia. Sympathetic activity increases capillary contraction and ischemia. The result is focal hardness in muscle, or taut band development. Muscle fiber injury releases bradykinin, K^+, cytokines, and other substances that activate and sensitize muscle nociceptors, causing pain.

Understanding this hypothetical model of the myofascial trigger point is important for a number of reasons. The model incorporates currently known muscle physiology, and explains clinical features and research findings that had not been understood before. For example, it describes a physiologic mechanism whereby the sympathetic nervous system modulates miniature end plate activity to produce what Simons called "end plate activity" at the trigger point. It challenges us to prove or disprove elements of the model, stimulating research into the nature of muscle pathology, biochemistry, and physiology. It challenges us to examine our clinical experience critically to better understand the nature of muscle dysfunction. We must ask whether this model meets the test of clinical relevance. We must ask whether our clinical findings are best explained by this model. We still do not fully understand the nature of the trigger point and how it develops and how it is inactivated. We do not know how needling the trigger point, compressing the trigger point, or stretching it, inactivates it and reduces pain. Nonetheless, the treatment principles described in the following chapters have been extremely useful in treatment.

Drs. Janet Travell and David Simons both combined the search for more effective treatment with persistent inquiry into the mechanism of trigger point formation and dysfunction. We attempt to do the same and hope that this volume contributes to that task.

Acknowledgments

Lucy and Bob: We would like to thank David Payne, our editor, who has patiently guided us in bringing the book together. Kim Battista's illustrations greatly enhance the text, and we are grateful for her suggestions that clarified many points.

Lucy: I would like to acknowledge the support and mentoring I received from Bob Gerwin and the other chapter authors, as well as Brian Whitfield, Mary Silvia, Mayer Burgan, Ben Daitz, Darcy Ward White, and Kirk Manson, colleagues who read my work and encouraged me. I would also like to acknowledge Janet Travell, who read and critiqued an article that later became the Shoulder chapter, and David Simons, who read and critiqued the Hip chapter. Ria and Ralynn Botzler, Dixie Chapian, and Melissa Tiernan provided daily assistance along the way. My children, Jason Russo, Blake, and Andrea Ferguson gave me encouragement and motivation, and Duncan Ferguson's memory was an incentive as well. I would like to thank my friend Dawn Redpath for her great support. Finally, my husband encouraged this creative endeavor every step of the way, over many years, with insight, patience, kindness, and loving support.

Bob: I wish to thank Jan Dommerholt, PT, MPS, who has worked with me for a decade, seeking better ways to understand our patients, to treat our patients, and to communicate these ideas through teaching our colleagues. Lawrence Funt, DDS, first raised the questions posed in this book more than 25 years ago, and introduced me to Drs. Travell and Simons. Ben Daitz, MD, further encouraged the teaching of this material. I have learned a great deal from teaching with Roberta Shapiro, DO. Dr. Siegfried Mense has made untold contributions to our understanding of the field of myofascial pain syndromes. Dr. Jay Shah continues to stimulate our thinking with his current studies into the nature of the trigger point. Drs. Ragi D. Wiygul and John Jarrell have expanded our thinking about chronic pelvic pain syndromes. Maria Giamberadino and Ursula Wesselmann introduced me to the concept of viscerosomatic pain. Many other clinicians, too numerous to name here, have stimulated my thinking or encouraged my continued endeavors in this field. Finally, my wife patiently saw this book develop over the years and encouraged me to continue. Her love and compassion, keen mind and insight, and the courage with which she overcame a life-threatening illness were my real inspirations in writing and editing this book.

Jeffrey Dann PhD, DiplAc
President, Traditional Japanese Acupuncture Foundation
Boulder, Colorado

Richard Finn, CMTPT
Director, Pittsburgh School of Pain Management
Pittsburgh, Pennsylvania

Diane L. Hoffman, PT, DPT
Flagstaff Medical Center
Flagstaff, Arizona

Paul D. Hooper, DC, MPH, MSc
Professor, Southern California University of Health Sciences
Whittier, California

David Scott Lynn
Trainer of Yoga/BodyWork Structural Therapists
Sedona, Arizona

Lucinda J. Mitchell, DC
Chiropractor
Silver Spring, Maryland

Cassandra E. Orem, BS, MS, MA Applied Psychology, RN, CMT
Consultant for Hospital Based Massage and Complimentary Care at St. Joseph's Medical Center
Towson, Maryland

Nancy L. Shaw, MTPT
Myofascial Pain Treatment Center
Springfield, Virginia

Janeen Wallace, DC
Assistant Professor, Clinical Sciences
New York Chiropractic College
Seneca Falls, New York

Contents

1   *Headache*

Robert Gerwin, MD

INTRODUCTION

Headache is a common complaint of patients in all general medical practices. Chronic, frequently occurring, intractable headache is a problem that plagues the patients of headache and pain clinics alike, as well as those seen in general medical clinics. The problem of acute or new headache, which demands urgent evaluation to exclude tumor, hemorrhage, arteritis, or infection, is not included in this discussion, but must be kept in mind as part of the differential diagnosis when there is a change in the pattern of headache. In general, any significant change in headache symptoms within the previous 6 months warrants investigation. Moreover, the possibility that a meningioma can produce chronic symptoms also must be kept in mind. Analgesic rebound headache is an important cause of headache, certainly in the chronic headache patient, and must be considered in every patient with a long history of headache and medication use. However, this chapter focuses on myogenic causes of headache, or headache of muscular origin, and in particular, the frequent, recurring headache, whether called migraine headache (MH) or chronic tension type headache (CTTH or TTH). The focus of this chapter is the contribution of the myofascial trigger point to the development of headache.

Most recurrent tension-type headaches, whether daily or episodic, have their origin in muscle trigger points, and migraine without aura is a frequent accompaniment of TTH. Dietary and emotional triggers of migraine are well known, but migraine without aura also can arise from myofascial trigger points in the muscles of the head, neck, and shoulder region, possibly by activation of the trigemino-vascular system (1). Understanding the nature of the trigger point and referred pain is the key to understanding and treating these headaches. The concept of referred pain best explains the clinical presentation of both tension-type and the migraine without aura headaches. An appreciation of the contribution of myofascial trigger points to the development of headache is central to the development of an effective treatment protocol for headache management. Treatment of myofascial trigger points in the muscles of the shoulder, neck, and head, and correction of the factors that lead to the development and maintenance of trigger points in these muscles, can provide effective management for these difficult headache problems.

BACKGROUND

Diagnosis and Headache Classification

Headache classification remains largely empirical, based on severity, frequency, duration, location, and the associated phenomena of photophobia and phonophobia, nausea, and vomiting. These distinctions break down in day-to-day clinical practice, because there is little to distinguish frequent migraine headache without aura from CTTH. Unilaterality of headache, aggravation of headache by routine physical activity, nausea and vomiting, and photophobia or phonophobia denote the headache as migraine. Unfortunately, these presentations also occur in persons with episodic or chronic tension-type headache, blurring the distinction. Marcus suggested the name *benign recurring headache* for these kinds of headaches (2), a term that is very apt and non-prejudicial as to origin of the headache. Differentiation of headache types for these very similar chronic headaches is found in the International Headache Classification of 1988 (3). The headache classification is an attempt to clarify headache types and to lead to proper treatment based on specific headache cause. This is largely successful. Proper naming or classification of headache certainly influences treatment of headache. However, some leading headache experts point out that epidemiologic studies have failed to find clinical features that distinguish TTH from migraine and have proposed a convergence hypothesis in which the premonitory symptoms can progress through TTH to migraine (4). Factors that are associated with the transformation of episodic migraine to chronic daily headache, including those patients in the chronic posttraumatic headache group, have been studied. They include allergies, asthma, hypothyroidism, hypertension, and alcohol or caffeine consumption (5). Unfortunately, the presence or absence of muscle trigger points that can refer pain to the head, thereby causing headache, have not been studied, and the role of referred pain in headache development and management has not been addressed. The exercise of understanding and naming a headache type is not an idle activity. In this regard, understanding the role of myofascial trigger points in chronic daily TTH adds to the ability to diagnose and manage these most common headache problems.

Migraine with aura stands alone as having very specific intracranial pathophysiologic abnormalities associated with the onset or prodromal phase of the headache, resulting in fortification **scotomata** (positive abnormal phenomena) or **aphasia** and **monoparesis** (negative abnormal phenomena). These phenomena are related to spreading cortical depression, now well demonstrated in humans, and are explained by the mechanism of trigeminovascular system activation and sterile neurogenic edema, a concept that has been well described (6,7). Migraine is complicated by neurologic deficits or aura in more than 30% of patients (8). Migraine with aura is not necessarily associated with myofascial trigger point headaches unless the trigger point activates the trigeminovascular system. Conversely, any severe and recurrent headache is most likely to be a form of migraine and to be responsive to anti-migraine therapy (9 [review article]). In keeping with this concept, frequent headache that has symptoms of both migraine and TTH has been called *transformed migraine* and may occur in as much as 5% of the U.S. population (10). Treatment of headaches that have characteristics of both TTH or muscular headache and migraine headache has largely been pharmacologic, although a recent study showed effectiveness of peripheral nerve stimulation of C1–C3 in refractory transformed migraine, a treatment based on the effect of modulating trigeminocervical complex activity through the upper cervical dorsal horn (11). The headache literature does not address the identification of myofascial trigger points in the muscles of the shoulder and neck region as a source of pain referred to the head and expressed as chronic daily headache and intermittent headache with migrainous features (without aura); nor does it suggest that treatment of the underlying trigger points should be an essential part of treatment.

The relationship of activation of the trigeminovascular system to the cause of chronic daily TTH with intermittent migrainous features (migraine without aura) is much less clear. That both types of headache, CTTH and MH, respond to similar drugs (ergotamine and the "triptans") is compatible with the concept that sterile neurogenic inflammation and edema may play a role in the final pathway to migraine phenomena without aura in the setting of TTH. Nevertheless, it may not be taken to mean that the initiating mechanisms of TTH are in fact related to the mechanisms of neurogenic edema and sterile inflammation, nor does it exclude the possibility that multiple ways exist to reach the final stage of mixed TTH with migrainous features.

Silberstein (12) discusses tension-type headache and commented on its overlap with migraine. He mentions the possibility that there could be a decreased pain threshold, suggesting that TTH is a form of localized fibromyalgia. He further speculates that myofascial input is interpreted as abnormal and that trigger points are produced. His recommended treatment is pharmacologic interruption of the headache cycle to desensitize the affected neurons. He evidently considers myofascial trigger points as secondary and not primary. He does not recommend inactivation of the trigger points whose pain referral patterns may have been the immediate stimulus for headache. Goadsby et al. (9) reject the concept of an overlap of headache types and state that TTH is characterized by the lack of associated features of nausea, vomiting, photophobia, or phonophobia, and that any severe and recurrent headache is most likely a form of migraine.

In a discussion of chronic daily headache, four categories of headache are offered: transformed migraine, CTTH, new daily persistent headache, and hemicrania continua (13). The pathogenesis of these headaches, including CTTH, is considered to include peripheral and central sensitization. Peripheral sensitization of muscle nociceptors in the pericranial muscles is specifically mentioned as a possible mechanism. The possibility that chronic daily headache or CTTH may be a manifestation of referred pain from muscle trigger points is not considered.

Another headache type that has been proposed, but which is controversial and not universally accepted, is cervicogenic headache as described by Sjaastad and Fredriksen (14). This headache type is described as a persistently unilateral headache that spreads to the frontal area about the eye, where it is maximal. It is a non-throbbing, continuous headache that is attributed to structures in the neck. Transient relief occurs with anesthetic blocks of the occipital nerve or the C2 nerve root. The designation has been criticized as attempting to identify a unique headache when there is little evidence for this position. It is also criticized because claims have been made that it is associated with myofascial trigger points, a concept not in the mainstream of current scientific thought (15). In truth, current concepts about the nature of the trigger point were not developed and the reliability of the diagnostic physical examination was not established when that was written. However, as will be pointed out in this chapter, the referral patterns of myofascial trigger points in the posterior cervical and suboccipital muscles reproduce the so-called cervicogenic headache.

Cervicogenic headache has been characterized as headache of cervical spinal origin; however, insofar as different structures in the neck have been implicated, different authors have proposed multiple definitions. Diagnostic blocks have been used to make the diagnosis, but attempts also have been made to identify clinical features that are characteristic of cervicogenic headache. Among the features that have been proposed are postural changes (head-forward posture) and decreased active range of neck motion. The difference in physical findings in persons with so-called cervicogenic headache who have been injured in motor vehicle accidents (MVA) compared with those who had no history of MVA has been looked at in an attempt to further characterize the unique features of cervicogenic headache. Those persons injured in MVA had decreased active range of motion in flexion/extension and rotation, decreased strength and endurance in the neck flexor muscles, and decreased strength of neck extensor muscles, whereas only the strength of the neck flexor muscles was reduced in non-MVA cervicogenic headache sufferers (16). No mention is made in this study of the presence of myofascial trigger points as a finding or as a contributing cause of headache.

Myogenic Headache

Headache caused by a trigger point in the sternocleidomastoid muscle was described by Travell in 1955 (17). Travell expanded this concept a dozen years later with a more comprehensive article that described headache caused by trigger points in the trapezius muscle, the sternocleidomastoid muscle, and the muscles of mastication, and noted the contribution of mechanical stress, including a variety of postural stresses, on the development of trigger points that could lead to headache (18). A full explication of the development of trigger point-induced headache patterns is found in the first volume of the text authored by Travell and Simons, *Myofascial Pain and Dysfunction: The Trigger Point Manual* (19). This text details the referred pain pattern of trigger points in each of the muscles of the head, neck, and shoulder region, doing so as descriptions of single-muscle syndromes. The second edition of this volume (20) clearly relates the trigger points to headache patterns and to current theories of headache genesis. Rogers and Rogers (21) reviewed the topic of headache and myofascial trigger points and stated that "myofascial trigger points in the face, scalp and neck may be a significant etiologic contributor to episodic or chronic tension-type headaches," but they added no new observations or data to further substantiate this position beyond their review of the literature.

Olesen and colleagues were the first to estimate tenderness in the pericranial muscles during a migraine attack, and they found that temporal, masseter, and neck muscles were tender (22–24). They also studied pericranial muscle tenderness in CTTH and correlated lower pressure pain thresholds and increased pericranial electromyographic activity with CTTH (25). Jensen studied 735 subjects from the general population and found 22 with CTTH. Muscle pressure pain thresholds were lower in persons, particularly women, with CTTH than in the general population (26). Central sensitization was considered a significant consequence in maintaining painful input from muscle. However, the concept that referred pain from tender muscles was important in the expression of CTTH was not specifically addressed. Central sensitization, based not only on the data that show that persons with CTTH have pericranial muscle tenderness, but also on the observation that the threshold to other painful stimuli (e.g., electrical pain threshold) also was reduced, has continued to be considered a critical aspect of the pathophysiology of tension-type headaches (27). Duckro (28) studied "myofascial irritation" in posttraumatic headache. He assessed muscle tenderness at seven predetermined sites, palpating muscle with 4-kg/cm² finger pressure for 1 minute, the subject standing throughout. He concluded that muscle tenderness or myofascial irritation was a significant contributing factor to headache, because it was present in a high percentage of migraine and TTH subjects. The study was uncontrolled, muscles were not selected on the basis of reproduction of relevant headache pain, and a standard palpation pressure was used, as has been described in the fibromyalgia literature, regardless of the firmness or depth of the muscle. This study used the term *myofascial* but did not apply the term to the myofascial trigger point as defined by Travell and Simons. It makes the point that many persons with posttraumatic headache have tenderness of cutaneous and subcutaneous tissues (including muscle), but does not relate tenderness to the cause of headache, consider the role of referred pain, or demonstrate that the incidence of muscle tenderness is different in posttraumatic headache than in non–posttraumatic headache.

A recent review of headache (29) mentions myofascial nociception and pericranial tenderness only in relation to TTH, even though it points out that TTH frequently coexist with migraine headache. It does not mention myofascial trigger points or referred pain phenomena in relation to headache. In general, myofascial trigger points have not been recognized as a cause of either TTH or migraine without aura. The most complete discussion of the relation of myofascial trigger points to headache is by Jaeger in the 2nd edition of volume 1 of the text by Simons, Travell, and Simons (20).

In another headache study, muscle hardness is used to describe muscle tension. Hardness was correlated with tenderness. The association of hardness with tenderness could be a description of the tender, taut band of the trigger point, although the authors did not use the term *trigger point*. Muscle hardness was greater in persons with CTTH than in controls and was not restricted to the period of headache, but was found even between headaches (30).

The focus of this chapter is on headache that is caused by muscular trigger points. The proposed mechanism is that the trigger point activates and sensitizes the dorsal horn neurons, resulting not only in hypersensitivity and allodynia, but a local spread of neuronal activation in the dorsal horn that refers pain to distant regions away from the trigger point in a segmental rather than dermatomal pattern. The referral patterns of pain are felt as frontal or parietal or vertex or behind-the-eye headaches. These headaches are very common and likely make up the bulk of the headaches in a community outpatient clinic.

Muscle Tenderness

Studies of tenderness in the pericranial muscles have been done in an attempt to identify the cause of migraine and TTH. As noted above, subjects with TTH have increased tenderness of pericranial muscles even between headaches, which increases during headache. EMG activity of pericranial muscles is also increased between headaches. Pressure pain tolerances and thermal tolerances, normal between headaches, are lowered during headache (31). Subjects with TTH who have myofascial tenderness of the pericranial muscles as determined by manual palpation have a lower pressure pain threshold and a lower pain tolerance than those with headache and no myofascial tenderness (25). These studies suggest that sensitization of the nociceptors occurs in pericranial muscles, and segmental central sensitization as well, which contributes to TTH.

Muscle tenderness in migraine, in episodic, and in chronic TTH have been examined in detail. Tenderness in pericranial muscles is increased in patients with TTH compared with normal subjects and with migraineurs (25,32). Pericranial temporal muscle tenderness is increased during migraine attacks, the increase being ipsilateral to the headache side when it is unilateral (24). However, there is no increase in pericranial, neck, and shoulder muscle tenderness in migraineurs between headache attacks, whereas pericranial muscle tenderness is increased in subjects with episodic and chronic TTH (32). The studies of pericranial muscle tenderness in various headaches have not examined the pericranial muscles for myofascial trigger points and referred pain in the sense that these terms are used and discussed in this chapter. Nonetheless, myofascial trigger points cause pericranial muscle tenderness and cause both TTH and MH directly, through referred pain, by causing central sensitization, and also by activating the trigeminovascular system.

Conventional Therapy

Recurrent TTH, or chronic daily headaches, are notoriously difficult to treat. Conventional treatment of these difficult headache problems can be divided into pharmacologic and nonpharmacologic therapies. Pharmacologic therapy is used for both acute and preventative treatment and consists of simple over-the-counter (OTC) analgesics such as acetaminophen and aspirin, nonsteroidal anti-inflammatory drugs (NSAID) such as ibuprofen, more specific drugs for acute headache such as the triptans and dihydroergotamine, and the prophylactic drugs such as the beta-blockers, calcium channel blockers, and anticonvulsant drugs such as valproic acid, gabapentin, and topiramate. CTTH are often treated with tricyclic antidepressant drugs similar to those used for the treatment of migraine headaches, and they also respond to the triptan drugs as migraine headaches do. Nonpharmacologic therapies include ice packs and heat to the head and neck, biofeedback to relax head and neck muscles and to change the skin temperature of the face and hands, cognitive behavioral therapy and stress management to decrease psychological stressors that result in headache development and persistence, and acupuncture to relax both muscle and psyche, relieve pain, and to eliminate headache.

Acute Headache Therapy

Acute headache treatment addresses both TTH, or headache accepted as muscular in origin, which we have referred to as "myogenic headache," and typical migraine without aura. Migraine in this discussion is limited only to migraine without aura and does not include migraine with aura, which is another type of headache altogether. Tension-type headache alone is more common, but when severe it displays many of the features of acute migraine without aura, namely, increased headache pain with activity, nausea and vomiting, and photophobia and phonophobia. In severe cases, TTH and migraine without aura blend into one headache type. The overlap is more striking when TTH begins unilaterally. In either case, however, the patient may want to lie down in a quiet, dark room, seeking emergency treatment only when the headache is incapacitating and when remedies at hand fail. Emergency treatment of severe CTTH usually consists of administration of an analgesic, either intramuscular ketorolac (an NSAID) or a rapidly acting opiate such as hydrocodone intramuscularly, plus an antiemetic. Emergency departments generally do not treat "muscle spasm" or trigger points that produce acute headache pain.

Acute therapies usually begin with NSAIDS and other simple non-narcotic analgesics. These include aspirin and other rapid-onset NSAIDS such as ibuprofen or naproxen sodium, and acetaminophen. Prescription drugs that are used in the acute treatment of TTH and migraine headache include the non-opiate combinations of aspirin or acetaminophen with caffeine and a sedative such as butalbital, a short-acting barbiturate. Another combination that is often used is isometheptene (a sympathomimetic), acetaminophen, and dichloralphenazone (Midrin, Carnrick Laboratories, Inc., Cedar Knolls, NJ). Muscle relaxants that act on the spinal cord, the brainstem, or the brain may be given. They include the GABA analog baclofen, diazepam (which is also a central nervous system depressant), and cyclobenzaprine, a centrally acting muscle relaxant that also inhibits the release of central nervous system noradrenaline. Their use is empiric, because there are no adequate studies of their efficacy. When these measures fail, the next drug that is used is often a triptan, a number of which are now available for prescription use in tablet form, in an orally disintegrating form, as a nasal spray, or as an injectable. Triptans were developed for treatment of migraine, for which they are very effective, but they are also effective in treatment of myogenic or TTH. Responsiveness of a headache to the triptans cannot be said to be diagnostic of migraine, because TTH also improves with triptan treatment. Triptan drugs have almost entirely replaced ergotamine drugs for the acute management of headache. Though their efficacy is great, they are expensive for use in frequently recurring headache. They also can lead to rebound headache with frequent use and, therefore, should not be used more than 2 or 3 times per week. Triptans are so effective, in fact, that when the headache is occasional, they are the drug of first choice, or the drug to use early in headache treatment if OTC drugs fail to provide immediate relief. Nausea or vomiting is treated symptomatically with anti-emetics such as promethazine or prochlorperazine given orally or by rectal suppository. Gastric motility is often reduced in the prodromal and acute phases of migraine, and a drug such as metoclopramide 10 mg given orally 20 to 30 minutes before other migraine medicine often improves absorption of the medication taken subsequently.

Opiates are frequently the next step in the management of headache. They are usually used as immediate-release, short-acting drugs (length of action, 4–6 hours), combined with aspirin, acetaminophen, or ibuprofen. Taken frequently, as they often are by persons with recurrent daily acute headache, they can cause rebound headache, cognitive impairment, constipation, and dependence. A more recent development in the pharmacologic treatment of recurrent daily acute headaches is the regular use of the slow-release, long-acting forms of oxycodone, morphine, methadone, or fentanyl to eliminate the problems of the short-acting opiates listed above, to eliminate the problem of opiate or drug rebound, and to avoid the complications of acetaminophen or salicylate toxicity. Nonetheless, the chronic use of opiates in any form in headache management remains highly controversial.

As described above, conventional treatment of CTTH or myogenic headache focuses on the elimination of the present headache (acute treatment) while reducing the likelihood of future headache recurrences (preventive treatment). In spite of their frequent occurrence in the population, these headaches are often resistant to treatment, and patients may resort to chronic analgesic drugs, both narcotic and non-narcotic. Current drug treatment, biofeedback, and stress management do not control headache in many persons. A review of treatment for recurrent TTH examined electromyography (EMG) biofeedback, cognitive therapy, and relaxation and found them to be more effective than no treatment (33). Specific trigger point inactivation was not considered in this study. The new interest in the use of botulinum toxin injections of the head and neck fits neatly into the paradigm of trigger point inactivation in CTTH that is the subject of this chapter, but more studies are needed to define the role of this potentially useful treatment. Botulinum toxin as used in the treatment of CTTH can be thought of as a long-lasting trigger point injection.

A practical problem arises when headaches occur almost daily. Many of the headache sufferers with mixed tension-type and migraine headaches have headache most days and treat each daily headache as an acute problem. Treatment of these headaches typically emphasizes drug therapy (34). None of the commonly used protocols for treatment of acute or chronic TTH emphasizes the identification and elimination of muscular trigger points or treatment of cervical spine articular dysfunctions.

Headache Prophylaxis

Prophylactic therapy first of all requires elimination of possibly offending drugs that can cause rebound headache. Conventional therapy of migraine without aura uses pharmacotherapeutic agents such as verapamil (a calcium channel blocker), tricyclic antidepressants, propranolol (a beta-blocker), or valproic acid, gabapentin, or topiramate (anticonvulsants) to prevent recurrences, and other agents as discussed above for acute headache management and to break the headache cycle. It is not yet clear whether these drugs also have a useful role to play in prevention of chronic daily TTH, but they are nevertheless frequently used for this purpose. Psychosocial or cognitive–behavioral therapy is also used (counseling, biofeedback, stress management). Dietary control to identify and avoid ingestion of foods known to trigger or aggravate headache is a common aspect of migraine treatment that has been used, but little studied, in CTTH treatment. Allergy-induced headache, however, is a potential problem in CTTH and deserves insightful questioning and allergy testing in selected cases. Botulinum toxin, currently being evaluated for the treatment of migraine headache, has been shown in preliminary studies to be effective in reducing TTH (35). Conventional headache protocols lack a clearly stated understanding of the need to address the myofascial trigger points in the head, neck, and shoulders that induce or perpetuate the headache in most cases, which are discussed in the next section.

MYOFASCIAL AND ARTICULAR APPROACH TO DIAGNOSIS AND TREATMENT OF HEADACHES.

Clinical observations of patients with chronic, recurrent headache, occurring most every week, and often most every day, have led us to the concept that the myofascial trigger point is the immediate cause of headache in many, if not in most, of these patients, regardless of whether the headache has features commonly associated with migraine without aura (nausea, vomiting, photophobia and phonophobia, dizziness, sweating). This concept has altered our approach to management, particularly to de-emphasizing drug therapy in favor of manual musculoskeletal therapies and biomechanical correction of postural dysfunction, with or without the addition of trigger point inactivation by needling or injection. This in no way implies that pharmacologic therapy, dietary considerations, allergies, and psychological factors need not be considered, but rather that the muscular basis of headache must be reconsidered as a potential treatable cause in every chronic headache patient. Thus, the evaluation of these patients must include a biomechanical assessment of posture and body structure (such as scoliosis), and a careful examination of the muscles of the head, neck, and shoulder for myofascial trigger points. The neck must be examined for segmental articular dysfunction such as an atlantoaxial dysfunction. The history must include evaluation of para-functional oral habits that lead to myofascial trigger point syndromes in the facial muscles (pencil chewing, fingernail biting). The temporomandibular joint (TMJ) must be examined as a source of facial muscle pain.

Overview of Myofascial and Articular Treatment of Headaches

Effect of Myofascial Trigger Point Treatment

Acute unilateral migrainous headache or acute band-like tension headache, with disabling headache, nausea, vomiting, photophobia, dizziness, diaphoresis, and faintness, the kind of headache that disrupts the clinic when the headache sufferer comes unexpectedly and in distress, can be eliminated within minutes by inactivation of the critical myofascial trigger points. This can be done by manual means (trigger point compression followed by stretching, or strain–counterstrain techniques) or by trigger point injection using lidocaine 0.25% (procaine no longer available), or by dry needling of the trigger point (insertion of a needle, commonly an acupuncture needle, into the muscle trigger

CASE 1-1

Patient History and Symptoms

A young woman in her 40s presented with intractable, recurrent migraine headaches that had both a chronic daily component of moderate or greater severity and a frequent disabling component that occurred one or more times each week. Headache was felt in the back of the neck, in the forehead, behind the eyes, and band-like around the head. She had multiple food sensitivities that triggered severe throbbing headache with photophobia and had learned to control her diet rigorously. She also had a chronic sensitivity to light and wore dark glasses and kept her home dimly lit. There was a family history of migraine. She had been given a trial of almost every prophylactic drug commonly used in headache prevention and had only modest benefit, but considerable adverse reactions, with each of them. Analgesics were of little benefit. She had TMJ dysfunction that had been treated with an oral splint. The patient had no history of head trauma, but she was experiencing ongoing severe stress over family issues involving her children.

Examination

She had a round-shouldered, head-forward posture, aggravated by her work as an editor. Myofascial trigger points were present in the pectoral muscles (major and minor) and the trapezius and upper back and shoulder region muscles. Trigger points that reproduced her headaches were found in the sternocleidomastoid, inferior capitis oblique, and the splenii and semispinalis muscles. Acute headache was immediately relieved by inactivation of the active cervical trigger points, and the headache could be reinstituted immediately by manual irritation of the trigger points.

Treatment

Treatment was manual therapy to the affected muscles, inactivation of facial, neck, and shoulder trigger points by trigger point injection with procaine 0.5%, instruction in self-stretching, and correction of the postural dysfunction to eliminate the head-forward posture. Manual therapy included trigger point compression, local muscle stretching, therapeutic stretching of the entire neck and shoulder functional muscle groups, post-isometric contraction/relaxation lengthening of muscle, and reciprocal inhibition. Therapy was given twice each week for 8 weeks. Stabilization and maintenance of a headache-free state was finally achieved by treating a contributing temporomandibular myofascial dysfunction that aggravated the cervical trigger points.

Follow-up

The headaches subsided after a dental specialist provided an oral appliance (mouth splint) to reposition the mandible and relax the muscles of mastication. The neck and shoulder muscles did not develop the trigger points recurrently as they had before use of the mouth splint. She continued with her therapy and exercises, decreasing the frequency of visits for office management. She became headache–free quite soon after the mouth splint was placed and adjusted. The round-shouldered posture could never be fully corrected. Stresses at home, particularly focused on her family, were not addressed. Despite this, she remained headache free, and did not require medication for headache as she had quite regularly before treatment. She did not return for 15 months, at which time she was seen for an acute headache of 3 days. She had stopped wearing her mouth splint and had not returned to the dental specialist. She had also stopped her home exercise program. Home family stresses had been substantially reduced, however. Trigger points that reproduced her headache were found in the sternocleidomastoid and splenius capitis muscles as well as the trapezius muscle. Inactivation of these trigger points by injection of local anesthetic followed by therapeutic muscle stretching eliminated the acute headache within 15 minutes. She was advised to resume her home exercise program and to consult the dental specialist again. Headache again subsided, but has recurred at greater intervals, reduced by about 50%. She later responded well to injections of botulinum toxin into neck and head muscle trigger points and into the corrugator muscle, with a further reduction in headache.

Discussion

This patient exemplifies the major points of muscular or myofascial headaches, or what may be termed "myogenic headaches," that is, headaches that have a major myofascial trigger point factor in their origin. Her headaches were of mixed origin, including a chemical (dietary) component that presumably had vasoactive consequences, a possible hereditary susceptibility, a partial response to acute headache drugs, intensification of her headaches by activation of myofascial trigger points, and the elimination of both the chronic daily headache and the episodic severe headache by treating the musculoskeletal dysfunction and trigger points.

CASE 1-2

Patient History

A 54-year-old woman with a long history of depression was evaluated for a 7-month history of diffuse headache that was disabling to the point that she could no longer work. She had chronic daily headache punctuated 2 or 3 times each week by intense focal headache accompanied by nausea, vomiting, photophobia, and phonophobia. The intense headaches could occur on either side, in the temple, the parietal region, or the frontal region. She had previously been evaluated with a neurologic examination, cervical spine x-rays, and a magnetic resonance imaging (MRI) scan, which were normal. The usual medications used to treat headaches failed to provide relief: tricyclic antidepressants, selective serotonin reuptake inhibiters, NSAIDs, and the triptans. Narcotic drugs also gave no relief. There was no history of trauma.

Examination Findings

The head was forward–positioned and the shoulders rounded, resulting in an exaggerated kyphotic posture with pronounced excessive cervical lordosis. Myofascial trigger points were found in the right trapezius muscle, the right sternocleidomastoid muscle, the right oblique capitis inferior muscle, and bilateral splenius capitis muscles. Trigger points in each of these muscles aggravated part of her headache when manually stimulated.

Treatment

She was treated at the initial evaluation with manual compression of each of the trigger points sequentially, followed by stretching of the neck and shoulder muscles. As the trigger points were inactivated one by one, her headache cleared. She informed the clinician when there was still one trigger point remaining that she could feel, and she indicated when that trigger point was released, and then announced that she was ready to leave. She was headache–free 15 minutes after the onset of treatment.

Follow-up

Her headache recurred approximately 7 hours later. She returned the next day and was treated with trigger point injections of procaine HCl into the trigger points of the muscles previously mentioned. The headache again resolved immediately and did not recur over the next 2 weeks. She complained of neck and shoulder pain, for which she was treated in physical therapy by trigger point compression, local stretching, therapeutic stretching, and assessment and correction of postural dysfunction (head-forward posture and rounded shoulders). Her depression was treated by a psychotherapist but had been resistant to both medication and counseling, and continued to be so. Daily headaches ceased, and she continued to have headaches at a reduced and manageable frequency of two or three each month, controlled with conventional therapy.

Discussion

This case is an example of the need to examine the muscles of the head, neck, and shoulders for trigger points that can refer pain to the head and that can produce both chronic tension-type and migrainous headache. The headaches can be aggravated by stimulating the appropriate trigger points and can be relieved by eliminating them.

---

point without injecting any substance.) The key to rapid elimination of acute headache is the identification of the triggering muscles so that the specific relevant trigger points can be inactivated. The reversal of headache, which occurs as rapidly as the trigger point is inactivated, speaks against neurogenic inflammation and edema as causes of the headache, as one would expect that more time would be needed to reverse those changes.

The chronic phase of treatment to maintain a headache-free-state goes beyond the acute treatment of headache, correcting those factors that perpetuate the trigger points in the relevant muscles. This means correcting mechanical imbalances such as leg length discrepancies, pelvic rotations, scoliosis, forward shoulder postures (with tight pectoral muscles), and addressing ergonomically stressful work conditions. Depression and anger often result in increased activity in myofascial trigger points of the shoulder muscles. In other words, the trigger points have to be eliminated, and steps must be taken to prevent their return.

Obtaining the History

Clues to important aspects of daily activities that stress muscles can be obtained by careful history taking. Cradling the telephone between the shoulder and the ear is a common muscular stress that can be alleviated by the use of hands-free speaker phones or headsets. Less obvious is the constant head-turning to the left by young women who travel on long trips sitting in the right front passenger seat, but who must turn to the left to deal with children in the back seat. Similarly, mothers who drive doing many errands with small children in the back seat stress the muscles of

Addressing Perpetuating Factors: Work Position in Relation to Eye Dominance

An office worker complained of chronic headaches that were present only on the days that she worked. She was found to be right-handed, but left eye dominant. Eye dominance is determined simply by having the patient make a circle of the index finger and thumb and holding it about 18 to 24 inches in front of the eyes. The patient is then asked to look at a target through the circle. By closing one eye at a time, the eye that sees the target through the circle is identified. That is the dominant eye. She had placed all of the written material to which she referred when at the computer on the right-hand side, causing a rotation of the head to the right and a tilt of the head to bring the dominant left eye closer to the reference material. Physical examination identified trigger points relevant to her headache in the left sternocleidomastoid muscle, the right splenius capitis, and right oblique capitis inferior. Moving the written reference material to the left of the keyboard under her dominant eye eliminated the need to rotate her head and resulted in a resolution of her headaches.

the right shoulder and those muscles that rotate the head to the right. Mixed eye–hand dominance can result in a "crooked" neck. Left eye dominance is not rare in right-handed persons, and results in rotation of the head to the right to bring the left eye over reading material or over material being written. Written material placed to the right of the keyboard at the computer produces the same stress on the neck muscles. Moving such material to the left, under the dominant eye, eliminates this kind of stress. (Identification of the dominant eye is discussed in Technique 1.1.) Activities associated with work or hobbies can initiate or perpetuate myofascial trigger points. A potter with left shoulder pain and trigger points in the upper trapezius, infraspinatus, and subscapularis muscles constantly turned her potter's wheel with the left hand. Similarly, a machinist repeatedly developed symptomatic trigger points in the right infraspinatus muscle as he turned a grinding wheel manually. Both of these individuals' conditions improved after alternative means of moving the potter's wheel and the grinding wheel were found. A brass horn musician was able to eliminate forearm pain by changing the angle at which he held his instrument, but he could not use abdominal breathing to lessen the pain of chronic scalene trigger points caused by chest breathing as he played.

Principles of History Taking

The history is critical in developing a diagnostic construct that directs the physical examination and treatment.

1. The frequency of headache is important, because headaches that occur frequently, for example, several times each week and last for one or several days, often have significant myofascial components. Headaches that occur once a month or less and last for 1 or 2 days are more likely to be typical migraine. A history of injury, particularly a whiplash-type injury, increases the likelihood that headache is myofascial in origin. Depression and psychological stress can lead to bruxism and clenching, activating the temporomandibular muscles, or aggravate upper trapezius muscle trigger points (36,37), and create secondary myofascial trigger point–induced headache.

2. Location of the headache is also useful for diagnosis. Unilateral headaches that remain one-sided and are pulsatile are considered characteristic of migraine. However, headache that includes the side of the head or the side of the face may arise from the temporomandibular muscles (masseter, temporalis, and pterygoids). Headache that is above or behind the eye, or that is in the frontotemporal region or in the parietal region, frequently indicates referred pain from trigger points that may be in the sternocleidomastoid, upper trapezius, or posterior cervical and suboccipital muscles. Posterior headache in the occipital region can be referred from trigger points in the sternocleidomastoid and semispinalis muscles, from facet joints in the upper cervical spine (38), and from nerve entrapment (greater occipital nerve) or from third "occipital" nerve (C3) irritation (39). Circumferential or band-like headache is typically TTH. When there is a posterior cervical component to

Addressing Perpetuating Factors: Position in the Auto

A young woman only had shoulder pain and migraine-like headaches on vacation. She always had trigger points in the right trapezius and left posterior cervical muscles, and headaches in the left parietal-frontal area, extending over the left eye, and pain in the right upper shoulder and right posterior neck, the referral pattern of the trapezius. She reported that her husband always drove on vacations, and that for the 5- to 7-hour drives she would constantly turn around to her left to tend to her children in the back seat. Our advice was that she ask her husband to let her share the driving, and stop more frequently to allow her to move and to stretch.

the headache, especially at the onset, or persistence between headache episodes, myofascial origin is likely.

3. Activities associated with headache are discovered by careful history taking.

Etiology

Common etiologies of muscle trigger points in the upper body that produce headache include all mechanical stresses that result in trigger point formation in the shoulder, head, and neck muscles. These include postural factors, biomechanical stresses such as leg length inequality, and pelvic rotation that results in shoulder muscle stress. Ergonomic stresses associated with work (e.g., computer operators, laborers) and any activity that is associated with prolonged static positions lead to the development of trigger points. Disorders of breathing (mouth breathers and chest breathers) promote head and neck trigger points. Whiplash injuries can lead to chronic pain (40). Virtually 100% of chronic whiplash patients in one community clinic had myofascial trigger points relevant to their pain (Gerwin, unpublished data, 2001). Family or work-related psychological stresses can aggravate myofascial trigger points in the head, neck, and shoulder.

Differential Diagnosis

Headaches that demand immediate attention may not be of myofascial origin, but they may have secondary myofascial trigger points associated with them. One important principle is that any headache that is distinctly different from prior headaches must be examined and fully evaluated, including imaging the brain. New-onset headaches (as opposed to an exacerbation of recurring headaches) also demand evaluation. A new headache of hours' or days' duration that is severe, and that may be associated with nausea and vomiting, must be evaluated for nuchal rigidity, because subarachnoid hemorrhage and meningitis are potential diagnoses. A progressively severe headache of weeks' or even of a few months' duration requires a detailed neurologic examination and imaging, because an intracranial mass lesion may present this way. There may be co-existent myofascial trigger points in the neck and shoulders, but they should not lead the examiner away from thinking of intracranial lesions. Any focal neurologic deficit or complaint of visual disturbance should be evaluated with a neurologic examination. Simple confrontation visual fields may indicate a hemianopsia. Funduscopic examination may disclose papilledema. Benign intracranial hypertension may be chronic but is usually progressive. When the patient with benign intracranial hypertension complains of visual disturbance, evaluation becomes urgent to preserve sight. Headache in the sixth decade of life and later is of particular concern because of temporal arteritis. Temporal arteritis is a distinct risk for unilateral blindness. It is characterized by unilateral headache and usually by temporal artery tenderness. The sedimentation rate is greatly elevated in 90% of cases, being near or over 100 mm/hr. It is a systemic illness, often associated with fever and weight loss.

Musculoskeletal pain in the neck, causing referred headache pain syndromes, generally improves with recumbency, whereas osteomyelitis or metastatic tumor–associated pain usually does not improve with rest. Brain tumors also may worsen when the head is lowered as the patient becomes recumbent.

In general, if the headache is at all suspicious in its presentation, or if the headache does not respond as expected in a short time such as 3 to 4 weeks, evaluation of causes other than musculoskeletal should be undertaken if they have not yet been done. A neurologist should be consulted if there is any doubt.

SYMPTOM PRESENTATION AS RELATED TO SPECIFIC MYOFASCIAL INVOLVEMENT

Trigger Point Referral Patterns and Headache

Each individual muscle of the head, neck, and shoulder that develops trigger points contributory to headache has a referral pattern that is characteristic of that muscle, and that is helpful in identifying the headache-producing muscle. In the clinical evaluation of headache, each of the muscles of the region is systematically examined for trigger points.

Muscle Trigger Point Referral Patterns

An annotated summary of the headache patterns associated with the referral patterns of head and neck muscles is provided in Figures 1-1 and 1-2. The trigger point or zone must be stimulated (firm, flat pressure or pincer grasp) for 5 to 10 seconds to elicit the referred pain pattern.

Upper trapezius muscle trigger points commonly refer pain to the back of the neck, base of the skull, temple, and jaw. Taut bands in the trigger point restrict full lengthening, potentially resulting in limited rotation to the side of pain, limited lateral bending, and limited neck flexion. The trapezius muscle is one of the most common muscles to harbor trigger points, and taut bands are easily discerned. Referral of pain to the upper neck and temple from these trigger points is frequently seen. Trigger points in the upper trapezius muscle are a common cause of persistent unilateral, and sometimes bilateral, headache. Trigger points are frequently found in the mid-portion of the upper trapezius but may be particularly active at the angle of the neck and shoulder where the trapezius muscle curves upward in the neck. This muscle always should be examined in persons with recurrent headache. When trigger points are found, the subject should be questioned for activities, stresses, or postures that result in trapezius overload.

The levator scapulae are not commonly thought to be associated with headache. However, the cervical attachment of the muscle is to the transverse processes of the upper four

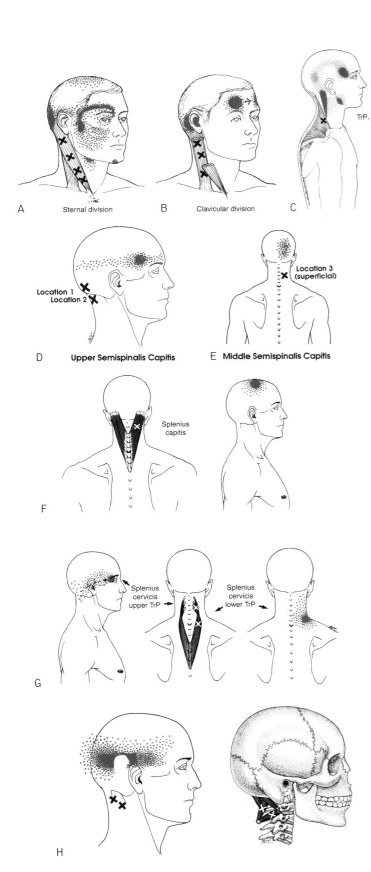

FIGURE 1-1. **Headache pain patterns referred from specific neck muscles.** The x's denote common trigger point (TrP) locations in each muscle, and the red zones indicate common patterns of referred pain. **A.** The more superficial sternal portion of the sternocleidomastoid muscle (SCM). **B.** The clavicular portion of the SCM. **C.** The upper trapezius portion of the trapezius muscle. **D.** The pain referral pattern from trigger points in the upper semispinalis capitis. **E.** The pattern referred from trigger points in the middle semispinalis capitis and the semispinalis cervicis. **F.** Splenius capitis. **G.** Splenius cervicis. **H.** The pain pattern referred from trigger points in the suboccipital muscles. Reprinted with permission from Simons DG, Travell JG, Simons LS: Travell & Simons' Myofascial Pain and Dysfunction: The Trigger Point Manual. Volume 1: Upper Half of Body. 2nd Ed. Baltimore: Lippincott Williams & Wilkins, 1999, Figs 7.1A & B (p. 310), 6.1 (p. 279), 16.1B & C (p. 447), 15.1A & B (p. 433), 17.1 (p. 473).

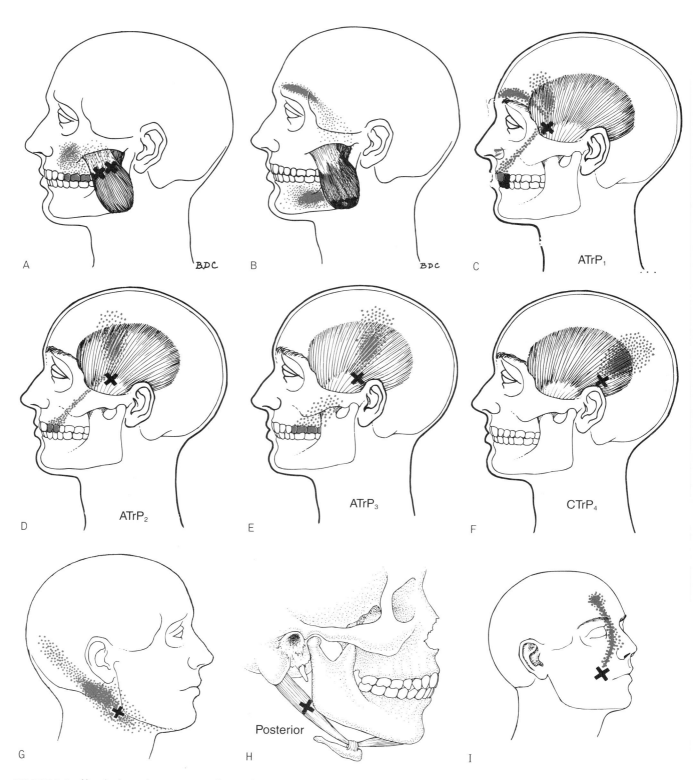

FIGURE 1-2. **Headache pain patterns referred from specific facial muscles.** The x's denote common trigger point locations. The red zones indicate common patterns of referred pain. **A.** and **B.** Patterns of referred pain from attachment trigger points in the upper and lower portions of the superficial masseter muscle. **C., D., E.,** and **F.** Referred pain patterns from trigger points in different portions of the temporalis muscle. **G.** and **H.** Pattern of referred pain from a trigger point in the posterior belly of the digastric muscle. **I.** Pain pattern referred from a trigger point in the zygomaticus major muscle. Reprinted with permission from Simons DG, Travell JG, Simons LS: Travell & Simons' Myofascial Pain and Dysfunction: The Trigger Point Manual. Volume 1: Upper Half of Body. 2nd Ed. Baltimore: Lippincott Williams & Wilkins, 1999, Figs. 8.1A & C (p. 331), 9.1A–D (p. 351), 12.1A & B (p. 398), 13.1B (p. 417).

cervical vertebrae. When trigger points in the levator cause it to be shortened, the muscle can pull the ipsilateral cervical vertebrae laterally. For example, if the left levator scapula muscle is shortened by trigger points, due to the shape of the lateral masses of C1 relative to the occiput, the lateral vertebrae will be side-bent to the right. Thus, dysfunction of the levator scapulae muscles may overload or create a somatic dysfunction of the left zygapophysial joints, causing tenderness and pain in the joints and potentially causing referred pain from the joints to the head, experienced as headache or pain typical of the referred pain of facet joint syndromes.

Sternocleidomastoid (SCM) muscle trigger points refer pain to the occiput, the vertex, the retroauricular area, the forehead, and the cheek. This muscle also is almost always involved with symptomatic trigger points in persons with recurrent headaches. Taut bands are common and frequently tender. They can occur in either or both of the two heads of the muscle, the sternal or the clavicular. The ventral sternal head trigger points refer to the forehead, whereas clavicular head trigger points refer to the ear and behind it. The initial response of many headache sufferers to palpation of the trigger points is to report that though the muscle is tender when firmly palpated, it does not refer to any headache site, and does not reproduce their headache. Maintaining pressure on the muscle for approximately 10 seconds allows the referral pattern to develop. The relevance of trigger points in this muscle to the usual headache can then be well appreciated. Persistent rotational dysfunction of the neck will cause chronic shortening of one SCM muscle and the development of an SCM myofascial syndrome. Moreover, if there is a C2–C3 dysfunction causing mechanical irritation of the overlying clavicular head of the SCM, it will be difficult if not impossible to resolve an SCM trigger point pain syndrome without first correcting the C2–C3 dysfunction.

Masseter muscle trigger points refer pain above the ipsilateral eye as well as to the ear, jaw, and teeth (see Figs. 1-1 and 1-2).

Temporalis muscle trigger points refer pain locally in the temporal–parietal area. Trigger points in the masseter and temporalis muscles are important because they are postural muscles that help control jaw position. The head always moves during chewing and speaking, closely linking jaw movement, jaw position, and the muscles of mastication. Trigger points in the muscles of the neck can be difficult to eliminate when trigger points in the masseter and temporalis muscles (and in the pterygoid muscles, which also contribute to control of jaw position) are not effectively treated. The jaw joint itself is usually normal, except for anterior displacement of the meniscus or joint disc that is the result of shortening of the pterygoid muscle. Dental specialists unfamiliar with the role of these muscle trigger points in maintaining headache may report that there is no internal derangement of the TMJ (which is correct) and that therefore there is no need to treat to relieve trigger points in these muscles (which is incorrect). Moreover, head position will alter the jaw joint relationships. A rounded-shoulder, head-forward posture will displace the jaw posteriorly, putting pressure on joint structures that do not normally bear such pressures. Reactive trigger points will form in the masseter, trapezius, and pterygoid. The jaw must be brought forward and downward to relieve the trigger points. This is usually done through an oral appliance or splint that is worn over the upper or lower teeth.

Zygomaticus muscle trigger points refer pain to the medial epicanthal region and to the forehead above the eye. Its participation in headaches in these locations is often overlooked, leaving the mistaken impression that the pain or headache originates in the frontal sinus.

Splenius capitis muscle trigger points refer pain to the vertex, and those in the splenius cervicis muscle refer pain along the side of the head in a band and behind the eye. Splenius cervicis trigger points also refer pain to the angle of the neck and shoulder and to the posterolateral neck. When trigger points occur bilaterally in these muscles, they produce a headache that is band-like about the head, or a squeezing, vise-like sensation. Unilaterally, they can be mistaken for the one-sided headache of migraine. Headaches precipitated by trigger points in these muscles are often preceded or accompanied by pain or stiffness in the neck.

Semispinalis cervicis trigger points refer pain to the occiput. Trigger points in the semispinalis capitis refer pain in a band-like distribution along the side of the head to the temple and forehead. Together, trigger points in these two muscles contribute to the circumferential headache that is so characteristic of TTH. However, these two muscles may develop trigger points unilaterally, and then the headache may be unilateral and migrainous. As trigger points activate unilaterally on either side, often moving from side to side, unilateral headache can shift sides, thereby mimicking common migraine or migraine without aura, which also affects each side of the head at one time or another. These two muscles are at risk for developing active trigger points when the neck is extended for long periods, or when it is tilted or cocked at an angle. The muscles that extend the neck, which include the semispinalis capitis and cervicis, the splenii, the trapezii, and the levator scapulae, act to stabilize the neck in flexion. That is to say, they act to check-rein flexion and prevent the head from falling forward when the neck is bent forward, as in writing or reading at a desk, or working at a computer. Prolonged reading with the neck bent or working at a computer or desk can activate trigger points in these muscles as they are contracted for prolonged periods to maintain a static forward head position.

Suboccipital muscle trigger points refer pain in a band-like distribution along the side of the head in the occipital, temporal, and frontal regions. These trigger points are frequently responsible in whole or in part for TTH symptoms, or cervicogenic headache. The suboccipital muscle that is palpable when it is shortened and contracted by taut bands is the oblique capitis inferior. It is identified by locating the first transverse process just below the mastoid process and the posterior process of C2. The oblique capitis inferior lies between these two points of attachment. The muscle can be tender, a taut band can be felt, and rotation of the head to the opposite side can be restricted when it has symptomatic trigger points. The other suboccipital muscles lie beneath the trapezius, the semispinalis capitis, and the splenius capitis and are difficult to palpate. They are most likely to be identified as the source of headache when they restrict forward head-bend or chin tuck, as they are more vertically directed than the oblique capitis inferior. Local tenderness and restriction of motion are physical examination signs of their involvement. Trigger points in these muscles are frequently associated with limitations of motion of the upper cervical spine caused by dysfunction of the occipitoatlantal joint, the atlanto-axis joint, or the C2–C3 joint. Diagnosis is made by examining the patient in the supine position with the neck flexed and relaxed in the operator's hands. Restrictions in rotation of the head signal dysfunction in these joints. They are also mobilized in this position, using post-isometric relaxation and contraction and relaxation techniques.

Trigger points in the muscles of mastication (the masseters, the pterygoids, and the temporalis muscles), and the related muscles of the anterior and posterior neck and shoulder region (that stabilize the head and neck against gravity and when talking and chewing), result in severe pain localized to the region of the TMJ and the side of the head. The resulting head pain can be acute and can be mistaken for an acute migraine headache. The focal point of the pain tends to be more localized to the side of the head in front of the ear and upwards into the temple. Headache may or may not occur. The pain can be persistent and dull, or sharp and stabbing. Increased pain caused by chewing or talking is a clue to involvement of the masticatory muscles. Elimination of the pain and headache can be accomplished by inactivation of the offending trigger points manually, or by trigger point injections, but stabilization and prevention of recurrent headaches requires treating the underlying causes of the acute TMJ dysfunction, most notably postural dysfunction and temporomandibular dysfunction.

Finally, trigger points in the muscles of the head, neck, and shoulder can act as sources of peripheral nociceptive stimuli that can activate the trigeminovascular system to initiate the events leading to neurogenic inflammation and sterile edema (e.g., release of substance P from perivascular trigeminal nerve endings) that are associated with classical migraine headaches, thus theoretically leading to the development of migraine headache with or without aura, in addition to chronic daily TTH that is primarily a muscular headache caused by referred pain from myofascial trigger points in the head, neck, and shoulder muscles.

Myofascial Entrapment of the Occipital Nerve

Entrapment of the greater occipital nerve by the semispinalis capitis and the cervical portion of the trapezius muscle can occur when trigger points cause compression of the nerve as it passes through these muscles. The greater occipital nerve arises from the second cervical nerve and supplies the sensory input over the ipsilateral occiput to the vertex, there overlapping the fibers of the trigeminal nerve. The nerve provides motor innervation to the semispinalis muscle before penetrating the trapezius muscle. Compression of the greater occipital nerve occurs most frequently as it penetrates the trapezius muscle, less often, but still commonly, as it penetrates the semispinalis capitis muscle, and least often where it wraps around the oblique capitis inferior muscle. The lesser occipital nerve travels more laterally, coming up the border of the sternocleidomastoid before supplying the posterolateral scalp behind the ear. It is not exposed to compression by the trapezius and semispinalis muscles. If it is symptomatic, it is more likely the result of osteoarthritis at C2–C3. Pain from compression of the greater occipital nerve is felt in the occiput and can be acutely exquisite. Patients say that they cannot lay the back of their head on the pillow. In the days when wearing a hat was common, patients would state that they could not wear them. The major symptoms are pain and extreme tenderness to touch and an intolerance of pressure. Sensory symptoms are surprisingly uncommon. Treatment of the underlying trigger points can release the nerve as it passes through the trapezius and semispinalis capitis muscles and relieve pain and tenderness. Trigger point inactivation can be accomplished by identification and injection of the trigger points by local anesthetic, or by manual techniques. Treatment may have to be repeated weekly for 3 to 4 weeks to sustain improvement in chronic cases.

Principles of Physical Examination

The neurologic examination should be normal for both migraine and TTH.

Evaluation of Muscle

Cervical and shoulder range of motion is always performed before muscle palpation because it gives clues to the presence of trigger points in neck and shoulder muscles. Restriction of neck movement is largely muscular rather than articular, in the absence of cervical fusion. Movements of the neck and jaw are complex, and each movement is the result of contraction and lengthening of several muscles at one time. Release of muscle trigger points almost always increases range of motion. It is for this reason that evaluating cervical range of motion has such utility. Rotation of the neck is tested as an unforced, guided movement, before palpation of the muscles. It is useful as a guide to determine which muscles may be in trouble, and as a means of evaluating the appropriateness of muscle trigger point examination.

Range of Motion and Joint Mobility. Muscles that are shortened as a result of contracted, taut bands associated with trigger points are unable to fully lengthen. This is seen dramatically in the muscles of the neck, whose trigger points refer pain to the head and cause headache, and in the muscles that control jaw movement.

Three directions of movement are assessed in the neck: lateral rotation, lateral bending, and flexion/extension. Active lateral rotation requires the simultaneous contraction of several pairs of agonist/antagonist muscles. The major muscles are the SCM and the splenius capitis. Others of importance are the splenius cervicis, the oblique capitis inferior, and the upper trapezius muscle. The SCM muscle is the only one of this group in which the contraction of the contralateral muscle is the prime rotator, rather than the ipsilateral muscle, although this is also true of the upper trapezius muscle. Restriction of lateral rotation should lead the examiner to consider which muscles are not able to lengthen fully. The same information can be gained from examination of passive range of motion. Active range of motion testing yields more information about the ability of the muscle to actively contract, or the limitation of contractile ability by active trigger points. In the case of restricted rotation of the head to the right, the examiner should think of shortening of the right sternocleidomastoid muscle, the left splenii, the left oblique capitis inferior, and the right upper trapezius. Lateral bending of the neck tests the medial and anterior scalene muscles and the upper trapezius muscles primarily, but also the SCM muscle. The splenius capitis is not active in lateral bending and does not play a role in restricting this movement. Muscle restrictions are all on the side contralateral to the direction of bending. Flexion/extension movement tests the stretching capacity of the anterior and posterior neck muscles: the SCM and the anterior scalene muscles that stretch during extension of the neck, and the upper trapezius, levator scapulae, splenii, semispinalis capitis, and the vertically directed suboccipital muscles that stretch in neck and head flexion. Another complex movement is head tilt, which evaluates restrictions of the scalenes and of the sternocleidomastoid. The scalenes bend the head obliquely forward and must lengthen in oblique backward movements. The SCM muscle not only rotates the head to the contralateral side, but also tilts the head upward.

The TMJ-related muscles are tested by examining interincisal mouth opening, lateral or side movement, and jaw protrusion. Mouth opening lengthens the masseters and temporalis muscles; side movement and protrusion (anterior and lateral) evaluates the pterygoid muscles.

Muscle Palpation. Palpation remains the most accessible examination technique for general clinical use. EMG identification of the characteristic spontaneous electrical activity of the trigger point (20) remains a research tool at this time, although it is being studied for use as a tool to guide therapeutic trigger point injections. Algometry (41) is a confirmatory tool that can be helpful in documenting the trigger point, but it does not find the trigger initially. Physical examination of trigger points by a skilled examiner is highly reliable for identification of the trigger point (42). Thus, it is possible to identify the responsible myofascial trigger points readily, simply by palpation, with instruction and with practice (43).

Muscle palpation identifies trigger points that reproduce pain, cause limitation of movement, and, most importantly, refer pain to the areas of headache. The tight bands of muscle that are tender are parallel to the long axis of the muscle and often feel like ropey cords in the belly of the muscle. Palpation is always done perpendicular to the direction of the muscle fiber axis, to feel the taut bands of muscle associated with the trigger point. The taut bands are easy to feel in the sternocleidomastoid, and the overlying sternal division can be separated from the underlying clavicular division that has a different distribution of referred pain. They can be felt as tight strands at the base of the mastoid process in splenius capitis. Palpation is performed for each muscle in the head, neck, and shoulder that can be related primarily or secondarily to headache. Muscles in the functional unit may contribute importantly to the maintenance of dysfunction and trigger points in the offending muscle that is finally responsible for the headache. Muscles that can contribute to any restricted movement must be examined carefully for trigger points. To assess the role that a particular muscle trigger point plays in the development of headache symptoms, the trigger point must be firmly compressed for as long as 10 to 15 seconds, as discussed previously, to elicit referred pain. A shorter period of palpation may not activate the referred pain pattern and may miss the role that a specific trigger point plays in that headache.

Examination for Perpetuating Factors

Perpetuating factors that interfere in the resolution of myogenic headache include both mechanical factors and more general medical factors. The mechanical factors are the same as those seen in other chronic myofascial pain syndromes, namely, scoliosis of any cause, and ergonomic and postural stresses that result in prolonged static shortening or loading of muscle. They must be identified and corrected. For example, scoliosis often produces an elevation of one shoulder, requiring the muscles of the neck on the side ipsilateral to the high shoulder to engage in static contraction that brings the head back to the midline. The various causes of scoliosis must be considered and corrected when possible: leg length inequality that requires a heel lift, myofascial trigger point shortening of the psoas or quadratus lumborum, which is corrected by stretching and lengthening the muscles, and pelvic torsion, or rotation of one ilium relative to the other. Correction is derotation of the hemipelvis by manual adjustment. Sloping shoulders can stress the trapezius muscles. A head-forward posture, often associated with rounded shoulders, produces several mechanical stresses. The effect of such a posture on the jaw has been discussed in association with the masseter muscle. The head-forward posture also results in changing the direction of the SCM from a slanting angle as the muscle runs from the sternum and clavicle anteriorly and inferiorly to the mastoid process posteriorly and superiorly, to a more vertical position as the mastoid process moves anteriorly with head. This shift of the head results in chronic shortening of the SCM muscle, promoting trigger points in the muscle that can produce headache symptoms. Postural factors and biomechanical stresses, such as leg length inequality and pelvic rotation that results secondarily in shoulder region muscle stress, are identified by physical examination. Work-related mechanical stresses such as repetitive strain syndromes or cumulative work-related trauma are identified by examination and by history taking.

Principles of Treatment

Treatment is directed toward the elimination of the specific cause of the headache, identification of the factors that have led to the headache and their correction, and identification and correction of the factors that perpetuate headache. These factors, identified through the history and physical examination, determine the type of treatment program that is developed for each patient.

Treatment of Muscle

1. Inactivation of the trigger point either manually or through a combination of trigger point injection of a local anesthetic, or intramuscular stimulation by a solid needle such as an acupuncture needle, followed by manual treatment, is the final proof that a trigger point is the critical factor in the genesis of the headache. It is also the first step in treatment. Trigger point compression for 30 to 60 seconds will alter the headache pain if the trigger point is responsible for part of the headache. Compression of the trigger point will initially increase pain, indicating to the patient and to the practitioner that the relevant "spot" has been found. Pain subsides in approximately 20 to 30 seconds, followed by palpable relaxation of the muscle in approximately 1 minute. This is usually evident to both the patient and the treating practitioner. Several muscles may need to be treated before the headache is relieved and the myofascial pattern becomes fully disclosed to the examiner. It is not unusual for a frontal headache to have components of referred pain from sternocleidomastoid, oblique capitis inferior, and splenius cervicis trigger points. There may be a temporary increase in pain until all of the relevant triggers are treated. The treated muscles are stretched after the trigger points are inactivated, the neck is mobilized to full range of motion, and moist heat is applied to complete the treatment.

2. Physical therapy is undertaken to treat the problems identified as relevant to the initiation and maintenance of the headache. This aspect of treatment is directed to repeated inactivation of specific trigger points in the muscles that refer pain to the head as headache, until they no longer recur spontaneously. Inactivation of the trigger points is done manually according to the techniques outlined below, and invasively by dry needling or by trigger point injection. Manual techniques follow the principle of first reducing the pain and then restoring full length to the muscle. When using intermittent cold and stretch, the two techniques are combined, the cold being used to reduce pain while the muscle is stretched. In another manual approach, pain is first reduced by means of direct compression of the trigger point, followed by a number of stretching procedures outlined in the following sections.

3. Corrective action is required to minimize the recurrence of the trigger point and the headache. This takes many forms and can take many weeks. Postural dysfunction that contributes to trigger point formation must be identified. A round-shouldered, kyphotic posture, associated with shortening of the pectoral muscles, promotes trigger point formation in the neck extensor muscles that must lift the head, and in the trapezius muscles. Corrective action in that case requires lengthening of the pectoral muscles and restoration of more normal head posture. Ergonomics of computer or telephone use need to be examined because static rotation or lateral bending of the head act as physical stressors of muscles that can cause headache. Chest breathers activate the SCM muscles with each breath. Teaching abdominal breathing is the correction, but it can take as long as 4 months to develop routine abdominal breathing patterns.

Dental assistance may be needed to treat headaches that include temporomandibular-related muscle dysfunction. Lack of adequate mechanical support in the mouth can lead to repositioning of the jaw and alteration of neck posture, and the persistence of trigger point pain. The masseter, pterygoid, and temporalis muscles are vulnerable in this circumstance. Head posture is responsive both to changes in the neck muscles and to the position of the jaw (try chewing or talking without moving the head). Hence, trigger points in the muscles that move the jaw are part of the functional muscle units of the muscles of the neck that control head posture. It is necessary to treat the muscles of the shoulder, neck, and face simultaneously when the muscles of the TMJ are involved. A dentist knowledgeable in this field can create a mouth splint that will support the jaw and alleviate the tension on the involved muscles. The jaw is a postural organ. When one chews or speaks, both the jaw and the head move. These movements require coordination of the muscles of mastication and the muscles of the neck and shoulder that control head and neck posture. Dysfunction in one part of this coordinated system promotes dysfunction in the rest of the system. Moreover, a retruded jaw, in which the mandible is pushed back into the joint, is associated with a forward head posture and forward shoulder displacement, both of which maintain head and neck trigger points. (See Jaeger B, Chapter 5, in Simons, Travell, Simons [20] for a more complete discussion of this subject.)

Examination of the range of motion of the joints in the region of interest identifies the muscle restrictions associated with myofascial trigger points. It is now obvious that the movements that test range of motion are the very movements that are incorporated into self and therapeutic stretching techniques.

Treatment Tips for Muscle Release. The patient must be relaxed, and the operator must have access to the muscles being treated.

1. The upper trapezius is treated by trigger point compression by the clinician, using either hand, with the patient in either the upright or the supine position. Approximately 30 seconds are required to eliminate the tenderness, and roughly 1 minute to relax the muscle. Local stretching by direct pressure on the muscle, exerted by flat or pincer pressure directed along the length of the taut band over a distance of approximately 1 to 2 inches, will further relax the trigger point. Self and therapeutic stretching of the trapezius requires that the shoulder be fixed so that it does not elevate during the lateral bend of the head. A lateral decubitus or prone position is convenient for the operator to apply most of the techniques except therapeutic stretching. The patient must be supine or upright to properly stretch the muscle. The stretch is a three-movement stretch. The first component is a lateral bend to stretch the side bend component of the muscle (the more anterior fibers). The second position is

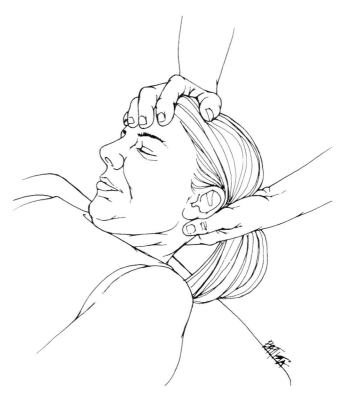

FIGURE 1-4. Therapist's stretch of the posterior cervical neck extensors. The therapist stands at the head of the seated or supine patient and flexes the neck forward.

forward, maintaining the lateral bend, to stretch the extension component of the trapezius (the more posterior fibers). The final movement is rotation of the back of the head away from the side being stretched, while maintaining the lateral-forward head position, because the trapezius inserts in the back of the head on the inion (Fig. 1-3). Positioning the head into a partial rotation facing the affected side, and then dropping the contralateral, forward-facing ear toward the chest, will accomplish the stretch. Rotating the inion adds more distance between the attachment of the upper trapezius medially to the inion and laterally to the acromion process.

2. The posterior neck muscles that extend the neck are stretched by flexing the neck (Fig. 1-4). The suboccipital muscles that extend the neck are stretched by keeping the neck straight and performing a chin tuck.

3. The posterior rotator muscles (the splenii and the oblique capitis muscles) are stretched by flexing the neck and slightly rotating the head (Fig. 1-5). The oblique capitis inferior is specifically stretched by fixing the transverse process of C2 with the operator's fingers while rotating the head 10° to 15° away from the affected side, to increase the distance between the origin and insertion on the muscle on the transverse process of C1 and the posterior process of C2, respectively.

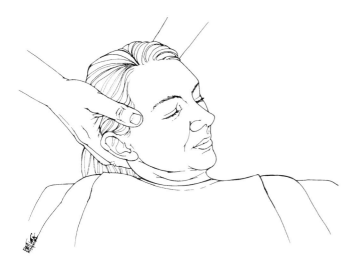

FIGURE 1-3. Therapist's stretch of the trapezius muscle. The operator stands at the head of the supine patient and side bends the neck away from the side to be stretched, flexes the neck, and finally rotates the head so the face is looking toward the side being stretched.

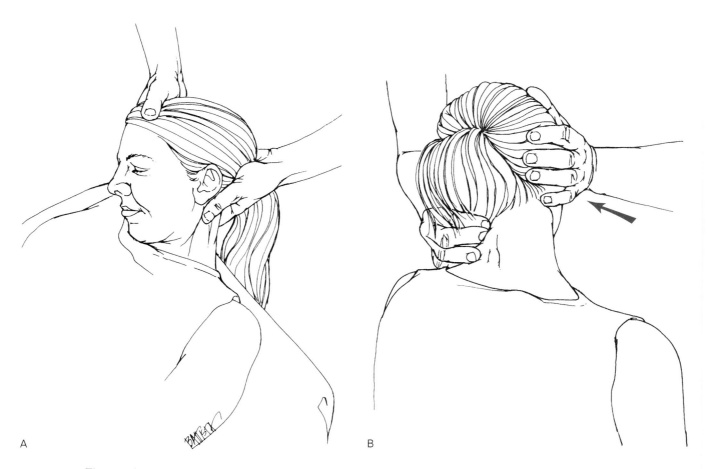

A   B

FIGURE 1-5. Therapist's stretch of the rotator muscles of the neck and the oblique capitis inferior muscle. A. Rotator muscles (the splenius capitis and cervicis and the oblique capitis inferior). The therapist stands at the head of the seated or supine patient. The head is flexed and rotated 30° away from the side to be stretched. **B.** Oblique capitis inferior muscle. The transverse process of C2 is fixed by the fingers of one hand while the other hand rotates the back of the head away from the C2 posterior process approximately 10°–15°.

4. The sternal head of the sternocleidomastoid muscle is stretched by combining extension of the neck and rotation to the ipsilateral side, while tilting the head upward (Fig. 1-6). The second position of the stretch is full turn of the head to the ipsilateral side and a downward tilt of the head, to increase the distance between the sternum and the mastoid process. The clavicular head of the sternocleidomastoid muscle is stretched by extension of the neck, upward tilt of the head, and rotation of the head to the contralateral side.

5. The scalene muscles are stretched by combining lateral bend to the opposite side (for the medial head) with rotation and upward head tilt to the opposite side (Fig. 1-7).

Treatment Techniques.

1. Intermittent cold and spray was used by Travell (20) extensively in her work with myofascial pain. The technique uses a cold stimulus such as a vapo-coolant spray (most commonly used), the sharp edge of ice inside plastic, or the edge of a half-round-head stove bolt that is kept in the freezer. The stimulus is both a thermal

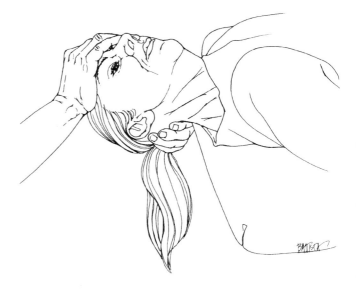

FIGURE 1-6. Therapist's stretch of the sternocleidomastoid muscle. The therapist sits at the supine patient's head. The head is side-bent away from the muscle to be stretched and extended. The face is rotated toward the side being stretched. The chin is then tucked downward.

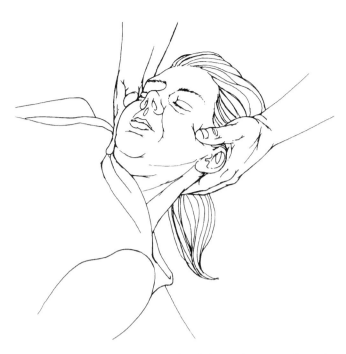

FIGURE 1-7. **Therapist's stretch of the scalene muscles.** The therapist sits at the head of the supine patient. The head is side-bent away from the muscles being stretched for the medial scalene muscle. The neck is put into extension, and the face is rotated toward the side being stretched.

(cold) stimulus and a tactile stimulus. Both stimuli activate the cutaneous A-beta fibers that inhibit the transmission of C and A-delta pain activity. The stimulus is applied from the trigger zone to the referred pain zone, sweeping approximately 10 cm/sec. Several linear sweeps are made, and the muscle is stretched. Care is taken to avoid cooling the muscle.

2. Beat Dejung (44) developed a protocol that is very useful in treating myofascial pain syndromes. The protocol combines several techniques that are well known to therapists. They are trigger point compression, with the important addition of short-excursion movements that contract and relax the muscle being treated. Short excursion manual stretching of the trigger point is performed by moving the fingers along the taut band, parallel to the fiber direction. Separation of fascial planes is performed by placing the fingers between muscles (when accessible, as between the upper trapezius and the upper levator scapula muscles). This movement also provides additional local stretch to the muscle. Large excursion movements of the limb or body part are performed by the subject during this maneuver. Intermittent cold may be applied, and then therapeutic stretching is performed. The patient is taught to do self-stretches. Trigger point injection, or intramuscular stimulation (a technique developed by Chann Gunn [45]) using acupuncture needles, or simply releasing the trigger point by dry needling the trigger zone with an

acupuncture needle, can be integrated into this treatment protocol.

3. Karel Lewit developed a technique called post-isometric relaxation or PIR (46). This technique is really an isometric contraction followed by relaxation and stretching. The muscle is stretched in the usual manner. When a barrier is reached, so that resistance is felt to further stretch, the patient is instructed to move the body part in a direction that contracts the muscle being treated. The examiner braces the body part so that no movement occurs and controls the effort exerted by instructing the patient to just "meet my force." The movement thus becomes isometric. Only approximately 10% to 15% of full effort is required to obtain relaxation during the stretching phase. The process is repeated until full stretch is achieved, or no further barrier can be overcome.

Treatment of Acute Headache. Patients sometimes present as an emergency and require acute treatment to relieve unrelenting headache. The subject can be placed supine on a treatment table in a darkened room. The muscles of the shoulder, neck, and head are palpated. When a tender trigger is found, particularly if it reproduces or worsens part of the headache, it can be treated manually by trigger point compression, and then gentle stretching. Trigger point injection with local anesthetic also can be used. These techniques can often eliminate a headache in 10 to 15 minutes. An optional additional treatment is the administration of ketorolac 30 to 60 mg intramuscularly.

Assessment and Treatment of Joint Dysfunction

Dysfunction of cervical spine movement, also referred to as restriction of cervical spine segmental movement, or segmental hypomobility, causes pain and is associated with shortening of cervical muscles caused by the taut bands of trigger points. In the osteopathic literature, these restrictions are referred to as somatic dysfunctions. Movement at cervical segments is limited by muscle length, ligamentous restrictions, and by the articular surfaces themselves. Movement is different at the occipitoatlantal joint, the atlantoaxial joint, and the 3rd through 7th cervical vertebral joints.

The occipitoatlantal (OA) joint moves primarily in a flexion–extension direction. Flexion is accompanied by a posterior translatory slide of the occiput on the atlas. Extension is accompanied by an anterior translatory slide of the occiput on the atlas. This means that the occiput slides posteriorly on the atlas in forward neck bending, and anteriorly when the neck extends. Rotation and side-bending at the OA joint always occur in opposite directions. Rotation of the occiput to the left on the atlas (face turning right) results in side-bending right as the occiput translates or slides to the left. An associated dysfunction occurs when the atlas also translates or slides left and becomes fixed, rather than freely moving and being capable of recentering. In this situation, myofascial trigger points can develop or be perpetuated by the persistent dysfunction of the atlas. This can result in severe ipsilateral headache, usually involving the occipital area.

Movement at the atlantoaxial (AA) joint is primarily rotational. The odontoid process of the axis limits flexion–extension at this joint. Also limiting are the articular surfaces of the joints. Likewise, lateral flexion does not occur at this joint. With rotation of the atlas (C1) on the axis (C2), there is sliding of the one articular facet upward and sliding of the opposite articular facet downward. This movement causes a slight wobble of the head. Movement of the two joints together, OA plus AA, results in a large range of extension–flexion and rotation. Segmental dysfunction at the AA joint occurs in rotation. Compensation for inferior (caudal) spinal segmental dysfunction occurs at these two suboccipital joints, the OA and the AA joints, to keep the eyes level. The transitional segment C2–3, between the rest of the cervical spine and the two suboccipital joints, sustains a great deal of mechanical stress and is a common site for segmental dysfunction. When there is significant rotational dysfunction at this level, SCM trigger points can be perpetuated.

The orientation of the facet joints in the cervical spine from C3 to C7 allows for a great deal of motion. The plane of the facet joints is oblique, part way between frontal and horizontal. This results in coupling side bending to rotation. Side bending and rotation are always to the same side in this part of the cervical spine, in contrast to the OA and AA joints. Functionally, the change in orientation of the facet joints with extension and flexion of the neck facilitates different motions of the neck. In extension, the articular joints are more vertical, facilitating side-bending. In flexion, the joints are more in a horizontal plane, facilitating rotation. Rotation and side-bending are the primary motions of this portion of the cervical spine, rather than flexion–extension. The unciform joints (of Luschka) lie on the lateral aspects of the vertebral bodies and limit lateral slide or translation of the cervical vertebrae during the coupled motions of side-bending and rotation. During coupled side-bending and rotation, the superior vertebrae slides laterally in the opposite direction. Segmental hypomobility in this section of the cervical spine occurs in the coupled motions of side-bending and rotation, and in lateral translation.

Examination for Segmental Dysfunction

Occipitoatlantal joint. The patient is seated. Place the examining fingers in the sulcus at either side of the base of the skull. Slide the fingers from the inion laterally and inferiorly until they rest in the posterolateral sulcus between the occiput and the atlas. As the patient flexes the neck to 30° at the occipitoatlantal junction only (not the whole cervical spine), feel the depth of the sulcus. An increased depth of the sulcus on one side compared with the other can indicate a dysfunction toward the shallow side. As the neck is then extended, assess the depth of the sulcus on each side. As above, increased

depth of the sulcus on one side indicates a side-bending dysfunction toward the shallow side.

Atlantoaxial joint. The patient lies supine, and the clinician is seated at the patient's head, hands placed so the fingers rest on the tips of the mastoid processes. The tips of the transverse processes of the first cervical vertebra (the atlas) lie just caudal to the mastoid processes. The fingers are moved dorsally to palpate the sulcus over the facet joints, and then ventrally to palpate the tips of the transverse processes. Asymmetries are noted, particularly bony prominence on one side and depression on the other, as well as relative posterior displacement of one transverse process compared with the other, indicating restricted segmental movement and rotational dysfunction. The fingers are kept on the transverse processes while the head is then flexed to 30° at the occipitoatlantal joint and rotated to one side and then to the other, until motion is felt at the transverse processes. A decrease in rotation on either side represents restriction of motion, whereas full rotation to one side represents unrestricted motion to that side. Posterior fullness and posterior rotation of the transverse process is associated with restriction of head rotation to the opposite side.

An associated myofascial trigger point syndrome at the atlantoaxial segment is that of the oblique capitis inferior. The muscle inserts superiorly and laterally on the transverse process of the atlas (C1) and inferomedially on the posterior process of the axis (C2). Trigger points in this muscle shorten it and restrict rotation of the head to the opposite side. Hardness in the muscle palpated between the two bony landmarks of the C1 transverse process just below the mastoid process and the posterior spinous process of C2 is the diagnostic finding on physical examination. To treat this restriction, the lamina of C2 must be fixed with the fingers to prevent it from moving with C1 when the head is gently and slightly rotated into the restriction to lengthen the muscle. A postisometric relaxation technique is often useful in this treatment.

Chiropractors often call this restriction an upper cervical fixation. Its persistence after usual cervical manipulations is the most frequent cause of postmanipulation headache. That headache usually can be prevented by assessing for and addressing this myofascial syndrome immediately after manipulation.

Lower cervical spine, C2–C7. The patient lies supine. The clinician sits at the patient's head, fingers on the posterior spinous process and the paraspinal muscles. The fingers are then moved over the posterolateral sulcus, marking the facet joints to the laterally positioned transverse processes, from C2 to C7. Rotate the head to evaluate restrictions in rotation, one hand on the head and one hand to fix (stabilize) the shoulder. Evaluate side bending in a similar manner. Limitation of rotation or side bending indicates a restriction in the direction of limitation of motion. Examine for the symmetry of the articular pillars with the patient supine. If one side is more posterior, the vertebrae may be rotated to that side. Flex the head while palpating the vertebrae. If the posteriorly rotated vertebrae becomes more posterior, it is restricted in flexion. It will either remain as is or improve in extension. Likewise, if the posteriorly rotated vertebrae becomes more posterior in extension, it improves in flexion (the motion being restricted in extension). Chiropractic nomenclature generally uses the spinous process rather than the vertebral body as the point of reference in designating the direction of rotation, but the principles are the same, and the designations are readily translated.

Similarly, lateral translation is evaluated for the C2–C7 segments of the cervical spine, but not at the atlantoaxial joint. Only rotation is evaluated at the atlantoaxial joint, because of the limitations of the odontoid ligament and the bony limitations to movement. Rotation at the AA joint is evaluated with the neck flexed to eliminate rotation in the lower cervical segments. A limitation of rotation in one direction is a restriction. Side bending restrictions of the lower (C2–C7) cervical segments are evaluated by sliding the articular pillar to one side, causing a lateral bend to the opposite side. The patient is supine. The operator sits at the head. The fingers are on the articular pillars of the vertebra of interest. The articular pillars are pushed to one side, causing the neck to bend to the opposite side. Both sides are evaluated, and any asymmetry is noted. The process is repeated with the neck in flexion and in extension. If the translation of the vertebra is decreased in flexion or in extension, then the restriction is exaggerated in that movement, and lateral bending to the opposite side will be limited. Finally, lateral translation at the occipitoatlantal joint is examined with the patient supine, the operator standing at the patient's head. The head is slightly forward bent, and sidebent on the neck, moving the occiput to one side. This side bending motion of the occiput to one side flexes the neck to the opposite side (sliding the occiput to the right bends the neck to the left). Side bending is coupled to rotation to the opposite side. Thus, lateral translation of the occiput to the right side-bends the head to the left and rotates the head to the right.

Identification of the C2–C3 dysfunction that aggravates the SCM muscle and perpetuates SCM trigger points is done with the patient lying supine, the operator at the patient's head. Palpation is over the anterior aspect of the neck bilaterally, the examiner's fingertips on the SCM, palpating the vertebral body through the muscle, comparing symmetry, tenderness, and joint play between the two sides. The prominence is appreciated on the affected (tender) side, and there is less anterior/posterior joint play or mobility on the affected side.

Treatment of Segmental Cervical Dysfunction

In general, treatment for cervical segmental dysfunctions follows the same principles at each level. The treatment described here uses the gentle mobilization technique of muscle lengthening to restore normal joint movement. The general principle is to move into the direction of restriction using contract–relax techniques to promote muscle relaxation and lengthening, thereby restoring normal mobility to the affected segment. For example, for treatment of a C3–4 restriction, the patient lies supine and the operator stands at the head of the table. The patient's head is held in the operator's hands and is rotated into the restriction until a barrier is reached. The head is held at the barrier, and the patient is instructed to rotate the head to the opposite side. The operator resists the contraction, keeping the head in place, not losing the gained rotation, creating an isometric contraction. The contraction need only be mild or gentle (10%–15% of full contraction). The muscle contraction is maintained for 4 to 5 seconds, then released, and the head is rotated through the barrier until a new barrier or restriction is reached. The process may be repeated until full rotation is achieved. Respiratory facilitation is achieved by holding the breath in inhalation (facilitating muscle contraction) during the isometric contraction, and lengthening the muscle during exhalation (facilitating relaxation). Eye movement facilitation is accomplished by looking toward the direction of movement or effort. When rotating into the restriction, the eyes look in that direction. When the muscles are isometrically contracted for head rotation in the opposite direction, the eyes are turned in that direction.

The atlantoaxial joint is unique in that the oblique capitis inferior has the potential to restrict its movement and requires a special release technique. Joint mobilization is facilitated by 2nd vertebral transverse stretching of the muscle. This can be done with the patient sitting, the operator standing to the side behind the patient. If the restricted movement is head turning to the left, the operator's right arm wraps about the patient's head, cradling the head. The operator's fingers are placed along the right side of the second posterior spinous process. The operator's left hand is held on the patient's forehead, fingers resting on the right temple. The head is gently rotated with the left hand approximately 10° to 15°, while the lamina is held in place. This maneuver keeps the second cervical vertebra from rotating with the atlas. If the second vertebral transverse process were not fixed in position, it would rotate with the atlas, and the muscle would not lengthen.

Medical Perpetuating Factors

Medical perpetuating factors are those conditions that tend to impair muscle metabolism directly or indirectly and prevent normal muscle response to the usual stresses of everyday activity. These factors are discussed in detail in Chapter 4 of Simons, Travell, and Simons (20). Four common medical perpetuating factors that occur in 10% to 16% of persons with chronic myofascial pain are iron deficiency, vitamin B12 and folic acid deficiency, and hypothyroidism. Iron deficiency is of special interest because by itself it can cause chronic headache. Iron deficiency is evaluated by measuring serum ferritin. Freely mobilizable iron stores in muscle, liver, and bone marrow are depleted at serum ferritin levels of 15 to 20 ng/mL. Microcytosis and anemia are seen at lower serum ferritin levels. Serum iron levels are too variable to be of practical value. Iron store depletion is associated with a sense of "coldness to the core," and lack of endurance or easy fatigability. Vitamin B12 deficiency is seen in at least 15% of persons with serum levels up to 350 pg/mL. Elevated methylmalonic acid confirms the diagnosis, but it may be normal in persons with metabolic abnormalities attributable to abnormal B12 utilization. Homocysteine elevation is suggestive of vitamin B12 deficiency but is elevated on a genetic basis so that it is a less specific marker for B12 deficiency. Fatigability is seen in B12 deficiency, along with loss of vibration sense in the toes. Folic acid evaluation requires the measurement of erythrocyte folate. In addition to peripheral neuropathy, it is marked by a sense of intense coldness, similar to iron deficiency, and loose stools. Hypothyroidism is characterized by tiredness, coldness, dry skin and coarsening of the hair, increased hair loss, and constipation. Thyrotropin assays (thyroid-stimulating hormone [TSH] and highly sensitive thyroid stimulating hormone [sTSH] are the most sensitive way of evaluating thyroid dysfunction. A second-generation TSH that can measure to 0.1 mIU/L is sufficient to screen for hypothyroidism, except when it is caused by pituitary gland failure. The sTSH and free T4 (FT4) must be done then. Other medical problems that appear to be associated with chronic myofascial pain syndromes that include headaches are recurrent candidiasis infections and parasitic infestations, particularly amoebiasis, estrogen deficiency, and fibromyalgia.

Hormonal causes of headache are associated with episodic headache, or more properly speaking, with menstrual migraine, and are beyond the scope of this discussion. Allergies, whether to food or to other substances, may cause either episodic or continuous headache. One woman, allergic to milk products, had chronic daily headaches with superimposed episodic headaches of increased sensitivity, until she eliminated all dairy products from her diet. Thereafter, her chronic daily headaches diminished. Analgesic-induced headache and analgesic rebound headache can present as chronic daily headache and are identified through the history of medication use. Psychological stresses may not be evident at first but may come to attention after repeated discussion of cause, or even after keeping a headache diary of events that occur in the hours or days preceding episodic headache. It was through such a diary that one woman discovered that her headaches, which occurred 3 to 4 days each week, always followed phone calls from her mother during which her mother belittled her. Mechanical perpetuating factors are discovered both through the history and by physical examination. History taking can uncover activities that result in ergonomic stresses as has already been discussed. Physical perpetuating factors are outlined in the preceding section on physical examination.

SELF CARE

General Principles

The patient is instructed in proper diet, for nutritional purposes, but also to avoid stress of the temporomandibular joint when that is involved. Hard or crunchy foods are to be avoided (nuts and hard, raw vegetables such as carrots or lettuce). Para-functional habits such as nail-biting and chewing pencils are avoided. Ergonomic factors are to be considered, such as the computer station, telephone habits such as tucking the phone between the ear and the neck, sleeping positions and pillows, and lifting and reaching activities associated with daily activities. Stress factors such as those associated with work or family must be addressed, and relaxation techniques and yoga or meditation can be used to decrease muscle tension. Physical exercise within the person's capability is encouraged. Specific self-stretches are discussed in the following section. They are prescribed both for therapeutic purposes and to maintain gains that have already been achieved.

Specific Self-Stretches

Self-stretching techniques that are related to headache address head and neck muscles and those shoulder muscles that control head movement (Fig. 1-8).

Self Shoulder Stretches. The patient is seated or standing. The ipsilateral shoulder is fixed by either sliding the hand

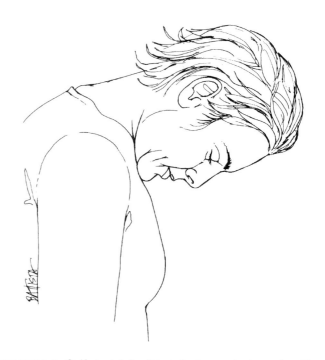

FIGURE 1-8. **Self-stretch for the posterior cervical muscles.** The patient rounds the torso forward and drops the head toward the chest. The posterior neck muscles often stretch further in the rounded position than when the patient starts from a more upright position.

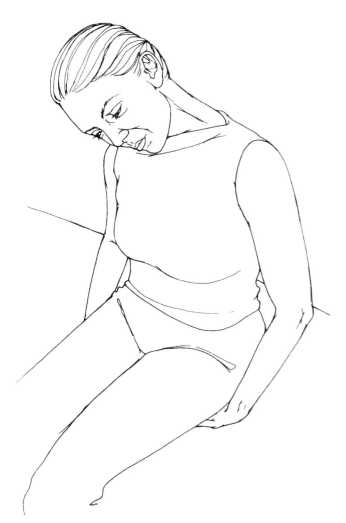

FIGURE 1-9. **Self-stretch for the trapezius muscle (then progressing to stretch the sternocleidomastoid muscle).** The patient is seated. For the right trapezius muscle, the head is allowed to fall to the left *and* is left side-bent. Keeping the side-bend, the head is allowed to fall forward into neck flexion. Finally, the face is turned to the left, rotating the posterior occipital insertion of the trapezius away from the shoulder. The right hand is tucked under the right thigh to keep the right shoulder from rising during the stretch. To self-stretch the right sternocleidomastoid, the head is then moved from the position of the trapezius self-stretch (side-bent to the left) and is rotated to the right, as if to look over the right shoulder, keeping the neck flexed. The chin is then tucked to elevate the occiput.

beneath the thigh (seated) or holding the hand behind the back (standing). The head is allowed to fall (by gravity) to the opposite side, head forward, while maintaining side bend. Finally, the face is turned partly toward the shoulder that is being stretched, away from the direction of side bend. This stretches the contralateral trapezius and sternocleidomastoid muscles (Fig. 1-9).

The patient sits or stands. The head is turned as if to look over the shoulder (the position that swimmers use to breathe when doing the crawl). The chin is then tucked in

to further flex the neck. This stretches the sternocleidomastoid muscle.

Self-Stretches of Neck Muscles. The patient is seated or standing. The head is rotated slightly (one third) to one side and the chin dropped. This stretches the splenii and the semispinalis muscles. Then the arm on the side opposite the direction of head turning (the right arm if the head is turned left) is brought over the head, rotating the glenoid fossa of the shoulder upward and the medial upper scapula insertion of the levator scapula downward. This stretches the levator scapula, which can refer pain to the neck (Fig. 1-10).

The neck is held straight. The chin is tucked down in the manner of the Buckingham Palace guards. This stretches the suboccipital muscles.

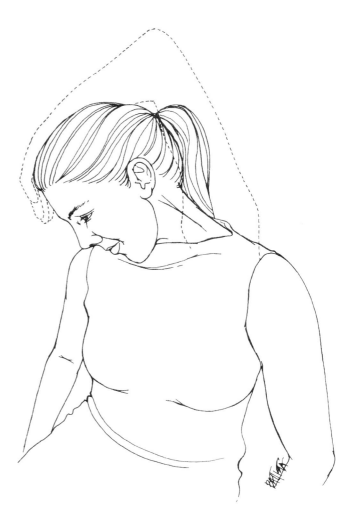

FIGURE 1-10. **Self-stretch for the splenius capitis and cervicis and for the semispinalis.** The stretch is performed sitting or standing, but not supine. The neck is flexed and rotated approximately 30° to the side opposite the muscles to be stretched. To stretch the levator scapula muscle, the ipsilateral arm is abducted to rotate the medial superior border of the scapula downward., thus lengthening the distance between the upper cervical attachments and the scapular attachment.

CONCLUSION

Frequent headache, whether called chronic daily headache, episodic tension-type headache, transformation migraine, or benign recurrent headache, is commonly caused by myofascial trigger points in the muscles of the shoulder, neck, and head. Treatment of the muscle triggers can be effective in relieving the acute headache. Treatment of chronic, recurrent headaches requires the inactivation of trigger points and identification of the factors that keep the myofascial pain syndrome active. The factors, whether they alter muscle metabolism as iron deficiency does, or produce a mechanical stress such as ergonomic stress and postural stress, must be corrected once identified. This treatment approach is integrated with the more traditional treatment of headache, including control of dietary factors and judicious use of pharmacologic agents.

HISTORY, EXAMINATION, AND TREATMENT PROTOCOL

History and physical examination are critical features of headache management. Therefore, protocols for history taking and for the important elements of the physical examination are outlined.

I. History

   A. The frequency, location, and triggers of headache

   B. Headache-associated symptoms (nausea, photophobia, etc.)

   C. Any family history of headache.

II. Examination

   A. Gait (look for pronated feet, scoliosis, imbalance)

   B. Sitting posture (look for head forward, rounded shoulders)

   C. General physical examination, including blood pressure and pelvic and hip function for restrictions that can influence spine and shoulder posture

   D. Neurologic examination

   E. Evaluate range of motion of neck and mouth opening

   F. Palpate the muscles of the shoulders, neck, and head for active trigger points and relevant taut bands

   G. Laboratory assessment of common perpetuating factors (e.g., thyroid function, iron deficiency)

III. Treatment

   A. Correct postural dysfunctions and restrictions.

   B. Correct associated medical problems.

   C. Address psychological stresses that affect muscles of the shoulder, head, and neck.

   D. Inactivate myofascial trigger points in the relevant muscles.

   E. Obtain dental consultation from a dental expert in myofascial-related headache if relevant.

   F. Instruct in a self-treatment program of stretches and of corrective techniques.

   G. Reassess if the headache persists.

Manual Myofascial Techniques for Release of Muscles Involved in Headaches

Editorial Note by Lucy Whyte Ferguson, D.C.

Manual myofascial release techniques are an integral part of the treatment of patients with headaches. Specific muscle releases for jaw muscles and anterior neck muscles are discussed in Chapter 2. Releases for the upper trapezius and splenius cervicis are discussed in Chapter 3. Releases of neck and shoulder muscles that affect head-on-neck posture are discussed in Chapters 4 and 9. When upper trapezius trigger points are recurrent, it is important to address muscles that refer pain and tenderness into the region of the upper trapezius.

The scalene, levator scapula, and lower trapezius muscle trigger points can refer pain and tenderness into the upper trapezius area. It is often very important to treat active trigger points in these muscles to obtain lasting improvement in headaches that are referred from upper trapezius trigger points.

A series of approaches can be used to release the splenius capitis, the semispinalis cervicis and capitis, and the suboccipital muscle group. Gentle passive stretch is often performed first with the patient seated.

A vapocoolant spray can be used over the muscles of the posterior neck and up onto the skull in the areas of referred pain during the stretches. The neck and head are taken forward and then forward with rotation slightly to either side, and then forward with slight lateral flexion to either side (Figs. 1-11 and 1-12). Thus, the clinician gently stretches the different portions of these muscles in their respective fiber directions. It is often difficult to stretch the fibers at the cervicocranial juncture in this position, because the clinician should not place too much pressure on the neck and head. It is helpful to follow the seated stretches with supine stretches. Here the clinician stands facing the patient and at the side of the table by the patient's left side. The clinician uses the left hand to reach under the right side of the patient's skull and lifts the head with gentle traction while using the vapocoolant spray (Fig. 1-13). The head is thus brought into flexion relative to the neck, and the clinician can use trigger point pressure release on the trigger points that are at the cervicocranial juncture. To address trigger points at the left side of the base of the patient's skull, the clinician stands at the patient's right side and reaches the right hand under the patient's left skull and lifts the head, gently stretching the involved muscles

and applying trigger point pressure to specific muscles as necessary. Often it is helpful to apply moist heat directly after these stretching procedures. If there is greater occipital nerve entrapment by the semispinalis capitis muscle, an ice pack can be folded over the top edge of a cervical hydrocollator before wrapping it around the patient's neck, and the combination of hot and cold will relax the muscles and decrease the nerve tenderness. The ice is also helpful when there is marked tenderness of upper cervical facet joints.

After the application of hot or hot and cold, further manual myofascial treatment can be performed. The clinician is seated at the head of the treatment table and cradles the head and neck of the supine patient. First, the clinician assesses patterns of mobility in the neck, to select the locations for further myofascial release efforts. Releases should be performed on areas in which there is restriction of normal patterns of mobility, rather than on areas in which there is muscle tenderness associated with hypermobility. The fingers of the clinician's hands can be gently cupped so that they create a ridge, and trigger point pressure release can be performed by letting the cervical spine slightly extend over the finger contacts (Fig. 1-14). As the muscles release, the clini-

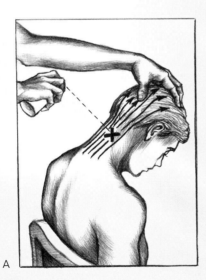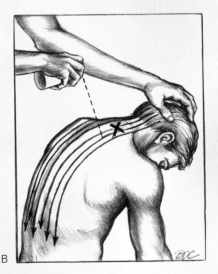

FIGURE 1-11. Posterior cervical muscle stretch (splenii and semispinalis) with application of vapocoolant spray. **A.** To stretch the upper posterior muscles, the patient's head and neck are bent forward while the spray is applied upward from the neck to the back of the head, to cover the referred pain pattern on the skull. **B.** To stretch the lower posterior muscles, the patient's upper back is rounded forward while the spray is directed from the lower neck downward into the referred pain region in the upper and middle back. The stretch is enhanced if the patient breathes out and looks down. Reprinted with permission from Simons DG, Travell JG, Simons LS: Travell & Simons' Myofascial Pain and Dysfunction: The Trigger Point Manual. Volume 1: Upper Half of Body. 2nd Ed. Baltimore: Lippincott Williams & Wilkins, 1999, fig. 16.6 A & B, p. 461.

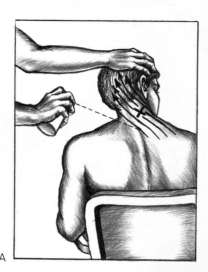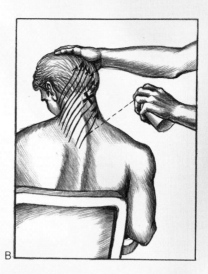

FIGURE 1-12. Spray pattern to stretch the more diagonal posterior cervical muscles. **A.** Passive stretch primarily of the right "Λ" diagonal muscles (i.e., multifidi and rotatores) and the left "V" diagonal (i.e., splenius) is performed by flexing the head and neck while turning head toward the right. **B.** Passive stretch primarily of the left " "Λ" diagonal muscles (i.e., multifidi and rotatores) and the right "V" diagonal muscles (e.g., splenius) is performed by flexing the head and neck while turning the face to the left. Reprinted with permission from Simons DG, Travell JG, Simons LS. Travell & Simons' Myofascial Pain and Dysfunction: The Trigger Point Manual. Volume 1: Upper Half of Body. 2nd Ed. Baltimore: Lippincott Williams & Wilkins, 1999, fig. 16.7 A & B, p. 462.

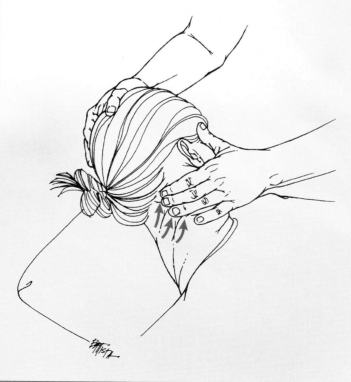

FIGURE 1-13. Passive stretch of the diagonal upper posterior cervical muscles combined with trigger point pressure release. The clinician contacts trigger points in the diagonal portions of the suboccipital muscles of the posterior neck at the cervicocranial juncture, or the splenius cervicis muscle slips as they cross the cervical facet joints. The clinician applies pressure to mobilize the joints and to perform trigger point pressure release of specific trigger points. The clinician simultaneously applies localized tissue traction to lengthen the taut muscle bands while rotating, or lifting and rotating, the head and neck of the supine patient. (The direction of the traction depends on what is required to lengthen the specific taut muscle bands in the posterior neck muscles.)

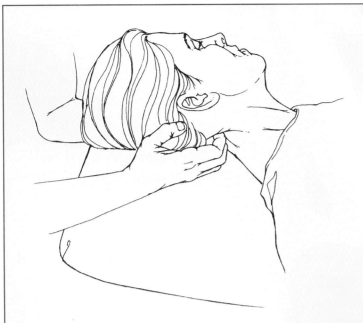

FIGURE 1-14. **Passive stretch of the vertical posterior cervical muscles combined with trigger point pressure release.** With the patient supine, the clinician's distal fingers are flexed or cupped to press between the vertebrae, or between the vertebrae and the occiput. The clinician's pressure combines localized traction to elongate muscle fibers with trigger point pressure release of specific trigger points. Mobilization of the vertebrae into increased ease of extension is also accomplished (if extension has been limited at the spinal level being treated.)

cian's contacts will gradually deepen. Then the clinician pulls the contacted portion of the neck into slight flexion. The patient can be instructed to gently extend the neck against the clinician's contact, and release into progressively greater flexion. This form of release can be performed at any level of the cervical spine at which movement is restricted. The specific direction of pressure for initial trigger point treatment and contract–relax technique can be tailored to the direction of greatest muscular restriction. Because of the many different directions of muscle fibers, especially at the cervicocranial juncture, these myofascial release techniques can be performed repeatedly in a variety of directions to address the most severely shortened muscle bands. As these release, the patterns of restriction are reassessed and the next taut bands are treated. These myofascial

techniques can be beneficial even after osseous manipulation of the cervical spine, or muscle energy techniques to address joint dysfunction have already been performed, to provide maximal relief from headaches.

After trigger points have released and taut bands have loosened, direct treatment of the entrapped occipital nerve can be performed. The clinician is seated at the head of the table and cradles the patient's head, with the fingertips contacting the point of greatest tenderness along the base of the occiput. The patient's head is slightly extended over the clinician's contact. The clinician exerts some pressure on the tender spot while the patient tucks the chin and flexes at the cervicocranial juncture and presses into the clinician's contact, stretching the muscles and nerve against the local resistance provided by the finger contact (Fig. 1-15). (A

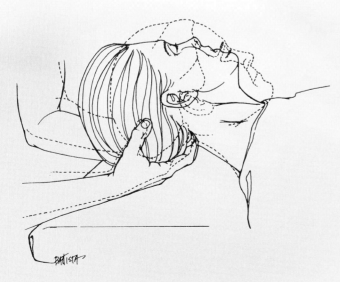

FIGURE 1-15. **Myofascial release of the semispinalis capitis with mobilization of the entrapped occipital nerve.** Initial position: The patient is supine, relaxed, with slight extension at the cervicocranial juncture. The clinician contacts the point along the base of the occiput that is most tender, pressing into the cervicocranial juncture at this point. The dotted lines show the ending position: The patient tucks the chin to the chest while pressing the base of the skull or the cervicocranial juncture into the clinician's contact. The clinician maintains the contact, offering local resistance to the tissue stretch, to mobilize the occipital nerve. (The concept of nerve mobilization is discussed in Chapter 6.)

fuller discussion of nerve mobilization is included in Chapter 6.)

It is often best to perform several treatments of more general myofascial release and joint care while avoiding direct contact and treatment of occipital nerve entrapment. The clinician should not treat the nerve entrapment if there is significant likelihood that the manual releases will not be sufficient to decrease symptoms. Stirring up the problem should be avoided. This is always a judgment call, and it is always helpful to have a medical doctor skilled in injection techniques available in case the patient's symptoms increase. Sometimes manual releases are followed by an increase in symptoms for 4 to 6 hours, and then a dramatic reduction of even long-standing pain thereafter. Even if injection techniques are used, it is beneficial to complete the process of releasing the muscular entrapment and facilitating the mobility of the nerve with manual techniques. This may lessen the likelihood of recurrence.

Sometimes, the manual treatment of trigger points will result in very rapid elimination of referred headache. In some patients, the tissues being treated are quite tender, and some headache lingers. Generally, if the relevant trigger points and joint dysfunctions or subluxations are treated, the patient will experience relief of the headache within 4 to 6 hours after the treatment has been completed.

References

1. Sanchez del Rio M, Moskowitz M. The trigeminal system. In: Olesen J, Tfelt-hansen P, Welch KMA, eds. The Headaches, 2nd Ed. Philadelphia: Lippincott Williams &Wilkins, 2000:141–149.
2. Marcus DA. Differentiating migraine from tension headaches: a real or artificial distinction. APS Bulletin 1991;1:1–9.
3. Classification and diagnostic criteria for headache disorders, cranial neuralgias and facial pain. Headache Classification Committee of the International Headache Society. Cephalalgia 1988;8(Suppl 7):1–96.
4. Cady R, Schreiber C, Farmer K, et al. Primary headaches: a convergence hypothesis. Headache 2002;42:204–216.
5. Bigal M, Sheftell F, Rappoport A, et al. Chronic daily headache: identification of factors associated with induction and transformation. Headache 2002;42:575–581.
6. Dostrovsky JO, Davis KD, Kawakita K. Central mechanisms of vascular headaches. Can J Physiol Pharmacol 1991;69:652–658.
7. Moskowitz MA. The neurobiology of vascular head pain. Ann Neurol 1984;16:157–168.
8. Launer L, Terwindt G, Ferrari M. The prevalence and characteristics of migraine in a population-based cohort: the GEM study. Neurology 1999;53:537–542.
9. Goadsby PJ, Lipton RB, Ferrari MD. Migraine: current understanding and treatment. N Engl J Med 2002;346:257–270.
10. Saper J. Daily chronic headache. Neurol Clin 1990;8:891–901.
11. Popeney C, Alo K. Peripheral neurostimulation for the treatment of chronic, disabling transformed migraine. Headache 2003;43:369–373.
12. Silberstein SD. Tension-type and chronic daily headache. Headache Q 1995;6:97–100.
13. Srikiatkhachorn A. Pathophysiology of chronic daily headache. Curr Pain Headache Rep 2001;5:537–544.
14. Sjaastad O, Fredriksen TA, Pfaffenrath V. Cervicogenic headache: diagnostic criteria. Headache 1990;30:725–726.
15. Edmeads J, Soyka D. Headache associated with disorders of the skull and cervical spine. In: Olesen J, Tfelt-Hansen P, Welch KMA, eds. The Headaches. New York: Raven Press, 1993:744–745.
16. Dumas J-P, Arsenault A, Boudreau G, et al. Physical impairment in cervicogenic headache: traumatic vs. nontraumatic onset. Cephalgia 2001;21:884–893.
17. Travell J. Referred pain from skeletal muscle: the pectoralis major syndrome of breast pain and soreness and the sternocleidomastoid syndrome of headache and dizziness. New York State Journal of Medicine 1955;55:331–340.
18. Travell J. Mechanical headache. Headache 1967;7:23–29.
19. Travell JG, Simons DG. Myofascial Pain and Dysfunction: The Trigger Point Manual, vol 1. Baltimore: Williams & Wilkins, 1983.
20. Simons DG, Travell JG, Simons LS. Myofascial Pain and Dysfunction: The Trigger Point Manual, vol 1, 2nd Ed. Baltimore: Williams and Wilkins, 1999.
21. Rogers EJ, Rogers RJ. Tension-type headaches, fibromyalgia, or myofascial pain. Headache Quarterly 1991;2:273–277.
22. Tfelt-hansen P, Lous I, Olesen J. Prevalence and significance of muscle tenderness during common migraine attacks. Headache 1981;21:49–54.
23. Clifford T, Lauritzen M, Bakke M, et al. Electromyography of pericranial muscles during treatment of spontaneous common migraine attacks. Pain 1982;14:137–147.
24. Jensen K, Tuxen C, Olesen J. Pericranial muscle tenderness and pressure-pain threshold in the temporal region during common migraine. Pain 1988;35:65–70.
25. Jensen R, Bendtsen L, Olesen J. Muscular factors are of importance in tension-type headache. Headache 1998;38:10–17.
26. Jensen R. Pathophysiological mechanisms of tension-type headache. In: Copenhagen: Foreningen af Danske Laegestuderendes Forglag, 1998:68.
27. Bendtsen L. Central sensitization in tension-type headache: possible pathophysiologic mechanisms. Cephalalgia 2000;20:486–508.
28. Duckro PN. Myofascial involvement in chronic post-traumatic headache. Headache Quarterly 1995;6:34–38.
29. Sandrini G, Nappi G. Primary headaches: diagnosis and treatment. Current Review of Pain 1999;3:100–108.
30. Ashina M, Bendtsen L, Jensen R, et al. Muscle hardness in patients with chronic tension-type headache: relation to actual headache state. Pain 1999;79:201–205.
31. Jensen R. Mechanisms of spontaneous tension-type headaches: an analysis of tenderness, pain thresholds and EMG. Pain 1995;64:251–256.
32. Jensen R, Rasmussen BK, Pederson B, et al. Muscle tenderness and pressure pain thresholds in headache: a population study. Pain 1993;52:193–199.
33. Bogaards MC, ter Kuile MM. Treatment of recurrent tension headache: a meta-analytic review. Clin J Pain 1994;10:174–190.
34. Cady R. Triptans and non-triptans: evaluation of migraine therapy. Headache Quarterly 2000;9:20–24.
35. Porta M. A comparative trial of botulinum toxin type A and methylprednisolone for the treatment of tension-type headache. Current Review of Pain 2000;4:31–35.
36. Lewis C, Gevirtz R, Hubbard D, et al. Needle trigger point and surface frontal EMG measurements of psychophysiological responses in

tension-type headache patients. Biofeedback & Self-Regulation 1994;3:274–275.

37. McNulty W, Gevirtz R, Berkoff G, et al. Needle electromyographic evaluation of trigger point response to a psychological stressor. Psychophysiology 1994;31:313–316.

38. Bogduk N, Simons DG. Neck pain: joint pain or trigger points. In: Vaeroy H, Merskey H, eds. Progress in Fibromyalgia and Myofascial Pain, vol 6. Amsterdam: Elsevier, 1993:267–273.

39. Lord SM, Barnsley Le, Wallis BJ, et al. Third occipital nerve headache: a prevalence study. J Neurol Neurosurg Psychiatry 1994; 57:1187–1190.

40. Barnsley L, Lord S, Bogduk N. Whiplash injury. Pain 1993;58: 283–307.

41. Fischer AA. New developments in diagnosis of myofascial pain and fibromyalgia. In: Fischer AA, ed. Myofascial Pain: Update in Diagnosis and Treatment, vol 8. Philadelphia: Saunders, 1997:1–21.

42. Gerwin RD, Shannon S, Hong C-Z, et al. Interrater reliability in myofascial trigger point examination. Pain 1997;69:65–73.

43. Simons D. Reply to M.I. Weintraub (Letter). Pain 1999;80:451–452.

44. Dejung B. Manuelle Triggerpunktbehandlung bei chronischer Lumbosakralgie. Schweiz Med Wochenschr 1994;124:82–87.

45. Gunn CC. The Gunn Approach to the Treatment of Chronic Pain. Edinburgh: Churchill Livingstone, 1996.

46. Lewit K: Manipulative Therapy in Rehabilitation of the Locomotor System. Oxford: Butterworth-Heinemann, 1991.

2 *Masticatory Myofascial Pain*

James Fricton, DDS

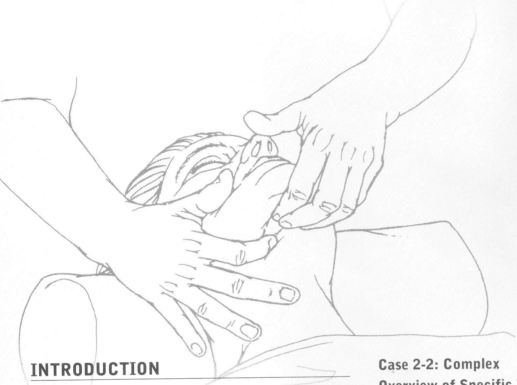

INTRODUCTION

MASTICATORY MYOFASCIAL PAIN: BACKGROUND

Diagnosis and Clinical Features

COMPREHENSIVE TREATMENT OF MASTICATORY MYOFASCIAL PAIN

Technique 2-1: Palliative self-care program for acute episodes of myofascial pain

Case 2-1: Simple

Case 2-2: Complex

Overview of Specific Treatment Issues

Explanatory Model in the Etiology and Progression of Myofascial Pain

CONCLUSION

Protocol for Managing Masticatory and Cervical Myofascial Pain

Technique Section: Manual Myofascial Release Techniques for Muscles Involved in Masticatory Myofascial Pain

INTRODUCTION

Masticatory myofascial pain (MMFP) is a regional muscle pain disorder in the head and neck, characterized by muscle tenderness in masticatory muscles and pain in the jaw, face, ear, teeth, head, or neck. This chapter introduces an etiologic model of MMFP that includes both peripheral and central pain mechanisms. Pain that is generated from peripheral neurologic mechanisms because of local biomechanical strain leads to the onset of early cases of MMFP, whereas central mechanisms associated with persistent psychosocial factors lead to increased chronicity of MMFP. Management of the syndrome naturally follows from this model with therapy to rehabilitate the trigger points while focusing effort on reducing all contributing factors. The purpose of this chapter is to discuss the most recent information on clinical characteristics, diagnostic criteria, and risk factors associated with development and progression of myofascial pain and how this information can be used in management of two example cases.

MASTICATORY MYOFASCIAL PAIN: BACKGROUND

Masticatory myofascial pain is the most common cause of persistent pain in the head and neck and often affects the muscles of mastication, facial muscles, and cervical muscles (1). Two studies of pain clinic populations have indicated that MFP was cited as the most common cause of pain, being reported in 54.6% of a chronic head and neck pain population (1) and 85% of a back pain population (2). In addition, Skootsky et al. (3) studied myofascial pain in a general internal medicine practice and found that, among those patients who present with pain, 29.6% were found to have myofascial pain as its cause. In one epidemiologic study of orofacial pain in a young female general population (ages 20–40), using specific criteria, Schiffman et al. (4) found that myofascial pain in the masticatory muscles occurred in approximately 50% of this general population, with 6% having symptoms severe enough to be comparable to patients seeking treatment. Although the exact cause of MMFP is unclear, recent research has improved our understanding of the clinical features and factors that contribute to the development and progression of MMFP. Understanding these will help in validating an explanatory model for the origin and treatment of MMFP.

Diagnosis and Clinical Features

The clinical characteristics of myofascial pain include trigger points in muscle bands, pain in a zone of reference, occasional associated symptoms, and the presence of contributing factors (Table 2-1). A trigger point is defined as a localized deep tenderness in a taut band of skeletal muscle that is responsible for the pain in the zone of reference and if treated will resolve the resultant pain (1,5–9). The zone of reference is defined as the area of perceived pain referred by the irritable trigger point. It is usually located over the trigger point or spreads out from the trigger point to a distant site. In the masticatory system, there are no neurologic deficits associated with the disorder unless a nerve entrapment syndrome with weakness and diminished sensation coincides with the muscle trigger points (8). This has occurred occasionally with the maxillary or mandibular nerve in the face. Results of blood and urine studies are generally normal unless the pain is caused by a concomitant disorder. Imaging studies including radiographs and magnetic resonance imaging do not reveal any pathologic changes in the muscle or connective tissue.

Because of this lack of objective findings and lack of diagnostic criteria, MMFP is often overlooked as a common cause of persistent pain (8,10–17). However, MFP, particularly in the head and neck, has numerous ancillary findings and common associations with joint disorders and other pain disorders. In addition, despite trauma being the major initiating factor, a multitude of other contributing factors perpetuate the condition and make it more difficult to treat (see Table 2-1). Each of these is discussed along with current knowledge of prevalence.

Symptom Presentation

The most frequent symptoms of MMFP include jaw pain, temple headaches, facial pain, ear pain, tooth pain, and oc-

---

TABLE 2-1

Clinical Characteristics of Masticatory and Cervical Myofascial Pain

Trigger Points in Taut Band of Muscle	Pain in Zone of Reference
Tenderness on palpation	Constant dull ache
Consistent points of tenderness	Fluctuates in intensity
Palpation alters pain locally or distally	Consistent patterns of referral Alleviation with extinction of trigger point
Associated symptoms	**Contributing factors**
Otologic tinnitus, plugged sensation	Macrotrauma and whiplash injuries
Paresthesias	Occupational and repetitive strain injuries
GI distress	Disuse
Visual disturbances	Oral para-functional muscle tension–producing habits
Dermatographia	Postural and repetitive strain Metabolic/nutritional Sleep disturbance Pacing problems Psychosocial stressors Depression Anxiety

cipital, frontal, or vertex headache. Because of the frequent convergence of **afferent** input from this area, referred pain is common and can confuse the diagnosis or location of trigger points. For example, myofascial pain frequently can cause pain in the teeth, often confusing dentists who do not find pulpal pathology as the cause of the pain. The pain is often continuous dull steady pain that is bilateral or unilateral. It can be accompanied by numbness, tingling, plugged ear, dizziness, or sensitivity in the teeth, confusing the diagnosis even further. When accompanied by a disk displacement, temporomandibular joint (TMJ) clicking and locking also can occur.

Trigger Points

A trigger point is a 2- to 5-mm diameter point of increased hypersensitivity in palpable bands of skeletal muscle, tendons, and ligaments with decreasing hypersensitivity as one palpates the band further away from the trigger point. The points may be active or latent (9). Active trigger points are hypersensitive and display continuous pain in the zone of reference that can be altered with specific palpation. Latent trigger points display only hypersensitivity with no continuous pain. This localized tenderness has been found to be a reliable indicator of the presence and severity of MMFP with both manual palpation and pressure algometers (18–20). However, the presence of taut bands appears to be a characteristic of skeletal muscles in all subjects regardless of the presence of MMFP (17). Palpating the active trigger point with sustained deep single-finger pressure on the taut band will elicit an alteration of the pain (intensify or reduce) in the zone of reference (area of pain complaint) or cause radiation of the pain toward the zone of reference. This can occur immediately or be delayed a few seconds. The pattern of referral is both reproducible and consistent with patterns of other patients with similar trigger points. Figures 1-1 and 1-2 illustrate the typical referred pain patterns from trigger points in the neck and facial muscles that are often involved in MMFP. Figure 2-1 illustrates the referred pain from trigger points in additional muscles. This enables a clinician to use the zone of reference as a guide to locate the trigger point for purposes of treatment. The patient's behavioral reaction to this firm palpation is a distinguishing characteristic of MMFP and is termed a "jump sign." This reaction may include withdrawal of the head, wrinkling of their face or forehead, or a verbal response such as "that's it" or "Oh, yes." The "jump sign" should be distinguished from the "local twitch response" that also can occur with palpation. This latter response can be elicited by placing the muscle in moderate passive tension and snapping the band containing the trigger point briskly with firm pressure from a palpating finger moving perpendicularly across the muscle band at its most tender point. This can produce a reproducible shortening of the muscle band (visible in larger muscles) and associated electromyographic changes characteristic of the "local twitch response" described later (12,21–23). In locating an active trigger point, the "jump sign" should be elicited

and if possible, alteration of the patient's complaint obtained through palpation.

Local and Referred Pain

In examining the basic concept of MMFP, namely, local and referred pain from trigger points, there must be evidence that supports the concept that the pain is related to or generated by the trigger point, particularly if it is distant from the trigger point. This evidence primarily stems from clinical observation and needs to be studied more rigorously in well-controlled scientific studies. First, clinical examination of trigger points demonstrates that in accessible muscles palpation of the active trigger points will alter the referred pain (usually with intensification). In addition, injections of local anesthetic into the active trigger point will reduce or eliminate the referred pain and the tenderness (24–26). Treatment such as spray and stretch, exercises, or massage, directed at the muscle with the trigger point also will predictably reduce the referred pain (27). Other evidence to confirm the relationship includes the use of pressure algometry to show a positive correlation between both the scope of tenderness and the severity of pain (28). In addition, the change in scope of tenderness in response to treatment correlates positively with the change in symptom severity ($r = 0.54$) (28).

Ancillary Findings and Relationship with Other Disorders

The affected muscles also may display an increased fatigability, stiffness, subjective weakness, pain in movement, and slight restricted range of motion that is unrelated to joint restriction (1,6–9). The muscles are painful when stretched, causing the patient to protect the muscle through poor posture and sustained contraction (29). For example, a study of jaw range of motion in patients with MMFP and no joint abnormalities indicated a slightly diminished range of motion of 35 to 45 mm (approximately 10% less than that of normal subjects) and pain in full range of motion. This is considerably less limitation than was found with joint locking caused by a TMJ internal derangement (20–35 mm) (17). This restriction may perpetuate the trigger point and develop other trigger points in the same muscle and agonist muscles. As mentioned earlier, this can cause multiple trigger points with overlapping areas of pain referral and changes in pain patterns as trigger points are inactivated. Other causes of diminished mandibular opening include structural disorders of the TMJ, such as ankylosis, internal derangements, coronoid hypertrophy, and gross osteoarthritis. These also must be ruled out with radiographs and clinical examination.

Although routine clinical electromyographic (EMG) studies show no significant abnormalities associated with trigger points, some specialized EMG studies indicate differences (12,21–23,30). The consistency of soft tissues over the trigger points has been found to be more than that for adjacent muscles (31,32). Skin overlying the trigger points in the masseter muscle appears to be warmer as measured

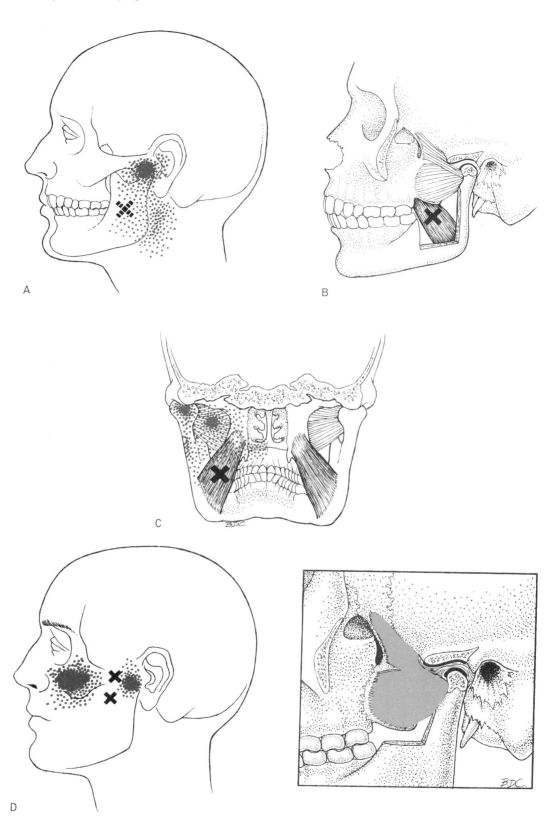

FIGURE 2-1. **Pterygoid muscles. A, B,** and **C.** Trigger points and referred pain patterns for the medial pterygoid muscle. **D.** Trigger points and referred pain patterns for the lateral pterygoid muscle. The x's denote the common trigger point locations, and the red zones are the common locations of pain referred from these trigger points. Note: Many other facial and neck muscles are involved in masticatory myofascial pain, and Figures 1-1 and 1-2 show many of these muscles.

Reprinted with permission from Simons DG, Travell JG, Simons LS. Travell & Simons' Myofascial Pain and Dysfunction: The Trigger Point Manual, vol 1: Upper Half of Body. 2nd Ed. Baltimore: Lippincott Williams & Wilkins, 1999, Figures 10.1 (p. 366) and 11.1 (p. 380).

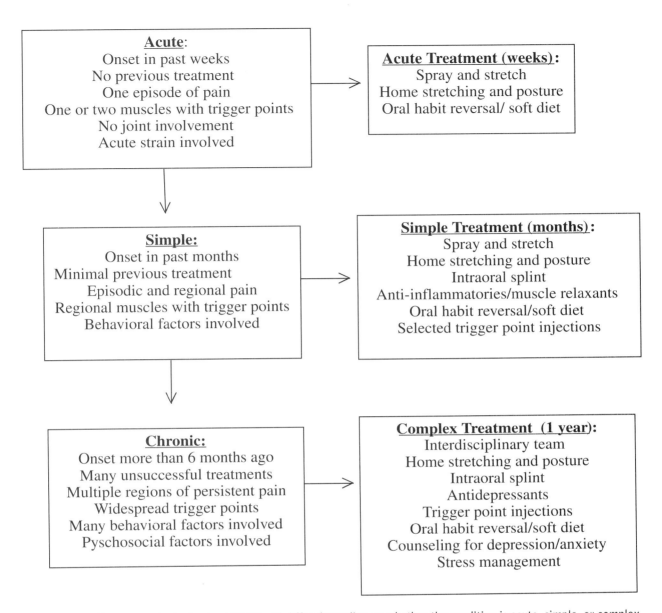

FIGURE 2-2. Treatment strategies for MMFP will differ depending on whether the condition is acute, simple, or complex.

by infrared emission (33). Although each of these findings is from a solitary study, they do provide preliminary evidence of a broad range of objective characteristics that may prove important in diagnosis of MMFP.

Many of the characteristics of MMFP are also found in other muscle pain disorders such as fibromyalgia, tension-type headaches, myositis, and muscle spasm. Perhaps the most pragmatic taxonomy related to differentiating muscle pain disorders is in the American Academy of Orofacial Pain's *Guidelines for Diagnosis and Management of Temporomandibular Disorders* (34). In this classification, muscle disorders are distinguished from each other by their clinical characteristics and not by pathophysiology or cause. Muscle pain disorders are classified as myofascial pain (regional pain and localized tenderness), fibromyalgia (widespread pain with localized tender points), myositis (regional pain and diffuse tenderness over the entire muscle), muscle spasm (brief painful contraction with limited range of motion), contracture (long-standing limited range of motion due to fibrosis), and muscle splinting (regional pain and localized tenderness accompanying a joint problem). Other terms used in the past for the broad category of muscle pain syndromes, such as *fibrositis, myofascial pain dysfunction (MPD), myelogelosen, interstitial myofibrositis, musculofascial pain dysfunction, TMJ dysfunction, nonarticular rheumatism,* and *myalgia,* are poorly defined and confusing and thus should be avoided.

In most recent classifications, the regional pain found with MMFP is distinguished from the widespread muscular pain associated with fibromyalgia (FM). These two disorders have many similar characteristics and may represent two ends of a continuous spectrum. For example, as Simons (35) points out, 16 of the 18 tender point sites in FM lie at well-known trigger point sites. Many of the clinical characteristics of FM, such as fatigue, morning stiffness, and sleep disorders, also can accompany MMFP. Bennett (36) compares these two disorders and concludes that these are two distinct disorders but may have similar underlying pathophysiology. The clinical significance of distinguishing between them lies in the more common centrally generated contributing factors in FM (sleep disorders, depression, and stress) versus the more common regional contributing factors in MFP (trauma, posture, and muscle tension habits) as well as the better prognosis in treatment of MFP as compared with FM.

COMPREHENSIVE TREATMENT OF MASTICATORY MYOFASCIAL PAIN

Many authors have found success in treatment of MMFP with the use of a wide variety of techniques, such as exercise, trigger point injections, vapo-coolant spray and stretch, intraoral splints, transcutaneous electrical nerve stimulation, biofeedback, posture correction, tricyclic antidepressants, muscle relaxant and other medications, and addressing perpetuating factors (5,6–9,34–38). However, the difficulty in managing MMFP lies in the critical need to match the level of complexity of the management program with the complexity of the patient's condition.

Thus, treatment strategies can differ depending on whether the condition is acute, simple, or complex (see Fig. 2-2). Acute cases of recent onset often can be managed with palliative care strategies designed to protect the muscles and encourage healing (Technique 2-1). Simple

---

BOX 2-1

Indicators of Case Complexity

Fulfilling any one of these criteria may suggest that this case is complex and may require the use of the team to improve outcomes.

1. Persistent pain (daily or regular) longer than 6 months in duration
2. Significant lifestyle disturbances such as loss of work, social activities, or home activities
3. High use of health care in the past, including medications for problem or related problems
4. Emotional difficulties related to problem, including depression, anxiety, or anger
5. Daily oral habits, such as clenching or grinding of the teeth
6. Significant stressful life events such as pacing problems, divorce, or recent death in family

---

cases with minimal behavioral and psychosocial involvement can be managed by a single clinician with home care, exercises, a stabilization splint, and spray and stretch. Results from clinical studies indicate that many patients with MMFP have complex conditions and have seen many clinicians and received numerous medications and other singular treatments for years without receiving more than temporary improvement (1). These complex cases can be most effectively managed within an interdisciplinary pain clinic setting that uses a team of clinicians to address different aspects of the problem in a concerted fashion. Failure to address the entire problem, including all involved muscles, concomitant diagnoses, and contributing factors, may lead to failure to resolve the pain and perpetuation of a chronic pain syndrome (Box 2-1). This complex team approach often requires shifting the paradigms implicit in patient care, listed in Table 2-2.

Regardless of complexity, evaluation of myofascial pain includes locating the trigger points and muscles involved as well as recognition of all contributing factors. Management of the syndrome follows with muscle exercises, splints, therapy to the trigger points, and reducing all contributing factors. The short-term goal is to restore the muscle to normal length, posture, and full joint range of motion with exercises and trigger point therapy (Box 2-2). This is followed over the long term with a regular muscle stretching, relaxation postural, and strengthening exercise program as well as control of contributing factors. Each of these major interventions is discussed in more detail as part of the two cases.

TECHNIQUE 2-1

Palliative self-care program for acute episodes of myofascial pain

1. Eat a soft diet and avoid caffeine.
2. Keep your tongue up and gently resting on the palate. Keep teeth apart as the rest position of the jaw.
3. Chew on both sides at the same time or alternate sides to minimize strain to muscles.
4. Avoid oral para-functional habits such as clenching and grinding the teeth, jaw tensing, or gum chewing.
5. Avoid excessive or prolonged opening of mouth.
6. Avoid stomach sleeping to minimize strain to the jaw during sleep.
7. Use over-the-counter analgesics or nonsteroidal anti-inflammatories as needed for pain.
8. Use heat or ice over the tender muscles.

TABLE 2-2

Shifting the Doctor/Patient Paradigms Involves Each Member of the Team Following the Same Concepts by Conveying the Same Messages Implicit in Their Dialogue with the Patient

Concept	Statement
Self-responsibility	You have more influence on your problem than we do
Self-care	You will need to make daily changes to to improve your condition
Education	We can teach you how to make the changes
Long-term change	It will take at least 6 months for the changes to have an effect
Strong doctor–patient relationship	We will support you as you make the changes
Patient motivation	Do you want to make the changes?

BOX 2-2

Short- and long-term goals in treatment of myofascial pain

Short-term goals
1. Reduce pain
2. Restore muscle to normal length with full joint range of motion
3. Restore muscle to normal posture
4. Reduce sustained muscle activity and tension

Long-term goals
1. Restore normal lifestyle activities
2. Reduce contributing factors
3. Regular stretching, postural, and conditioning exercises
4. Proper use of muscles

CASE 2-1

Simple

Kim S. was a 26-year-old white married high school band director who was referred to the clinic by her orthodontist and physician.

Symptoms

Her chief complaints included:

1. Bilateral temporal headaches. These occurred two to three times per week and were of constant duration. The pain fluctuated in intensity.

2. Bilateral jaw pain, particularly on chewing and use of the jaw. It occurred on a daily basis and lasted only a few minutes beyond the use of the jaw.

She also noted that other recent symptoms included TMJ noises and difficulty chewing, and her bite was unstable. She denied any other dental symptoms, neurologic symptoms, ear, nose, and throat symptoms, or other sinus symptoms.

History of Illness

The onset of these symptoms occurred 1 month before presenting to the clinic after a motor vehicle accident. She had no direct trauma to the face or head. She gradually developed jaw pain and temple headaches after the accident. She has taken acetaminophen and ibuprofen for the pain. This helped the pain somewhat, but she continued to have symptoms that bothered her. In addition, the bite had shifted and became unstable. Overall, her pain condition had improved, but her orthodontist referred her to the clinic to evaluate and treat the jaw symptoms and evaluate the cause of the bite instability.

Medical History

A review of her medical history indicated that she had a routine physical examination recently, and everything was within normal limits. Her blood pressure was 112/76 mm/Hg, and her pulse was 76 beats/min. She was approximately 8 weeks pregnant and had some morning nausea because of this. Family history was noncontributory. There was no history of infectious diseases. Past surgeries included third molar removal with minor complications associated with general anesthesia. She was not currently using any prescription medications.

Personal History

She was a 26-year-old woman who was working full-time as a band director at the local grade schools and high school. She was the first child of two in her family, with a younger brother. She denied any abuse or other stress in her family as a child. She was recently married, with no children. The relationship with her family and husband has been good. She found that her teaching responsibilities were large, and, because of the pain, work was somewhat stressful. The pain interfered with normal jaw activities including chewing, eating hard foods, playing musical instruments, and continuous talking as a school teacher. She admitted to being anxious because of the persistent pain. She noted some weekly **oral parafunctional habits**, including clenching and grinding her teeth at night, thus waking up with sore jaws, holding the jaw forward, and unilateral chewing.

(continues)

CASE 2-1 Continued

Examination

Stomatognathic examination showed a normal maximum jaw opening of 45 mm with a passive stretch opening of 48 mm from incisal edge to incisal edge. There was pain bilaterally in the preauricular area on opening. There was no deviation on opening. There was slight limitation of 6 mm with protrusion and 6 mm with right laterotrusion and a normal 10-mm left laterotrusion. There was pain in the jaw in all excursive movements. Inspection of the temporomandibular joints showed no locking open or closed. Palpation of the TMJs on opening showed normal translation and fine **crepitus** bilaterally.

Palpation of the masticatory and cervical muscles for tenderness indicated tenderness in the following muscle sites: anterior, middle, and posterior temporalis bilaterally duplicating her headaches superior, and middle masseter bilaterally duplicating her jaw pain, posterior mandibular area on right, submandibular area at the angle of the mandible bilaterally, insertion of the sternocleidomastoid bilaterally, and upper trapezius bilaterally. She was not tender in the parietal or occipital reference sites. Palpation of the temporomandibular joints for tenderness was unremarkable.

Occlusal examination showed 28 teeth with a **class II division 1 occlusion** of the right and a **class I occlusion** on the left. She had a 3 mm horizontal overlap and 3 mm vertical overlap. She also had some crowding of the teeth. She had orthodontic treatment in the past. Examination of the functional occlusion indicated that she had an unstable occlusion with **posterior prematurities** bilaterally in **postural rest closure** and guided position. She had a significant slide from guided position of the jaw to full **intercuspal position** of 2 mm anteriorly, 2 mm vertically, and 2 mm to the left. She had **canine guidance** in lateral excursions and no working or non-working side interferences. Vertical dimension was within normal limits. Intraoral examination showed no evidence of dental caries, periodontal disease, gingivitis, tooth wear, or soft tissue disease. However, some maxillary posterior teeth were tender to percussion. Results of a review of general appearance, mental status, and cranial nerve evaluation were within normal limits. Head and neck inspection showed no abnormalities in the skull, skin, eyes, ear, nose, throat, hair, and vascularity. Sinus percussion was normal. There were no masses, swellings, or enlarged nodes palpated.

Diagnoses

Based on this evaluation and using guidelines of the American Academy of Orofacial Pain, the primary physical diagnosis responsible for the chief complaints included myofascial pain of the masticatory (masseter and temporalis) and some posterior cervical muscles with associated pain and muscle tenderness. Contributing factors included the occlusal or bite instability, stressful life events, mild anxiety reaction, and oral para-functional habits.

Treatment Approach for Simple Case

This case was relatively acute, of recent onset, and having few behavioral and psychosocial factors, and thus was considered simple. Initial treatment over the first month consisted of palliative home care to protect the muscles from repetitive strain and encourage relaxation and healing (see Technique 2-1). There were no active treatments provided during this period while pre-authorization was obtained from the insurance company. The patient complied well with the home care recommendations, and at her follow-up appointment 1 month later, she had a decrease in the jaw pain intensity. However, with some persistent pain, the patient desired continued care. Thus, the dentist initiated care over next 2 months at biweekly intervals. The treatment included masticatory muscle exercises primarily focusing on stretching and tongue posture, an intraoral stabilization splint, and spray and stretch. At this second visit, impressions were taken for the splint while the dentist reviewed the exercises for the jaw. The splint was inserted at the third visit with a review of compliance with exercises and reduction of oral habits by the dentist. The splint was then worn over the next 3 months, primarily at night, whereas the exercises and oral habit reduction were continued during the day.

Exercises

Masticatory muscle stretching, relaxation posture, and strengthening exercises were provided. A home program of active and passive muscle stretching exercises was designed to reduce the activity of trigger points, whereas relaxation and postural exercises were designed to reduce susceptibility to trigger point reactivation. Conditioning exercises also were reviewed to improve circulation, strength, and durability of the muscles.

One of the goals of the set of jaw exercises was to restore the normal range of jaw motion. A slightly limited jaw opening and palpation of the masticatory muscles indicated that there were trigger points within the elevator muscles: temporalis, masseter, and medial pterygoid. Mandibular opening was measured as the **inter-incisal distance** with a normal maximum range of opening between 45 and 60 mm or approximately three knuckles' width (nondominant hand). Her mandibular opening with trigger points in the masseter was 40 mm or two knuckles width. This patient had a borderline limitation in range of motion of the jaw.

CASE 2-1　Continued

The patient was instructed to perform active stretching at home and in the office 6 times per day for a few minutes each time as illustrated in Figure 2-3. Active stretching of the muscles increased the opening to the normal range as well as decreased the pain. It was emphasized to avoid rapid, and relaxation jerky stretching or over stretching of the muscle to reduce potential injury to the muscle. Postural and relaxation exercises for MMFP also were provided to the patient to teach her mental reminders to hold the body in a balanced, relaxed

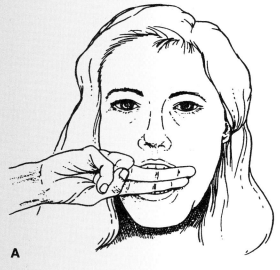

FIGURE 2-3. **Exercises to improve jaw range of motion and correct posture.** These exercises can be used for initial postural correction and range of motion restoration for masticatory myofascial pain. They can restore normal joint function, and mobility and a more comfortable and normal jaw position. They are performed gradually and gently six times daily for about 1 minute each. **A.** Jaw should be stretched slightly beyond the point of tightness and pain, usually 2 to 3 fingers width. Precaution should be made to avoid over-stretching with acutely strained jaws or severe capsulitis of the temporomandibular joint. **B.** The following six exercises are performed to correct posture and hold the body in a balanced and relaxed position that affords the best mechanical advantage for the jaw. In the first exercise, the tongue is held gently on the roof of the mouth with the teeth slightly apart, to reduce oral habits and relax the jaw.

Modified with permission from Rocabado M, Iglarsh Z: Musculoskeletal Approach to Maxillofacial Pain. Philadelphia: Lippincott, 1991, figs 7–3 (p. 49) and 16–17 through 16–22 (p. 188–191).

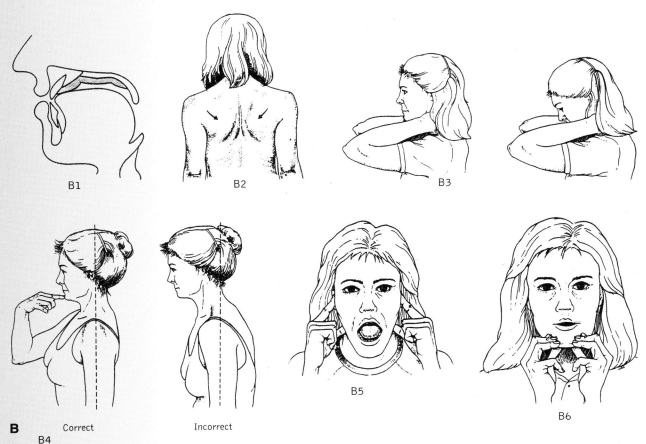

continues

CASE 2-1   Continued

position and use the body in positions that afford the best mechanical advantage. She was also instructed to place the tongue gently on the roof of the mouth and keep the teeth slightly apart. Sleeping posture on the side or back with the head (but not jaw) supported by the pillow was also suggested to avoid waking up with soreness. Improved posture was facilitated by regular physical conditioning. This patient was placed on a regular conditioning program to facilitate increased aerobic capacity and strength. Aerobic programs such as an exercise class, regular running, walking, biking, or swimming are recommended to improve comfort, endurance, and functional status of patients with MMFP.

Intra-oral Splint

In this case, the full-arch stabilization splint was used at night and as much as possible during the day to protect the teeth, muscles, and joints from oral habits such as clenching and reduce the biomechanical strain to the muscles. Impressions, taken at the second visit, were sent to the laboratory for construction of a mandibular heat-cured hard acrylic splint. The splint was inserted at the third visit and adjusted. This splint, also called a flat-plane, **gnathological**, or full-coverage splint, was designed to provide postural stabilization and to protect the TMJ, muscles, and teeth. For this reason, the patient was asked to wear it most of the day and all night long. The splint's occlusal surface was adjusted to provide a stable occlusal posture by creating single contacts in all posterior teeth in **centric relation** and **centric occlusion**. Anterior guidance was provided by the incisal plane, and lateral guidance was provided by a canine ramp. Complications and problems with the splint were monitored at the next visit 2 weeks later. Possible complications that were evaluated included difficulty speaking from thickness, a tight-fitting splint, plaque and caries, gingival inflammation, bite shifting, and mouth odors attributable to poor oral hygiene. In this case, the splint was too thick in the lingual, making it difficult to pronounce the "s" sound. This was adjusted. At each of the subsequent visits every 2 weeks, the splint was adjusted again to ensure the splint was still hitting evenly on both the posterior teeth in centric occlusion and centric relation. Over the next month, the bite instability that had plagued her was reduced, because the jaw shifted posture as the splint was adjusted.

Spray and Stretch

In this case, the spray and stretch technique for reducing myofascial pain trigger points was used to provide stretching with repetitive counter-stimulation. With the spray and stretch technique, vapo-coolant was applied over the muscle with simultaneous passive stretching. This provided her immediate reduction of pain at the visit, whereas the overall management program helped obtain longer-lasting relief. The technique involved directing a fine stream of vapo-coolant spray from the finely calibrated nozzle toward the skin directly overlying the muscle with the trigger point. A few sweeps of the spray were first passed over the trigger point and zone of reference before sufficient manual stretch to the muscle was added to elicit pain and discomfort. The masticatory muscles were put on a progressively increasing passive stretch with three fingers, to a minimum of 45 mm incisal opening. The jet stream of spray was directed at an acute angle 30 to 50 cm (1–1.5 feet) away. It was applied in one direction from the trigger point toward its reference zone in slow, even sweeps over adjacent parallel areas at a rate of approximately 10 cm/sec. This sequence was repeated up to four times. The patient's muscle was warmed with the warm hand after each sequence to prevent over cooling. Frosting the skin and excessive sweeps were avoided because the underlying skeletal muscle temperature may lower, thus aggravating trigger points. The range of passive and active motion were tested before and after spraying as an indication of responsiveness to therapy. Her range of motion from incisal edge to incisal edge was 45 mm before and 48 mm without pain after the procedure. If spray and stretch had failed with repeated trials, the causes for this failure would have been evaluated, including 1) inability to secure full muscle length because of bone or joint abnormalities, muscle contracture, or the patient avoiding voluntary relaxation; 2) incorrect spray technique; or 3) failure to reduce perpetuating factors. In this case, the problem was corrected. If the pain persisted despite this, manual therapy (described later) or direct needling with trigger point injections would have been indicated.

Results

The results in this case were typical of most patients with simple histories and straightforward problems as treated by a single clinician. Changes in each of her presenting symptoms were carefully monitored. By the end of the three visits over 2 months, the patient felt the following changes in her chief complaints:

1. The bilateral temporal headaches that had originally occurred 2 to 3 times per week were gone during the

CASE 2-1 Continued

last 2 weeks of the treatment period. At follow-up 3 months after the last visit, she reported that the headaches were no longer a problem.

2. The bilateral jaw pain that had occurred during chewing and use of the jaw was also gone. At follow-up she did, however, report occasional stiffness of her jaw when she chewed too hard or persisted in clenching her teeth.

Objectively, range of motion was normal with only minimal tenderness in the muscles of mastication. Subjectively, she reported excellent satisfaction in achieving pain relief and had more stability in her bite.

Follow-up

She was placed on an aftercare program to maintain her progress. This included avoiding overuse of the jaw with normal daily activities. She was asked to tell her dentist and dental hygienist about the temporomandibular disorder and to ask them to be careful in opening the mouth too wide or for too long. She was also asked to maintain the home program that she had used to initially improve the problem. Finally, because many patients do have occasional flare-ups, she was asked to try to identify any factors that might contribute to this if it occurred. She was able to maintain her symptom progress at the 5-month follow-up with minimal flare-ups and was quite satisfied with care.

CASE 2-2

Complex

Anita was a 39-year-old white married law clerk and graduate student who was referred to the clinic by her physician.

Symptoms

Her chief complaints included:

1. Bilateral jaw and facial pain that was greater on the right than the left side. It occurred on a daily basis and was constant. It fluctuated in intensity during the course of a day.

2. Occipital pain that she described as pain in the "pillar" of her neck radiating up to the head. It also occurred on a daily basis and was constant.

3. Headaches bilaterally in the temples that occurred twice per week.

She also noted other recent symptoms that included TMJ cracking, earaches, difficulty chewing, weakness in the right jaw, tingling in the right face, her bite was off, blurred vision, teeth sensitive to cold, congested nose, dizziness, fatigue, generalized joint pain, generalized weakness, shoulder pain, and arm pain. She denied any other dental symptoms, neurologic symptoms, ear, nose, and throat symptoms, or other sinus symptoms.

History

The onset of the symptoms occurred in the 1980s when they gradually came on with no initiating events.

She was seen at that time by an otolaryngologist who ruled out significant ear, nose, and throat disease and a neurologist who ruled out neurologic disorders. No treatment or medications were recommended. In 1985, she had a head injury at work that aggravated her symptoms. Since 1990, the symptoms had been getting worse, so she sought care with her dentist. He recommended a splint but it was not made because of insurance problems. She was referred to another neurologist, who prescribed muscle relaxants that helped somewhat. She was also referred to a rheumatologist who diagnosed her with fibromyalgia and prescribed amitriptyline and ibuprofen. Subsequently, she was also referred to a physical therapist for exercises and modalities, primarily for the neck pain. Anita sought help with a massage therapist on her own and had some improvement in the pain. Overall, her pain condition had improved slightly, but she continued to have daily constant jaw pain. Thus, she was referred to the clinic to evaluate and treat the persistent jaw symptoms. She had no diagnostic tests or radiographs of the jaw before the referral.

Medical History

A review of her medical history showed that she had a routine physical examination 3 years previously that was normal. She was diagnosed with fibromyalgia 2 years ago. In a review of family medical history, she noted that her brother also had a TMJ problem. Past surgeries included removal of a lipoma from her left arm and wis-

continues

dom teeth extraction several years ago. The only trauma she had was the injury to her head at work, as noted earlier. This trauma did aggravate the jaw and head pain. Her current medications included terfenadine and beclomethasone dipropionate on occasion for sinus congestion and amitriptyline 20 to 30 mg at bedtime, and ibuprofen, 1 tablet 2 to 3 times per day. She also noted being allergic to codeine.

Personal History

She was a 39-year-old woman who was working 80% time as a law clerk and was attending graduate school for a Ph.D. in counseling. She was the third child of four in her family. She denied any abuse in her family, but her mother was chemically dependent on alcohol. She was recently married with no children. The relationships with her family and husband were good. Significant stress existed because of her recent wedding, remodeling of her new house, and attending school and working at the same time. She reduced her work schedule to 80% because of the pain. In addition, the pain interfered with other daily activities, including vigorous exercise, sleeping, and driving, and interfered with normal jaw function, including chewing, eating, and speaking. She admitted to being occasionally depressed and anxious because of the pain and its restriction of daily activities. She reported a significant number of regular oral parafunctional habits, including clenching when awake and at night, biting tongue and lips, tongue thrust, unilateral chewing, holding her teeth together and her jaw tense, and cradling the phone with her shoulder. She consumed caffeinated coffee and tea 3 times per day and noted some difficulty sleeping.

Examination

Stomatognathic examination showed a maximum jaw opening of 39 mm with a passive stretch opening of 48 mm from incisal edge to incisal edge. There was restriction on opening but no pain. There was an "s" deviation on opening. There was 8 mm of protrusion, 8 mm of right laterotrusion, and 13 mm of left laterotrusion. There was pain in the left jaw on right laterotrusion. Inspection of the temporomandibular joints indicated no locking open or closed. Palpation of the temporomandibular joints (TMJs) on opening showed a normal translation and a faint opening click of the left side.

Palpation of the joint for tenderness found none. Palpation of the masticatory and cervical muscles for tenderness showed tenderness in the following muscle sites: right anterior, middle, and posterior temporalis, superior, middle and inferior masseter bilaterally, pos-

terior mandibular area bilaterally, middle body of sternocleidomastoid bilaterally, and splenius capitis bilaterally. She was not tender to palpation in the parietal or occipital reference sites used to evaluate excessive pain response.

Occlusal examination showed 28 sound teeth and class I occlusion bilaterally with 2 mm horizontal overlap and 2 mm vertical overlap. She had good interdigitation and intercuspal position stability. She had no crossbites, open-bite, crowding, occlusal plane problems, or midline shift. She had not had orthodontic treatment in the past. Examination of the functional occlusion indicated that she had posterior prematurities on the left side in both postural rest closure or guided position. She had no slide from guided position of the jaw to full intercuspal position. She had canine guidance in lateral excursions and no working or nonworking side interferences. Vertical dimension was within normal limits. Intraoral examination showed no evidence of dental caries, periodontal disease, gingivitis, tooth wear, or soft tissue disease. However, there was significant ridging on the tongue, suggestive of tongue thrust. No teeth were tender to percussion.

A review of general appearance, mental status, and cranial nerve evaluation was within normal limits. Head and neck inspection indicated no abnormalities in the skull, skin, eyes, ear, nose, throat, scalp, and vascularity. Sinus percussion was normal. There were no masses, swellings, or enlarged nodes palpated.

Radiographic Examination

Radiographic examination included Panorex and TMJ tomograms. Interpretation of TMJ tomography indicated normal-appearing condyles bilaterally with no degenerative changes. There was normal anterior translation bilaterally. Joint spaces were slightly narrow bilaterally. Interpretation of Panorex radiographs showed no dental, periodontal, or bony pathologic conditions. Sinuses and nasal passages were intact and clear.

Diagnoses

Based on this evaluation, the primary physical diagnosis responsible for the chief complaints included:

1. Myofascial pain of the masticatory and cervical muscles with associated pain and muscle tenderness using guidelines of the American Academy of Orofacial Pain

2. Fibromyalgia associated with widespread pain, fatigue, and tenderness as diagnosed by the criteria of the American Rheumatology Association

3. Nasal rhinitis associated with nasal congestion and drainage as diagnosed by the otolaryngologist

Contributing factors in this case were numerous and included long duration of the problems, oral parafunctional habits, significant stressors, dietary issues, and emotional difficulties.

General Approach to Treatment

In this case, numerous criteria for determining complexity were evident, including chronicity, lifestyle interference, high health care use, and significant stressors; thus, a team approach was recommended. Although a single clinician may have had success in managing this type of complex patient alone, the assumption behind a team approach was that it was vital to address different aspects of the problem with different clinicians to spend the time and care necessary on each problem. This enhanced the overall potential for success as exemplified in this case. The decision to use a team was made at the time of evaluation. It was important to have made this decision at the beginning of treatment and not partially through a uni-dimensional treatment plan that was failing after a few months. As noted earlier, it was important to set the patient up from the start with the treatment plan that had the highest potential for success.

Once team care was selected, a long-term management program was implemented that both treated the physical diagnosis and reduced contributing factors. In this case, we used a splint and trigger point injections by the dentist, exercises and postural rehabilitation with the physical therapist, and cognitive–behavioral therapy with the health care psychologist to reduce oral habits and manage the stressors. Appointments were about 1 per week with the entire team for 4 to 6 weeks, and then monthly for 4 months of aftercare with the dentist. The splint was inserted at the first treatment appointment and adjusted at each subsequent visit. The patient was evaluated and then instructed in the exercises at the first physical therapy visit, and the patient's compliance and technique was monitored at subsequent visits. The health psychologist evaluated the patient for further contributing factors and implemented a habit reversal program for the oral habits. Subsequent visits included addressing the stress, dietary factors, and emotional issues. The trigger point injections to the masseter, temporalis, and splenius capitis muscles were performed by the dentist later, at appointments 5, 6, and 7. The goals of trigger point injection were to help break up resistant trigger points and gain more long-term relief than had

been achieved in the first weeks of the program. (Trigger point injections are not always used in every case.)

In this case, team management for MMFP involved a dentist, health psychologist, and a physical therapist meeting about weekly for 4 visits initially. The dentist was responsible for establishing the initial physical diagnosis, providing initial home care, placing and adjusting a splint, injecting myofascial trigger points, and monitoring patient progress. The splint was inserted as described in case 1 at the first of these visits and adjusted at subsequent visits. The trigger point injections were completed at visits 5, 6, and 7. The psychologist was responsible for providing instruction about contributing factors and stress and habit management, and for establishing a program to support the patient and family in making changes. The psychologist evaluated the patient at the first visit and provided follow-up support at visits 2, 3, and 4. The physical therapist was responsible for providing support and instruction on an exercise and posture program, and also performed spray and stretch of the affected muscles much as was described in the care of Case 2-1. The physical therapist evaluated the patient at the first visit and instructed on all of the stretching and postural exercises for the jaw and neck. At visits 2, 3, and 4, the physical therapist reviewed the progress and compliance with the exercises. Each clinician was also responsible for establishing a trusting, supportive relationship with the patient while reaffirming the self-care philosophy of the program, reinforcing change, and assuring compliance. The patient was viewed as responsible for making the changes. The team met weekly from 8:30 AM to 9:00 AM to review the patient's progress.

Trigger Point Injections

In more chronic myofascial pain cases such as this, trigger point injections (TPI) have also been shown to reduce pain, increase range of motion, increase exercise tolerance, and increase circulation in muscles (24–26). The patient met the criteria and reviewed the precautions for use of TPI, and proper patient consent was obtained. Procaine (1.0%), a local anesthetic, was used without vasoconstrictors in this case. A series of three sets of TPIs were performed in the masseter, temporalis, and splenius capitis muscles. At the end of each visit, the patient left virtually free of pain. The pain gradually returned, but the level of pain was reduced. By the end of the third set of injections, the patient had significantly less pain. This was maintained by the exercises, postural changes, and behavioral changes.

continues

CASE 2-2   Continued

Cognitive–Behavioral Therapy to Control Contributing Factors

One of the common causes of failure in managing MMFP is failure to recognize and subsequently control contributing factors that may perpetuate muscle restriction and tension. Correcting poor oral habits and lifestyle interference through education and long-term reinforcement was essential to preventing a treated trigger point from returning. A cognitive–behavioral therapy (CBT) strategy is the most common technique used to change habits and was used in this case. CBT can include a range of techniques, such as habit reversal, massed practice, and overcorrection. Although many simple habits can change by making the patient aware of them, changing the persistent oral habits in this case required a structured program that was facilitated by the health psychologist. The patient was made aware that the habits will not change by themselves and that she was responsible for initiating and maintaining the behavior change.

With this knowledge, combined with monitoring of the habits by the patient, the habits changed readily, resulting in continued improvement in pain. Progress with changing habits was addressed at each of four appointments with the patient. The habits changing need to be addressed in this manner for more than 6 months for the change to be maintained over the long term. For this reason, the health psychologist followed up with the patient for several monthly visits as part of the aftercare program.

Biofeedback was also helpful at two of the visits (37,38,40). Biofeedback is a structured therapy based on the theory that when an individual receives information about a desired change and is reinforced for making it, the change is more likely to occur. Generally, biofeedback training uses equipment to measure biologic activity (e.g., surface electromyography to measure muscle activity). The equipment was designed with a "feedback" loop so that the patient received immediate information or feedback about biologic activity. When this information was available to the patient, she was able to see and feel the change in jaw muscle function, of which she had been previously unaware. Muscle tension in the jaw was reduced on receiving information from EMG measures about how postural changes in the jaw (tongue up and teeth apart) can reduce muscle activity.

In some cases, patients may have significant psychosocial problems that accompany MMFP, and they may benefit from antidepressant or antianxiety medication, counseling, or psychotherapy with a mental health professional. In this case, the patient was on tricyclic medication, and a decision was made to continue this.

Results

The results in this case were typical of those of most patients with complex histories and contributing factors. Changes in her original presenting symptoms were carefully monitored. By the end of the initial 4 weeks of the treatment program, she felt the following changes:

1. The incidence of bilateral jaw and facial pain was reduced to 1 per week, and the intensity of pain was much reduced. Duration was also shortened, with the pain lasting only a few hours, and this could be further reduced with the exercises and relaxation of the jaw.

2. The frequency of the occipital headache pain that she described as pain in the "pillar" of her neck radiating up to the head was also reduced. Although these headaches had been daily and constant, after treatment they occurred only 2 to 3 times per week and lasted only a few hours. They could also be further reduced with ibuprofen.

3. Headaches bilaterally in the temples that had occurred twice a week had subsided by the last week of the 4-week treatment program. In follow-up aftercare, she reported the headaches occurred only once every 2 to 3 weeks and only when she was under stress.

Follow-up

Over the next 6 months, the patient continued to maintain progress but had periodic flare-ups. When aggravations of the pain occurred, we asked the patient to try to identify those factors that caused the increase. The patient discovered that, when her driving time was increased, she clenched her teeth, and this aggravated her condition. In addition, when she did not sleep well, she often developed a headache the next day. These issues were addressed in follow-up sessions. Long term, the patient was quite satisfied with the outcomes and care provided.

Overview of Specific Treatment Issues

Although the interdisciplinary team program provided a broader framework for treating this patient, it added another dimension to the skills needed by the clinicians: working as part of a coordinated team. Failure to adequately integrate care can result in poor communication, fragmented care, distrustful relationships, and eventually confusion and failure in management. In this case, team coordination was facilitated by a well-defined evaluation and management system that clearly integrated team members.

A prerequisite to this team approach was the use of an inclusive medical model and conceptual framework that placed the physical, behavioral, and psychosocial aspects of illness on an equal and integrated basis. With an inclusive theory of human systems and their relationship to illness, the patient was assessed as a whole person by different clinicians from diverse backgrounds. For example, a dentist evaluated the physical diagnosis and dental causes of pain, the physical therapist evaluated poor postural habits and biomechanical musculoskeletal problems, and the psychologist evaluated behavioral problems, emotional issues, and social stressors.

Each factor identified as a contributing factor became a part of the problem list that was addressed in the treatment plan. In the process, the synergism of addressing each factor in the etiology of the disorder became apparent to clinicians. For example, the social stressors led to anxiety, the anxiety led to sustained muscle tension behaviors such as clenching, which contributed to the myofascial pain. The pain subsequently resulted in forward head posture, shoulder shrugging, and masticatory muscle tension, which again perpetuated the myofascial pain. When sleep was disturbed, the patient became more fatigued and consumed more caffeine. At times, this caused rebound pain and further disturbed sleep, and thus perpetuated the cycle. The pain contributed to more anxiety, and the cycle continued. Likewise, a reduction of each factor worked synergistically to improve the whole problem. Treatment of only one factor may improve the problem, but relief may be partial or temporary. Treatment of all factors simultaneously added a cumulative effect that was greater than the effects of treating each factor individually.

Changing behavioral factors can be relatively effective in reducing pain but may need to be supplemented by dealing with the emotional and social stressors that may generate them. Change of tension-producing habits, such as repetitive clenching, using a habit reversal technique was accomplished in this case by use of several steps:

The patient was instructed to become more aware of the habits, using a kitchen timer set to beep every 30 minutes or visual stickers placed in frequently observed locations in her daily environment, to remind her to check whether a habit was present. The most common repetitive strain habits include clenching when awake and at night, biting tongue and lips, tongue thrust, unilateral chewing, holding her teeth together and her jaw tense, and cradling the phone with her shoulder. The behavioral approach to addressing these habits included the following steps:

1. The patient was instructed on how to correct it (for example, what to do with the teeth and tongue) and

2. The patient was instructed on why to correct the habits (to reduce strain on the injured muscles.)

Habits can change relatively rapidly with this approach but will return if a more comprehensive approach is not used. The patient was also advised to reduce intake of caffeinated beverages and improve her sleep.

Numerous other methods are available for providing the repetitive stimulation to myofascial trigger points that may be just as effective as spray and stretch. These included manual therapy massage, acupressure, and ultrasound to provide noninvasive mechanical disruption; moist heat applications, ice pack, and diathermy to provide skin temperature change; and transcutaneous electrical nerve stimulation, electroacupuncture, and direct current stimulation to provide electric current stimulation. Spray and stretch was chosen in the above cases because of the simplicity and effectiveness in the hands of the treating clinician. Invasive approaches to treating trigger points include acupuncture or dry needling, trigger point injections of local anesthetic, or trigger point injections of corticosteroids or saline. These methods cause direct mechanical or chemical alteration of trigger points in complex cases. In more chronic myofascial pain cases such as the case 2, trigger point injections have been shown to reduce pain, increase range of motion, increase exercise tolerance, and increase circulation of muscles. Because the critical factor in relief is the mechanical disruption of the trigger point by the needle, the precision in needling of the exact trigger point and the intensity of pain during needling were the major factors in inactivating trigger points. Trigger point injections with local anesthetic are generally more effective and comfortable than dry needling or injecting other substances, such as saline, although acupuncture may be helpful for patients with chronic trigger points in multiple muscles. The effect of needling can be complemented with the use of local anesthetics in concentrations less than those required for a nerve conduction block. This can markedly lengthen the relative refractory period of peripheral nerves and limit the maximum frequency of impulse conduction. Precautions to the use of trigger point injections include allergy, bleeding disorders, liver disease, uncontrolled heart disease, anxiety, young children, and pregnant women. Complications from injections include hematoma, peripheral nerve injury from needle, allergic reaction to anesthetics, flare-up of muscle or joint pain if too tender, accelerated degeneration from excessive steroid injections, and systemic reaction from intravascular injections. Failure to achieve results with TPI may be caused by incorrect diagnosis, poor technique, excess tenderness and inflammation if present, muscle causing referred pain to joint, failure to gain normal range of motion, presence of excessive joint dysfunction from disc displacement, and complications from the injection.

Explanatory Model in the Etiology and Progression of Myofascial Pain

As with all chronic pain conditions, concomitant social, behavioral, and psychological disturbances often precede or follow the development of MMFP (44). Patients report psychological symptoms such as frustration, anxiety, depression, and anger if acute cases become chronic. Maladaptive behaviors such as pain verbalization, poor sleep and dietary habits, lack of exercise, poor posture, muscle tension–producing habits, and medication dependencies also can be seen when pain becomes prolonged. Oral para-functional muscle tension–producing habits such as teeth clenching, jaw thrust, gum chewing, and jaw tensing can add strain to the masticatory system and lead to MMFP. These habits can be generated as a form of tension release as well as a learned behavioral response (44–47). Postural strain caused by a forward head posture, increased cervical or lumbar lordosis, occlusal abnormalities, and poor positioning of the head or tongue also have been implicated (35,48). Each of these may complicate the clinical picture by perpetuating the pain, preventing compliance with the treatment program, and causing self-perpetuating chronic pain cycles to develop. Because this broad number of factors can complicate management, a psychometrically derived instrument has been designed to facilitate assessment of these contributing factors (44).

A study was conducted to determine which factors among physical, demographic, behavioral, and psychosocial factors were significant in delaying the recovery of patients with masticatory myofascial pain (44,49). In this study, 94 subjects with a chronic myofascial pain disorder were studied before their entering an interdisciplinary treatment program to determine which factors were most predictive of outcome (40). Treatment outcome was determined based on significant decreases in the Craniomandibular Index and the Symptom Severity Index from pretreatment to posttreatment. Stepwise multiple regression analysis yielded a total of 10 potential predictors of poor treatment response for chronic temporomandibular subjects. These items included poor attitude about success of treatment, low self-esteem, low energy, feeling worried, low level of sexual activity, poor eating habits, poor sleep, feeling confused, unrealistic expectations of reducing problem, and frequent use of the problem as an excuse to avoid activities. Low self-esteem, feeling worried, low energy, and poor sleep were identified as the most important useful predictors of treatment outcome for the group studied. Each are correlates of depression. These findings suggest that pretreatment psychosocial information is particularly important in mediating treatment response for chronic pain patients.

The results of this research suggest that an explanatory model can account for the development of MMFP from its onset to increasing severity in chronic cases. Specific initiating factors for acute MMFP include both macrotrauma and microtrauma. Macrotrauma includes those events that initiate the pain, including a direct or indirect injury to the jaw from trauma such as a motor vehicle accident (both with and without a direct blow to the jaw), yawning excessively, opening wide at a dental visit, over-chewing, or getting hit in the jaw. Microtrauma can also initiate the problem, but the patient may report no specific initiating event. This can occur from behavioral factors such as clenching and grinding of the teeth that place repetitive strain on the masticatory muscles and lead to the early development of MMFP. Despite these traumatic events leading to early MMFP, previous research suggests that psychosocial factors such as depression play a key role in leading to progression from acute to chronic.

The nature of the peripheral neuropathologic or dysfunctional processes of MMFP trigger points, and the central nervous changes associated with the regional pain when it progresses from acute to chronic are still not fully understood. A number of histologic and biochemical studies have been completed on biopsy specimens of tender points in patients with both generalized and regional muscle complaints (50–59). These studies have shown no specific anatomic changes in the muscle but do suggest localized progressive increases in oxidative metabolism, depleted energy supply, and resultant changes in the muscle nociception. This may be particularly true of type I muscle fiber types associated with static muscle tone and posture.

Studies of muscle energy metabolism found a decrease in the levels of adenosine triphosphate (ATP), adenosine diphosphate (ADP), and phosphoryl creatine and abnormal tissue oxygenation in muscles with trigger points (50–52). It has been hypothesized that these changes represent localized progressive increases in oxidative metabolism and depleted energy supply in type I postural muscle fiber types. This may result in progressive abnormal muscle changes that initially include nociceptive activation occurring within the muscle, particularly muscle fiber type I and surrounding connective tissue (53).

Localized tenderness and pain in the muscle involve types III and IV muscle nociceptors activated by noxious substances such as potassium, histamine, kinins, or prostaglandins that are released locally and cause tenderness (54–60). These afferent inputs converge with other visceral and somatic inputs in the cells such as those of the lamina I or V of the dorsal horn on the way to the cortex, resulting in perception of local and referred pain. These inputs may be inhibited by multiple peripherally or centrally initiated alterations in neural input to this "central biasing mechanism" of the brain stem through various treatment modalities such as cold, heat, analgesic medications, massage, trigger point injections, and transcutaneous electrical stimulation. These inputs also may be facilitated by multiple peripherally or centrally initiated alterations in neural input. Further sustained neural activity such as clenching, poor postural habits, or central nervous system (CNS) alterations such as depression will support the reverberating circuit, further perpetuating the problem. This explains the multiple contributing factors that can be responsible for the progression from acute to chronic pain and points to the need for a sophisticated management strategy for both acute and chronic MMFP.

CONCLUSION

As discussed earlier, treatment strategies should differ, depending on whether the condition is acute, simple, or complex (see Fig. 2-2). Although palliative care strategies with a single clinician can readily improve simple acute cases (see Technique 2-1), complex cases require treatment with a team of clinicians. When the choice of treatment strategy is made during the initial evaluation, this helps to maximize the potential for success by matching the complexity of the patient with the complexity of the care needed (Fig. 2-4). This implies that a behavioral and psychosocial evaluation should be conducted on all patients with persistent pain. This includes querying the patient about each oral habit, sleep problems, postural problems, pacing problems, repetitive strain activities, emotional issues such as anxiety, depression, and anger; cognitive issues such as poor understanding; and social issues such as stress or secondary gain. On completion of this evaluation, correct decisions can be made regarding the level of care required. Also, the contributing factors that need to be addressed are identified at the outset. A pain questionnaire that is completed before the first visit can be useful in saving time during the evaluation and allows for a more thorough review of all possible factors before seeing the patient for the initial evaluation. Once identified, the contributing factors are addressed within the treatment plan. With more contributing factors present, the necessity for the use of a team approach becomes clear.

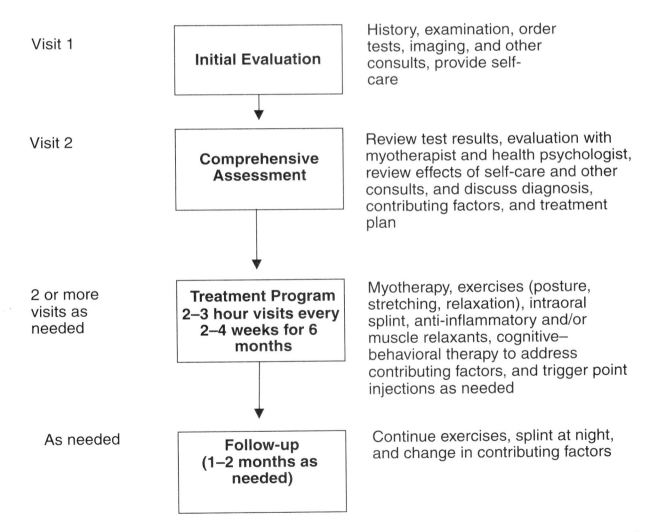

Visit 1 — **Initial Evaluation** — History, examination, order tests, imaging, and other consults, provide self-care

Visit 2 — **Comprehensive Assessment** — Review test results, evaluation with myotherapist and health psychologist, review effects of self-care and other consults, and discuss diagnosis, contributing factors, and treatment plan

2 or more visits as needed — **Treatment Program 2–3 hour visits every 2–4 weeks for 6 months** — Myotherapy, exercises (posture, stretching, relaxation), intraoral splint, anti-inflammatory and/or muscle relaxants, cognitive–behavioral therapy to address contributing factors, and trigger point injections as needed

As needed — **Follow-up (1–2 months as needed)** — Continue exercises, splint at night, and change in contributing factors

FIGURE 2-4. **Flow chart of an outpatient pain program.** This illustrates that the patient flow, from evaluation to assessment to treatment, includes many components. The key to successful management lies in matching the patient's needs with the unique combination of active treatment, education on contributing factors, and self-care appropriate for that patient.

Evaluation of MMFP includes locating the trigger points in the muscles of the jaw and neck, as well as recognizing the contributing factors and correctly identifying the complexity of the case (See the Treatment Protocol section, following). Management of MMFP involves selection of palliative care strategies, including the use of a stabilization splint, muscle exercises, the use of TPI, and physical therapy modalities applied to the trigger points. Depending on the complexity of the case, cognitive–behavioral therapy with a health psychologist is included in the treatment plan, to reduce the contributing factors. The short-term goal is to restore the muscles to normal length, to improve posture, and to achieve full range of joint motion. The long-term goals include reducing the symptoms and their negative effects while helping the patient to return to normal function and minimizing the need for future care. The difficulty in managing MMFP lies in the critical need to match the level of complexity of the management program with the complexity of the patient. Failure to address the entire problem through a team approach in complex cases may lead to failure to resolve the pain and perpetuation of a chronic pain syndrome.

PROTOCOL FOR MANAGING MASTICATORY AND CERVICAL MYOFASCIAL PAIN

I. Evaluation

A. Identify trigger points in masticatory and cervical muscle

B. Identify each area of pain

1. Frequency

2. Duration

3. Intensity

C. Identify contributing factors

1. Direct macrotrauma (e.g., blow to jaw)

2. Indirect macrotrauma (e.g., whiplash injuries)

3. Repetitive postural strain (e.g., phone bracing)

4. Oral para-functional habits (e.g., clenching and grinding of teeth)

5. Dietary factors (e.g., caffeine)

6. Sleep disturbance

7. Psychosocial stressors

8. Anxiety and depression

D. Determine simple versus complex

1. Simple: single-clinician evaluation and treatment

2. Complex: team evaluation, including dentist, physical therapist or chiropractor, psychologist

II. Management

A. Acute care with palliative self-care

B. Simple case management with single clinician

1. Self-care

2. Splint

3. Jaw exercises

4. Spray and stretch and/or manual therapy

5. Oral habit instruction

C. Complex case management

1. Self-care

2. Splint

3. Trigger point injections and/or manual therapy

4. Medications (muscle relaxants as needed)

5. Exercises with physical therapist or chiropractor

6. Cognitive–behavioral therapy with psychologist

7. Counseling as needed

Manual Myofascial Release Techniques for Muscles Involved in Masticatory Myofascial Pain

Editorial note by Lucy Whyte Ferguson

Manual myofascial release techniques are an integral part of combined dental and myofascial care of the patient with masticatory myofascial pain. It is helpful to perform some myofascial release before the patient has impressions taken for the making of an oral splint. Some patients have limited range of motion and may flare-up from the process of taking impressions. Follow-up visits of myofascial release are helpful as well. Some patients experience immediate increased muscle relaxation as they start to wear the oral splint, but others experience some increased hypertonicity, and myofascial care enhances their adaptation to the splint. A decrease in hypertonicity should be a direct result of the use of the splint. Furthermore, as the muscles relax, the bite may change somewhat, and the splint will need to be adjusted. Myofascial care of the muscles of the jaw and neck will often help with the adaptation to the changes in the splint. Care to address joint dysfunction, particularly in the upper cervical spine, often also helps the patient attain maximum benefit from the use of the splint. Care of the neck and shoulder muscles to improve head on neck posture also enhances the response to the splint. The splint therapy is thus a very dynamic process that often requires a good coordination of care between the dentist and the clinician providing the manual myofascial care.

The muscles of the jaw can be stretched by having the patient use two fingers to contact over the lower teeth and gently traction the mouth open. The patient closes the eyes while vapo-coolant spray is applied in sweeps along the length of the muscles of mastication, from the lower jaw to the anterior, middle, and posterior portions of the temporalis. The clinician can contact trigger points in the masseter and temporalis with some pressure, as the patient gently pulls the jaw progressively further open, thus enhancing localized tissue stretch and trigger point release (Fig. 2-5). Both the medial and lateral pterygoid muscles release during this stretch process as well, and the stretch can be enhanced by having the patient resist the manual traction on the jaw, and then release and relax the jaw muscles several times in succession. After moist heat is applied to these muscles, the clinician can perform trigger point pressure release on the remaining trigger points in the tem-

poralis muscle. It is helpful to have the patient again provide gentle traction while the clinician contacts the trigger points. Because the temporalis is a thin muscle stretched over the temporal bone, it is most effective to perform the trigger point contact while also tractioning the muscle tissue away from the jaw joint. (Trigger point pressure release is usually performed on thicker muscles, and the clinician goes deeper as the more superfi-

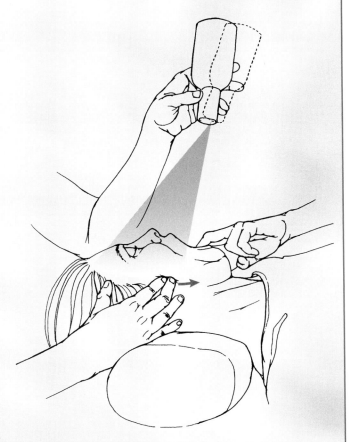

FIGURE 2-5. Stretch of temporalis muscle (and other muscles). The patient stretches the jaw open gently with two fingers placed over the lower teeth. The patient is supine with the head tipped back slightly. The clinician uses trigger point pressure and local stretch of taut bands to enhance effectiveness of stretch. Vapocoolant spray also may be applied, to improve the stretch.

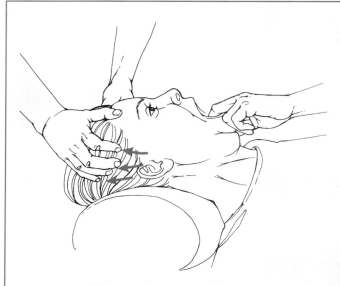

FIGURE 2-6. Trigger point pressure release while stretching temporalis muscle. The clinician performs local tissue stretch away from the TMJ and applies specific pressure on trigger points in the temporalis muscle. The patient is supine, and the clinician sits at the head of the treatment table.

cial tissues release.) A light cream can be used, and the clinician's fingers slowly progress along the taut bands from the jaw joint to the distal portion of the temporalis muscle as the more proximal trigger points release and the muscle bands elongate (Fig. 2-6).

To treat the masseter, buccinator, and medial pterygoid muscle trigger points, the clinician contacts the medial pterygoid muscle in the posterior lateral mouth (inside), between the upper and lower molars with the thumb. The fingers (outside) contact the masseter or the buccinator (Fig. 2-7). This pincher contact can be used to provide static compression, or to stretch the muscle group to increase spacing between the upper and lower teeth by pressing or tractioning tissue laterally with the pincher contact. The fingers can compress and move along the length of the muscle fibers, or across the fibers, however the clinician finds most effective for release of taut muscle bands and trigger points. This release can be quite painful if the patient has very tender trigger points, but the release and elongation of the medial pterygoid and masseter is very important to improve both joint and

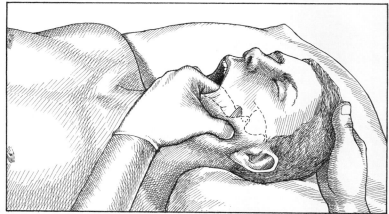

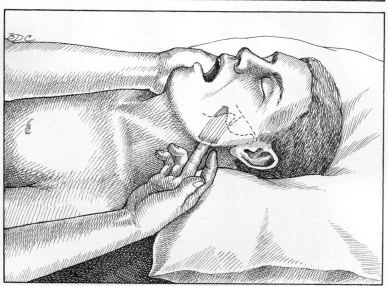

FIGURE 2-7. Pincher position for treatment of trigger points in the medial pterygoid muscle. The clinician's gloved thumb contacts the muscle behind the last molar, and the mouth is opened wide enough for the finger to contact between the molar teeth. Trigger point pressure release can be combined with localized tissue stretch performed in a medial to lateral direction. Reprinted with permission from Simons DG, Travell JG, Simons LS. Travell & Simons' Myofascial Pain and Dysfunction: The Trigger Point Manual, vol 1: Upper Half of Body. 2nd Ed. Baltimore: Lippincott Williams & Wilkins, 1999, fig. 10.3 (p. 370).

muscle function. The clinician needs to be in good communication with the patient about the patient's tolerance to the pain and the subsequent relief of pain and improved bite. The clinician should avoid direct contact pressure on the jaw joint itself, particularly if there is a degree of tenderness in the joint suggestive of capsulitis. However, the clinician can apply gentle but firm contact just medial and anterior to the jaw joints with the index finger of each hand as the patient is instructed to slack the jaw. By palpating through the masseter muscle and tractioning anteroinferior on the deep tender muscle tissue in this location and passively inducing some jaw opening, the clinician probably can effect trigger point pressure release on a small portion of the lateral pterygoid muscles (Fig. 2-8). Myofascial release techniques are always performed bilaterally, to maintain balance of the muscles of mastication.

After there has been progressive release of tender trigger points and taut bands in the muscles of mastication, joint dysfunction in the TMJ can be addressed by either gentle osseous adjustment (high velocity but very low amplitude and very low force) or by muscle energy techniques. Further muscle tension reduction often results from improved joint function.

The neck muscles that have the most direct effect on the function of the TMJ and the associated muscles are the sternocleidomastoid and digastric muscles, because they are an integral part of the functional unit with the jaw muscles, and because they both can produce pain referral into the jaw area and thus increase muscle hypertonicity and trigger point activity in the muscles of mastication. Passive stretch of the sternocleidomastoid (SCM) muscle is readily performed on the seated patient, turning the head away from the right shoulder, and dropping

the head back while resting the patient's head on the clinician's chest or abdomen to stretch the right clavicular portion of the SCM (see Fig 1-6). The head is turned to the right, dropped back and away from the right shoulder, to elongate the right sternal portion of the SCM, and then the right occiput is elevated at the end of the stretch to complete the release. The left SCM is released by performing these same maneuvers to the opposite side. The clinician can hook the index finger around the front of the sternal portion of the SCM, just inferior to the lateral mandible and the ear, to increase the stretch of the SCM as the occiput is lifted (Fig. 2-9). Pinching other lower segments of the SCM during the seated stretch is not recommended, because of the possibility of inadvertently compressing the carotid sinus and causing a rapid change in blood pressure, and possibly affecting the patient's heart rhythm and consciousness. But pincher palpation of the SCM in the seated patient when the muscle tissue is not being stretched taut is quite safe, because the

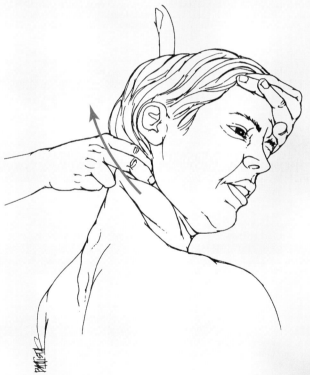

FIGURE 2-9. Final position for stretch of the sternal portion of the SCM muscle. The patient's chin is dropped and the mastoid process on the same side is lifted. The clinician can enhance local muscle stretch by hooking a finger around the upper SCM just under the ear, and pulling posteriorly as though to take the neck and head further into rotation toward the shoulder. Vapo-coolant spray can be applied in successive upward sweeps over the areas constituting the referred pain pattern, including the posterior skull, the temple, the forehead, and the jaw.

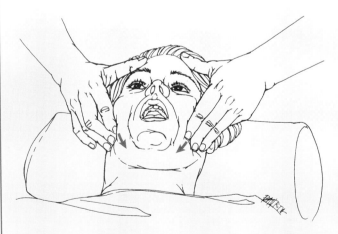

FIGURE 2-8. Trigger point pressure release with tissue traction anteroinferior, to treat lateral pterygoid trigger points as well as overlying muscle tissue. The supine patient is instructed to slack the jaw while the clinician contacts and presses as though to open the jaw further.

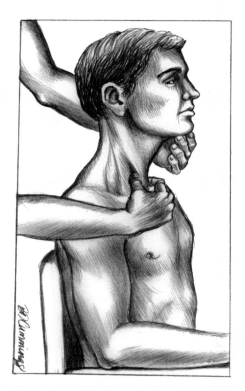

FIGURE 2-10. **Pincher palpation of the SCM muscle in the seated patient.** Trigger point pressure release is performed while placing a slight pull on the muscle, away from the underlying neck tissues. Reprinted with permission from Simons DG, Travell JG, Simons LS. Travell & Simons' Myofascial Pain and Dysfunction: The Trigger Point Manual, vol 1: Upper Half of Body. 2nd Ed. Baltimore: Lippincott Williams & Wilkins, 1999, fig. 7.4A (p. 318).

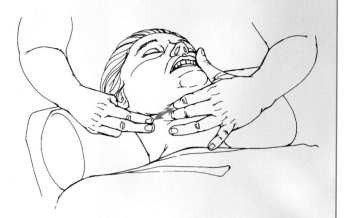

FIGURE 2-12. **Double trigger point pressure release with traction between the contacts, to treat trigger points in the posterior belly of the digastric muscle.** The patient is supine with the head tilted back slightly. With one hand, the clinician contacts the lateral border of the hyoid and tractions medially, while contacting with the other hand the trigger points all along the posterior belly as it passes toward the mastoid process. While contacting each trigger point in the posterior belly, the clinician applies trigger point pressure release. This may be combined with tissue traction laterally or posteriorly to simultaneously elongate taut bands.

muscle is tractioned away from underlying neck tissues (Fig. 2-10). Pincher palpation and local tissue traction is also effective when the patient is supine (Fig. 2-11); it is helpful to perform this procedure all the way along both the superficial and deep portions of this muscle, from origin to insertion.

The digastric muscle is most readily treated in the supine patient with the head tilted back so that the throat area is prominent. The posterior belly of the digastric muscle is palpated and compressed just inferior to the angle of the jaw, and the taut bands in this portion of the muscle can be traced to the mastoid process of the temporal bone, and it can be treated all along its length (Fig. 2-12). The anterior bellies of this muscle

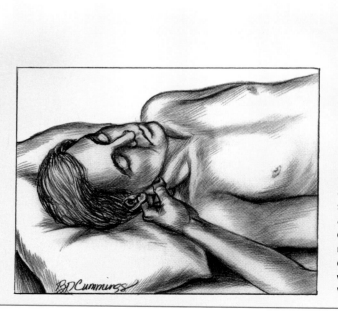

FIGURE 2-11. **Pincher palpation of the SCM in the supine patient.** The patient's head is turned slightly toward the side being treated to create some slack of the muscle. The clinician uses pincher palpation to address multiple trigger points along the entire length of the muscle, while pulling the more superficial sternal portion or the deeper clavicular portion away from underlying neck tissues and thus simultaneously elongating taut bands. Reprinted with permission from Simons DG, Travell JG, Simons LS. Travell & Simons' Myofascial Pain and Dysfunction: The Trigger Point Manual, vol 1: Upper Half of Body. 2nd Ed. Baltimore: Lippincott Williams & Wilkins, 1999, fig. 7.4B (p. 318).

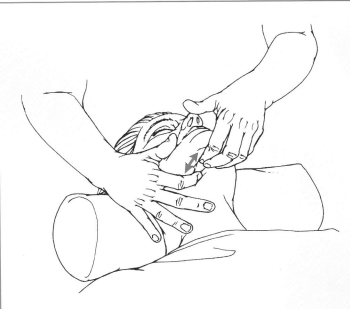

FIGURE 2-13. **Myofascial release of trigger points in the anterior belly of the digastric muscle.** Patient lies supine with the head tilted slightly back. The clinician performs double trigger point pressure release, and applies traction between the contacts. The clinician contacts the superior border of the lateral portion of the hyoid bone and applies traction inferiorly, while contacting trigger points in the anterior belly with the other hand. The latter hand performs trigger point pressure release on all of the trigger points between the hyoid bone and the attachment at the mandible, while stretching upward on the muscle tissue to simultaneously lengthen the taut bands.

are attached just to the right and left of the center of the underside of the mandible, and the trigger points can be palpated and compressed all the way from the mandible to the fibrous loop that connects the digastric muscle indirectly to the hyoid (Fig. 2-13).

The infrahyoid muscles are part of the functional unit with the SCM and the digastric muscles. Pressure on trigger points in these muscles is performed by pressing under the medial border of the SCM and just lateral to the thyroid and cricoid cartilages (Fig. 2-14). Pressure on these trigger points deep in the throat can be of help with patients who have difficulty swallowing, and who have a muscular sore throat (a sore throat with no evidence of other pathology or illness.) One of the most interesting muscles in this group of deep throat muscles is the omohyoid muscle. The superior belly attaches superiorly to the hyoid and inferiorly to the clavicle by a fibrous expansion connected to its central tendon. The lateral belly passes posterior to the SCM but superficial to the anterior and middle scalene muscles and attaches laterally to the scapula near the scapular notch (Fig. 2-15). To palpate and trace the lateral belly, one hand can contact the superior belly just medial to the SCM, and above the clavicle (Fig. 2-16). Intermittent medial traction, pressing toward the throat cartilages, can create gentle traction that can be felt by the fingers of the other hand, in the lateral belly of the muscle as it runs laterally just above the clavicle. Because this thin muscle is the only muscle that runs from medial to lateral and attaches to the scapula while the deeper muscles have more vertical fibers, the tension induced by medial pressure on the superior belly makes identification and treatment of the lateral belly possible. The muscle also stands out prominently when the head is tilted toward the contralateral side and can be mistaken for the upper trapezius or the scalene muscles. When this muscle is

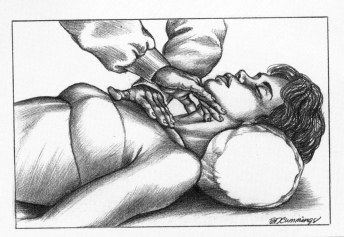

FIGURE 2-14. **Trigger point pressure release and applying tissue traction to treat trigger points in the infrahyoid muscles.** The clinician applies trigger point pressure while reaching under the medial border of the SCM and treating muscles lateral to the thyroid and cricoid cartilages while pressing down (inferiorly) on the clavicle, sternum, or chest. This can be performed with the clinician standing above the supine patient, or with the clinician seated at the head of the treatment table while contacting the patient in the same locations. Reprinted with permission from Simons DG, Travell JG, Simons LS. Travell & Simons' Myofascial Pain and Dysfunction: The Trigger Point Manual, vol 1: Upper Half of Body. 2nd Ed. Baltimore: Lippincott Williams & Wilkins, 1999, fig. 12.7C (p. 409).

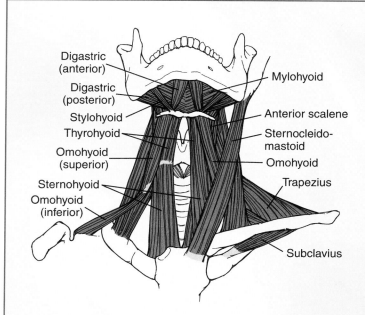

FIGURE 2-15. **The omohyoid muscle has two bellies.** The superior belly attaches to the inferior body of the hyoid bone and extends toward the clavicle. A fibrous slip attaches the omohyoid to the clavicle. From this slip, the inferior belly of the omohyoid muscle extends laterally and inferiorly and attaches to the cranial border of the scapula, near the scapular notch. Reprinted by permission from Hendrickson T. Massage for Orthopedic Conditions. Baltimore: Lippincott Williams & Wilkins, 2003, fig. 5.8 (p. 167).

shortened, it can constrict across the brachial plexus, and it is often difficult to fully stretch the scalene and upper trapezius muscles if this muscle remains abnormally taut (61). The omohyoid muscle is often very tender when there is injury to jaw, neck, and shoulder muscles in auto accidents. Trigger point pressure release is effective to treat both taut bands and trigger points in each of these throat muscles. Treatment of other neck muscles and of shoulder muscles is discussed in Chapters 2, 3, 4, and 9.

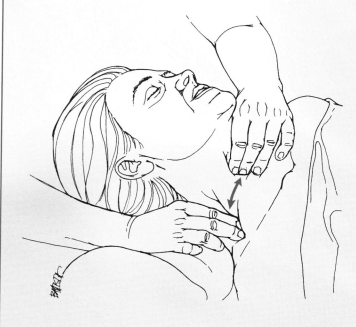

FIGURE 2-16. **Supine treatment of trigger points in the omohyoid muscle.** The head is tilted slightly back and the neck is laterally flexed somewhat away from the side being treated. The clinician places gently lateral-to-medial intermittent traction on the superior belly of the omohyoid (medial to the SCM and above the clavicle.) The other hand palpates the changes in muscle tension of the inferior belly of the omohyoid that result from the intermittent traction, as a way of identifying and differentiating the omohyoid's more horizontal fibers from the more vertical surrounding muscles. Trigger point pressure is used to treat the tender trigger points all the way from the medial portion of the inferior belly to its attachment on the superior border of the scapula. Gentle tissue traction also can be applied from medial-to-lateral, to simultaneously elongate taut bands.

References

1. Fricton JR, et al. Myofascial pain syndrome of the head and neck: a review of clinical characteristics of 164 patients. Oral Surg Oral Med Oral Pathol 1985;60:615–623.

2. Fishbain DA, Goldberg M, Meagher BR, et al. Male and female chronic pain patients categorized by DSM-III psychiatric diagnostic criteria. Pain 1986;26:181–197.

3. Skootsky SA, Jaeger B, Oye RK. Prevalence of myofascial pain in general internal medicine practice. Western Journal of Medicine 1989; 151:157–160.

4. Schiffman EL, Friction JR, Haley DP, et al. The prevalence and treatment needs of subjects with temporomandibular disorders. J Am Dent Assoc 1990;120: 295–303.

5. Bonica JJ. Management of myofascial pain syndrome in general practice. JAMA 1957;164: 732–738.

6. Simons DG. Traumatic fibromyositis or myofascial trigger points. Western Journal of Medicine 1978;128:69–71 [correspondence].

7. Simons DG. Muscle pain syndromes—Part I. [Review]. American Journal of Physical Medicine 1975;54:289–311.

8. Travell J. Myofascial trigger points: clinical view. In: Bonica JJ et al., eds. Advances in Pain Research and Therapy. New York: Raven Press, 1976:919–926.

9. Simons DG, Travell JG., Simons LS. Myofascial Pain and Dysfunction: The Trigger Point Manual, Volume 1, 2nd edition, 1999:94–177.

10. Arlen H. The otomandibular syndrome: a new concept. Ear Nose Throat J 1977;56:60–62.

11. Aronoff GM, Evans WO, Enders PL. A review of follow-up studies of multidisciplinary pain units. Pain 1983;16:1–11.

12. Arroyo P Jr. Electromyography in the evaluation of reflex muscle spasm. Simplified method for direct evaluation of muscle-relaxant drugs. Journal of the Florida Medical Association 1966;53: 29–31.

13. Awad EA. Interstitial myofibrositis: hypothesis of the mechanism. Arch Phys Med Rehabil 1973;54:449–453.

14. Bengtsson A, Henriksson KG, Larsson J. Reduced high-energy phosphate levels in the painful muscles of patients with primary fibromyalgia. Arthritis Rheum 1986;29:817–21.

15. Braun B, et al. A Cross-sectional study of temporomandibular joint dysfunction in post-cervical trauma patients. Journal of Craniomandibular Disorders, Oral and Facial Pain, 1992;6:24–31.

16. Bengtsson A, Hennksson KG, Jorfeldt L, et al. Primary fibromyalgia: A clinical and laboratory study of 55 patients. Scand J Rheumatol 1986;15:340–7.

17. Fricton J, Dall' Arancio D. Myofascial pain, a controlled outcome study of interdisciplinary management. Journal of Musculoskeletal Pain 1994;2:81–99.

18. Fricton JR, Schiffman EL. Reliability of a craniomandibular index. J Dent Res 1986;65:1359–64.

19. Reeves JL, Jaeger B, Graff-Radford SB. Reliability of the pressure algometer as a measure of myofascial trigger point sensitivity. Pain 1986;24:313–21.

20. Schiffman E, et al. A Pressure Algometer for MPS: Reliability and Validity. Pain, 1987. 4(suppl): p. S291.

21. Fricton JR, et al. Myofascial pain syndrome: electromyographic changes associated with local twitch response. Arch Phys Med Rehabil 1985;66:314–317.

22. Lewit K. The needle effect in the relief of myofascial pain. Pain 1979;6:83–90.

23. Simons DG. Electrogenic nature of palpable bands and "jump sign" associated with myofascial trigger points. In: Bonica JJ, et al., ed. Advances in Pain Research and Therapy. New York, Raven Press, 1976:913–918.

24. Cifala JA. Myofascial (trigger point pain) injection: theory and treatment. Osteopath. Med 1979;31–36.

25. Cooper AL. Trigger point injection: its place in physical medicine. Rehabil Arch Phys Med 1961;42:704–709.

26. Jaeger B,. Skootsky SA. Double blind, controlled study of different myofascial trigger point injection techniques. Pain 1987; 4(suppl):S292.

27. Jaeger B, Reeves JL. Quantification of changes in myofascial trigger point sensitivity with the pressure algometer following passive stretch. Pain 1986;27:203–10.

28. Fricton JR, Schiffman EL. The craniomandibular index: validity. J Prosthet Dent 1987;58:222–228.

29. Travell J. Identification of myofascial trigger point syndromes: a case of atypical facial neuralgia. Arch Phys Med Rehabil 1981;62: 100–106.

30. Dexter JR, Simons S. Local twitch response in human muscle evoked by palpation and needle penetration of trigger point. Arch Phys Med Rehabil 1981;62:521–522.

31. Fischer AA. Documentation of myofascial trigger points. [Review]. Arch Phys Med Rehabil 1988;.69:286–291.

32. Fischer AA. Tissue compliance meter for objective, quantitative documentation of soft tissue consistency and pathology. Arch Phys Med Rehabil 1987;68:122–125.

33. Berry DC, Yemm R. A further study of facial skin temperature in patients with mandibular dysfunction. Journal of Oral Rehabilitation, 1974;1:255–264.

34. Ohrson, J (ed.). Guidelines for Diagnoses and Management of Temporomandibular Disorders. Quintessence, 1999.

35. Simons D. Muscular pain syndromes, in Fricton J, Awad EA, eds. Myofascial Pain and Fibromyalgia. New York: Raven Press, 1990:1–43.

36. Bennett R. Myofascial pain syndromes and the fibromyalgia syndrome: a comparative analysis, in Fricton J, Awad EA, eds. Myofascial Pain and Fibromyalgia. New York: Raven Press, 1990:43–66.

37. Clarke NG, Kardachi BJ. The treatment of myofascial pain-dysfunction syndrome using the biofeedback principle. J Periodontol 1977;48:643–645.

38. Graff-Radford SB, Reeves JL, Jaeger B. Management of chronic head and neck pain: effectiveness of altering factors perpetuating myofascial pain. Headache 1987;27:186–190.

39. Miehlke K, Schulz G. So called muscular rheumatism. Internist 1961;2:447–453.

40. Fricton J, Hathaway K, Bromaghim C. Interdisciplinary management of patient with TMJ and craniofacial pain: characteristics and outcome. J Cranio Disord Facial Oral Pain, 1987; 1:115–122.

41. Ng K, Lorenz, eds. New approaches to treatment of chronic pain: a review of multidisciplinary pain clinics and pain centers. NIDA Research 36 Monograph Series. Washington, DC: U.S. Government Printing Office, 1981.

42. Rodin J. Biopsychosocial aspects of self management, in Karoly P, Kanfer FH, eds. Self Management and Behavioral Change: From Theory to Practice. New York: Pergamon Press, 1974.

43. Schneider F, Kraly P. Conceptions of pain experience: The emergence of multidimensional models and their implications for contemporary clinical practice. Clin Psych Rev 1983;3:61–86.

44. Fricton JR, Nelson A, Monsein M. IMPATH: microcomputer assessment of behavioral and psychosocial factors in craniomandibular disorders. Cranio, 1987;5:372–381.

45. Berry DC. Mandibular dysfunction pain and chronic minor illness. Br Dent J 1969;127:170–175.

46. Gold S, et al. Sites of psychophysiological complaints in MPD patients: II. Areas remote from orofacial region. J Dent Res 1975;480: 165 [abstr].

47. Evaskus DS, Laskin DM. A biochemical measure of stress in patients with myofascial pain-dysfunction syndrome. J Dent Res 1972;51: 1464–1466.

48. Kendall HO, Kendall F, Boynton D, in Posture and Pain. Huntington, NY: R.E. Krieger, 1970:15–45.

49. Fricton J, Oleson T. Predictors of outcome for treatment of temporomandibular disorders. Journal of Orofacial Pain 1996;10:54–66.

50. Yunus MB, Kalyan-Raman UP, Kalyan-Raman K, et al. Pathologic changes in muscle in primary fibromyalgia syndrome. Am J Med 1986;81:38–42.

51. Lund N, Bengtsson A, Thorborg P. Muscle tissue oxygen pressure in primary fibromyalgia. Scand J Rheumatol 1986;15:165–73.

52. Ibrahim GA, Awad EA, Kottke FJ. Interstitial myofibrositis: serum and muscle enzymes and lactate dehydrogenase-isoenzymes. Arch Phys Med Rehabil 1974;55:23–28.

53. Simons DG, Travell J. Myofascial trigger points, a possible explanation [letter]. Pain 1981;10:106–109.

54. Kniffki KD, Mense S, Schmidt RF. Responses of group IV afferent units from skeletal muscle to stretch, contraction and chemical stimulation. Exp Brain Res 1978;31:511–522.

55. Lim RKS, Guzman F, Rodgers DW. Note on the muscle receptors concerned with pain, in Barker D, ed. Symposium on Muscle Receptors. Hong Kong: Hong Kong University Press, 1962: 215–219.

56. Mense S. Nervous outflow from skeletal muscle following chemical noxious stimulation. J Physiol 1977;267:75–88.

57. Mense S, Schmidt RF. Muscle pain: which receptors are responsible for the transmission of noxious stimuli? In Rose FC, ed. Physiological Aspects of Clinical Neurology. Oxford: Blackwell Scientific Publications, 1977;102:265–278.

58. Pomeranz B, Wall PD, Weber WV. Cord cells responding to fine myelinated afferents from viscera, muscle and skin. J Physiol 1968;199:511–532.

59. Selzer M, Spencer WA. Convergence of visceral and cutaneous afferent pathways in the lumbar spinal cord. Brain Res 1969;14:331–348.

60. Melzack R. Myofascial trigger points: relation to acupuncture and mechanisms of pain. Arch Phys Med Rehabil 1981;62:114–117.

61. Simons DG, Travell JG, Simons LS. Myofascial Pain and Dysfunction, The Trigger Point Manual, vol 1, 2nd Ed. Baltimore: Lippincott Williams & Wilkins, 1999:397–415.

3 — Neck Pain and Dysfunction Following Whiplash

Jan Dommerholt, PT, MPS, Margaret W. Royson, DO
and Lucy Whyte Ferguson, DC

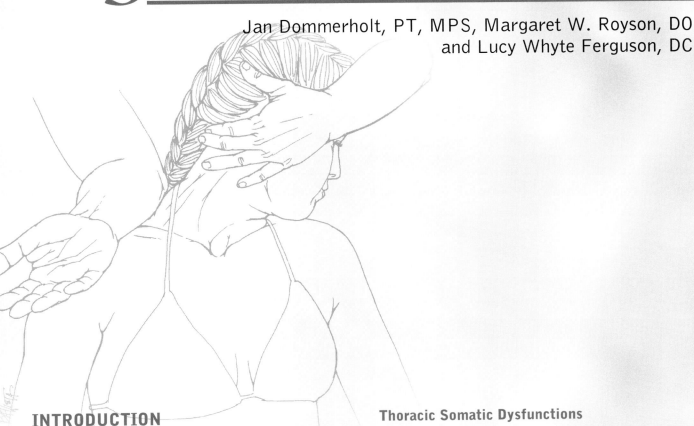

INTRODUCTION

Few injury patterns are surrounded by as much controversy as whiplash. The exact mechanisms of whiplash are still debated, and disagreement exists as to which anatomic structures are involved (1,2). Some authors feel strongly that low-speed collisions cannot cause complaints of chronic pain, and they advocate nonorganic factors such as "compensation or litigation neurosis" or "chronic illness behavior," whereas others are convinced that there is a direct correlation between collisions and chronic pain (3–5). The subject of whiplash concerns many different disciplines, including medicine, engineering, biomechanics and biomechanical trauma, epidemiology, psychology, economics, law and law enforcement, insurance, health policy, ergonomics, and so on. Medical specialties involved in the treatment of patients with whiplash-associated-disorders (WAD) include physiatry, neurology, orthopaedic surgery and neurosurgery, rheumatology, internal medicine and family practice, ophthalmology, radiology, psychiatry, dentistry, psychology and clinical social work, chiropractic, and occupational and physical therapy.

Although the scientific literature does not provide any substantial evidence for the relevance of myofascial pain syndrome (MPS) following whiplash injuries, clinicians familiar with MPS and its treatment find that myofascial trigger points commonly contribute to complaints of persistent pain and dysfunction (6–8). In a retrospective review of patients, Gerwin and Dommerholt reported that clinically relevant trigger points were found in 100% of patients involved in whiplash accidents, with the trapezius muscle most often involved (9). After treatment emphasizing the inactivation of trigger points and restoration of normal muscle length, close to 80% of patients experienced little or no pain, even though the average time following the initiating injury was 21/2 years at the beginning of the treatment regimen. A recent German study of 1,096 cases of low-velocity collisions indicated that myogelosis was found in 80% of all cases (10). The concept of "myogelosis" in the European literature is considered synonymous with the term "trigger point" used in the United States (11).

NECK PAIN FOLLOWING WHIPLASH: BACKGROUND

The actual cost of whiplash is difficult to determine, because of assumed underreporting and many other factors. The costs associated with whiplash include medical expenses, lost income to the family, the cost of property damage, police expenses, and even more obscure factors, such as the cost of delays to road users as a result of congestion caused by traffic accidents (12). The economic cost alone of motor vehicle crashes in the year 2000 was $230.6 billion (13). The most thoroughly investigated motor vehicle accidents are fatal crashes, which in the United States are doc-

umented by the National Highway Traffic and Safety Administration. In 1998, motor vehicle accident crashes ranked eighth behind cardiac disease, cancer, and cerebrovascular accidents as the leading causes of death in the United States. In the year 2002 alone, 2,926,000 people were injured and 42,815 people were killed in an estimated 6,316,000 police-reported motor vehicle traffic crashes, or an average of one person every 12 minutes (13). However, the actual number of injured individuals is probably substantially higher. In general, police officers are not well trained in traffic accident reporting, and in many jurisdictions, the police do not even come to the scene of an accident unless immediate medical attention is required (14). People may develop delayed injuries after crashes that at the time of the accident may not be recorded. Many studies have documented that the onset of symptoms, such as neck pain, may be delayed by several hours or even days, thereby excluding these individuals from being included in police reports (15–18).

The threshold for injury is usually much lower than the damage threshold for vehicles (19). In 1955, Severy and colleagues showed that in experiments with human volunteers involved in an 13-kph rear-impact crash, the head and neck were exposed to acceleration forces up to 2.5 times the acceleration forces of the vehicle (Fig. 3-1) (20). Many more recent studies have confirmed that the damage thresholds for various vehicles may vary between 13 and 20 kph, whereas injuries may occur at speeds of less than 10 kph (21–28). In other words, the argument used so commonly by defense attorneys and medical "expert witnesses" that individuals could not possibly have sustained any injuries in the absence of property damage is not necessarily supported by scientific evidence. There is no doubt that acute neck injury can occur after low-speed collisions. Whether chronic pain can develop as a direct consequence of a low-speed crash continues to be debated in the literature and in court rooms, with strong opinions on both sides (2,22,29,30).

Although 97% of all rear-end collisions do not result in fatal or serious injuries (Table 3-1), approximately 5% to 15% of whiplash injuries are reported to lead to permanent disability (31–34). Whiplash can occur in all collision types. Rear-end collisions with a change of velocity after impact of less then 16 kph were found to account for 45% of reported injuries, compared with only 2% in frontal collisions (31). When considering all neck injuries irrespective of impact mechanics and velocity changes, the number of occupants injured in frontal collisions was twice as high as those involved in rear-end impacts (Fig. 3-2) (35).

The severity of injuries depends on a number of variables. These include the type of impact (frontal, rear-end, side impact, rollovers, or combinations); the impact height; the relative speed, acceleration, and mass of the vehicles involved in the accident and the resultant velocity change; the position of the occupant within the vehicle (front seat or back seat, driver or passenger); the seat-rebound characteristics; head position at the time of impact (including the dis-

Phase III

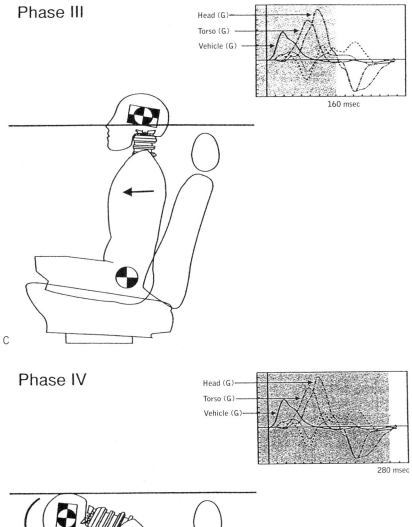

Head (G)
Torso (G)
Vehicle (G)

160 msec

C

Phase IV

Head (G)
Torso (G)
Vehicle (G)

280 msec

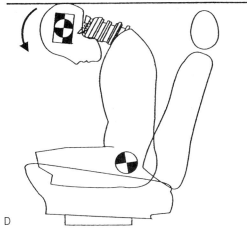

D

FIGURE 3-3. *(Continued)*

junction, the lower cervical spine, and the craniomandibular complex are exposed to high rotational and shear forces and are therefore at increased risk for injury.

During phase III, the head and trunk are at peak acceleration forces, whereas the vehicle is decelerating, which results in increased flexion rotation forces for the head and trunk (Fig. 3-3C). During phase IV, the vehicle no longer accelerates, and the head and trunk are at full deceleration. The seatbelt may restrain the trunk from forward flexion, but the head will continue in forceful flexion, causing sudden high levels of torque at the cervicothoracic junction (Fig. 3-3D). Whether the head actually goes into a hyperextended position during low-speed collisions is questionable, but there is little doubt that this occurs with higher velocities and greater force patterns (2,4,24,49).

Panjabi and colleagues conducted multiple biomechanical studies of whiplash and proposed that the initial phase of whiplash is a two-stage response of the neck to a forward acceleration of the thoracic spine (50). In the first stage, the cervical spine develops an S-shaped curvature, with lower-level extension and upper-level flexion. The second stage involves extension of the entire cervical spine. They suggested that especially the S-shaped curvature that precedes full cervical extension may potentially be most damaging, as it stretches the anterior elements of the lower cervical spine beyond their normal yield limits. Resulting injuries would be consistent with AIS-1 injuries. Panjabi and colleagues described increased segmental flexibility at the corresponding lower cervical levels (51). The S-shaped curvature may result in lengthening of the sternocleidomastoid and longus colli muscles, thereby causing a contraction-induced muscle injury of these muscles (52,53).

Diagnosis and Clinical Features

The term *whiplash* was first used in 1928 to describe the motion of the head and neck in a motor vehicle crash, and it has had many definitions since (54). It is often used to describe the symptoms and signs that follow an impact, usually a motor vehicle collision. The report of the Quebec Task Force on Whiplash Associated Disorders suggested the following definition: an acceleration-deceleration–induced mechanism of energy transfer to the neck, which may result in bony or soft tissue injury to the neck, which in turn may lead to a variety of clinical manifestations (55).

The Quebec Task Force graded whiplash-associated disorders (WAD) from 0 to 4. Although this classification has not been validated, it is often quoted and used in the literature. Grade 0 is characterized by a whiplash exposure without pain or other signs and symptoms. Grade 1 is characterized by a delayed onset of pain, minor neck stiffness, nonfocal tenderness only, and no abnormalities found on examination. Grade 2 features an early onset of neck pain and focal neck tenderness, reduced spinal range of motion, spasms, and radiating symptoms. Grade 3 includes all the features of grade 2, as well as signs of neurologic deficits. Grade 4 includes all of the features of grade 3, as well as a fracture or dislocation (55).

WAD include musculoskeletal lesions, peripheral and central nervous lesions, neurologic and vestibular lesions, and otorhinolaryngologic and audiologic lesions (56). The cardinal musculoskeletal symptoms are neck pain and headache, but also include shoulder and arm pain, paresthesia, weakness, low-back pain, and craniomandibular pain (57,58). Nearly all cervical structures can be involved in a whiplash, such as the cervical zygapophyseal joints, the vertebrae, the intervertebral discs, muscles, ligaments, as well as the nervous system (57).

Considerable evidence exists that cervical and lumbar zygapophyseal joints are frequently damaged in many whiplash patients, although it remains difficult to determine whether a true causal correlation exists between chronic zygapophyseal joint pain and involvement in a previous collision, and whether these injuries occur even with low-velocity impacts (2,4,59–63). In a sample of 92 cases of a total of 273 subjects with chronic neck pain after whiplash, the estimated speed of impact was as much as 48 kph according to police records. Eighty-eight percent of the 92 cases were diagnosed with zygapophyseal joint dysfunction (64). During low-velocity impacts, it is very unlikely that the lumbar zygapophyseal joints and associated soft tissues are injured, but it is unknown which minimum impact velocity or change in velocity is required to cause zygapophyseal joint dysfunction (62). During the initial phase after impact, the vertebral bodies are separated anteriorly, while the zygapophyseal joints are impacted posteriorly because of an extension motion (65). The diagnosis is made with fluoroscopically guided diagnostic blocks of the painful joints (65). In autopsy studies of the cervical and lumbar regions in victims of fatal crashes, which in itself suggests that the impacts occurred at higher impact velocities, traumatic injuries were associated with clefts in the cartilage plates of the intervertebral discs, posterior disc herniations, hemarthrosis in facet joints, fractures of the superior articular process and subchondral bone plate, and tears of the articular capsule not visible on standard medical imaging (60,66–68).

Injuries to muscles have been associated primarily with muscle tears or sprains, usually classified as grade 1 or grade 2 WAD (69). Several studies have shown that persons involved in whiplash have greater difficulty relaxing their muscles in between tasks, especially when exposed to low biomechanical loads (70,71). Baker established that the splenius capitis, semispinalis capitis, and sternocleidomastoid muscles developed symptomatic trigger points in 77%, 62%, and 52% of 52 patients, respectively (72). Others have reported the development of trigger points as well, although none of the studies were done prospectively (9,10,17). It is noteworthy that the referred pain patterns of the cervical zygapophyseal joints are nearly identical to the referred pain patterns of the cervical muscles (73).

Chronic Pain Following Low-Velocity Collisions

The greatest controversy in any discussion of WAD is the question of whether low-speed collisions can result in chronic pain and disability. Several studies have demonstrated that most patients recover fully (31–34). Only 5% to 15% of whiplash patients become chronic pain patients, a percentage that is remarkably similar to the development of chronic pain after other musculoskeletal injuries (74–76). Whether the hyperextension and hyperflexion movement patterns actually occur during low-speed collisions, and, therefore, whether the various musculoskeletal structures are really exposed to forces beyond their biomechanical yield capacity, is questionable. Are the anterior neck muscles truly exposed to eccentric contractions and subsequent injury if the head does not move into a hyperextended position? Do injuries to the cervical zygapophyseal joints occur at such low-impact speeds?

Litigation, Insurance and Cultural Aspects

Some have argued that the development of chronic symptoms after low-speed collisions is driven by litigation and compensation potential, but the scientific literature does not support this notion (3,77). Many studies have shown that there is no correlation between settlement and reports of pain and dysfunction (78–82). In a recent study, 34% of the subjects involved in a rear-end collision experienced pain and dysfunction 24 months after the collision. Only 7.7% of the subjects sought financial compensation, whereas none received any compensation for pain and suffering (83).

Conversely, changing the structure of the insurance reimbursement system did have significant consequences in Canada and Australia. The Canadian province Saskatchewan experienced a 28% drop in the incidence of whiplash claims after changing from a tort system to a no-fault system, with an average decrease of more than 200 days to the closure of claims (84). Similar trends were seen in the state of Victoria, Australia, where claims for whiplash were reduced from 17% to 10% after new legislation was introduced in 1994 that made it more difficult to file a claim and get compensation (85). Although the lack of compensation may reduce the display of disability, the levels of expressed pain are not necessarily reduced (86).

Ferrari and Russell argued that cultural differences between countries are of critical importance in understanding chronic pain phenomena following whiplash, illustrated by studies that demonstrated that in Lithuania and Greece, chronic pain problems did not seem to develop (87–92). Whereas cultural differences are certainly likely, it is difficult to make this conclusion, especially from the Lithuanian studies. In a detailed analysis of the initial Lithuanian research by Schrader and colleagues, Foreman and Croft described critical methodological flaws and concluded that only 1% of the subjects were selected appropriately for inclusion in the study, making it and its follow-up studies flawed as well (19,90,91).

Current Insights in Chronic Pain Development

It is somewhat surprising that so many years after the initial introduction of the gate-control theory of pain, which provided the basis for an integrated model of physiologic and psychological factors for the development of chronic pain states, some researchers continue to depend primarily on the biomedical model of pain (93). As Turk summarized: "The biological model . . . assumes that an individual's complaints should result from a specific disease state represented by disordered biology, the diagnosis of which is confirmed by data from objective tests of physical damage and impairment" (94). The conclusion that complaints of chronic pain after a collision would only be conceivable if there were evidence of "persistent damage after the acute injury" reflects the unidimensional biomedical model and negates more up-to-date pain research and perspectives. Chronic pain after whiplash is neither somatic nor psychogenic; the development of hypersensitivity must be understood from the biopsychosocial perspective of the pain sciences, and consider not only the initial whiplash injury, but also the psychological and social factors that influence the pain experience (94–96). Hypersensitivity may include hyperalgesia (spontaneous pain or an exaggerated response to noxious stimuli), allodynia (pain following normally innocuous stimuli), and hyperpathia (pain that is excessively amplified) (97).

Another important factor to the development of chronic pain after low-velocity collisions lies in the possible involvement of the sympathetic nervous system and the plasticity of the central nervous system (98). Sympathetic dysfunction after whiplash (e.g., vasomotor symptoms and complaints of burning pain) has been described by several researchers and may be related to the sprouting of sympathetic fibers in the dorsal root ganglia (99–105). In addition, the anterior cervical intervertebral discs have a sympathetic nerve supply, which may be activated during whiplash injuries, further contributing to sympathetic dysfunction (106). The role of the central nervous system (CNS) in whiplash patients has only recently been studied. It is conceivable that the persistent pain after whiplash injuries is due to nociceptive changes secondary to tissue damage. After tissue injury, excitatory transmitters (e.g., glutamate and substance P) acting though N-methyl-D-aspartate and neurokinin 1 receptors initiate a cascade that may activate secondary messengers (e.g., calcium, nitric oxide, and prostaglandins) and nociceptive terminals, which in some individuals can result in persistent physiologic and morphologic alterations in the central nervous system (86,107).

A long-term increase in the excitability of wide-dynamic-range neurons in the dorsal horn may influence the processing of both noxious and non-noxious stimuli and eventually lead to hypersensitivity and the development of chronic pain disorders (108). The nociceptive barrage from joint and muscle nociceptors during injury has been shown to cause central hyperexcitability in animals, and it is likely that this phenomenon occurs in patients with chronic whiplash pain as well (109–112). In fact, a recent study supported this notion. Patients with chronic whiplash pain featured muscular hyperalgesia, not only in the neck and shoulder regions, but also in distant areas, such as the anterior tibialis muscle, in which patients usually do not experience any pain (113). Although the exact mechanisms of the persistent hyperexcitability are not known, sensitization of the peripheral terminal and a central facilitation evoked by persistent small afferent input are necessary (107). It is hypothesized that the ongoing nociceptive input from myofascial trigger points and the cervical zygapophyseal joints is sufficient to maintain the central hypersensitivity, which would also provide an explanation for the immediate relief of pain after trigger point inactivation or percutaneous radiofrequency neurotomy.

Central sensitization may lead some physicians to diagnose fibromyalgia in patients with chronic whiplash pain; however, caution must be exercised in giving patients a diagnosis of fibromyalgia, especially when other objective diagnoses account for the pain, including MPS and joint dysfunction (114–118). Once the patient has reached a chronic pain state, there is usually no more evidence of the initiating tissue injury, because normal tissue healing would have occurred. Therefore, there are no valid indications for medical imaging studies after whiplash except in the presence of neurologic findings, including central disc herniations, or to screen for fractures (60,119–122). Linking persistent damage or injury to chronic pain or disability after whiplash is no longer considered a valid construct against the background of the pain sciences.

Several studies have confirmed that cognitive and psychological dysfunction is common after whiplash injuries (123–125). The psychosocial symptoms, such as depression, anxiety, and fear-avoidance behavior, are triggered by the initial injury and develop as the result of the development of chronic pain and subsequent adjustment problems to the somatic symptoms (126–128). When the pain complaint is resolved, the psychological distress disappears (129,130). Patients may become increasingly concerned about the persistent nature of the chronic symptoms and the prospects of long-term suffering and disability (33). Other psychological problems may include problems with behavioral control, sleep, sexuality and libido, depression, anxiety, and anger; however, these were not found to be significant in predicting the outcome after injury (124,128,130,131). Neuropsychological evaluations of cognitive functioning indicated significant and persistent age-adjusted cognitive deficits, primarily in the areas of executive functioning and working memory, that are not detectable by positron emission tomography (PET) and single photon emission computed tomography (SPECT) scanning (132,133).

Conventional Treatment Approaches

Although the report of the Quebec Task Force has been criticized for methodologic flaws, it did illustrate the lack of scientific studies on the management of patients with WAD (55,134,135). Conventional treatments often consist of muscle relaxants, anti-inflammatories, rest, and the use of a cervical collar, even though several studies have indicated that rest and immobilization tend to retard the recovery period (136–138). In a critical review of the literature, Bogduk concluded that during the acute phase, few strategies are scientifically grounded. Patients may be prescribed simple analgesics or nonsteroidal anti-inflammatory drugs, whereas during the first 8 weeks, a home exercise program appeared to be more effective than passive mobilization, ice, or rest and analgesics.

Very few treatment approaches have been scientifically validated for patients with chronic whiplash pain as well, other than radiofrequency neurotomies (134). Others were more optimistic in their conclusions and established that during the subacute phase, multimodal interventions consisting of postural training, manual technique, and psychological support were significantly more effective than the use of physical agents only, such as electrotherapy and ultrasound. In many instances, such a multimodal approach prevented the onset of chronic pain symptoms (139). The combination of proprioceptive exercises, a lecture, and an active home program was found to be more efficacious than an educational lecture with a few recommendations alone (140).

INTEGRATED MYOFASCIAL AND ARTICULAR TREATMENT APPROACH

Once the pain has become chronic, the role of central sensitization in maintaining whiplash-associated pain becomes paramount, and emotional and psychological aspects of the pain response also figure more prominently (141). Persistent articular, neural, and muscular dysfunction contribute to both central sensitization and to immediate pain. Therefore, each of these factors must be assessed when evaluating the patient with chronic whiplash symptoms. Although there is little published evidence that myofascial trigger point therapy and joint manipulation or mobilization is effective in treating chronic whiplash pain, the studies on the treatment of cervical zygapophyseal joint dysfunction suggest that these therapies would be beneficial.

How and when the joint mobilizations are performed are influenced by the clinician's background and experience. Within chiropractic, the emphasis is usually placed on high-velocity–low-amplitude thrust manipulations to treat the somatic dysfunctions. Within osteopathy, the focus may be on more gentle osteopathic mobilization, whereas in physical therapy the general consensus seems to avoid early spinal mobilizations, but to encourage restoration and maintenance of full movement of the cervical spine.

An interdisciplinary program combining medical interventions, injection therapy, dry needling, and physical therapy was found to return close to 80% of patients to a functional life, even though all patients had failed previous therapeutic programs and were not seen until an average of 2 1/2 years after the whiplash (9). Others have confirmed that the inactivation of myofascial trigger points after whiplash significantly improves the patient's status (17,141–144). Su and Su described the successful use of acupuncture in so-called "oh yes"-points, which, on closer examination, appeared to be myofascial trigger points as well (145,146). The following case histories illustrate how myofascial treatments may be included in the overall treatment approach. It should be obvious that there is an urgent need to advance the scientific basis of the existence and treatment of myofascial pain syndrome after whiplash.

Case history 3-1 illustrates early myofascial care, initiated within 48 hours after an auto accident. Case history 3-2 was more complex and involved numerous treatment regimens that failed or that were only provided partial and transitory relief. Eventually, an epidural block was used to treat nerve root involvement, and facet injections were used to treat capsular injury. In this case, the care of the myofascial and joint dysfunctions were an integral part of the treatment plan and helped to localize the sources of pain and decrease the mechanical stresses affecting both the nerve root and the cervical facets, and thus helped bring about resolution of long-standing pain with minimal invasive intervention.

CASE 3-1

Patient History

Ms. S was a 56-year-old woman who was examined and treated approximately 48 hours after an auto accident in which a truck struck the right front of her vehicle. Within a couple of hours after the accident, her neck and back stiffened, her neck started to ache, and she had lower back pain.

Her medical history included three significant auto accidents with neck injuries 5 years, 3 years, and 1 year before the current accident. She had been treated for 6 to 8 months for injuries sustained in each of these accidents. As a result of the accident 5 years before, she had developed significant pain in her right arm and weakness of finger extension. She was found to have significant foraminal stenosis, with osteophytes bilaterally at C6–C7 and on the left at C5–C6. She had a radial tunnel syndrome with entrapment of the radial nerve with a posterior interosseus syndrome treated surgically. Some residual weakness persisted. She also received chiropractic care, including gentle osseous manipulation with myofascial release to her neck and back, on four occasions in the 3 months before the accident, with improvement in joint function and movement.

Examination

Cervical range of motion was limited and painful, with flexion limited to 90% of normal. Right and left lateral flexion, right rotation, and left rotation were each limited to two thirds of normal. Biceps and triceps tendon reflexes were normal. Cervical compression alone as well as right lateral flexion with compression produced left-sided neck pain. Cervical muscles were tense, including the scalene, sternocleidomastoid, upper trapezius, and levator scapulae muscles bilaterally. There was joint tenderness and restriction of cervical spine intersegmental mobility at C1–C2 and C6–C7–T1. Thoracolumbar

movement was normal, but painful. Knee and ankle tendon reflexes were normal, and there were no signs of lumbar radiculopathy.

Jaw muscles were tense bilaterally, including the left masseter and temporalis muscles. Jaw protrusion and lateral excursions were limited, suggesting shortened pterygoid muscles. Other muscles that showed increased muscle tone included the pectoralis major, the biceps, the infraspinatus, the paraspinal muscles in the middle and lower back, the bilateral quadratus lumborum, right iliopsoas, and adductor muscles. There was a stripe of increased muscle tone and tenderness across the abdominal muscles, consistent with seatbelt compression. Spinal intersegmental mobility at T8–T9 and L5–S1 was restricted, and these levels were tender.

Treatment

Treatment consisted of gentle spray-and-stretch myofascial release technique (described later in the chapter), gentle spinal mobilization, and light massage to the tendons of each injured muscle to slightly spread the origin and insertion apart (also described later). Brief moist heat therapy was applied, and the patient was instructed in gentle home stretches. She was seen every other day over the next week and was referred to a massage therapist for massage and manual myofascial release. The muscles relaxed somewhat, but discreet taut bands and trigger points were readily palpated. Gentle high-velocity/low-amplitude adjustment of the restricted areas of the cervical spine was performed, resulting in improved joint function and reduced tenderness, as well as decreased localized paraspinal muscle tightness. The taut bands and trigger points in the neck localized to the left side, particularly persisting in the posterior scalene and splenius cervicis muscles. Other neck and shoulder muscles became more relaxed, and head, neck, and shoulder

(continues)

CASE 3-1 Continued

posture began to normalize. There was an increase in mid-back pain a few weeks later associated with the postural readjustment of the shoulders. Treatment was then directed toward improving mid-back spine and rib flexibility to accommodate the shift of the shoulders. She was instructed to lie on a tennis ball once a day, the ball applied to specific tender spots in the paraspinal muscles, which also mobilized the restricted costovertebral joints. The ball was positioned at a specific spot for 30 seconds to 2 minutes and then moved to another tender spot. The mid-back pain largely subsided within the week, and there was increased costovertebral mobility.

Massage frequency was reduced to once weekly while she continued neck, back, and shoulder stretches. The trigger points in the left splenius capitis and cervicis diminished, and right cervical rotation improved markedly. She was discharged from care 2 months after the accident.

Follow-up

Ms. S had one recurrence of neck pain 11 months later associated with a flu-like illness. This responded well to trigger point therapy and mobilization of the facet joints.

CASE 3-2

History

Ms. T, age 31, complained of chronic, severe neck pain, daily headaches, right shoulder and forearm pain, and right hand numbness, especially of her thumb, index, and middle fingers, 1 year after a motor vehicle accident. She also reported symptoms of temporomandibular joint dysfunction and of a sleep disorder. She had been seen by her primary care physician, a physiatrist, a neurologist, a chiropractor, and a psychologist without effective resolution of her symptoms.

Ms. T. was returning home from the emergency department on the evening of the accident, after having been treated for a migraine headache. She had been given meperidine and a cervical collar because her "head felt too heavy to hold up." At the time of the accident, she was seated in the right front seat and seat-belted. She was turned slightly to the left when the van was struck on her side by a vehicle estimated to be traveling about 35 mph. She had no loss of consciousness, did not strike her head, and did not have any lacerations or contusions. She felt immediate neck pain. Damage to her vehicle was such that she had to be "cut out of the van" and removed from the driver's side. She returned to the same emergency department where she had been previously seen. She had no fractures and was treated with muscle relaxants and anti-inflammatory medications and released.

Her symptoms developed over 3 days after the motor vehicle accident. She had six physical therapy sessions in which she received cervical mobilization and stretching, which was painful and of minimal help. Chiropractic adjustments to her cervical spine were extremely painful and were stopped. Her chiropractor then used only heat and gentle mobilization techniques once per week for the next 6 months, giving her transient relief.

Myofascial trigger point therapy was given once per week for 3 months, giving her brief pain relief, but the trigger points in her neck and upper back always returned. She was treated by a physiatrist after 8 months of continued headaches, neck pain, and right hand numbness. He added opiates, a selective serotonin receptor inhibitor (SSRI), and a muscle relaxant to her drug regimen. A magnetic resonance imaging (MRI) scan of her neck showed a central disc protrusion at C5–6 with spinal cord impingement. An orthopedic surgeon told her that surgery was not needed. Electrodiagnostic studies showed no evidence for a cervical radiculopathy. She was treated with cervical traction. which exacerbated her symptoms. Her primary care physician diagnosed fibromyalgia syndrome and sent her to a psychologist, who diagnosed posttraumatic stress disorder (PTSD). She was treated with psychotherapy for 18 months, including eye movement desensitization and reprocessing (EMDR) and cognitive therapy. However, her therapist thought that the headaches, neck pain, and hand numbness were not psychologically induced. The psychologist referred her to an osteopathic physician for further evaluation.

Examination

The patient had decreased range of motion of the cervical spine and point tenderness in the cervical and upper thoracic paravertebral muscles. The right shoulder was painful to touch at the acromioclavicular joint and at the proximal biceps tendon. She had tenderness in her upper back muscles, especially on the right side. The right sacroiliac joint was tender, and there was a trigger point in the right piriformis muscle.

The neurologic examination was normal, despite her complaint of right hand numbness.

CASE 3-2 Continued

There was 60 degrees of neck flexion, 30 degrees of cervical extension, 45 degrees of rotation to each side, 20 degrees of side-bending to the left, and 40 degrees of side-bending to the right. There were no signs of rotator cuff tear or of shoulder dislocation. The right biceps tendon stability was intact, although she experienced pain during the examination. (Certain injuries and mechanical dysfunctions of the shoulder, as well as aging, can result in some slippage of the biceps tendon relative to the bicipital groove. The examination did not show this to be a significant feature of this patient's condition.)

She had left temporomandibular joint (TMJ) tenderness, with masseter and temporalis muscle trigger points. Medial pterygoid trigger points were also palpable intraorally. There were trigger points in the right sternocleidomastoid, anterior and medial scalene muscles, upper trapezius muscles, right splenius capitis, splenius cervicis, and suboccipital muscles. She had bilateral sternoclavicular and acromioclavicular joint tenderness, the right side being more tender than the left. Moreover, there were trigger points in both pectoralis major and pectoralis minor muscles and in the right subscapularis, rhomboid, teres minor, latissimus dorsi, and quadratus lumborum muscles.

Osteopathic Examination

The osteopathic examination showed the following:

1. Left posterior ilial somatic dysfunction (SD)

2. Right-on-right forward sacral torsion

3. L2–4 group SD, side-bent right, rotated left (L2–4 N Sr Rl)

4. T4–T9 group SD, side-bent left, rotated right (T4–9 N Sl Rr)

5. T7 SD, side-bent left, rotated left, in flexion (T7 F Sl Rl)

6. T3 SD, side-bent right, rotated right, in extension (T3 E Sr Rr)

7. C6 SD, side-bent right, rotated right, in extension (C6 E Sr Rr)

8. C4 SD, side-bent right, rotated right, in flexion (C4 F Sr Rr)

9. C3 SD, side-bent left, rotated left, extension (C3 E Sl Rl)

10. Occiput-on-atlas, side-bent right and rotated left, in extension (O-A E Sr Rl).

See Box 3-1 for discussion of these diagnostic terms.

Treatment and Clinical Course

The muscle trigger points were treated with manual trigger point therapy, trigger point injections, and muscle energy techniques (see Chapter 10). Cervical, thoracic, and lumbosacral trigger points improved with therapy, except that she could not tolerate manipulation or muscle energy techniques to her neck. Cervical zygapophyseal joint injection from C3 to C7 reduced her pain and allowed muscle energy techniques to be used in the cervical and thoracic region (see Technique boxes 3-1 and 3-2). These techniques were then effective in treating the somatic dysfunctions found in the cervical and thoracic spine. Bilateral epidural blocks at the C5–6 level eliminated her neck and shoulder pain and her arm numbness. The trigger point injections and myotherapy were given concurrently with the cervical zygapophyseal joint injections and epidural blocks. She was treated with tricyclic antidepressant drugs that reduced pain, improved sleep, and reduced headache frequency. She also was treated with a short course of rapidly tapered steroids that decreased symptoms of neuropathy and of neck pain. Posttraumatic stress disorder was treated with psychotherapy. Treatment extended over 3 months at weekly intervals and monthly for an additional 3 months.

Follow-up

She had a difficult course but finally experienced her first relief from chronic pain in 2 years. She is now fully recovered and has only occasional headaches that she treats with acetaminophen or nonsteroidal anti-inflammatories.

Discussion

Ms. T. had severe right neck and shoulder pain, headaches, and right hand numbness without neurologic deficit. Her condition had failed medical management with anti-inflammatories, muscle relaxants, SSRI antidepressants, and opiate pain medications. Her symptoms were exacerbated by chiropractic cervical adjustments, osteopathic muscle energy techniques, and cervical traction. She had seen multiple physicians and therapists. She was diagnosed with fibromyalgia syndrome by her primary care physician. This was an unfortunate but typical scenario for a whiplash injury. A closer look at her symptoms gave important clues to their cause.

Diagnostic manipulation of each cervical segment disclosed individual somatic dysfunctions at C6 E Sr Rr,

(continues)

CASE 3-2   Continued

C4 F Sr Rr, C3 E Sl Rl, and an OA E Sr Rl (occipitoatlantal, type I somatic dysfunction described in Technique 3-1.) An ideal technique for treating this type of problem is with osteopathic muscle energy techniques. She was initially intolerant of even gentle osteopathic manipulation of her cervical spine. However, these techniques were easily tolerated after cervical zygapophyseal joint injections. Trigger point therapy initially gave only temporary relief. Trigger points recurred in response to somatic articular dysfunctions or segmental cervical or thoracic spine dysfunction. Cervical epidural blocks relieved most of the remaining neck and shoulder pain. Osteopathic muscle energy techniques could then be used and were effective in improving cervical spine joint function. Myofascial care also became effective at this point, further reducing the patient's pain level and allowing for full return of function to her neck and upper back.

Myofascial care was important in helping to address sources of persistent pain and in reducing the stresses on the cervical joints. For example, the splenius capitis and splenius cervicis muscles insert on the lower cervical and upper thoracic vertebrae. Active trigger points in these muscles refer pain to the occiput and behind the eye, causing chronic headache. They also can force the cervical spine to side-bend and rotate, creating multiple sites of somatic dysfunction resulting in restricted movement and neck pain. The affected suboccipital muscles (the rectus capitis posterior minor and the oblique capitis superior) attach to the occiput and the atlas (C1).

These muscles are also a common source of headache. They can pull eccentrically on the occiput to create occiput-atlas (OA) somatic dysfunction. Once injection procedures had controlled the facet and nerve root pain, the myofascial care was effective in reducing neck and head pain, and in allowing for the restoration of normal cervical joint mobility.

Ms. T experienced thoracic and lumbosacral muscular pain relief with trigger point injections, spray and stretch techniques, heat, and myotherapy. The scalene muscles that were holding the right first rib in an elevated position were released, allowing the first rib to drop, and relieving pressure on the brachial plexus that was contributing to hand numbness. The shortened left subscapularis muscle held the scapula cephalad and forward, thus elevating the distal clavicle, and this resulted in tenderness and dysfunction at the left sternoclavicular joint. Subscapularis release resulted in a change in scapulohumeral mechanics and a reduction of stress to the sternoclavicular joint. (Scalene and sternocleidomastoid muscle trigger points also can refer pain and tenderness into the clavicular region and the sternoclavicular joint.) Her TMJ symptoms were corrected by temporalis, medial pterygoid, and masseter trigger point releases. A home stretching program was prescribed by her physical therapist. She was able to sleep through the night for the first time in over 2 years. Her psychologist noted a more optimistic outlook and greater problem-solving abilities. She was able to return to her usual life activities.

Overview of Neck Pain and Dysfunction following Whiplash

Treatment of myofascial trigger point pain syndromes and muscle restrictions, and treatment of cervical and thoracic joint dysfunctions are successful strategies in the care of patients who have had acute whiplash-associated injuries. The goal of these therapies in early management is to reduce acute symptoms and restore normal range of motion and function early so as to diminish the likelihood of developing a chronic pain condition.

Treatment of myofascial and joint dysfunction often can contribute to improving the status of individuals with chronic pain after whiplash injuries. Chronic whiplash-associated pain may be related to myofascial trigger points and dysfunction, it may be related to joint dysfunction, and it can be the result of nerve entrapment (that may be the result of myofascial trigger points). A combined myofascial and articular approach can decrease the severity of nerve entrapment syndromes. Myofascial and articular therapy have the potential of decreasing chronic pain and improving function and the quality of life.

Etiology

Most soft tissue neck injuries that are seen in a general pain practice occur as the result of motor vehicle accidents. Other incidents that can produce similar injuries include slip and fall injuries, sports injuries that involve falls (e.g. water skiing and snow skiing injuries), and assaults. Persons are at risk for whiplash-type injuries when there has been excessive and rapid neck movement from any cause. The dynamics of each of these types of accidents are different, but each involves a **strain** of the neck muscles and a **sprain** of the ligaments. In whiplash injuries, induced movement is beyond the normal compliance of the muscles and ligaments of the neck and often beyond the tolerance of the cervical zygapophyseal joints. Other regions of the body are

BOX 3-1

Osteopathic Diagnostic Nomenclature

An osteopathic somatic dysfunction (SD) is named for the "dysfunctional" position in which the vertebral segment(s) and related muscular, neural, vascular, lymphatic components are found. Single vertebrae can be fixed in flexion or extension and according to physiologic laws of motion, side-bending and rotation must then be in the same direction. This is considered a type II somatic dysfunction. If there is a group curve, in which multiple vertebra are involved, according to the laws of physiologic motion, the curve is in a neutral position, neither flexed nor extended, and side-bending and rotation are in opposite directions. This is considered a type I somatic dysfunction.

An example of a type II SD would be if C4 were palpitated and found in extension, side-bent right, and rotated right. This would mean that C4 moved easily into extension and had difficulty moving into flexion. In fact, its barrier to motion would be flexion. This is also true for side-bending and rotation. C4 would be found to side-bend and rotate better to the right than to the left. This would be called a C4, extension, side-bent right and rotated right somatic dysfunction. The abbreviation for this dysfunctional vertebra would be C4 E Sr Rr, to indicate the position of ease of motion of the dysfunctional vertebral unit.

A somatic dysfunction is therefore named for the position of its freedom or ease of motion. However, this is a dysfunctional or altered position and not one that is physiologically balanced. To treat this condition, the vertebra or vertebral curve needs to be moved through its barriers toward normal physiologic motion and reposition to its normal physiologic position.

To treat the SD described above, the C4 vertebra would be placed into its barriers to motion, that is C4 E Sl Rl. At the level of C4, the vertebra would be positioned in extension, left side-bending and left rotation, so that the vertebra could be felt up against its barriers to motion. A muscle energy technique would be used to progressively return the vertebra back to its physiologically functional position. In other words, the vertebra would be slowly brought through its barriers to motion until full functioning was returned to it and it no longer moved more easily into a painful and dysfunctional position. (Muscle energy principles and practices are explained in the Low Back chapter in Box 10-5). How muscle energy techniques are applied to cervical and thoracic somatic dysfunction is illustrated in the Technique boxes in this chapter. Specifically, the muscle energy techniques for C6 E Sr Rr, C4 F Sr Rr, C3 E Sl Rl, and OA E Sr Rl, for the cervical spine and T4–T9 N Sr Rl, T7 F Sl Rl, and T3 E Sr Rr for the thoracic spine are described.

Note that osteopathic nomenclature is not identical to chiropractic nomenclature but can be readily translated. For example, the point of reference for osteopathic designation of rotation is the body of the vertebra, whereas the chiropractic reference is the spinous process. Thus, if the body rotates toward the right, the spinous process rotates toward the left and the terms can be translated.

---

also frequently injured in whiplash, and those injuries may affect the level of pain of the whiplash-associated disorder and can retard recovery.

Cautions

Before initiating manual therapy of significant traumatic neck injury, assessment should address:

1. Any sign of brain injury, including concussion or changes in memory, concentration, balance, or coordination

2. The level of pain, the history of onset of the pain and its location, and joint mobility. A determination is made as to whether the cervical spine is stable or unstable (listhesis with movement), or whether there are throat symptoms indicating bleeding in the anterior cervical tissues. In the rare cases in which movement is extremely guarded, and in which there is unusually extreme localized spine tenderness, the clinician must consider and rule out spinal fracture.

3. Signs of cervical nerve root injury

4. Vertebral artery sufficiency if treatment will include putting the neck into extension and rotation during the course of treatment

Symptoms/Pain Presentation

The patient with a whiplash-associated disorder often has sustained injuries to other areas of the body as well. Neck-related symptoms include neck pain, head pain, jaw joint and muscle pain, upper back pain, and arm and hand pain. Other symptoms include paresthesias, dizziness, nausea, blurred or double vision, ringing in the ears, conjunctival infection, difficulty swallowing, and sore throat. Although there can be other causes of these symptoms, specific myofascial trigger points can account for or contribute to the

TECHNIQUE 3-1

Muscle Energy Techniques for Cervical Somatic Dysfunctions

For theC6 SrRr SD, the patient is placed in a supine position, and the practitioner is seated at the patient's head. In this case, C6 is found to move easily into extension, right side-bending, and rotation. This is the *name* or the position of the ease of motion of this somatic dysfunction, (Each position is tested for ease or difficulty of motion at C6; flexion and extension, left and right side-bending, and rotation.) To apply a muscle energy technique, the operator would place the cervical spine, at the C6 vertebra, into flexion, left side-bending and left rotation until the barriers to motion were met in all three planes of motion. The patient would then be asked to either extend or right side-bend or rotate the head to the right against the practitioner's resistance, with 3 to 5 pounds of pressure, for 3 to 5 seconds (only one plane of motion is necessary to gain the full effect of the muscle energy technique). The patient is then asked to relax while the practitioner repositions the patient's head into a new, but less pronounced, position of motion resistance. The procedure is repeated three to four times until the barriers to motion have been eliminated and joint function has been restored (**A**).

The C3 E Sl Rl and C4 F Sr Rr SDs would be managed much the same as C6 SD already discussed except that the positions needed to treat these dysfunctions would be modified (**B and C**).

In fact, the only cervical somatic dysfunction that is treated differently with a muscle energy technique is the occipitoatlantal somatic dysfunction. This is a specific type I dysfunction, found only at the junction between the occiput and the first cervical vertebra. The mechanics of this joint dictate that the motions of side-bending and rotation are in *opposite* directions and the primary movement of this joint is in flexion or extension.

In the case given, the occipitoatlantal (OA) somatic dysfunction is in extension, side-bent right, and rotated left (OA E Sr Rl). This would mean that the sulcus or depression made by the occiput as it joins with the first cervical vertebra, the OA joint, would feel *deeper* on the left or *fuller* on the right, as the patient extended her head. This would mean that the OA joint had a right side-bending dysfunction. According to the physiologic laws of motion at the OA joint, if there is *right* side-bending there is *left* rotation.

To treat this patient, her head would be placed into flexion at the OA joint, side-bent left, and rotated right. And she would be asked to extend her head and hold for 3 to 5 seconds with a pressure of 3 to 5 pounds. In so doing, the chin would automatically press up into the practitioner's resistance. This technique, like the other muscle energy techniques, would be repeated 3 to 5 times until the OA joint was restored to its normal physiologic motion (**D**).

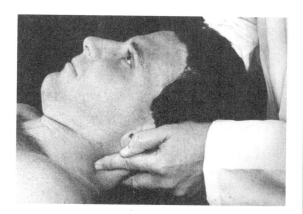
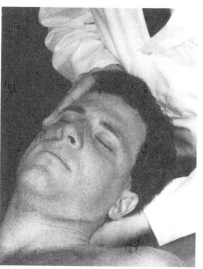

(A) Somatic Dysfunction C6 E Sr Rr. This means that C6 is in extension and is sidebent right and rotated right. Thus, the position in which muscle energy technique is performed is with C6 taken to the end range of motion into flexion, sidebent left, and rotated left. (ME position: C6F Sl, Rl.) Reprinted with permission from DiGiovanna EL, Schiowitz S. An Osteopathic Approach to Diagnosis and Treatment, 2nd Ed. Philadelphia: Lippincott-Raven, 1997, Fig. 7.13A and B (p. 118).

TECHNIQUE 3-1

Muscle Energy Techniques for Cervical Somatic Dysfunctions (*Continued*)

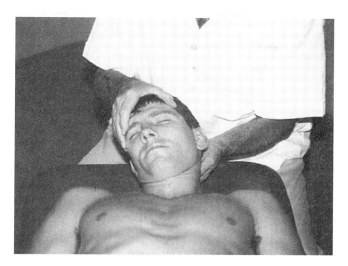

(B) Somatic Dysfunction C3 E Sl Rl. This means that C3 is in extension and is sidebent left and rotated left. Thus, the muscle energy position is C6 in flexion, sidebent right and rotated right. (ME position C6 F Sr Rr.) Reprinted with permission from Greenman PE. Principles of Manual Medicine, 2nd Ed. Baltimore: Lippincott Williams & Wilkins, 1996, Fig. 13.44 (p. 191).

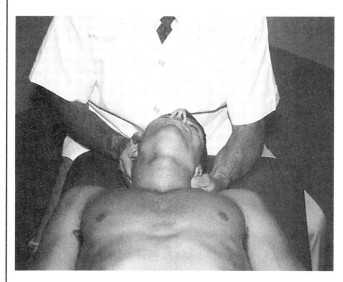

(C) Somatic Dysfunction C4F Sr Rr. This means that C4 is in flexion and is sidebent right and rotated right. Thus, the muscle energy position is C4 in extension, sidebent left and rotated left. (ME position C4E SlRl.) Reprinted with permission from Greenman PE. Principles of Manual Medicine, 2nd Ed. Baltimore: Lippincott Williams & Wilkins, 1996, Fig. 13.40 (p. 190).

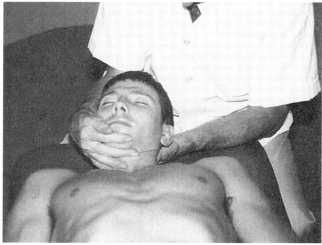

(D) Somatic Dysfunction OAE SrRl. This means that the occiput–atlas joint is in extension and is sidebent right and rotated left. Thus, the muscle energy position is with the occiput–atlas joint taken into flexion, sidebent left and rotated right. (ME position OAF Sl Rr.) Reprinted with permission from Greenman PE. Principles of Manual Medicine, 2nd Ed. Baltimore: Lippincott Williams & Wilkins, 1996, fig. 13.53 (p. 194).

TECHNIQUE 3-2

Muscle Energy Techniques for the Thoracic Somatic Dysfunctions

The patient had two types of thoracic SDs, a single dysfunction at T3 E SrRr and a single dysfunction at T7 F Sl Rl, which was found in the middle of the group SD between T4–T9 N Sr Rr. This means that there was a type II SD (T7) at the apex of the group type I SD (T4–9), which is not an unusual finding.

The single SD, T7 F Sl Rl, would be treated by having the patient seated with the practitioner behind her. The patient would be extended at T7, side-bent right, and rotated right. She would then be asked to either side-bend to the left or rotate to the left against the practitioner's resistance, and hold the position for 3 to 5 seconds with 3 to 5 pounds of pressure for a total of 3 to 5 times (A).

For the group SD, T4–T9 N Sr Rl, the position for treatment would be T4–T9 N Sl Rr with the patient sitting. The concavity of the group curve would be on the right. The rotational component would to the left according to the physiologic laws of motion for a type I SD. To straighten this functional curve, the patient would be positioned to side-bend to the left and asked to side-bend to the right against the practitioner's resistance for 3 to 5 seconds, 3 to 5 times (B).

The T3 E Sr Rr dysfunction would be treated similarly to the single T7dysfunction (C).

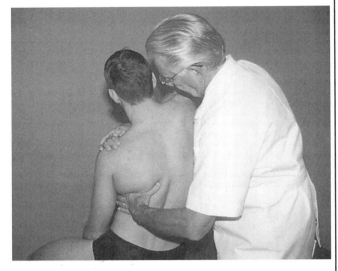

(B) Group Somatic Dysfunction T4–T9N Sr Rl. This means that T4–T9 are in neither flexion nor extension, but are sidebent right and rotated left. Thus, the muscle energy position is T4–T9 in neutral, sidebent left and rotated right. (ME position T4–T9N Sl Rr.) Reprinted with permission from Greenman PE. Principles of Manual Medicine, 2nd Ed. Baltimore: Lippincott Williams & Wilkins, 1996, fig. 14.35 (p. 219).

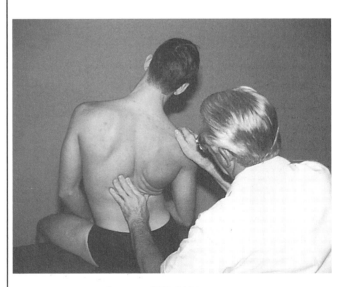

(A) Somatic Dysfunction T7F Sl Rl. This means that T7 is in flexion and is sidebent left and rotated left. Thus, the muscle energy position is T7 in extension, sidebent right and rotated right. (ME position T7E Sr Rr.) Reprinted with permission from Greenman PE. Principles of Manual Medicine, 2nd Ed. Baltimore: Lippincott Williams & Wilkins, 1996, fig. 14.30 (p. 217).

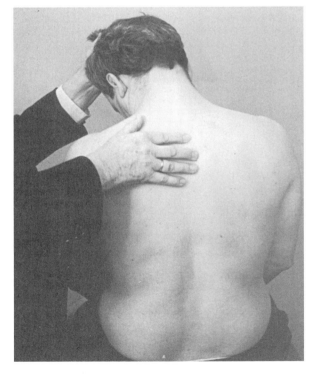

(C) Somatic Dysfunction T3E Sr Rr. This means that T3 is in extension and is sidebent right and rotated right. Thus, the muscle energy position is T3 in flexion, sidebent left and rotated left. (ME position T3F Sl Rl.) Reprinted with permission from Ward RC, ed. Foundations for Osteopathic Medicine. Baltimore: Williams & Wilkins, 1997, fig. 57.3 (p. 886).

severity of most of the symptoms listed. Injury to the mid-back, lower back, and pelvis and associated musculature is common. There also may be extremity injuries.

Myofascial Entrapments

The commonest entrapments associated with neck injuries include occipital nerve entrapment contributing to headaches (see Chapter 1) and brachial plexopathy, causing a thoracic outlet syndrome (see Chapter 4.)

Treatment

Rehabilitation of the patient who has had a whiplash injury includes appropriate care during the acute phase and a planned progression of care once the acute phase is over. It also includes identification of correction of perpetuating factors that continue to cause pain, even after many years.

Evaluation and Treatment of Muscles during the Acute Phase

The release of shortened hypertonic muscles and associated trigger points should be performed within 24 to 48 hours after a traumatic whiplash injury. The release of taut muscles can be started as soon as the muscles begin to shorten. The severity of the injury may be underestimated if the patient is examined and treated on the same day as the accident. The patient's muscles may be even more tense the following day, and unless the patient is treated on that day as well, muscle tightness will increase. The severity of the injury is assessed, and a determination is made as to whether the areas to be treated are stable. If there is dislocation or fracture, movement must be limited in the areas where those injuries occurred. The neck of the patient who has fractured ribs, for example, can be treated.

The technique for performing myofascial release and lengthening hypertonic muscles in a patient who recently suffered a traumatic injury is dramatically different from that usually used to treat patients with a chronic myofascial disorder. First, a technique must be chosen that does not involve much handling of the muscles. The use of a vapocoolant (spray and stretch) is quite appropriate for this application and can dramatically increase the ability to lengthen taut tender neck muscles. The patient is very gently taken through passive stretch positions, and much of the stretch takes place with gravity providing the impetus and only very gentle pressure on the part of the clinician. The patient is told that the muscles are traumatized and there is no benefit to be derived from further stressing them, and that the clinician will try to coax the muscles out of their shortened and tender state, but will not want to force movement. The patient is then asked to say when the end of the range of reasonably comfortable movement has been reached. The patient says "Stop" as soon as a significant increase in pain is felt in each stretch, and that stretch procedure is immediately ended. Stretching is performed on all of the muscles in which there is palpable muscle tightness,

even in areas where the patient has no perceived pain. The usual areas of muscle injury and hypertonicity include:

- Neck muscles: anterior and posterior and lateral muscle groups.
- Jaw muscles: interior and exterior muscles are often hypertonic even when there has been no direct impact to the jaw. The whipping movement of the head on the neck during the accident often forces the mouth open and closed very quickly and forcefully.
- Chest muscles: often worse on the side of shoulder belt impact.
- Shoulder and arm muscles: there is often increased tone of the muscles that pull the humerus and the scapulae forward, including the pectoral, subscapularis, and anterior serratus muscles. The tightness often extends into the upper arms, affecting the biceps and brachialis muscles, and sometimes extends into the lower arms, especially if the steering wheel was gripped during impact.
- Upper and lower back muscles: including muscles between, on, and under the scapulae. The paraspinal and quadratus lumborum muscles are often hypertonic in the lower back.
- Abdominal muscles: often there is a stripe of muscle hypertonicity across the abdomen corresponding with seat belt impact.
- Groin muscles: if there has been significant back muscle injury, the groin muscles will often shorten and develop trigger points as well. This will be accentuated if there was impact between the knees and the dashboard.
- Leg muscles: hypertonicity of these muscles depends on patterns of impact and whether there was a forceful attempt to brake during the accident.

After performing all of the stretches, moist heat can be applied very briefly. The day after the accident, moist heat is applied for no more than 5 minutes, barely enough to induce relaxation, and ice may be used simultaneously over localized areas of exquisite tenderness. Ice may be applied for 10 minutes after the heat has been removed. After the heat and ice application, very gentle origin–insertion massage is performed (Technique 3-3) on each muscle that was found to be hypertonic. This procedure is generally only performed on the first visit and is quite time-consuming, but it appears to produce significant clinical benefit.

Home Care of Muscles. The patient who can be trusted to perform stretches *very gently* is given instructions in gentle stretching of the injured muscles, to be performed every 1 to 3 hours, but never to the point of pain (Fig. 3-4). Neck stretches (see Figs 1-8, 1-9, and 1-10) are performed very gently with the help of gravity, by dropping the head and torso forward, drawing the head directly to the side, and then turning the head toward the axilla and again drawing it

TECHNIQUE 3-3

Origin–Insertion Massage

The clinician places gentle contact at opposite ends of each muscle, at the tendons of origin and insertion. Pressure is applied toward the bone, and away from the belly of the muscle, providing gentle stretch of the muscle fibers, and gentle compression at the location of the **Golgi tendon apparatus**. This pressure may help to "reset" the tendon apparatus that had been stretched in the accident, so it will not continue to upregulate the muscle tension as a protective mechanism. It may be simply that some compression at a potential site of attachment trigger points helps avert their formation. Because we do not know the mechanisms involved in the formation of attachment trigger points, it is difficult to speculate. But this technique has been found to be very clinically useful in the early treatment of patients with traumatic injuries. Each injured muscle is addressed in this manner.

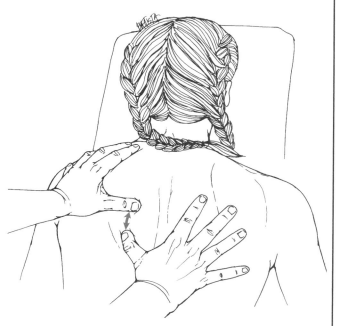

(B) Origin insertion massage on the paraspinal muscles. The clinician contacts the tendons of origin and insertion, gently pressing toward the respective bones, and the process is repeated for multiple portions of the paraspinal muscles.

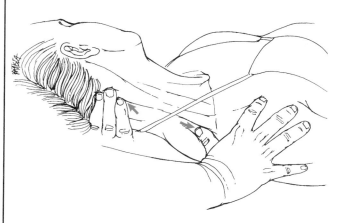

(A) Origin insertion massage on upper trapezius muscle. The clinician contacts the tendons of origin and insertion, gently pressing toward the respective bones, and allowing the shoulder to drop as the muscle releases.

In some cases, it is easy to perform the treatment while elongating the muscle gently, as in the case of the upper trapezius. As the muscle releases, the shoulder of the supine patient can be gently dropped, and the head and neck can be gently shifted away from the shoulder (**A**). The superficial paraspinal muscles comprise bands of muscle that are made up of a series of fibers that originate at different levels and attach several spinous or rib levels away from their origin. It is important to contact the muscle at multiple locations, to address the origin and insertion of each portion of these muscles (**B**).

laterally and inferiorly toward the axilla. The hand can be used to gently increase stretch. For example, while stretching the posterior neck muscles, one or both hands can be placed on the posterior head to gently aide the forward movement. Then, to stretch the right upper trapezius, the left hand can contact the right side of the head, above the ear, and gently draw the head away from the right shoulder. To stretch the right levator scapula, the head is turned toward the left axilla and the left hand is placed on the right posterior skull to gently pull the head away from the right shoulder and down toward the left axilla. The patient is instructed not to overstretch because the muscles will worsen if too

much pull is exerted in the stretches. Ice is used at home for the first 24 to 48 hours, and only brief hot showers are allowed. Then the application of alternating hot and cold is recommended for the next several days: 10 to 15 minutes of moist heat, 10 to 15 minutes of ice, then 10 to 15 minutes of moist heat (this sequence can be reversed if it is better tolerated.) As the acuteness of symptoms subsides, heat can be used alone. Besides the gentle stretches, lying on the ball (or a roll of socks or a hackey sack if the ball is too hard to start with,) is often instituted as well, to reduce paraspinal muscle tension and improve rib–spinal joint mobility. If there has been an injury to the jaw muscles, the patient is instructed

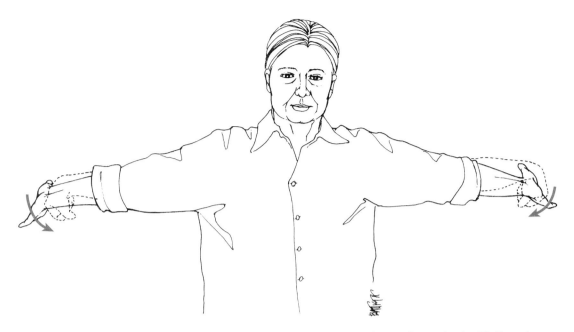

FIGURE 3-4. **Shoulder and upper extremity stretches.** Reach the shoulders and arms back with the palms up and the wrists tilted back. Then reach the shoulders and arms back with the palms facing down and the wrists and fingers curled under.

in pincer massage of the jaw muscles, to be performed once or twice per day (Fig. 3.5).

As the patient improves, more vigorous stretches can be introduced; the patient should perform these without pain (Figs. 3-6–3-8). Although stretches of the anterior neck muscles can be introduced, posterior neck muscle stretches should be continued. Strengthening activities should definitely not be initiated during the acute phase, particularly during the first 2 to 3 weeks. Thereafter, the tendency for muscles tightness and pain to increase in the course of normal activity should be assessed. As the patient has fewer flare-ups in the course of normal activity, more vigorous exercise will be tolerated. When strengthening activities are initiated, care should be taken not to work the muscles that have active trigger points, because this will simply aggravate the remaining trigger points.

If strengthening is undertaken when there is still significant trigger point activity in the muscles being exercised, one of two possible outcomes usually results: (1) the muscles will not strengthen despite good effort at exercise; or (2) the muscles will strengthen but pain will increase. Therefore, muscles that still have significant myofascial trigger points should be monitored to see whether each new exercise causes increased pain. If so, the exercise must be modified or discontinued, and the exacerbation of pain should be treated.

The gentle resistance of water in pool exercise is often tolerated well at the beginning of a strengthening program. Exercise of the middle and lower trapezius muscles, shoulder retraction, and other activities to improve posture are also often well tolerated at this stage. In fact, postural

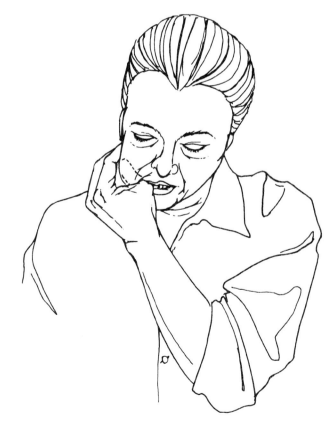

FIGURE 3-5. **Jaw muscle self-massage.** Reach the thumb inside the cheek, near the back teeth, and grab the jaw muscles between the thumb and the index finger. Strum, press, and pull on the taut bands to elongate them.

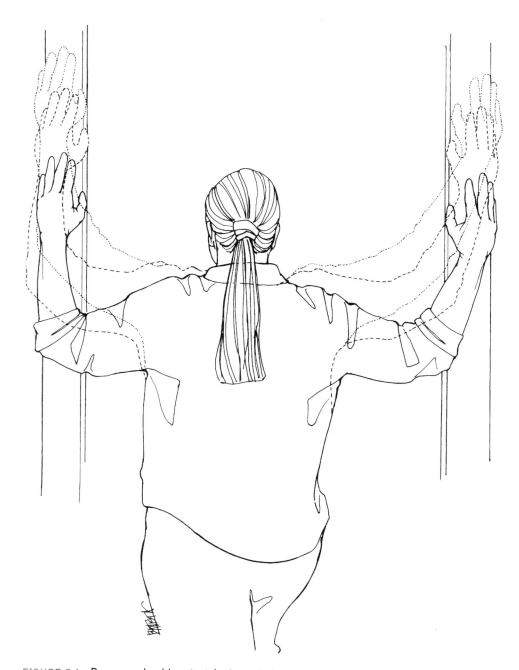

FIGURE 3-6. **Doorway shoulder stretch.** Stretch the pectoral muscles by standing in a doorway with the flat of the forearms against the door frame, and one foot through the door and in front of the other foot. Shift the body weight forward from the back foot to the front foot, stretching the chest and shoulders with the arms below, at, and above shoulder height. Only stretch within a reasonably comfortable range.

stabilization activities undertaken to improve postural control in the upper and lower back can often make a positive contribution to the rehabilitative effort.

General Muscle Treatment Plan Although the treatment described in this chapter has been developed from clinical experience and is consistent with current research on the benefits of early mobility, there has been no significant research to directly validate its benefits. The basic treatment approach is based on the hypothesis, presented by Simons, Travell, and Simons (146), that development and continuation of myofascial trigger points develops from an energy crisis in which compressed capillaries lessen the availability of nutrients and oxygen to the mus-

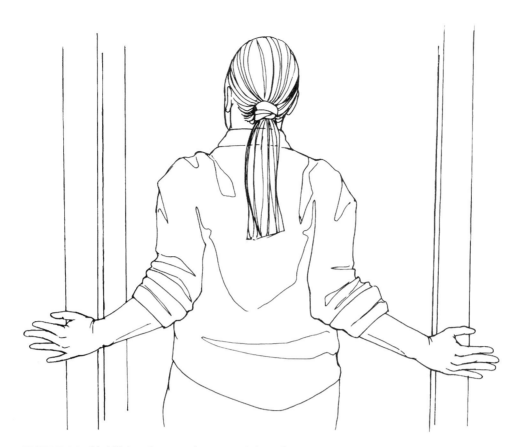

FIGURE 3-7. **Mobilizing the scapulae toward the spine.** With one foot forward, place the hands against the doorframe at waist level. Shift the torso forward until the scapulae approximate.

cle, which leads to the release of sensitizing substances that activates peripheral nociceptors and causes pain. It is hypothesized that the release of excessive amounts of acetylcholine initiates muscle contraction. Thus, it is possible that the further development of trigger points is more likely, and they are more likely to be numerous and severe, if the muscle tightness or initial trigger point formation from the initial injury is sustained, and if it decreases local muscle circulation and therefore impairs recovery of injured muscle tissue.

It is explained to the patient that goal of acute care is to "keep a lid on" the degree of muscle shortening and pain so that the patient will be in a better state when the acute phase is over. Therefore, the patient is encouraged to use whatever other modalities will reduce the pain level, particularly to help attain restful sleep. Although it is not the purpose of this chapter to discuss the use of medications and nutritional supplements, nor to review the analgesic effects of various physical therapy modalities, it is clear that early treatment of the muscle and joint injuries often reduces pain sufficiently for the patient to be comfortable, but that supplemental therapy may nevertheless be helpful in achieving patient comfort. During the acute phase, generally the first 2 to 3 weeks after an accident involving

whiplash, the patient is treated approximately every other day. When the injuries are more severe, daily treatment may initially be necessary. The goal of treatment is to repeatedly gently release muscle tightness and to improve circulation and joint mobility. Our experience suggests that some of the symptoms from whiplash injuries come about because there is sustained muscle shortening and tightness. Muscle relaxants and anti-inflammatory drugs do not necessarily decrease the muscle tightness adequately. Instead, muscles often may become progressively shortened, tight, and painful, particularly through the development of additional myofascial trigger points, so that the patient's symptoms and restricted mobility become progressively worse several weeks after the injury. Therefore, if treatment repeatedly relaxes muscle and restores normal muscle length, a measure of control or mitigation of this progressive sequence may be achieved. The frequency of treatment depends on what is necessary to prevent progression in the injured muscles. When the acute phase of injury is over, treatment often can be reduced to twice per week. Trigger point myotherapy or neuromuscular therapy is also often recommended to help restore normal muscle tone throughout the layers and the entire length of the injured muscles.

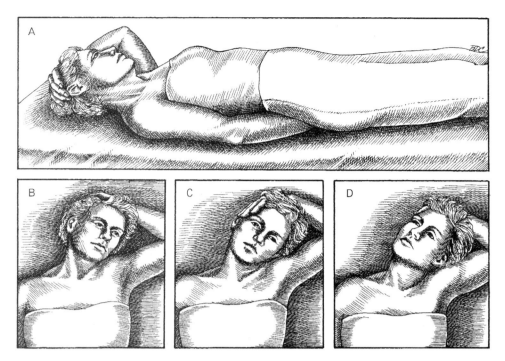

FIGURE 3-8. **Scalene stretch.** The scalene stretch can be performed seated or supine. Each position passively stretches one of the three major scalene muscles. The exercise should always be done bilaterally. **A.** The hand of the side to be stretched is anchored under the buttock. **B.** To stretch the posterior scalene, the face is turned toward the direction of pull. **C.** To stretch the middle scalene, the face looks forward. **D.** To stretch the anterior scalene, the face looks away from the direction of pull. Reprinted with permission from Simons DG, Travell JG, Simons LS. Travell & Simons' Myofascial Pain and Dysfunction: The Trigger Point Manual, vol 1: Upper Half of Body, 2nd Ed. Baltimore: Lippincott Williams & Wilkins, 1999, fig. 20.14 (p. 531).

Evaluation and Treatment of Joint Dysfunction during the Acute Phase

There is invariably joint subluxation or somatic dysfunction in the areas in which muscles are shortened and tender. This is particularly apparent in the spine, but also at rib–spinal junctures, and across other major joints where the initial trauma has caused muscle shortening that has altered the normal patterns of mobility. Almost invariably, the scapulae and humerus are initially moved forward by shortened pectoral muscles. The development of trigger points in the pectoral, subscapularis, and anterior serratus muscles are associated with shortened taut bands that continue to hold the humerus and scapula forward. In the course of muscle treatment, gentle joint mobilization can be performed. The areas of most significant joint restriction are assessed, and they are gently rocked or pressed to increase mobility. Gentle manual traction also can be effectively performed (Technique 3-4).

If there has been significant trauma to the neck or back muscles, the quick movements of osseous high-velocity spinal manipulation are not performed during the first several sessions. As abnormal muscle tone reduces and mobility increases, it may be apparent that localized facet and joint tenderness is a prominent feature of the continuing pain and restriction. A judgment can be made regarding

whether the patient can tolerate the quick, gentle maneuvers involved in osseus adjustments, but the patient's judgment is the deciding factor. After the maneuvers are described, the patient may say, "I don't think I am ready for that yet." Even before the clinician brings up the subject, often the patient may say, "It just feels as though my back needs to be popped and would then feel better." After the muscle releases are performed and heat is applied (or ice when indicated), and the tissues are in a relatively relaxed state, the maneuvers can be successfully completed with very little impulse (thrust) and very short amplitude.

Rotational forces also can be minimized by addressing rotational restrictions in the position the neck is placed into before the lateral to medial thrust is applied. For example, if the vertebral body of C3 is rotated to the left, which means that the spinous process rotates to the right, the head and neck can be turned to the right, thus bringing the spinous process back toward the center. A specific lateral-to-medial thrust can then be gently applied to the left C3 facet or zygapophyseal joint. This maneuver is termed a **lateral break**, but there is a rotational component in positioning before the thrust. When osseous maneuvers are performed, a reflexive decrease of local muscle tone occurs within seconds, so effective treatment of the spinal subluxations assists in further release of taut muscles. The goal of this treatment is to

TECHNIQUE 3-4

Simultaneously Combining Myofascial Treatment and Articular Mobilization Techniques

In the course of performing passive stretches to treat myofascial involvement, a series of techniques can be combined to achieve maximum benefit, and these techniques can be applied in multiple body positions. They can be employed with more specificity and slightly more vigorously after the acute phase of patient care. Whereas joint mobilization always accompanies stretching, the effectiveness of care can be enhanced by specifically palpating for joint restriction and localizing the stretch procedures and trigger point pressure to simultaneously improve joint function. For example, a sequence of treatment for the patient with a whiplash injury can start with the patient seated. The posterior neck muscles can be stretched first by taking the patient's head gently forward. Then the right upper trapezius can be stretched by taking the head away from the right shoulder. Then the head can be drawn away from the shoulder and also back toward the examiner's body to stretch the posterior and middle scalenes and the clavicular portion of the sternocleidomastoid. Then the head can be rotated back toward the right shoulder to stretch the sternal portion of the right sternocleidomastoid and the anterior scalene. The head is then dropped forward to complete the sternocleidomastoid stretch. After this, the head can be turned toward the opposite shoulder and taken forward and away from the right shoulder to stretch the levator scapula and the splenius muscles. While the muscles are being passively stretched, the trigger points within the muscle can be compressed. Also, the same pressure can be used to increase joint mobility of restricted joints. For example, the trigger points in the levator scapula often lie right over restricted rib–spinal joints, so the same pressure that is used to press on the trigger points can also be directed to increasing the mobility of the stiff joints (A).

If a taut band of muscle is not releasing well, postisometric relaxation or contract relax techniques can be used. For example, if the anterior portion of the right upper trapezius is not releasing fully with the passive stretch, even when compression is added, the clinician takes the head to the end of the range of motion, and stabilizes the head and shoulder while asking the patient to gently press the head toward the right shoulder, hold for a slow count of 4, and then release and drop the head toward the left shoulder. The head and neck will usually move farther from the right shoulder, and the procedure can be repeated. Percussion also can be used to encourage better release of deep trigger points. (The percussion technique is discussed in Chapter 4.)

In a seated position, the pectoral muscles also can be stretched by bringing the arms up and back, one at a time. Biceps and brachialis muscles, brachioradialis,

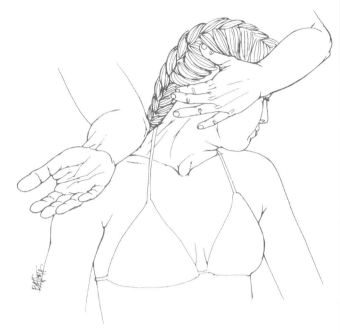

(A) Combining muscle stretch and joint mobilization. During passive stretch of the levator scapula muscle, the clinician uses the pressure of the flat of the forearm, just above the elbow, to *gently* depress the 1st rib and mobilize the rib–thoracic joint.

wrist extensors, and wrist flexors also can be stretched in this position, simply by bringing the arm back, stretching across the elbow with the palm facing forward and back, curling the fingers under to close the hand, or tipping the fingers back to open the hand. (For more detail regarding shoulder releases, see Chapter 4.)

With the patient in a side-lying position, the clinician can place downward pressure on the top of the shoulder, placing specific digital pressure on trigger points in the scalenes, sternocleidomastoids, upper trapezius, and levator scapula muscles (combining trigger point pressure release with gentle traction). At the same time, this may release tension and improve the mobility of the clavicle, scapula, humerus, and cervical spinal joints, and pressure can be specifically directed to release and mobilize joints that have been found to be restricted.

When the patient is prone, pressure can be directed to again drop the shoulder away from the head and neck (B). The clinician also can reach the fingers to the front of the patient's neck, contacting both ends of the scalenes and stretching them apart. In this position, it is not difficult to feel the bony restriction of the cervical spine if there are extension subluxations. If so, the bone will feel more prominent and more anterior under the

(continues)

TECHNIQUE 3-4

Simultaneously Combining Myofascial Treatment and Articular Mobilization Techniques *(Continued)*

muscle and more resistant to anterior to posterior pressure. By drawing the fingers gently from anterior to posterior (upward from the treatment table), these restricted joints can be mobilized. Sometimes it is helpful to ask the patient to let the chin drop slightly toward the chest, to reduce the postural tension on this area so that it will be easier to mobilize these joints (**C**). With the patient in the prone position, stiff rib/spinal joints also can be gently pressed on to increase mobility.

When the patient is supine, the neck can be lifted, and the suboccipital muscles can be stretched and compressed manually at the same time. Deep paraspinals and posterior joint restrictions can also be addressed in a similar fashion, simply by localizing pressure and creating a fulcrum at the level of restriction. The neck and head are pulled away from each shoulder while performing any form of trigger release. The head is turned, the splenius muscles are compressed over the restricted cervical joints, and the restricted cervical joints are gently rocked to release restriction. If the first rib is restricted, it is gently depressed while stretching the levator scapula and upper trapezius. In this position also, the extension subluxations in the neck, which cause a feeling of hard

tension under the scalenes or sternocleidomastoid muscles, can be mobilized from anterior to posterior.

It would not be necessary to use all of these treatment modalities and perform all of these maneuvers on every patient. But the clinical assessment should identify locations of significant trigger points and taut bands and significant joint restriction. It is helpful to access and treat muscle and joint dysfunction in multiple positions. Different parts of the dysfunctional muscle will be palpable in different positions, with slightly different angles of stretch. When these procedures are performed before osseous adjustments, the clinician can focus the adjustments very specifically on those joints that have not already released. Also, the thrust employed can be gentler. When low-force, high-velocity, short-amplitude osseous adjustments are performed, there is immediate decrease in paraspinal muscle hypertonicity and trigger points. However, often other areas of joint and muscle restriction persist, or there may still be some residual restriction in the joint already manipulated. The techniques of mobilization, compression, and stretch, when used after osseous adjustment, are a valuable step to further enhance response.

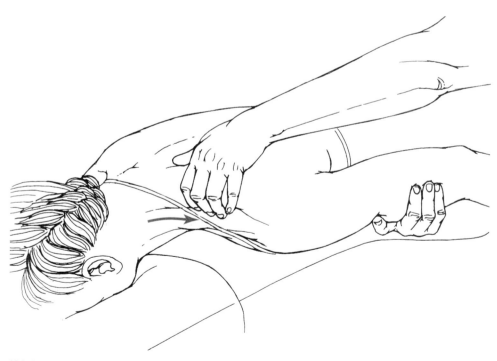

(B) **Combining traction and trigger point pressure release.** With the patient in a prone position, the clinician can combine gentle traction on the arm with trigger point pressure release, to accomplish muscle elongation and treat remaining trigger points in the anterior border of the upper trapezius muscle.

TECHNIQUE 3-4

Simultaneously Combining Myofascial Treatment and Articular Mobilization Techniques (*Continued*)

This amount of handling of muscle and joint tissue should never be performed on the patient with an acute whiplash injury. When the trauma of a whiplash is fresh, the focus is on gentle release of muscles and joints with minimal handling. (More detailed discussion of myofascial release and joint release regarding areas other than the neck will be found in the appropriate chapters.)

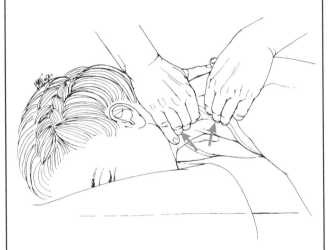

(C) Combining traction stretch with joint mobilization. With the patient prone, the clinician can reach both hands to the anterolateral neck and can contact portions of the shortened scalene muscles, performing a sustained stretch release by performing *gentle* traction between the contact hands. The underlying joint restrictions (extension subluxations) can be mobilized by adding a *gentle* anterior to posterior traction or rocking motion to this maneuver.

restore normal patterns of joint mobility and muscle function, and to promote healing.

When damage to vertebral facet joints is likely, or when there is disc herniation with lateral extrusion rather than cord compression, osseous manipulation may be an appropriate and beneficial treatment approach, and the myofascial release techniques may produce sufficient decrease in muscle tone that very little thrust is required to perform these adjustments. In such cases, rotational forces must be particularly avoided to minimize the chances of causing any further damage to the injured tissues. Also, the patient's progress must be monitored to assess whether there is any progression of the nerve deficit, or an increase rather than decrease in pain related to the facet joint. Other treatment techniques, including osteopathic joint muscle energy tech-

niques, are very appropriate and may be tolerated better by some patients, whereas osseous manipulation may be tolerated better by others. Obviously, other interventions will be required to address the problems of patients whose conditions do not respond to the myofascial and articular approach.

When there is facet joint injury, shortening of the splenius muscles that wrap around the facets can increase pressure across the facet joint, so it is imperative to lengthen the splenius muscle as well as improve the mobility of the joint. When a disc disorder or nerve root disorder is being treated, particular attention should be paid to those muscles that exert vertically compressive forces on the cervical spine. Both the scalenes and the levator scapulae, because they lie in a plane close to the vertical, can exert a compressive force like a vise grip across the involved cervical spinal segments. Efforts to release these muscles will not be successful if the nerve root irritation is severe enough to reinitiate muscle shortening so soon that there is no effective period of decompression. In these circumstances, manual techniques are often combined with trigger point injection or dry needling of trigger points. If this is not sufficient to allow the nerve root to heal, an epidural injection may be given. When myofascial care is instituted after an epidural has been given, it is often possible to make significant gains in reducing muscle and joint dysfunction and reducing the compressive forces across the nerve root. Although a series of three epidural injections is often recommended by pain specialists, it is rare that more than one epidural is required, because the pain is much less likely to recur if the compressive forces have been reduced by the myofascial and joint care. This is an example of the enhanced effectiveness that arises from a comprehensive team approach to pain management.

Chronic Care and Completing Rehabilitation

One of the clinician's main challenges is to successfully complete rehabilitation so that normal joint and muscle mechanics are restored, leading to less chronic complaints in the injured neck. Often treatment progresses at a good pace during the early stages of rehabilitation, only to reach a plateau in the later stages. The patient continues to experience discomfort, and symptoms can be easily reaggravated in the course of normal activity. Certainly every effort must be made to rule out more serious complications, such as a cervical disc injury or persistent facet joint irritation, and to select other appropriate treatment modalities if these are the problems that are preventing further improvement. If these problems are not preventing the patient's progress, then the clinician needs to carefully reassess the patient's muscle and joint dysfunctions and plan the means of completing rehabilitation. At this point, it is also essential to identify and address perpetuating factors that reaggravate the patient's condition.

Another challenge is patients who have had a whiplash injury years ago and have continuing pain and other symptoms. These patients may have nondermatomal patterns of pain and numbness in the extremities, as well as dizziness, headaches, and tinnitus, and neck pain and stiffness. Their course of care with other practitioners has often been unproductive because standard imaging methods do not delineate a pathologic condition responsible for their symptoms. A myofascial approach provides tools for assessing whether myofascial trigger points are largely responsible for each of these chronic symptoms.

Whiplash-associated disorders are not limited to the neck but can affect the entire body. Besides the neck, they commonly affect the thoracic and lumbar spine, the pelvis, and extremities, and multiple muscles and muscle groups, the brain, balance, hearing, vision, and chronic pain also can affect hormonal function. The jaw is often affected as well. The nervous system is affected, and many motor vehicle accident victims have PTSD and depression. Whenever there has been long-standing myofascial involvement, it is invariably accompanied by joint dysfunction—a complex of SD that should be fully assessed and treated. One approach to combining myofascial release techniques and joint care is detailed in Technique 3-5.

If muscles do not improve with comprehensive trigger point myofascial therapy or injection therapy and treatment of the subluxations or joint dysfunction within 3 months, there is usually nerve impingement or facet joint involvement. There also may be arthritic changes from previous neck injuries or from aging. Imaging and referral for evaluation by a neurologist, orthopedist, or anesthesiologist are appropriate.

Epidural, facet, and selective nerve root blocks, and so on, are useful adjuncts to therapy for patients with whiplash injuries, but there can be residual trigger points and SDs or subluxations that also need to be cleared before the whiplash "total body" trauma is healed. Combining treat-

---

TECHNIQUE 3-5

Supine Release of the Splenius Cervicis Muscle as It Passes over the Cervical Facets

To complete treatment of myofascial involvement from a whiplash injury, even one that took place many years ago, it is helpful to fully release the splenius muscles. The deep trigger points in these muscles often cannot be palpated in a supine position with the head straight. But as soon as the head is rotated to the end of cervical range of motion with the patient still supine, the taut splenius muscles can be palpated in the posterolateral neck, as they cross each cervical facet or zygapophyseal joint. Joint mobility will also feel restricted, and although there may be actual joint restriction, the stiffness and resistance felt may simply be caused by the tethering of the splenius muscle across the joint. After the splenius muscle is released, the joint mobility can be reassessed. As the patient's condition improves, only certain portions of the splenius cervicis will be palpably taut and tender.

To perform the palpation, the last two joints of the index or third finger are held in a hook and the muscle is strummed, while also trying to feel for space and mobility at the underlying joint (see Fig. 1-13). When the muscle fibers are taut, it will feel as though the fingers cannot "get into" the joint area. It will feel as though several joints move as a block, rather than being able to feel each vertebra lifting up, moving forward, and rotating slightly at the facet joint relative to the vertebra below.

Once the locations of taut bands have been located in the splenius muscle, a variety of techniques can be used to release them, including trigger point pressure release, percussion, cross-fiber massage, etc. If these taut bands will not release fully with manual techniques, trigger point injection or dry needling can be performed, but again the taut bands will be missed unless the patient is put in the appropriate position that places the muscle fibers in a partial stretch. The patient also can be instructed to perform stretches by turning the head, while using the contralateral hand to hook around the restricted locations, thereby helping to release the taut bands.

When the deep splenius trigger points have been released, and the taut bands have been elongated, generally there will be an increase in cervical rotation. It also feels as though the neck will more readily go into a curve when the splenius muscle has been released, with the facets gliding forward rather than being tethered posteriorly by the taut muscle bands. Thus, this procedure may help restore a more normal cervical lordosis. When these releases have been performed, incidents causing a stiff neck with little provocation, such as "sleeping wrong," stiffening after driving, or after other nonstrenuous activities, occur less often. Thus, this procedure is an essential part of restoring neck function to close enough to normal that the patient will be more independent of future care and intervention.

Many patients do not really feel a problem with the neck when only the deep splenius trigger points remain. The clinician can locate the taut tender splenius muscles and demonstrate for the patient that there is still a lingering myofascial problem that affects joint function and may warrant further attention to prevent future flare-ups; the patient may later say that the "neck was never the same after the whiplash." The choice can be left to the patient, and usually these last trigger points can be addressed and released over the course of 2 to 6 weeks, and treatment can be brought to a close at that point, with the patient at a better level of joint and muscle function.

ments for myofascial and joint dysfunction with these other procedures is more likely to successfully address the sources of chronic pain and to minimize the need to repeat the procedures.

Evaluation and Treatment of Joint Dysfunction in Patients with Chronic Neck Pain. The assessment and treatment of subluxation or joint dysfunction involves understanding the normal mechanics of spine function, developing the skill to assess restrictions in normal spinal mobility, and applying treatment techniques to restore more normal joint mobility. Some patients respond very well to low-force, short-amplitude specific spinal manipulation, usually performed by chiropractors. Such manipulations involve taking a restricted joint into the position in which it is restricted and, knowing the appropriate angles of normal joint function and mobility, thrusting gently to create a gap in the cervical facets and pass through the restricted range of motion to restore a fuller range of motion. The gapping of the facets generally is accompanied by a gaseous release into the joint space, where a vacuum has been created by the manipulation, thus producing the typical popping sound. There is generally an immediate reduction in joint tenderness and in paraspinal muscle hypertonicity after the cervical manipulation. Although this is the technique most widely used by chiropractors and probably most fully researched, there are other techniques such as activator technique and positional release technique that chiropractors also employ that do not involve significant thrust. Osteopaths most often use muscle energy techniques to restore normal spinal mobility. These techniques are described in some detail in relation to Case History 2. The detail is presented because the practitioner can gain some appreciation of palpating joint restriction and palpating changes in joint mobility achieved by applying muscle energy techniques. Cervical manipulation techniques used by chiropractors are not described in detail, because they are of a complexity such that it is not worthwhile to teach them in this format, nor in brief courses. But in the hands of well-trained chiropractors, these techniques are generally safe and effective (147,148.) Furthermore, when combined with myofascial release techniques, the cervical spinal manipulations can be gentler, with less thrust or impulse required to achieve the desired results. If the practitioner learns to appreciate the presence and importance of joint restriction in the patient with chronic pain after a whiplash injury, then appropriate referral can be made to a health practitioner experienced in the various ways of restoring normal joint mobility, as part of a comprehensive treatment plan to address the sources of dysfunction and pain.

Treatment of Muscles and Joints to Complete Rehabilitation or to Treat Chronic Neck Problems. Clinical experience indicates that three major muscular factors can keep the patient from successfully completing rehabilitation from a cervical soft tissue injury:

1. *Head on neck posture as it is affected by shoulder position and function.* When the shoulders are pulled forward, the head and neck will necessarily be carried forward, and there will be excessive gravitational stresses on the upper trapezius and levator scapulae, in the course of normal activity. The humerus may be held forward by shortened pectoral muscles, or occasionally by the coracobrachialis. The patient also may suffer from a condition that could be called "shoulder blades in the armpits syndrome." The scapula may be pinned close to the axilla by shortened subscapularis or anterior serratus muscles. If the scapula cannot glide toward the spine readily, then these muscles need to be released to improve posture and restore more normal muscle and joint function at the cervicothoracic juncture. Sometimes reasonable progress can be achieved in releasing muscles in the pectoral area and about the scapula, but there is weakness or inhibition of the middle and lower trapezius (149). Therefore, in the course of normal activity, it is likely that the muscles that pull the shoulders upward and forward will continue to overpower the muscles that hold the shoulders down and back. It is remarkable how quickly some patients can progress when they perform resistive exercise directed at strengthening the middle and lower trapezius muscles. But the exercise regimen needs to be carefully designed to avoid muscle shortening in the pectorals and the upper trapezius, as this will only prolong the patient's rehabilitation and delay recovery. (For a fuller discussion of shoulder release techniques and managing joint and muscle dysfunction in the shoulder area, see Chapter 4.)

A variant of myofascial involvement in the shoulder area that affects rehabilitation of the neck is shortening of the latissimus dorsi. The latissimus dorsi that is implicated may have active trigger points that contribute to pain in the interscapular region and pain down the arm. The trigger points also may be latent, which means that they are tender and there are numerous taut bands in the muscle, but there is no spontaneous pain associated with them. Postural analysis is a key to the presence of active or latent latissimus dorsi trigger points that are impeding rehabilitation of the neck. For example, if the right levator scapula, upper trapezius, and scalene muscles are a site of recurrent and persistent trigger points with their associated pain, one would ordinarily expect that the right shoulder blade and perhaps the clavicle would be raised. If they are level with the left or even depressed relative to the left, then it is very likely that some muscle is shortened sufficiently to pull the right scapula inferiorly. The latissimus dorsi is a prime candidate, and once the trigger points in it have been released and the muscle has been well elongated, the mechanical tension on the neck muscles will be reduced, and their rehabilitation will be enhanced. It is easy to miss latent trigger points in the latissimus dorsi in the usual myofascial examination, but it is relatively easy to appreciate the shortening of this muscle when the patient is prone and the relative tension of the right and left posterior axillary (armpit) fold is compared (Fig. 3-9).

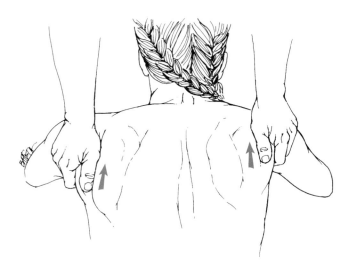

FIGURE 3-9. **Assessing shortness of the latissimus dorsi muscles.** The clinician grasps one posterior axillary fold in each hand and feels the relative tension between each shoulder and the ipsilateral hip. In this case, the patient's left latissimus dorsi muscle is shortened.

Forward head and shoulders are also affected by persistence of taut bands in the rectus abdominis muscle. Again, latent abdominal trigger points may be depressing the rib cage and altering posture, but this can be easily missed because the clinician is concerned with persistent neck pain, and there may be no persistent back pain typically caused by active abdominal trigger points.

2. *Deep splenius shortening and the alteration of cervical joint mechanics.* Although patients may have made good progress in rehabilitation, they may not have achieved full cervical rotation and continue to have easy aggravation of the neck with activity or when sleeping. Although all of the muscles of the neck may feel fairly relaxed in a neutral supine position, when the neck is rotated, tension may be felt in the posterolateral neck, and trigger points in the deep muscles that pass over the facets or zygapophyseal joints may be palpated and treated. The anterior neck muscles, including the sternocleidomastoid and the scalenes, also may need to be addressed to achieve full rotation, and the more superficial posterior neck muscles as well. However, trigger points in these muscles are easier for the experienced clinician to palpate, whereas the deep splenius trigger points are easy to overlook but are paramount in importance. Even though the scalene muscles have little or no function in rotation, significantly shortened scalene muscles are an important factor in the forward neck and head posture that characterize patients with chronic myofascial pain after a whiplash injury. A neck that is fixed in a forward position does not rotate as far as a neck that is in a more anatomically normal or erect position. Thus, the shortened scalenes will need to be addressed as well. The anterior colli muscles also have been suggested as muscles responsible for straightening of the normal cervical lordosis (150).

One way to evaluate range of cervical motion and the relative importance of achieving specific muscle releases is to take the neck to the end of motion in one direction and palpate which muscles are specifically restricting further motion in this direction. For a muscle to participate in restriction of motion, it has to be at tension at the end of the movement. If the muscle is somewhat slack at the end of the movement, then it cannot be a limiting factor. Again, the release of the deep splenius seems to be very important in restoring normal joint mobility and range of motion after a whiplash injury. This is the case even when we are dealing with chronic residuals from a whiplash that occurred years or even decades before the current treatment. Performing manipulation or mobilization procedures for the cervical facets or zygapophyseal joints is also important at this stage of rehabilitation, and goes hand in hand with the splenius release in achieving normal patterns of joint and muscle function.

3. *Continuing TMJ dysfunction perpetuating joint and muscle dysfunction in the neck.* Sometimes the injury to the muscles of the jaw was not apparent on initial evaluation, soon after the injury. But it is worthwhile to check muscle and joint function in the jaw area at intervals, because dysfunction can be delayed. Often the only symptoms a patient will experience from the disorder in the jaw joint and associated muscles are headache and neck pain, the same symptoms that can be caused by myofascial and joint dysfunction in the neck. When there is TMJ area myofascial dysfunction, with or without joint dysfunction, trigger points in the sternocleidomastoid, the levator scapula and upper trapezius, or the suboccipitals may continually reset, despite what would otherwise be adequate treatment. Appropriate treatment of the TMJ dysfunction can dramatically improve muscle and joint function in the neck, so that rehabilitative efforts in this area become much more productive.

These three considerations are the most important in bringing muscle and joint rehabilitation to a successful conclusion. By assessing and treating these dysfunctions, the patient can move beyond a plateau and achieve reasonably successful rehabilitation. These three factors come into play throughout the course of rehabilitation, and the more successfully they can be addressed, the less likely that the patient will reach a plateau with an unacceptable level of continuing pain. Often these three factors still come into play years and even decades after the original whiplash injury. With patients whose necks have "never been the same" for years after such an injury, assessing and treating these three factors can often bring them to a significantly better level of rehabilitation, where they can much more easily control reaggravation with home exercise and self-care techniques.

Where manual techniques have not proved successful in restoring normal joint and muscle function in the neck, and the patient continues to suffer from neck-related pain, diagnostic evaluation with zygapophyseal or facet blocks has demonstrated usefulness and good clinical outcome (151).

Perpetuating Factors. Other factors—such as emotional stress, repetitive stresses in the workplace, sleep position, hormonal factors, allergies and their affects on trigger point activity, nutritional status—also can play an important role in perpetuating chronic pain after a whiplash injury. These and other factors are discussed very thoroughly by Simons, Travell, and Simons (152). Restoration of normal joint and muscle function is often very helpful in the detective work involved in identifying perpetuating factors. If the patient is in a constant level of pain, it is difficult to know what factors need to be addressed. However, if treatment techniques can address muscle and joint function and bring about a significant level of relief, then there is variability in the patient's symptoms, and the clinician can help the patient track down the source of the variability or worsening of symptoms. Does the neck and head pain recur whenever the patient has a stressful encounter at work or at home? Is the pain increased when the patient is having other signs of allergy? Is the pain worse when the patient increases intake of caffeine or sugar? Here the patient can take increasing levels of responsibility for rehabilitation, by increasing self-awareness and using coping strategies to deal with reaggravations. This is also the circumstance in which it is very useful for the clinician to work with an interdisciplinary group of health practitioners who can help assess any biopsychosocial factors that are retarding or complicating rehabilitation.

Patient Exercise during the Late, Chronic Stage of Rehabilitation. Exercise in the latter stages of rehabilitation is designed to address the specific remaining areas of joint and muscle dysfunction. Earlier in rehabilitation, the patient was achieving improvements with general neck and shoulder stretches; in the later stages, the clinician must assess which specific muscles or portions of muscles are still shortened, and whether the patient's stretches are addressing these specific muscles. The clinician can review the exact angle of stretch used in each of the neck muscle stretches. The clinician also often will find that the patient is stretching portions of the pectoral muscle that have already elongated well but is not specifically stretching certain portions that remain shortened. The clinician can put the patient in the appropriate position and specifically stretch the remaining portion of the muscles, so that the patient is aware of what should be felt during the stretches. Figure 3-10 provides one example of a localized stretch. The key to effective stretching during the later stages of rehabilitation is specificity. No matter how well the patient appeared to be performing stretches 2 months ago, there is no substitute for careful reevaluation of the stretches to ascertain how to achieve the remaining releases that are necessary.

At this stage also, it is helpful for the patient to perform postural exercise and increase aerobic activity. It has not been demonstrated, however, that strengthening exercises of the neck itself are required. Clinical experience indicates that strengthening exercises performed by the neck muscles

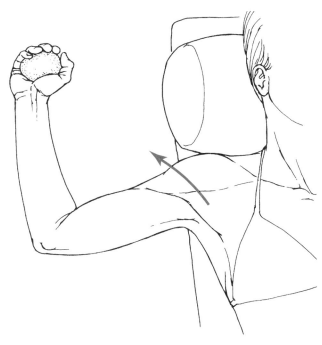

FIGURE 3-10. **Focused external rotation stretch.** The pectoralis minor and the outer border of the pectoralis major often stay taut after the rest of the pectorals have released. A focused external rotation stretch using a small weight is performed supine with the arm extended off the side of a couch or bench. To repeat, the weight is taken through adduction toward the waist and then is lifted from the waist to again drop the arm into external rotation (rather than simply lifting the weight using the same muscles that were just stretched.)

can cause reaggravation in some patients, even in those whose rehabilitation had been almost complete. Thus, the clinician must carefully assess whether the desired neck muscle strength may be adequately achieved by stretching activities that will result in greater available contractile function because of the greater muscle length. Strengthening exercises for the postural muscles in the back and shoulders are often productive and help relieve the chronic strain on the neck muscles.

CONCLUSION

Effective early treatment of patients with WAD to reduce the level of muscle hypertonicity appears to reduce the degree of myofascial dysfunction later in the course of care and also to significantly reduce the length of rehabilitation. Gentle restoration of normal muscle and joint function is initiated as soon after the injury as the patient can tolerate, preferably within the first 48 hours after the accident. Certainly well-designed comparative treatment trials will need to be conducted to establish the actual reduction of rehabilitation time, but most clinicians cannot fail to notice a dramatic change in their ability to treat the WAD patient in apparently shorter periods when they become skilled in the treatment of myofascial pain and dysfunction. Furthermore, clinicians who use these treatment methods will find that they can help patients with complex injuries to a better level of rehabilitation and a fuller recovery.

Effective completion of rehabilitation and effective treatment of patients with neck-related complaints that persist years after the initial injury require increasing specificity in assessing, treating, and restoring normal patterns of joint and muscle function. Also, addressing muscle and joint dysfunction can help to identify other pain-generating disorders that are complicating rehabilitation, such as persistent facet or nerve-related pain, and appropriate care can be recommended for these disorders. Furthermore, treatment of these disorders appears to be more likely to successfully reduce the patient's chronic pain disorder if the muscle and joint dysfunction are being concurrently treated. Specificity is also required in identifying and addressing perpetuating factors. A thorough myofascial approach together with effective treatment of joint dysfunction generally significantly improves the patient's pain status, increases the tolerance of normal activity, and reduces the frequency of reaggravation.

Although treatment recommendations presented in this chapter are the result of clinical experience, and the refinement of clinical approaches over many years, the authors hope that the treatment models described for both acute and chronic WAD patients will become the subject of further research.

TREATMENT PROTOCOL

1. **Treat trigger points and accomplish muscle elongation of both anterior and posterior neck muscles, including the upper trapezius, levator scapula, sternocleidomastoid, and scalene muscles.**

2. **Treat joint restrictions associated with myofascial involvement in the above muscles, such as first and second rib–spinal joint restrictions affecting the release of trigger points in the upper trapezius and the levator scapula, and extension or rotational restrictions that are palpable under the sternocleidomastoid and the scalene muscles.**

3. **Treat trigger points in the deeper paraspinal muscles and suboccipital muscles.**

4. **Treat the associated joint restrictions involving all of the cervical facets and restrictions of joint play at the occiput, C1, and C2.**

5. **Treat the muscles affecting humerus and scapula position, particularly the subscapularis, anterior serratus, pectoralis minor, and outer border of the pectoralis major, as well as the latissimus dorsi, and address postural retraining so that the head on neck posture will improve. Lengthen abdominal muscles if they are not allowing the rib cage and chest to lift.**

6. **Mobilize the scapula back toward the spine, and the humerus back and down (but in the case of the depressed scapula accompanying the shortened latissimus, mobilize the scapula cephalad).**

7. **Address any muscle weaknesses that are perpetuating a head-forward posture, particularly weakness of the middle and lower trapezius.**

8. **Periodically evaluate the muscles of the jaw, to identify whether these muscles and any TMJ dysfunction are a part of the myofascial disorder.**

9. **Focus on identifying perpetuating factors, and any pain disorder that does not resolve with myofascial and articular care, so that appropriate measures (including facet and epidural injections) may be taken to address remaining problems.**

References

1. Luan F, Yang KH, Deng B, et al. Qualitative analysis of neck kinematics during low-speed rear-end impact. Clin Biomech (Bristol, Avon) 2000;15:649–657.
2. Tencer AF, Mirza S. Whiplash mechanics in low speed rear-end automobile collisions. J Musculoskel Pain 2000;8:69–86.
3. Croft AC. The case against "litigation neurosis" in mild brain injuries and cervical acceleration/deceleration trauma. J Neuron Musc Sys 1993;1:149–155.
4. Ferrari R. The Whiplash Encyclopedia: The Facts and Myths of Whiplash. Gaithersburg, MD: Aspen, 1999.
5. Berry H. Chronic whiplash syndrome as a functional disorder. Arch Neurol 2000;57:592–594.
6. Fricton JR. Myofascial pain and whiplash. Spine 1993;7:403–422.
7. Teasell RW. The clinical picture of whiplash injuries: An overview. Spine 1993;7:373–389.
8. Covey MC. Posttraumatic myofascial pain syndrome. Physical Medicine and Rehabilitation 1998;12:73–84.
9. Gerwin RD, Dommerholt J. Myofascial trigger points in chronic cervical whiplash syndrome [Abstract]. J Musculoskel Pain 1998;6:28.
10. Schuller E, Eisenmenger W, Beier G. Whiplash injury in low speed car accidents. J Musculoskel Pain 2000;8:55–67.
11. Simons DG. Triggerpunkte und Myogelose. Manuelle Medizin 1997;35:290–294.
12. Galasko CSB. (1998) The costs of whiplash-associated disorders. In: Gunzburg R, Szpalski M, eds. Whiplash Injuries: Current Concepts in Prevention, Diagnosis, and Treatment of the Cervical Whiplash Syndrome. Philadelphia: Lippincott-Raven, 1998:283–290.
13. Traffic safety facts 2002. Washington, DC: U.S. Department of Transportation, National Highway Traffic Safety Administration, 2003.

14. Compton CP. The use of public crash data in biomechanical research. In: Nahum AM, Melvin JW, eds. Accidental Injury; Biomechanics and Prevention. New York: Springer, 1993:49–65.

15. Hildingsson C, Toolanen G. Outcome after soft-tissue injury of the cervical spine. A prospective study of 93 car-accident victims. Acta Orthop Scand 1990;61:357–359.

16. Balla JI. The late whiplash syndrome. Aust N Z J Surg 1980;50:610–614.

17. Evans RW. Some observations on whiplash injuries. Neurol Clin 1992;10:975–997.

18. Radanov BP, Sturzenegger M, De Stefano G, et al. Relationship between early somatic, radiological, cognitive and psychosocial findings and outcome during a one-year follow-up in 117 patients suffering from common whiplash. Br J Rheumatol 1994;33:442–448.

19. Freeman MD, Croft AC. The controversy over late whiplash: Are chronic symptoms after whiplash real? In: Gunzburg R, Szpalski M, eds. Whiplash Injuries: Current Concepts in Prevention, Diagnosis, and Treatment of the Cervical Whiplash Syndrome. Philadelphia: Lippincott-Raven, 1998:161–165.

20. Severy DM, Mathewson JH, Bechtol CP. Controlled automobile rear-end collisions, an investigation of related engineering and mechanical phenomena. Can Services Med J 1955;11:727–758.

21. Bailey MN, Wong BC. Data and methods for estimating the severity of minor impacts. In: Proceedings of the Forty-First Stapp Car Crash Conference. Warrendale: Society of Automotive Engineers, 1995; 139–174.

22. Brault JR, Wheeler JB, Siegmund GP, et al. Clinical response of human subjects to rear-end automobile collisions. Arch Phys Med Rehabil 1998;79:72–80.

23. Foret-Bruno JY, Dauvilliers F, Tarriere C. Influence of the seat and head rest stiffness on the risk of cervical injuries. Proceedings of the 13th International Technical Conference on Experimental Safety Vehicles 1991;S-8-W-19:968–974.

24. McConnell WE, Howard RP, Guzman HM. Analysis of human test subjects kinematic responses to low velocity rear end impacts. In: Proceedings of the Forty-First Stapp Car Crash Conference. Warrendale: Society of Automotive Engineers, 1993:21–31.

25. Meyer S, Weber M, Castro W, et al. The minimal collision velocity for whiplash. In: Gunzburg R, Szpalski M, eds. Whiplash Injuries: Current Concepts in Prevention, Diagnosis, and Treatment of the Cervical Whiplash Syndrome. Philadelphia: Lippincott-Raven, 1998: 95–115.

26. Olsson J, Bunketorp O. An in-depth study of neck injuries in rear end collisions. 1990 International IRCOBI Conference. Lyon: IRCOBI, 1990:269–280.

27. Szabo TJ, Welcher J. Dynamics of low speed crash tests with energy absorbing bumpers. In: Proceedings of the Forty-First Stapp Car Crash Conference. Warrendale: Society of Automotive Engineers, 1992;1–9.

28. Thomson RW, Romilly DP, Navin FPD, et al. Energy attenuation within the vehicle during low speed collisions. Vancouver: Transport Canada, 1989.

29. Ferrari R, Russell AS. Development of persistent neurologic symptoms in patients with simple neck sprain. Arthritis Care Res 1999;12:70–76.

30. Nielsen GP, Gough JP, Little DM, et al. Human subject responses to repeated low speed impacts using utility vehicles. In: Proceedings of the Forty-First Stapp Car Crash Conference. Warrendale: Society of Automotive Engineers, 1997:189–212.

31. Kahane CJ. Evaluation of head restraints: Federal motor vehicle safety standard 202. Washington: Department of Transportation; National Highway and Traffic Safety Administration, 1982.

32. Nygren A (1984) Injuries to car occupants—some aspects of the interior safety of cars. A study of a five-year material from an insurance company. Acta Otolaryngol Suppl 1984;395:1–164.

33. Radanov BP, Sturzenegger M, Di Stefano G. Long-term outcome after whiplash injury: A 2-year follow-up considering features of injury mechanism and somatic, radiologic, and psychosocial findings. Medicine (Baltimore) 1995;74:281–297.

34. Satoh S, Naito S, Konishi T, et al. An examination of reasons for prolonged treatment in Japanese patients with whiplash injuries. J Musculoskel Pain 1997;5:71–84.

35. Jakobsson L. Automobile design and whiplash prevention. In: Gunzburg R, Szpalski M, eds. Whiplash Injuries: Current Concepts in Prevention, Diagnosis, and Treatment of the Cervical Whiplash Syndrome. Philadelphia: Lippincott-Raven, 1998:299–306.

36. Ryan GA, Taylor GW, Moore VM, et al. Neck strain in car occupants: injury status after 6 months and crash- related factors. Injury 1994;25:533–537.

37. Evans L. Age dependence of female to male fatality risk in the same crash: an independent reexamination. J Crash Prevention Injury Control 2000;2:111–121.

38. Soderstrom CA, Dischinger PC, Kerns TJ. Alcohol use among injured sets of drivers and passengers. Accid Anal Prev 1996;28: 111–114.

39. Soderstrom CA, Smith GS, Dischinger PC, et al. Psychoactive substance use disorders among seriously injured trauma center patients. JAMA 1997;277:1769–1774.

40. Sturzenegger M, Radanov BP, Di Stefano G. The effect of accident mechanisms and initial findings on the long-term course of whiplash injury. J Neurol 1995;242:443–449.

41. Bring G, Bjornstig U, Westman G. Gender patterns in minor head and neck injuries: An analysis of casualty register data. Accid Anal Prev 1996;28:359–369.

42. Mackay M, Hassan AM, Hill JR. Current and future occupant restraint systems. Physical Medicine and Rehabilitation 1998;12: 29–38.

43. (1995) Special issue: Whiplash injuries. Status report. Arlington: Insurance Institute for Highway Safety, pp.1–7.

44. Jakobsson L, Lundell B, Norin H, et al. Whips–Volvo's whiplash protection study. Accid Anal Prev 2000;32:307–319.

45. Wiklund K. Saab active head restraint system; seat design to reduce the risk of neck injuries. In: Gunzburg R, Szpalski M, eds. Whiplash Injuries: Current Concepts in Prevention, Diagnosis, Treatment of the Cervical Whiplash Syndrome. Philadelphia: Lippincott-Raven., 1998:307–313.

46. Chapline JF, Ferguson SA, Lillis RP, et al. Neck pain and head restraint position relative to the driver's head in rear-end collisions. Accid Anal Prev 2000;32:287–297.

47. Maher J. Report investigating the importance of head restraint positioning in reducing neck injury in rear impact. Accid Anal Prev 2000;32:299–305.

48. Foreman SM, Croft AC. Whiplash Injuries: The Cervical Acceleration/Deceleration Syndrome, 2nd Ed. Baltimore: Williams & Wilkins, 1995.

49. Castro WH, Schilgen M, Meyer S, et al. Do "whiplash injuries" occur in low-speed rear impacts? Eur Spine J 1997;6:366–375.

50. Panjabi MM, Grauer JN, Cholewicki J, et al. (1998) Whiplash trauma injury mechanism: a biomechanical viewpoint. In: Gunzburg R, Szpalski M, eds. Whiplash Injuries: Current Concepts in Prevention, Diagnosis, Treatment of the Cervical Whiplash Syndrome. Philadelphia: Lippincott-Raven, 1998:79–87.

51. Panjabi MM, Nibu K, Cholewicki J. Whiplash injuries and the potential for mechanical instability. Eur Spine J 1998;7:484–492.

52. Brault JR, Siegmund GP, Wheeler JB. Cervical muscle response during whiplash: evidence of a lengthening muscle contraction. Clin Biomech (Bristol, Avon) 2000;15:426–435.

53. Jull GA. Deep cervical flexor muscle dysfunction in whiplash. J Musculoskel Pain 2000;8:143–154.

54. Crowe HE. Injuries to the cervical spine. In: Meeting of the Western Orthopaedic Association, San Francisco, 1928.

55. Spitzer WO, Skovron ML, Salmi LR, et al. Scientific monograph of the Quebec Task Force on whiplash-associated disorders: redefining "whiplash" and its management. Spine 1995;20:1S–73S.

56. Cesarani A, Alpini D, Boniver R, et al. Whiplash Injuries: Diagnosis and Treatment. Berlin: Springer, 1996.

57. Barnsley L, Lord S, Bogduk N. Whiplash injury. Pain 1994;58: 283–307.

58. Cote P, Cassidy JD, Carroll L. The factors associated with neck pain and its related disability in the Saskatchewan population. Spine 2000; 25:1109–1117.

59. Lord SM, Barnsley L, Wallis BJ, et al. Chronic cervical zygapophysial joint pain after whiplash: a placebo-controlled prevalence study. Spine 1996;21:1737–1744.

60. Jonsson H, Jr., Bring G, Rauschning W, et al. Hidden cervical spine injuries in traffic accident victims with skull fractures. J Spinal Disord 1991;4:251–263.

61. Barnsley L, Lord SM, Wallis BJ, et al. The prevalence of chronic cervical zygapophysial joint pain after whiplash. Spine 1995;20:20–25.

62. Banks R, Martini J, Smith H, et al. Alignment of the lumbar vertebrae in a driving posture. J Crash Prevention Injury Control 2000;2: 123–130.

63. Winkelstein BA, Nightingale RW, Richardson WJ, et al. The cervical facet capsule and its role in whiplash injury: a biomechanical investigation. Spine 2000;25:1238–1246.

64. Gibson T, Bogduk N, MacPherson J, et al. Crash characteristics of whiplash associated chronic neck pain. J Musculoskel Pain 2000;8:87–95.

65. Bogduk N, Teasell R. Whiplash: the evidence for an organic etiology. Arch Neurol 2000;57:590–591.

66. Taylor JR, Twomey LT. Acute injuries to cervical joints. an autopsy study of neck sprain. Spine 1993;18:1115–1122.

67. Twomey LT, Taylor JR, Taylor MM. Unsuspected damage to lumbar zygapophyseal (facet) joints after motor-vehicle accidents. Med J Aust 1989;151:210–212, 215–217.

68. Taylor JR, Twomey LT, Corker M. Bone and soft tissue injuries in post-mortem lumbar spines. Paraplegia 1990;28:119–129.

69. Barnsley L, Bogduk N. Medial branch blocks are specific for the diagnosis of cervical zygapophyseal joint pain. Reg Anesth 1993;18: 343–350.

70. Fredin Y, Elert J, Britschgi N, et al. A decreased ability to relax between repetitive muscle contractions in patients with chronic symptoms after whiplash trauma of the neck. J Musculoskel Pain 1997;5: 55–57.

71 Nederhand MJ, MJ IJ, Hermens HJ, et al. Cervical muscle dysfunction in the chronic whiplash associated disorder grade II(WAD-II). Spine 2000;25:1938–1943.

72 Baker BA. The muscle trigger: evidence of overload injury. The Journal of Neurological & Orthopaedic Medicine and Surgery 1986;7: 35–44.

73 Bogduk N, Simons DG. Neck pain: joint pain or trigger points. In: Værøy H, Merskey H, eds. Progress in Fibromyalgia and Myofascial Pain. Amsterdam: Elsevier, 1993:267–273.

74. Elliott AM, Smith BH, Penny KI, et al. The epidemiology of chronic pain in the community. Lancet 1999;354:1248–1252.

75. Zondervan K, Barlow DH. Epidemiology of chronic pelvic pain. Baillieres Best Pract Res Clin Obstet Gynaecol 2000;14:403–414.

76. Buskila D, Abramov G, Biton A, et al. The prevalence of pain complaints in a general population in Israel and its implications for utilization of health services. J Rheumatol 2000;27:1521–1525.

77. Pearce JM. Whiplash injury: a reappraisal. J Neurol Neurosurg Psychiatry 1989;52:1329–1331.

78. Maimaris C, Barnes MR, Allen MJ. 'Whiplash injuries' of the neck: a retrospective study. Injury 1988;19:393–396.

79. Hodgson SP, Grundy M. Whiplash injuries: their long–term prognosis and its relation to compensation. Neurol Orthop 1989;7:88–91.

80. Pennie B, Agambar L. Patterns of injury and recovery in whiplash. Injury 1991;22:57–59.

81. Watkinson A, Gargan MF, Bannister GC. Prognostic factors in soft tissue injuries of the cervical spine. Injury 1991;22:307–309.

82. Parmar HV, Raymakers R. Neck injuries from rear impact road traffic accidents: prognosis in persons seeking compensation. Injury 1993;24:75–78.

83. Brison RJ, Hartling L, Pickett W. A prospective study of acceleration-extension injuries following rear-end motor vehicle collisions. J Musculoskel Pain 2000;8:97–113.

84. Cassidy JD, Carroll LJ, Cote P, et al. Effect of eliminating compensation for pain and suffering on the outcome of insurance claims for whiplash injury. N Engl J Med 2000;342:1179–1186.

85. Fildes B, Vulcan P. Injury outcome and crash characteristics. In: Griffiths M, Brown J, eds. The Biomechanics of Neck Injury. Adelaide: Institution of Engineers, 1995:1–10.

86. Munglani R. Neurobiological mechanisms underlying chronic whiplash associated pain: the peripheral maintenance of central sensitization. J Musculoskel Pain 2000;8:169–178.

87. Ferrari R, Russell AS. Epidemiology of whiplash: an international dilemma. Ann Rheum Dis 1999;58:1–5.

88. Ferrari R, Schrader H, Obelieniene D. Prevalence of temporomandibular disorders associated with whiplash injury in Lithuania. Oral Surg Oral Med Oral Pathol Oral Radiol Endod 1999;87:653–657.

89. Obelieniene D, Bovim G, Schrader H, et al. Headache after whiplash: a historical cohort study outside the medico-legal context. Cephalalgia 1998;18:559–564.

90. Obelieniene D, Schrader H, Bovim G, et al. Pain after whiplash: a prospective controlled inception cohort study. J Neurol Neurosurg Psychiatry 1999;66:279–283.

91. Schrader H, Obelieniene D, Bovim G, et al. Natural evolution of late whiplash syndrome outside the medicolegal context. Lancet 1996;347:1207–1211.

92. Partheni M, Constantoyannis C, Ferrari R, et al. A prospective cohort study of the outcome of acute whiplash injury in Greece. Clin Exp Rheumatol 2000;18:67–70.

93. Melzack R, Wall PD. Pain mechanisms: a new theory. Science 1965;150:971–979.

94. Turk DC. Biopsychosocial perspective on chronic pain. In: Gatchel RJ, Turk DC, eds. Psychological Approaches to Pain Management. New York: The Guilford Press, 1996:3–32.

95. Heikkila H, Heikkila E, Eisemann M. Predictive factors for the outcome of a multidisciplinary pain rehabilitation program on sick-leave and life satisfaction in patients with whiplash trauma and other myofascial pain: a follow-up study. Clin Rehabil 1998;12:487–496.

96. Gifford LS, Butler DS. The integration of pain sciences into clinical practice. J Hand Ther 1997;10:86–95.

97. Woolf CJ, Decosterd I. Implications of recent advances in the understanding of pain pathophysiology for the assessment of pain in patients. Pain Suppl 1999;6:S141–147.

98. Koltzenburg M. The changing sensitivity in the life of the nociceptor. Pain Suppl 1999;6:S93–102.

99. Hinoki M. Vertigo due to whiplash injury: a neurological approach. Acta Otolaryngol Suppl 1984;419:9–29.

100. Khurana RK. Oculocephalic sympathetic dysfunction in posttraumatic headaches. Headache 1995;35:614–620.

101. McLachlan EM, Janig W, Devor M, et al. Peripheral nerve injury triggers noradrenergic sprouting within dorsal root ganglia. Nature 1993;363:543–546.

102. Khurana RK, Nirankari VS. Bilateral sympathetic dysfunction in post-traumatic headaches. Headache 1986;26:183–188.

103. Shinder V, Govrin-Lippmann R, Cohen S, et al. Structural basis of sympathetic-sensory coupling in rat and human dorsal root ganglia following peripheral nerve injury. J Neurocytol 1999;28:743–761.

104. Jones MG, Munson JB, Thompson SW. A role for nerve growth factor in sympathetic sprouting in rat dorsal root ganglia. Pain 1999;79:21–29.

105. Adeboye KA, Emerton DG, Hughes T. Cervical sympathetic chain dysfunction after whiplash injury. J R Soc Med 2000;93:378–379.

106. Stolker RJ, Vervest AC, Groen GJ. The management of chronic spinal pain by blockades: a review. Pain 1994;58:1–20.

107. Yaksh TL, Hua XY, Kalcheva I, et al. The spinal biology in humans and animals of pain states generated by persistent small afferent input. Proc Natl Acad Sci U S A 1999;96:7680–7686.

108. Rygh LJ, Svendsen F, Hole K, et al. Natural noxious stimulation can induce long-term increase of spinal nociceptive responses. Pain 1999;82:305–310.

109. Sessle BJ, Hu JW. Mechanisms of pain arising from articular tissues. Can J Physiol Pharmacol 1991;69:617–626.

110. Maixner W, Fillingim R, Sigurdsson A, et al. Sensitivity of patients with painful temporomandibular disorders to experimentally evoked pain: evidence for altered temporal summation of pain. Pain 1998;76:71–81.

111. Hoheisel U, Sander B, Mense S. Myositis-induced functional reorganization of the rat dorsal horn: effects of spinal superfusion with antagonists to neurokinin and glutamate receptors. Pain 1997;69:219–230.

112. Mense S, Hoheisel U. New developments in the understanding of the pathophysiology of muscle pain. J Musculoskel Pain 1999;7: 13–24.

113. Koelbaek Johansen M, Graven-Nielsen T, Schou Olesen A, et al. Generalized muscular hyperalgesia in chronic whiplash syndrome. Pain 1999;83:229–234.

114. Buskila D, Neumann L, Vaisberg G, et al. Increased rates of fibromyalgia following cervical spine injury: a controlled study of 161 cases of traumatic injury. Arthritis Rheum 1997;40:446–452.

115. Dommerholt J. Muscle pain syndromes. In: Cantu R, Grodin A, eds. Myofascial Manipulation. Gaithersburg, MD: Aspen, 2000.

116. Dommerholt J and Issa T. Differential Diagnosis: Myofascial Pam Syndrome, in Fibromyalgia. Edinburgh: Churchill Livingstone, 2003.

117. Gerwin RD. Myofascial pain and fibromyalgia: diagnosis and treatment. J Back Musculoskeletal Rehab 1998;11:175–181.

118. White KP, Ostbye T, Harth M, et al. Perspectives on posttraumatic fibromyalgia: a random survey of Canadian general practitioners, orthopedists, physiatrists, and rheumatologists. J Rheumatol 2000;27:790–796.

119. Bonuccelli U, Pavese N, Lucetti C, et al. Late whiplash syndrome: a clinical and magnetic resonance imaging study. Funct Neurol 1999;14:219–225.

120. Davis SJ, Teresi LM, Bradley WG, Jr., et al. Cervical spine hyperextension injuries: MR findings. Radiology 1991;180:245–251.

121. Ronnen HR, de Korte PJ, Brink PR, et al. Acute whiplash injury: is there a role for MR imaging?—a prospective study of 100 patients. Radiology 1996;201:93–96.

122. Borchgrevink GE, Kaasa A, McDonagh D, et al. Acute treatment of whiplash neck sprain injuries: a randomized trial of treatment during the first 14 days after a car accident. Spine 1998;23:25–31.

123. Bring G, Westman G. Chronic posttraumatic syndrome after whiplash injury: a pilot study of 22 patients. Scand J Prim Health Care 1991;9:135–141.

124. Wallis BJ, Lord SM, Barnsley L, et al. The psychological profiles of patients with whiplash-associated headache. Cephalalgia 1998;18:101–105.

125. Radanov BP, Dvorak J, Valach L. Cognitive deficits in patients after soft tissue injury of the cervical spine. Spine 1992;17:127–131.

126. Lee J, Giles K, Drummond PD. Psychological disturbances and an exaggerated response to pain in patients with whiplash injury. J Psychosom Res 1993;37:105–110.

127. Radanov BP, Begre S, Sturzenegger M, et al. Course of psychological variables in whiplash injury: a 2-year follow-up with age, gender and education pair-matched patients. Pain 1996;64:429–434.

128. Radanov BP, Dvorak J. Spine update: impaired cognitive functioning after whiplash injury of the cervical spine. Spine 1996;21:392–397.

129. Wallis BJ, Lord SM, Bogduk N. Resolution of psychological distress of whiplash patients following treatment by radiofrequency neurotomy: a randomized, double-blind, placebo-controlled trial. Pain 1997;73:15–22.

130. Radanov BP, di Stefano G, Schnidrig A, et al. Role of psychosocial stress in recovery from common whiplash. Lancet 1991;338:712–715.

131. Henry GK, Gross HS, Herndon CA, et al. Nonimpact brain injury: neuropsychological and behavioral correlates with consideration of physiological findings. Appl Neuropsychol 2000;7:65–75.

132. Bicik I, Radanov BP, Schafer N, et al. PET with 18fluorodeoxyglucose and hexamethylpropylene amine oxime SPECT in late whiplash syndrome. Neurology 1998;51:345–350.

133. Radanov BP, Bicik I, Dvorak J, et al. Relation between neuropsychological and neuroimaging findings in patients with late whiplash syndrome. J Neurol Neurosurg Psychiatry 1999;66:485–489.

134. Bogduk N. Whiplash: why pay for what does not work? J Musculoskel Pain 2000;8:29–53.

135. Freeman MD, Croft AC, Rossignol AM. "Whiplash associated disorders: redefining whiplash and its management," by the Quebec Task Force: a critical evaluation. Spine 1998;23:1043–1049.

136. McKinney LA. Early mobilization and outcome in acute sprains of the neck. BMJ 1989;299:1006–1008.

137. Borchgrevink GE, Smevik O, Nordby A, et al. MR imaging and radiography of patients with cervical hyperextension-flexion injuries after car accidents. Acta Radiol 1995;36:425–428.

138. Rosenfeld M, Gunnarsson R, Borenstein P. Early intervention in whiplash-associated disorders: a comparison of two treatment protocols. Spine 2000;25:1782–1787.

139. Provinciali L, Baroni M, Illuminati L, et al. Multimodal treatment to prevent the late whiplash syndrome. Scand J Rehabil Med 1996;28:105–111.

140. Taimela S, Takala EP, Asklof T, et al. Active treatment of chronic neck pain: a prospective randomized intervention. Spine 2000;25:1021–1027.

141. Turk DC, Okifuji A. Assessment of patients' reporting of pain: an integrated perspective. Lancet 1999;353:1784–1788.

142. Byrn C, Borenstein P, Linder LE. Treatment of neck and shoulder pain in whip-lash syndrome patients with intracutaneous sterile water injections. Acta Anesthesiol Scand 1991;35:52–53.

143. Freund BJ, Schwartz M. Treatment of chronic cervical-associated headache with botulinum toxin a: a pilot study. Headache 2000;40:231–236.

144. Freund BJ, Schwartz M. Treatment of whiplash associated with neck pain with botulinum toxin-a: a pilot study. J Rheumatol 2000;27:481–484.

145. Su HC, Su RK. Treatment of whiplash injuries with acupuncture. Clin J Pain 1988;4:233–247.

146. Simons DG. Myofascial trigger points and the whiplash syndrome (letter). Clin J Pain 1989;5:279.

147. Howe DH, Newcomb RG, Wade MT. Manipulation of the cervical spine: a pilot study. J R Coll Gen Pract 1983;33:564–579.

148. Vernon HT, Aker P, Burns S, et al. Pressure pain threshold evaluation of the effect of spinal manipulation in the treatment of chronic neck pain: a pilot study. J Manipulative Physiol Ther 1990;13:13–16.

149. Janda V in Liebenson C. Rehabilitation of the Spine: A Practitioner's Manual. Baltimore: Williams & Wilkins, 1996:97–112.

150. Foreman SM, Croft AC. Whiplash Injuries, The Cervical Acceleration/Deceleration Syndrome. 3rd Ed. Baltimore: Lippincott, Williams & Wilkins; 2002:1–129.

151. Bogduk N, Marsland A. The cervical zygapophysial joints as a source of neck pain. Spine 1988;13:610–617.

152. Simons DG, Travell JG, Simons LS. Myofascial pain and dysfunction. In: The Trigger Point Manual, vol 1., 2nd Ed. Baltimore: Williams & Wilkins; 1999:178–235.

4

Shoulder Dysfunction and "Frozen Shoulder"

Lucy Whyte Ferguson, DC
Thoracic Outlet Syndrome
section by Robert Gerwin, MD

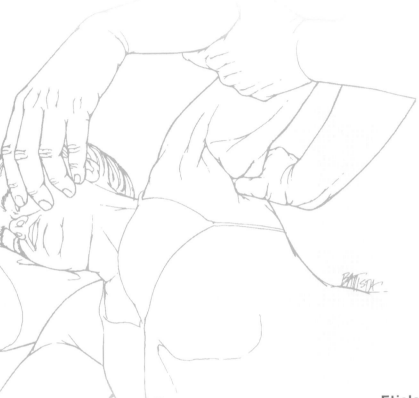

INTRODUCTION

"Frozen shoulder" is an enigmatic condition and a challenge to the treatment skills of any practitioner. As described in this chapter, conventional treatment approaches have drawbacks and are based on some false assumptions about the nature of the pathologic condition involved. A functional musculoskeletal treatment approach that identifies and treats a set of muscles involved with myofascial trigger points and an interrelated set of dysfunctional joints generally results in quicker recovery with less intensive treatment and much less pain during rehabilitation. An increased range of pain-free motion automatically results from restoration of good scapulohumeral joint mechanics, elimination of trigger points, and restoration of normal muscle length.

Thoracic outlet syndrome is a closely related condition. A special section regarding evaluation and treatment of this condition follows the frozen shoulder protocol.

FROZEN SHOULDER: BACKGROUND

Frozen Shoulder is a general term used to describe severe shoulder dysfunction, with flexion, abduction, and internal and external rotation limited to half the normal range of motion (1). Pain, which is also a defining criterion, is most pronounced in the anterior or middle deltoid region, and is worsened by attempts to move the arm beyond the easily accessible range. External rotation is considered the most limited movement in most cases (2–4). Although some frozen shoulders develop secondary to trauma and enforced immobility, other cases frequently occur with no specific known injury or instigating event.

The lifetime incidence of frozen shoulder in the general population is approximately 2%. The condition affects 10% to 20% of diabetics, and 36% of insulin-dependent diabetics (5).

Diagnosis and Clinical Features

The term *frozen shoulder* is used only when other conditions such as cervical radiculopathy and rotator cuff tears have been ruled out. In fact, some researchers have pointed out that other conditions account for shoulder immobility and pain in a high percentage of supposed frozen shoulder cases (4). The diagnostic process involves taking a careful history to identify trauma to the neck or shoulder. The clinician assesses the limited range of motion and identifies the location of pain at the end of motion. If provocative tests such as cervical compression produce pain in the shoulder, it is worthwhile to perform a full evaluation of the cervical spine. Imaging to evaluate the integrity of the rotator cuff is warranted if the patient has a history of trauma and focal weakness of rotator cuff muscles. Minor avulsion fractures are easily missed during clinical evaluation, and other factors such as tumors must be considered and ruled out as well.

Frozen shoulder can accompany other conditions, including rheumatoid arthritis and Lyme disease. The clinician needs to identify any systemic diseases as well as address the shoulder dysfunction and pain.

Several authors have identified three stages of frozen shoulder (3,6–8):

- *Stage 1.* The initial stage is characterized by a great deal of pain that limits movement. Nighttime pain is often severe in this stage. This initial painful phase usually lasts 2.5 to 9 months.

- *Stage 2.* The second stage is characterized by stiffness but decreased levels of general pain. In fact, pain is experienced primarily when the individual tries to move at the ends of the restricted range of shoulder mobility. This second stage typically lasts 4 to 12 months.

- *Stage 3.* The third stage is the recovery or "thawing" phase, and generally lasts from 5 to 26 months. The average duration of the whole condition is 30 months.

Some studies have shown that many patients, with or without treatment, are able to return to normal activity and show no signs of significant shoulder pathology 2 to 3 years after the onset of frozen shoulder. Other longitudinal studies have shown longer-lasting pain and limitation in one third to half of the subjects followed, even 5 to 7 years after onset.(3,6,9,10).

Conventional Treatment Approaches

Many attempts have been made to define the nature of frozen shoulder and the specific pathologic conditions involved to develop effective treatment strategies. Most of the treatment strategies employed today were developed to deal with a hypothetical pathology of inflammation and adhesion. Nevaiser and Nevaiser (6) described the appearance of inflammation and the fact that the joint capsule adhered tightly to the humerus. Consistent with this theory of pathology is the fact that whereas a normal joint holds 25 to 30 mL fluid on arthroscopic injection, a frozen shoulder capsule holds only 5 to 10 mL (8). Recently, however, several thorough and well-designed imaging studies involving frozen shoulder patients have shown *no adhesions* in the shoulder joint capsule. Wiley (4) performed arthroscopic evaluation of frozen shoulder patients before and after manipulation under anesthesia and could locate no adhesions. Rizk et al. (11) found no intracapsular or extracapsular structural adhesions on arthroscopy or during open surgical release. Ozaki et al. (12) observed what they called intraarticular adhesions but considered them to be the result of pathology and not a cause. In fact, their description of the surgical appearance of the joint is quite instructive: The term *adhesive capsulitis* was coined to describe the pathologic condition and, by implication, the cause of so-called frozen shoulder. However, we never found the synovial tissue to be adherent to the humerus. Rather, it had shrunk until it tightly embraced the humeral head. As the humeral head was mobilized, it readily peeled from the humeral articular cartilage (12).

Although the tearing or popping sounds resulting from manipulation of the frozen shoulder have been interpreted as the tearing of adhesions, studies of premanipulation and postmanipulation arthrograms showed that *tearing of the joint capsule and synovium* were the demonstrable changes after manipulation under anesthesia (7,9,13). Several studies have shown that the capsule is also torn during arthroscopic distension of the joint capsule, but some researchers disagree (5,11).

The theory of inflammation also has been challenged. Histologic studies have been performed on tissues removed from patients requiring open release or arthroscopic release because of failure to respond to manipulation under anesthesia. Bunker (14) studied tissues removed from the rotator interval and arising near the subscapularis bursa, and Ozaki et al. (12) studied tissues removed from the coracohumeral ligament and the rotator interval. Both teams of researchers found extensive fibroblasts and myoblasts and dense fibrous tissue characteristic of fibrinoid degeneration. There were no inflammatory cells, and the tissue was not distinguishable from that found in Dupuytren's contracture (12,14,15).

Recent studies have changed the theories about the pathologic condition involved in frozen shoulder, but the same basic treatment approaches have continued, although with new rationales. Aggressive physical therapy programs involving repetitive stretching were formerly performed to break adhesions; these same regimens are now used to stretch the contracted joint capsule. Various physical therapy modalities are used to decrease pain during the performance of these exercises (16–18). However, for some patients, the pain cannot be reasonably controlled during the exercises. Even when the pain can be tolerated during the therapy session, it often increases that night and the next day. Therefore, some therapists have recommended gentler methods to avoid pain (8,19). However, the lengthy nature of the rehabilitation process by traditional means, with either an aggressive program or a gentle program, is a significant concern. It is not unusual for physical therapy to be performed for up to 6 months.

Mao et al. (20) studied the impact of this sort of physical therapy for a period of 4 to 6 weeks to see whether arthrography would show an increase in joint capacity. They found that range of motion improved in both acute and chronic frozen shoulder patients, but the improved mobility was accompanied by only a 2.82-mL increase in joint capacity in acute patients (with pain for less than 2 months), and there was no change in joint capacity in chronic cases (with pain for more than 2 months.) These studies suggest that extracapsular tissues change during therapy, and muscles, tendons, and ligaments that become shortened may be a factor in the restricted motion of chronic frozen shoulder patients (20).

Corticosteroids administered both orally and by injection also have been used to treat the frozen shoulder patient, with no demonstrable effect on treatment outcome (16,21). This is not surprising, because the condition has not been shown to involve significant inflammation. Cortisone injection, guided by fluoroscopy to ensure intracapsular placement, might result in decreased pain, particularly during the early acute period. However, this procedure is not yet established as having any application in the treatment of frozen shoulders.

When months of conservative measures fail to result in improvement, manipulation under anesthesia is often performed (3,22). This procedure was formerly used to rupture adhesions but is now used with the express purpose of rupturing the contracted joint capsule. Several authors warn that care must be taken not to break the humerus or tear the subscapularis tendon (4,10,23). Manipulation under anesthesia does not work in approximately 20% of cases and has less effectiveness with diabetic patients than with other patients (9,24). Frozen shoulder recurs after manipulation under anesthesia in some cases (23,25). A major concern regarding this procedure is pain, not just immediately after the procedure, but during the following 2 to 3 weeks. In one study, 95.4% rated this treatment method as good or excellent, but 34.9% said that they would not recommend the treatment to a friend in the same situation, because of the pain during the first 2 weeks after mobilization (1).

Arthroscopic distention of the joint capsule is also a painful treatment, and comparative studies do not indicate that this method of treatment improves results (5).

For patients who fail to achieve results with manipulation under anesthesia or arthroscopic distention of the capsule, arthroscopic sectioning of the coracohumeral ligament, excision of tissue in the rotator interval, or a z-plasty elongation of the subscapularis tendon may be recommended (13,15,24). The efficacy of these procedures has not been established. Examination of the tissues excised during these surgeries has shown fibrinoid, rather than inflammatory, tissue changes. It is not clear, however, whether fibrinoid degeneration is a uniform characteristic of frozen shoulder, or whether it occurs primarily in this particular population that was unresponsive to other treatments, and therefore such tissue changes would characterize only a late and unresponsive stage of this disorder.

In summary, conventional therapies for frozen shoulder leave much to be desired. The physical therapy regimen is prolonged and usually painful, and manipulation under anesthesia is painful, has certain dangers, and fails to help a significant portion of patients. Comparative outcomes of other surgical procedures have not been fully evaluated. It is certainly possible that clinicians overlook extracapsular factors that may cause the protracted restriction and pain of frozen shoulder. Whereas scapular dyskinesia has been recognized as a feature of shoulder dysfunction, the central importance of restoring normal scapular mobility and contribution to shoulder range of motion has probably not been fully appreciated. It is worthwhile, therefore, to investigate other approaches to recovery in which rehabilitation is faster, more easily tolerated, and more likely to bring about successful outcomes. It is also possible that fibrinoid degeneration, as seen in frozen shoulder patients who have experienced repeated treatment failure, may be minimized by successfully completing rehabilitation in a shorter period.

MYOFASCIAL AND ARTICULAR APPROACH TO THE DIAGNOSIS AND TREATMENT OF SHOULDER DYS-FUNCTION AND FROZEN SHOULDER

In Volume 1 of *Myofascial Pain and Dysfunction*, Janet Travell and David and Lois Simons propose a muscular dysfunction model rather than an inflammation, adhesion, and fibrosis model of frozen shoulders, although they acknowledge that adhesions may be present in a very small number of cases (25). They point out that the subscapularis muscle, if shortened because of myofascial dysfunction, can account for the characteristics of a frozen shoulder, and that frozen shoulders can successfully be treated by addressing the shortened subscapularis.

Frozen shoulder involves a functional unit or group of shortened neck and shoulder muscles, each with myofascial trigger points. In most patients, the primary limiting muscle is the shortened subscapularis, but successful rehabilitation entails identifying and successfully treating the other dysfunctional muscles as well. Frozen shoulder is also characterized by a series of interrelated dysfunctional joints. Clinically, a series of joint dysfunctions typically occur in the patient with frozen shoulder, but the position and function of the scapula is most critical in understanding the pathomechanics of this disorder. In a frozen shoulder, the scapula is often held close to the axilla and elevated, and thus the glenoid fossa, into which the humerus articulates, is in an abnormal location. The scapula and humerus tend to move as a unit, and when movement is attempted, it is as though the humerus hits a painful "roof" or barrier far short of normal range of motion. According to this model, extracapsular factors press the humerus upward against the capsule, folding it, reducing its fluid capacity, and causing the appearance of a "shrunken capsule closely embracing the head of the humerus" (12). If the restrictions affecting the scapula can be released and the scapula can be moved posteromedially and inferiorly toward the spine, a full range of humeral motion can usually be readily restored. The focus of this therapy is dramatically different from that of conventional physical therapy, because the humerus is *not* repeatedly stretched to the end of its range of mobility, where traditional therapy produces the most pain. Rather, efforts are made to release the extracapsular muscle and joint factors that restrict movement of the humerus, and the resultant increased available range of motion is then *gently* explored.

A myofascial approach to frozen shoulder not only contributes to alternative methods of restoring mobility; it also provides an alternative understanding of the patient's pain. Some inflammation may occur, particularly during the early, painful stage of frozen shoulder. The pain and tenderness in later stages appears to be referred from active trigger points or is a result of the shearing and compression forces on joints, tendons, or bursae resulting from shortened muscles, particularly the powerful subscapularis muscle. Referred tenderness from active trigger points has given rise to the concepts of pseudotendinitis and pseudobursitis, discussed later.

The three case histories that follow provide clear examples of the pattern of joint and muscle dysfunction that is typically present in patients with frozen shoulder. They also present a course of treatment for both acute and chronic frozen shoulder that is based on the myofascial and joint dysfunction model as an alternative to the inflammation, adhesion, or fibrosis and shrunken capsule model. Because the same myofascial and joint dysfunction is present to a degree in many other shoulder conditions, the treatment model described has very broad application.

CASE 4-1

Acute Shoulder Injury—No Progression to Frozen Shoulder

Patient History and Symptoms

F.B., a 17-year-old football player, was injured when a tackle resulted in his arm being wrenched backward. He left the playing field in obvious pain, shaking his arm repeatedly. Within minutes, a slightly anterior humerus subluxation was manipulated, which dramatically reduced the pain. He returned to the field and played the rest of the game without incident, and without appearing to favor the shoulder. He was instructed to ice the shoulder that evening, even though he noticed little pain or soreness after the game. The next morning, however, the young athlete was unable to lift his arm and was experiencing considerable pain in the deltoid region of the shoulder.

Examination Findings

Examination showed hypertonic upper trapezius, levator scapula, pectoralis major, anterior serratus, teres minor,

CASE 4-1   Continued

teres major, and infraspinatus muscles, all on the left side. Marked tenderness was present at the subdeltoid bursa and the tendons in the bicipital groove. Normal spinal joint mobility was restricted at C7, T1, and the first rib on the left, and rib–thoracic restriction was found at T4, T5, T6, also on the left. (None of this joint dysfunction or subluxation had been present before the football game, when the patient was treated for an unrelated complaint.) F.B. could actively flex the shoulder to 70°, and passively flex to 100°. Internal rotation was somewhat restricted; external rotation was normal, though painful.

Treatment

Treatment consisted of spray-and-stretch myofascial release, first of the neck muscles, then of the shoulder muscles. Some manual traction of muscle fibers and pressure on trigger points was applied during the spray procedures, to maximize muscular release without overstressing irritated joint areas. Particular attention was paid to releasing the anterior border of the upper trapezius, which inserts onto the clavicle, because of the contribution of clavicle rotation to scapulohumeral movement in normal shoulder biomechanics (26). After the upper trapezius muscle was released, and before the release of shoulder muscles, active flexion of the humerus had already improved by 20° (from 70° to 90°). Shoulder muscles were then treated and elongated.

In addition, a standing maneuver with anterior to posterior thrust against a wall was used to release the left rib–thoracic restrictions, and a cervical lateral break, with slight rotational component in the set-up positioning, was used to restore left lateral flexion and extension at C7, T1. Moist heat was applied to the neck and shoulder area.

After one treatment, a full range of shoulder movement had been restored, although mobility was still somewhat painful. There was a marked reduction in tenderness in the bursa area and in the biceps tendon region. Approximately 70% to 80% of the tenderness subsided within the course of one treatment. Because the biochemical processes involved in true inflammation and the associated tenderness would not allow such a quick improvement, true inflammation could not have

---

TECHNIQUE 4.1

Percussion Technique

This technique was taught by Janet Travell in her seminars, and she used the technique for over 40 years. It is mentioned in some osteopathic literature and was described by John Loeser for the treatment of stump and phantom limb pain (44).

The technique involves the use of a standard triangular reflex hammer to lightly tap or bounce on a trigger point in a rhythmic fashion. Travell performed the tapping approximately every other second, but other rhythms, such as a heartbeat-like rhythm, are also effective. Eight to twelve taps are usually required to release a trigger point, after which the trigger point area can be repalpated to determine when the point has been extinguished. Stretching of the muscle follows, to complete the procedure. The mechanism responsible for the effectiveness of this technique remains unknown.

---

been the primary cause of this patient's tenderness. Instead, the tenderness appears to have been primarily referred from active myofascial trigger points, a condition known as pseudobursitis and pseudotendinitis.

Two days later, a second treatment resulted in greater ease of shoulder movement and further reduction of pain on movement. Percussion Technique (Technique 4-1) was used to fully release the trigger points in the pectoral muscle that were still present after the spray-and-stretch release techniques and trigger point pressure release. Moist heat was then applied to the treated muscles. The patient performed a home stretching program.

Follow-up

The shoulder was checked 3 weeks later, and no further treatment was required. At that time, there was no recurrence of the shoulder dysfunction, active trigger points, or subluxations in the treated areas of the cervical and thoracic spine.

CASE 4-2

Acute Injury—With Progression to Frozen Shoulder

Patient History and Symptoms

A.F., age 45, fell on the ski slope, fracturing his right wrist (a chip fracture of the distal radius) and spraining his left shoulder. The fall happened so fast that he could not describe the manner of impact or how he landed. After x-rays were taken at the emergency health service at the ski area, the medical doctor molded a splint with ace wrap to stabilize the wrist. Ice was applied to the injured wrist and shoulder, and A.F. was advised to use a sling if supporting the weight of the arm caused too much pain in the sprained shoulder.

Examination Findings

A.F. was examined later on the day of the injury. Examination showed restriction of normal spinal mobility at C7, T1 with a reduction of left lateral flexion and extension at this level, and rib–thoracic restriction at T3, T4, T5, and T6 on the left. There was restriction of normal joint play of the humerus, with reduction of anterior-to-posterior and cephalad-to-caudad mobility. The scapula was pulled laterally and anteriorly along the posterior rib cage, with reduced independent movement between the scapula and humerus. The upper trapezius, levator scapula, pectoralis major, teres major, teres minor, infraspinatus, supraspinatus, anterior serratus, and subscapularis muscles, all on the left, were hypertonic. Subsequent evaluation indicated active trigger points and twitch response in these same muscles after the acute hypertonicity had subsided. Latent trigger points and muscle shortening were noted on the right side of the neck and the right shoulder. (Travell and Simons have encouraged bilateral treatment of muscle groups to address the affected members of the functional unit.) There were 25° of internal rotation and 10° of external rotation of the left humerus. Severe pain limited passive flexion to 50° and passive abduction to 40°. Pain was primarily in the region of the sub-deltoid bursa and lower portions of the deltoid muscle. (Some authors use the term *frozen shoulder* to refer only to chronic cases of severe shoulder dysfunction, lasting for several months, whereas others recognize an acute frozen shoulder characterized by severe limitation of movement and pain. Case 2 can be viewed as either an acute frozen shoulder or as a severe shoulder dysfunction that very likely would have progressed to become a chronic frozen shoulder in the absence of successful intervention.)

Treatment

A.F. was seen daily for 4 days, then every other day for 2 weeks, then twice per week for a month, with a 2-week hiatus during that month. Initial treatment involved spray-and-stretch release of hypertonic muscles and myofascial involvement of the neck, then of the shoulder muscles. Ice was used for the first week over the tender areas of the shoulder joint, and moist heat was applied on the surrounding treated muscles after each treatment. An activator and mobilization were used to release the thoracic spine and rib subluxations. A cervical lateral break, with slight rotational component in the set up positioning, was used to restore left lateral flexion and extension at the C7, T1 juncture.

This treatment was intended to reduce pain and restore some mobility, but the restrictions recurred during the initial week of treatment. Trigger point activity was then also noted in the deltoid, proximal triceps, biceps, and brachialis muscles. The shortened position of these upper arm muscles from the use of a sling was probably a factor in the development of these additional trigger points. Furthermore, some of the primary trigger points in the neck and shoulder muscles tend to refer pain into the arm and set off additional trigger points in the muscles located within the referred pain regions (27). A.F. used aspirin during this period, performed gentle stretches, used ice, and took hot baths, and was able to dispense with the sling by the fifth day.

Gradual improvement in shoulder function and reduction of pain was achieved with each treatment. However, pain increased and mobility decreased between treatments despite his performing gentle stretches, and lying on a tennis ball to enhance rib–thoracic mobility in the interscapular region. The humerus was adjusted during the third treatment, with a gentle but painful maneuver. No recurrence of the loss of joint play at the humerus occurred. Percussion technique with the reflex hammer was particularly effective in releasing the pectoral and anterior serratus trigger points. Before the hiatus in treatment, flexion to 130° was achieved before pain limitation, and there was full internal rotation and 25° of external rotation. Scapular dysfunction was still present, apparently because of the shortened subscapularis. With the scapular dysfunction, the subscapularis is capable of forcing the humerus upward in the shoulder capsule, thereby contributing to anterior shoulder pain on shoulder flexion. The subscapular treatment approaches used up to this point in the patient's treatment involved stretching the arm away from the scapula, but these release techniques did not result in sufficient

CASE 4-2   Continued

release of the subscapularis to alter mobility of the shoulder blade. As long as the scapular function was disordered, the loss of mobility between treatments complicated progress.

During the 2-week hiatus in treatment, in spite of self-care techniques, A.F.'s external rotation decreased to 15° and his flexion to 100°. Computer use and driving seemed to be particularly aggravating activities, and the patient needed to stretch during and after these activities.

On resumption of treatment, percussion technique was used to release the subscapularis muscle. With the patient lying on his side, percussion was applied to the tendon of the subscapularis, where it passes through the axilla. As the subscapularis released, the scapula was progressively mobilized away from the humerus and toward the spine. After release of the subscapularis and mobilization of the scapula, a marked increase in the cephalad-to-caudad humeral glide and a significant improvement in flexion and external rotation occurred. In the course of that single treatment, passive flexion increased from 100° to 180°, and full external rotation was restored with discomfort but minimal pain. From this point on in treatment, there was no loss of range of motion between sessions.

The focus of the next treatment changed because the location of pain and the pattern of joint restriction had shifted. A.F. now complained of nocturnal pain in the shoulder, traveling down the arm to the lateral epicondyle, and sometimes producing an ache in the wrist. This is the characteristic referred pain pattern of the supraspinatus muscle (28). Treatment therefore focused on the release of this muscle, plus remaining trigger points in the deltoids and teres major and minor. At the T7, T8, and T9 levels, a lack of accommodation to the shift in the scapular position, with reduced extension and lateral flexion at these same levels, was found. These restrictions were adjusted with a prone maneuver, as well as activator and mobilization. Joint restriction in this area may have been caused by compensation for the former position of the scapula.

The stabilization phase of A.F.'s treatment involved addressing muscle weakness. Resistive manual muscle testing (29) indicated weakness of the middle and anterior deltoid and supraspinatus, as well as the rhomboid and middle and lower trapezius muscles. The first three muscles were actively involved in the myofascial disorder; therefore, exercise focused on stretches to continue to lengthen them and thereby restore their normal strength. The weakness of the other three muscles apparently resulted from their being in a prolonged stretched state secondary to the forward position of the scapula and humerus. Gentle resistive exercise of these muscles was prescribed, performed in the middle range of muscle activity, using rubber tubing. The patient was instructed to stretch before and after these exercises to prevent reactivating trigger points. Goading techniques, including neurolymphatic points and origin–insertion massage (30), also were used to stimulate normal function in each of these muscles.

Follow-up

After the stabilization phase of rehabilitation, A.F. was able to perform normal strenuous activity, including taking a spill onto his left shoulder on the ski slopes, without reaggravating his condition.

CASE 4-3

Chronic Frozen Shoulder
Patient History

E.C., a 56-year-old overweight female Native American, taking medication for diabetes and a thyroid condition, was treated for a long-standing frozen shoulder. Eighteen years earlier, her right arm had been wrenched during an altercation, and that arm, in her words, "has not been right since." The arm had been a major source of pain during the last 5 years (before treatment in 1992), and she had been unable to move it normally since 1989. She was examined and treated with pain medication at the Indian Health Service and was diagnosed with "arthritis" of the shoulder. She also had a course of acupuncture treatment but continued to have pain. X-rays taken in 1987, and again in 1989, showed a progression of degenerative changes in the shoulder joint.

Symptoms

E.C.'s major pain and tenderness were located in the anterior shoulder area and the subdeltoid bursa, as well as the anterior and posterior deltoid. She also complained of pain radiating down the arm, with tenderness to palpation just proximal and distal to the elbow, and at the radial aspect of the wrist. She tended to carry the arm, flexed at the elbow, close to her side.

(continues)

CASE 4-3 Continued

Examination Findings

On initial examination, passive flexion was 70° and passive abduction 80°, both limited by severe pain. Internal and external rotation were entirely absent. There was restriction of normal cervical flexion joint play on the right at the C5, C6 levels, and reduction in right lateral flexion and extension at the C7, T1 levels. Rib–thoracic restrictions were present in the right interscapular region, most severely at the T3 level. Reduction of the cephalad-to-caudad and anterior-to-posterior joint play of the right humerus was seen. The right scapula was drawn forward, upward, and lateral along the right rib cage. Restriction of normal joint play at the right radius at both the radio-humeral joint (elbow) and the radio-ulnar joint (wrist) also was noted. Major myofascial trigger point activity and muscle shortening were evident in the right scalene, upper trapezius, pectoralis major, subscapularis, anterior serratus, teres major and minor, infraspinatus, biceps, brachialis, and wrist extensor muscles. Latent trigger points and some muscle shortening of some of the same muscles on the left side were present.

Treatment

E.C. was treated 12 times over the course of 4 months. Treatment consisted of mobilization of the cervical and thoracic spine, with use of the activator to mobilize the right ribs in the interscapular region. Osseous manipulation of the humerus was performed twice, with gentle manual traction and mobilization on the other visits. Osseous manipulation of the right radius at the elbow and wrist was performed once. Spray-and-stretch myofascial release was performed with the neck, shoulder, and arm muscles on each visit. Percussion technique was used to treat trigger points in the pectoralis, biceps, and brachialis muscles. On the last two visits, percussion technique was applied to the subscapularis and associated muscles in the posterior fold of the axilla.

With the exception of some reaggravation of the shoulder from an instance of kneading bread, the patient made steady progress. After 10 visits and before the subscapularis release, she had achieved 150° of shoulder flexion and a similar degree of abduction and normal internal rotation, although external rotation was still absent. On the next visit, when the percussion subscapular release and mobilization of the scapula toward the spine were introduced, flexion and abduction increased to 180° and external rotation improved from 0° to 35°. With the final treatment and the benefit of home stretches, the patient's external rotation was restored to 45°.

Follow-up

When E.C. was examined some months later for a low back complaint, no deterioration in the right shoulder function was evident.

Overview of Shoulder Dysfunction and Frozen Shoulder

These case histories illustrate common patterns found in patients with acute shoulder dysfunction and chronic frozen shoulders. In Case 4-1, the football player developed the pattern of muscle and joint dysfunction very quickly, after a relatively minor injury. He did not have these muscle and joint problems before the injury; however, the body apparently reacted to the minor injury by developing subluxation in the same joint areas and myofascial involvement in the same set of muscles as those found in patients with much more severe sprains, or more chronic frozen shoulders. (However, the powerful subscapularis muscle was not involved, in contrast to the two other cases.) An interesting subject for further investigation is determining how the body institutes such changes and the sequence of muscle and joint reactions. Simons, Travell, and Simons have noted similar patterns that seem to arise from overuse rather than trauma, causing a myofascial disorder that progresses to frozen shoulder (25).

The second case shows a treatment sequence for an individual with a more traumatic injury, and an accompanying need to vary the treatment and home exercise as the clinical picture changes. Cases 4-2 and 4-3 also demonstrate the critical importance of releasing the powerful subscapularis muscle and freeing up scapular movement. The dramatic improvement in humeral range of motion after the use of these techniques illustrates the importance of the role of the shortened subscapularis in the compromise of shoulder function and the compression syndrome involved in frozen shoulder. Treatment is more efficient and far less painful if the practitioner treats joint disorders and myofascial dysfunction, rather than trying to force the shoulder into greater movement. The clinician will find that, once the proper myofascial restrictions are addressed, the body will respond by allowing greater movement. After one area of trigger points is released, passive movement of the humerus is checked, and the remaining muscle bands causing restricted movement can be palpated and sequentially treated, layer by layer, until full movement has been achieved.

The third case illustrates the fact that even a long-standing shoulder dysfunction, with arthritis and very restricted movement, can be successfully approached as a myofascial disorder. Adhesions or a shrunken capsule clearly have not limited progress. The patient has achieved normal movement and elimination of pain, yet treatment approaches involved little pain and no attempts to force restricted movement.

In all three cases, a large portion of the pain and tenderness appears to have been attributable to referral from myofascial trigger points or the effects of compression forces generated by muscle shortening and joint dysfunction. It is remarkable that, after the acute stage of this condition, the level of pain can be significantly and quickly lowered by the release techniques just discussed. Identifying and treating *all* muscles that contain active trigger points, which are capable of referring pain and tenderness to the involved tissues, is important. True inflammation will not abate quickly from the use of the techniques described, but "pseudo-inflammation" (pseudotendinitis, pseudobursitis) will decrease with each step of myofascial and joint release. To distinguish true inflammation from pseudo-inflammation, myofascial release and joint mobilization/manipulation become an essential part of the diagnostic process. By making this distinction, the clinician can assess how much of the treatment procedures and home care (if any) should be focused on treating inflammatory reaction, and how much should be focused on treating joint and muscle disorder.

Etiology

Shoulder dysfunction and frozen shoulder can arise from any of the following:

- A fall on the shoulder or hand
- A sprain of the shoulder (wrenching overstretch)
- Overuse of shoulder muscles (lifting, pulling, throwing, repeated cross-body movements)
- Repeated minor strains (such as repeated yanks from a dog on a leash)
- Lack of movement because of pain (brachial plexus neuropathy, shingles)
- Immobilization because of fracture or surgery (including mastectomy)
- Shoulder replacement

The abnormal mechanics related to the pain, limitation of movement, and weakness in the patient with a shoulder replacement are identical to the abnormal mechanics of the more typical frozen shoulder patient. A shrunken capsule cannot be the underlying pathologic condition, because the capsule has been removed in the course of the surgery. These patients respond very well to the treatment of extracapsular factors as described in this chapter.

In addition, some aspects of shoulder dysfunction can occur in a whiplash-type auto accident, even without direct impact to the shoulder (although trauma arising from shoulder seatbelt restraint may be a factor). In such instances, the restoration of normal shoulder mechanics and posture is often critically important in reducing the stress on the cervical spine and musculature so that spinal rehabilitation can progress satisfactorily. Shoulder dysfunction and frozen shoulder also may arise for unidentifiable reasons.

Cautions

Patients should be evaluated carefully for cervical or brachial neuropathy, a major tear in the rotator cuff, or neoplasm or other underlying medical disorder that refers pain into the shoulder. These patients require different care directed at the specific pathology involved.

X-rays of the shoulder also are important to evaluate for conditions that would require other treatment. An outlet view should be taken to identify whether bone spurs are causing impingement. Significant degenerative change, in terms of roughening of the joint surfaces, does not preclude the successful use of a myofascial and articular approach to restoring shoulder mobility. Even some patients with the appearance of bone-on-bone can achieve reasonable range of motion and reduction of pain and discomfort. If a patient is not making good progress in treatment, the clinician should not persist without investigating whether there are sizable bone spurs affecting shoulder mechanics. Sizable spurs probably preclude successful treatment, and significant degenerative changes usually slow the patient's progress; the clinician should be alert to whether further treatment is expected to be productive.

Symptom/Pain Presentation

The patient presents with pain in the anterior or middle deltoid on movement of the humerus, and significant restriction of normal range of motion. Abnormal scapulohumeral rhythm is evidenced by the fact that the scapula elevates markedly and moves whenever there is an attempt to flex or abduct the humerus. If the patient is in an acute stage of injury, the pain may be more diffuse and may be present even when the patient is not moving. Finding a comfortable position for sleep is often difficult, and generally the patient is prevented by pain from sleeping on the affected shoulder. Even after pain levels have been reduced and other functions have returned, throwing overhand is often impossible. Pain may be part of the problem, but even if pain is not present, the alteration in scapulohumeral rhythm can make the coordination necessary for throwing impossible. Full rehabilitation has not been completed until the patient is able to move the arm normally, sleep on the affected shoulder, throw a ball, or use the arm in a satisfactory functional manner.

Shoulder impingement is a form of shoulder dysfunction that commonly involves the same set of muscle and joint dysfunctions as those found in the frozen shoulder patient. In shoulder dysfunction, the myofascial involvement of the subscapularis and the supraspinatus are of primary importance. In shoulder impingement, only certain movements cause pain—usually a reaching movement toward the side, whereas pure shoulder flexion is often painless. The same treatment model presented in this chapter has been used successfully in the treatment of this related disorder.

Myofascial Entrapments

The most common muscular entrapment of a nerve that occurs with shoulder dysfunction involves the scalene and the pectoralis minor muscle entrapments of the brachial plexus, and both are discussed fully in the section on thoracic outlet syndrome that follows. A less common entrapment of the suprascapular nerve may result from trigger points in the infraspinatus muscle, with profound infraspinatus weakness, and eventual atrophy if the condition persists.

Treatment

To successfully treat the joint and muscle dysfunction involved in frozen shoulder and related conditions, myofascial releases must be performed on a series of muscles, particularly the important subscapularis. In fact, the rate of improvement in the subscapularis generally determines the rate of progress of rehabilitation. Proper mobility of the joint structures must be restored. For results to last, posture also must be improved. Figure 4-1 shows the pattern of muscle and joint dysfunction that must be addressed.

The primary point in treatment, however, is that *very little treatment time is spent directly trying to press the humerus to greater range of movement.* The notion of "no pain, no gain" should be thrown out the window. In fact, progress often reverses when patients are treated by traditional methods that emphasize pressing against the end barrier to increase range of motion, either during treatment sessions or in home exercise. This is not to say that these treatment methods do not sometimes achieve the desired effect. How-

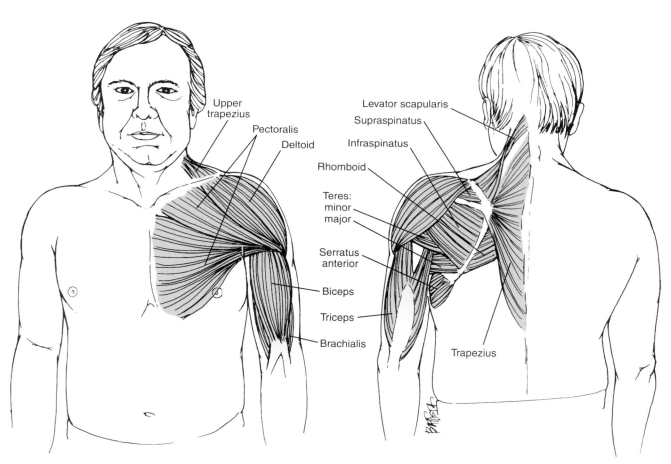

FIGURE 4-1. **Relationship between muscle and joint dysfunction in a patient with frozen shoulder.** Viewed from the front, the patient's dysfunctional shoulder appears further forward (protracted) than the opposite shoulder, and the clavicle is often higher. Viewed from the back, the scapula on the side of dysfunction is further from the spine and may wing more than the opposite scapula. The line of the upper trapezius or top of shoulder is often higher on the dysfunctional side, and the rib–thoracic joints medial to the scapula may be more prominent. This pattern of functional alignment would be normal if the patient were reaching forward, but is maintained even at rest. Some patients may have aspects of dysfunction in both shoulders.

ever, a simpler, easier, quicker, and less painful course of rehabilitation is effected when the clinician takes an indirect approach rather than continually trying to breach the barrier directly. The approach is based on a thorough understanding of myofascial treatment methods and gentle restoration of joint mobility.

A typical treatment sequence will demonstrate the elements of myofascial and joint release. Although it is certainly not the only treatment sequence, it will illustrate typical treatment methods and the fact that the barrier to movement is explored but not repeatedly directly challenged.

Seated Releases

The clinician performs systematic stretching of all of the major neck muscles with the patient seated. The scalene, upper trapezius, and levator scapula are the most important neck muscles involved in these shoulder disorders. In fact, the patient with a frozen shoulder often exhibits dramatic overuse of the upper trapezius and levator scapula, as these muscles work to gain additional lift of the restricted humerus to reach objects above shoulder level. The attempt in treatment is to lower the clavicle and the scapula relative to the neck. (The humerus will also lower, as the glenoid fossa in the scapula lowers.)

Next, an initial stretch is performed on the pectoral muscles, flexing and abducting the humerus in a range that may be uncomfortable, but taking care to avoid a painful range. The biceps is also stretched at this time. As the biceps releases, it is often possible to discern the extent to which the shortened biceps has contributed to shoulder pain with movement. Biceps involvement makes abduction with retraction painful, but it usually has little effect on direct flexion. Because the range of humeral movement is restricted, it is often helpful for the clinician to stretch the patient's pectorals directly by hooking the clinician's hands under the pectoral muscles at the anterior axilla with the patient's arms resting at the sides of the torso. The clinician can lean back and pull and stretch the pectoral muscles, using the chair to support the patient's torso (Fig. 4-2). Thus, significant stretching of the pectoral muscles can be achieved in a focused manner without flexing the humerus.

To release muscles about the scapula in a seated position, the clinician can abduct the humerus and support the involved arm at the elbow, and then hook the fingers of the other hand along the inferolateral border of the scapula. The clinician then exerts gentle traction to release the scapula medially and away from the humerus. The scapula position also can be addressed by cupping the fingers of each hand around the upper humerus, and pressing the thumbs against the flat portion of each scapula, stretching the shoulders back, and attempting to flatten the scapulae against the torso. Major changes in scapula mobility do not usually occur in these maneuvers, but they are warm-ups for the side-lying maneuvers described below.

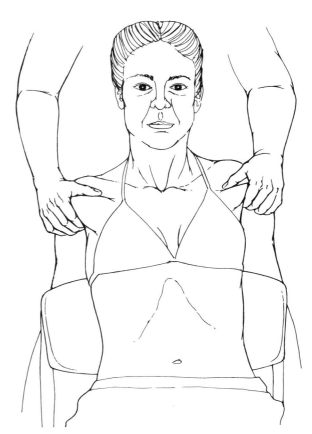

FIGURE 4-2. The clinician stretches the pectoral muscles of the seated patient. The clinician hooks both hands under the lateral border of the pectoral muscles. The chair and the muscle shortness provide the resistance, and the clinician leans back and maintains a gentle but firm upward and anterior to posterior pull on the muscles as they stretch.

Finally, the seated position is also a good position for release of the paraspinal, trapezius, and posterior serratus superior muscles. The patient rounds the chest and shoulders forward and draws first one and then the other arm forward across the torso, while the clinician assists the stretch. Some pressure with the flat of the clinician's elbow can help with the trigger point releases and can increase rib–spinal mobility in the restricted areas.

Side-Lying Releases

With the patient side-lying, the clinician abducts the arm to the point of slight discomfort but not pain. Two muscles that generally are pulled to tension in this position are the pectoral muscles, particularly a deep portion at the lateral border of the pectoralis major, and the subscapularis. In the patient with frozen shoulder, the subscapularis tendon is actually raised within the axilla and can be readily treated in this position. Percussion technique is particularly helpful in achieving these releases. The anterior serratus muscle also may be taut, holding the scapula toward the axilla, and it, too, can be readily treated in this position.

Next, the clinician can place caudad pressure on the clavicle and the scapula and can see which neck muscles are still taut and restricting the "drop down" of these bones. Remaining trigger points in the scalene, levator scapula, and upper trapezius can thus be addressed at this time.

Once a good release in these groups of muscles has been achieved, the clinician can proceed to perform more mobilization of the scapula. With the humerus abducted until tension is felt, but not pain, the clinician presses the lateral border of the scapula away from the humerus and toward the spine (Fig. 4-3). Then the clinician can place the thumb of one hand parallel to the scapula and under the lateral border of the scapula, as deeply as the muscles will allow, and gradually glide the thumb toward the spine. Some cephalad pressure can be exerted to release the deep upper subscapularis trigger points, and some caudad pressure can be exerted to release shortened bands of the anterior serratus muscle and guide the scapula inferomedially toward the spine. The clinician's other hand or arm can assist this process by drawing the humerus caudad and posterior, either by contacting the humerus just below the clavicle or by hooking the thumb under the pectoral muscle and stretching it to allow the humerus to move back. By using the other hand to shift the position of the humerus, the clinician creates slack for the scapular motion, which then can be advanced by the main treating hand. (Fig. 4-4). Another aspect of scapular mobility can be treated in this position as well, by gently pressing the knee against the scapula and trying to flatten it against the torso and toward the spine, while stabilizing the anterior shoulder and arm with both hands, one hand at the elbow and the other at the head of the humerus (Figure 4.5). A gentle rocking motion can be used to mobilize the scapula, and this same motion can be used to rock the restricted rib–thoracic joints, just medial to the scapula.

It is often useful to give patients a rest after these procedures. The clinician should allow the patient to rest with moist heat all around the shoulder, neck, upper back, and upper arm for 10 minutes, before proceeding with the prone releases.

Prone Releases

With the patient prone, the clinician may be able to easily determine the amount of restriction that is still present in the anterior shoulder. A paradox may be apparent in this position. The humerus may be held too closely proximate to the clavicle, so the humerus needs to be mobilized in a caudad direction. However, the pectoral muscles, particularly the pectoralis minor, may be pulling the humerus caudad and anterior. Therefore, what we really want to achieve is posterior and caudad mobility of the humerus, with the accompanying pectoralis release and sometimes subclavicular release as well, freeing the tip of the humerus so that it can move up (cephalad), back (retraction), and down (caudad.) The movement thus described is an arc. This can be achieved by hooking the fingers of one hand under the pectoral muscle at the anterior axilla and applying traction cephalad on the muscle, while holding the lower humerus with the other hand and applying traction gently in a caudad direction (Fig. 4.6). If shortened neck muscles are still elevating the clavicle and scapula, the clinician can address them again in this position.

The myofascial releases necessary for throwing can be assessed in this position, by externally rotating the humerus and retracting the shoulder. Sometimes the taut pectoral muscles are the limiting factor, but even after good pectoral release, the teres muscles and posterior deltoid often are still shortened and can be felt to restrict the mobility between the humerus and scapula necessary for performing a throwing movement. Stretches and compression can be performed until it is easier to retract and externally rotate the humerus. The clinician is thus apparently trying to create slack or a groove between the scapula and the externally rotated and retracted humerus (Fig. 4-7). The slack that is achieved will facilitate the independent movement of the scapula and humerus necessary for the cocking-back motion that gives impetus to throwing.

Repeat of Side-Lying Releases

Repeating some of the scapular and muscle releases in the side-lying position often is worthwhile. This is because these releases are critical to increasing the range of shoulder motion, and because the relaxation after the moist heat often allows additional progress within the same treatment session.

Supine Releases

In the supine position, the clinician can access the subscapularis trigger points, and can hold and press them

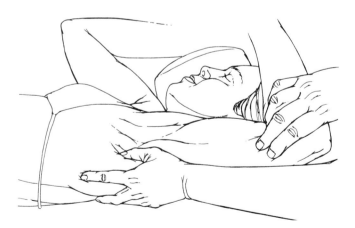

FIGURE 4-3. **With the patient side-lying, the clinician presses the lateral border of the scapula down and toward the spine.** The humerus is supported and abducted close to the end of comfortable range of motion, and the clinician exerts pressure on the scapula away from the humerus, medially and inferiorly. This is one of a series of maneuvers to increase space between the humerus and scapula and decrease the linkage between the two in normal movement.

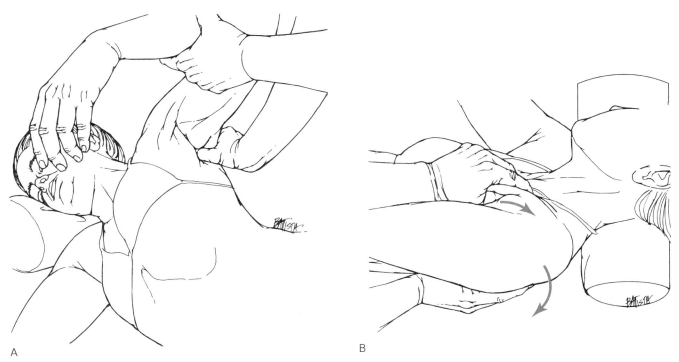

A   B

FIGURE 4-4. **With the thumb under the scapula, the clinician mobilizes the scapula toward the spine. A.** The humerus is elevated to insert the thumb under the lateral border of the scapula. The length of the thumb is parallel to the vertical lateral border of the scapula and slides under it toward the spine along the rib cage, until muscular resistance is encountered in the subscapularis or anterior serratus muscles. The thumb then provides sustained pressure against the trigger points and taut bands that are resisting the mobilization, until they release sufficiently to allow some gain in translating the scapula medially and inferiorly toward the spine. **B.** The other hand may simultaneously stretch the taut pectoral muscles. The thumb is inserted under the lateral inferior border of the pectoral muscle. The myofascial treatment involves some pinching pressure on the trigger points as well as using the web between the clinician's thumb and index to provide upward and backward pressure to elongate taut bands. The net effect is that the humerus translates up and back and eventually down in a semicircular motion while the scapula translates inferiorly and toward the spine.

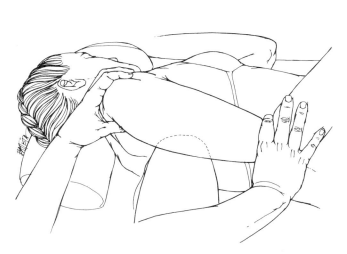

FIGURE 4-5. **Using the knee as a fulcrum to flatten the scapula toward the spine.** The clinician uses one hand to contact the shoulder and the other to contact the elbow and stabilize the humerus at the side of the body. The knee is then placed against the flat of the scapula to retract it while extending the upper back, and gently pulling back the humerus at the shoulder.

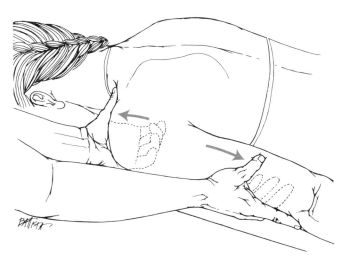

FIGURE 4-6. **Prone traction release of the pectoral muscle.** The clinician holds the humerus with one hand and exerts traction caudad, away from the clavicle. The other hand is inserted from the top of the shoulder under the pectoral fold of the axilla and traction is applied upward, cephalad, to lengthen the shortened bands of pectoral muscle.

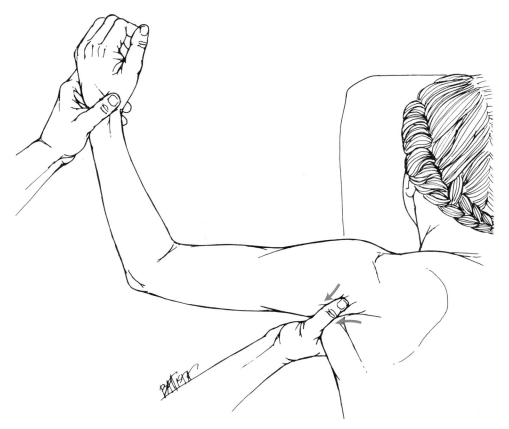

FIGURE 4-7. Freeing up external rotation of the shoulder and the posterior axillary fold. The humerus is abducted and externally rotated with the patient prone. With shoulder dysfunction, the posterior axillary muscles are shortened, and there is insufficient give or play between the scapula and the humerus in this position. The clinician presses between the scapula and the humerus as though to restore a fold. This myofascial release and mobilization is an essential step to restore the patient's ability to cock the arm back to throw a ball.

against the scapula while gently abducting and flexing the humerus. In later stages of treatment, the patient can go through passive and active flexion and abduction of the humerus, while the clinician holds the trigger points (Fig. 4-8). (Levels 3 and 4 of myofascial release techniques are discussed in more detail in Chapter 6.) If the humerus is still being held anterior relative to the other shoulder, the clinician can take a broad contact with one hand against the front of the shoulder, with the thumb in the axilla; the patient's elbow is supported with the clinician's other hand so that the arm position does not encourage the anterior position of the shoulder. Then the patient gently presses the shoulder anterior with only partial effort (10%), holding for 4 seconds, and then releasing (Fig. 4-9). This may be repeated, with reduction of the anterior position of the humerus.

Only after all of this preliminary work, designed to create more space for shoulder movement, *is the mobility of the shoulder directly challenged.* Usually the patient can flex and abduct the humerus at least 20 more degrees than he or she could at the beginning of the treatment session, with *no pressure exerted on the humerus to increase the flexion and ab-*

duction. In other words, gentle passive movement generally increases significantly as a result of the procedures described. Then, the clinician can hold the humerus at the limit of movement, and the patient can exert pressure (10% effort) to decrease flexion or abduction, holding for 4 seconds and then releasing (post-isometric relaxation). After full relaxation, the clinician can then advance the movement of the humerus into flexion or abduction until a new barrier is reached. This can be repeated. *At no time is the mobility of the humerus forcibly advanced.* Similar procedures can be used to increase external and internal rotation.

General Tips Regarding Treatment

Although the procedures described are the primary ones for treating shoulder dysfunctions, other techniques also can be useful and appropriate. Specific treatments may be necessary to address spinal involvement, clavicular restriction, anterior ribs in the chest, and so on. Furthermore, not all of these procedures would be vigorously performed on someone in the acute stage of frozen shoulder. Even with a patient who has a chronic condition, the clinician must assess exactly how much can be done in each session without generating excessive pain after treatment. Pain is usually counterproductive because it encourages the body to replace the myofascial involvement, which is precisely what is being treated. Some soreness and discomfort are expected, but pain should be avoided. Trigger point injection of the subscapularis, anterior serratus, and outer deep pectoralis muscles can be a helpful adjunct to the manual procedures in those patients who are making slower than normal progress, and those who reach a plateau in their rehabilitation without acceptable function and pain levels.

Patient Exercise and Home Care

Exercise During Acute Phase. Initially, the clinician encourages the patient to perform simple stretches in a pain-free range. The humerus can be stretched backward at a pain-free height, with the elbow straight and the forearm supinated and then pronated. The humerus also can be drawn forward across the torso, also at a pain-free height. Codman's exercises are often helpful as well—gentle swinging figure-eights performed with the humerus, while the patient's upper body is horizontal and the arm is dependent. Shoulder muscle stretches are performed every couple of hours during the waking day. Neck stretches are also important (see Chapter 3.)

The patient gently explores range of motion once or twice per day. Good relaxation for pain-free movement often is easier to achieve with a passive stretch. The patient raises the arm and supports the hand on a shelf or piece of furniture and then lowers his/her torso, and turns the torso so that the arm abducts as well as flexes. The patient should feel only slight discomfort during these procedures while attempting to maintain relaxed movement. If the patient can roll the scapulae back toward the spine without pain, then these shoulder retractions are performed every couple of hours, along with the stretches.

The clinician also instructs the patient to think about lifting the chest and letting the shoulders drop down and back, frequently throughout the day. Even if the patient only feels pain during the performance of certain movements, the shoulder is often unconsciously held in an elevated and forward guarded position during much of the day. The clinician often has to encourage the patient to voluntarily relax the shoulder down and back during the treatment procedures described above, and then encourages the patient to develop this awareness throughout the day.

Sleep position is an important feature of home care. Because patients are generally in significant pain when lying on the affected shoulder, they usually sleep with the involved shoulder up, and the arm dropping forward across

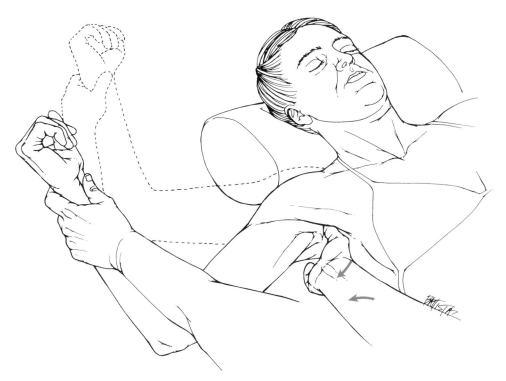

FIGURE 4-8. **Myofascial release 3 and 4 of the subscapularis muscle. A.** The beginning position for levels 3 and 4 myofascial release of the subscapularis muscle (indicated by the arm in solid line). The clinician contacts or pinches the subscapularis trigger points against the anterior surface of the scapula. **B.** The completion position for level 3 & 4 myofascial release of the subscapularis muscle (indicated by the arm in dotted line). While the trigger point contact is maintained, the patient actively or passively abducts the humerus. This procedure is repeated 3 or 4 times.

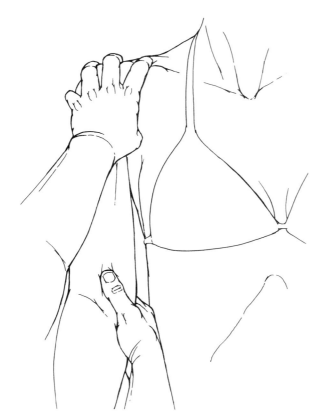

stretch the subscapularis. The patient lies supine on a bed or other flat surface and abducts the arm along the surface. When the patient hits the "catching" or painful point, the shoulder is relaxed and the scapula is dropped and retracted as much as possible, to allow further movement. When shoulder impingement is part of the clinical picture, the noninvolved arm reaches across the torso and raises the involved arm at the "catching" point and then lowers the arm again above the pain point, and the abduction movement is continued. This abduction exercise should become smoother and smoother over time until the pain and "catching" subside altogether.

Another advanced stretch is the bucket-seat stretch for elongating the pectoralis minor and coracobrachialis. The stretch is performed when the humerus continues to tilt forward and caudad, even after the other pectoral muscles have loosened and shoulder retraction has become easier. To stretch the right shoulder muscles, the patient sits in the driver's seat of a car with bucket seats, then reaches the right forearm behind the passenger seat (Fig. 4.11). The humerus is thus in an externally rotated and abducted position, with retraction. The combination of the stabilization of the back by the driver's seat and the stretch of the

FIGURE 4-9. Post Isometric Relaxation to release the anterior posture of the humerus. The clinician contacts the front of the shoulder with the thumb under the pectoral muscle. Gentle pressure is exerted toward the treatment table, to take up the tissue slack and retract the shoulder to its initial limit. The elbow is stabilized so that it is horizontal, along the side of the torso rather than dropping toward the table. The patient is instructed to press toward the ceiling with the shoulder for 4 seconds, against the clinician's resistance. When the patient releases pressure, the clinician's hand at the upper humerus drops further toward the table, taking up the tissue slack. This sequence is repeated 2 or 3 times.

the chest. The elbow also may be flexed. The patient thereby accentuates the postural and positional distortions during sleep and shortens many of the muscles the clinician is working to lengthen. To change this pattern, the clinician instructs the patient to keep the arm straight along the side of the body, or to drape the arm over a pillow just in front of the torso, with the arm extended at the elbow.

Advanced Exercises. As the patient's condition improves, stretching further into flexion and abduction will be possible while still keeping pain at a minimum. At this point, the clinician may want to introduce doorway stretches (Fig. 4-10). These stretches usually need to be performed one side at a time, because of the disparity in mobility of one side compared with the other. The clinician also can suggest specific stretches for the specific shoulder muscles that need to be elongated. For example, supine abduction of the humerus with external rotation can be a helpful way to

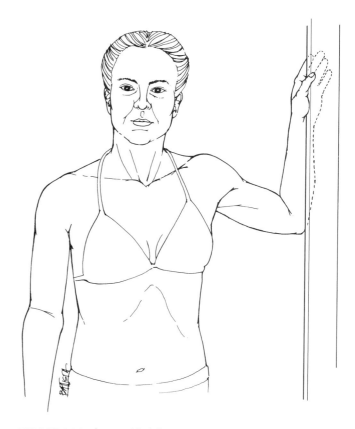

FIGURE 4-10. A one-sided doorway stretch to lengthen the pectoral muscles. Bilateral shoulder stretches are often too difficult to perform initially, but the patient can perform the stretches with one arm at a time, at several heights, taking care not to stretch into significant pain.

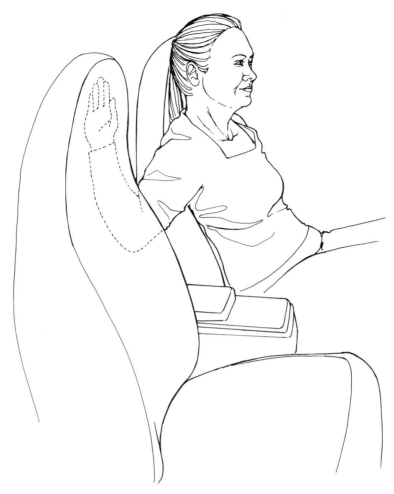

FIGURE 4-11. **A bucket-seat stretch to elongate the pectoralis minor and coracobrachialis.** The flat of the forearm is placed behind the bucket seat next to the patient. The combination of the stabilization behind the patient's back, and the position of the forearm, creates a good stretch.

shoulder muscles using the passenger's seat is quite effective. Once the patient feels the effect of this exercise in the car, it can be performed at home using regular household furniture.

In the later stages of rehabilitation, the middle and lower trapezius muscles frequently require strengthening exercise to counteract weakness and disuse. For example, a reverse pushup is performed standing, with the back leaning into the corner of a room, with the elbows at approximately shoulder height. The retraction of the shoulders lifts the back of the torso further from the corner (Fig. 4.12). At the gym, a reverse fly machine also can be used to strengthen these muscles. Another effective exercise is a prone arm raise performed on a bench with the arms abducted to 90° (for exercising the middle trapezius) and to 135° (for the lower trapezius) and with the thumbs pointing toward the ceiling (forearms supinated) (Fig. 4.13). The arms are raised and lowered in relation to the floor, 20° to 30°. Initially, the weight of the arms is often sufficient ex-

ercise. Later, the patient can hold a 3-lb. or 5-lb. weight in each hand. The patient should be careful to keep the neck relaxed. This exercise also can be performed with the patient erect, using various types of horizontal pulley apparatuses and counterweights.

A patient often can assist with treatment by lying on a ball to put pressure on trigger points and mobilize restricted rib–spinal joints. A tennis ball, handball, or racquetball is placed under the erector muscle, at the rib–spinal juncture while the patient lies supine and simply breathes and relaxes the shoulders back for 1/2 to 2 minutes until the tenderness decreases. The ball is then moved up or down the back to the next tender spot, and the procedure is repeated. This procedure for self-care is performed once daily. The upper rib–spinal joints may require mobilization during the early stages of treatment, and the lower rib–spinal junctures may require mobilization to accommodate the retraction and lowering of the scapula during later stages of treatment. The patient also

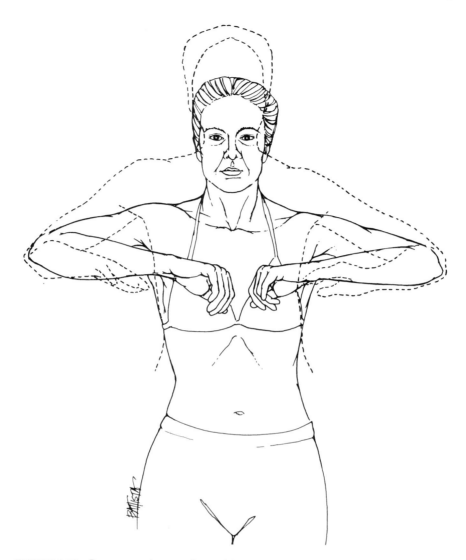

FIGURE 4-12. Reverse push-up performed in a corner to strengthen muscles of shoulder retraction. Initially the patient stands with the torso dropped into the corner, feet 12 to 18 inches from the corner, and elbows at shoulder height. Then the muscles between the scapulae: the rhomboid, middle, and lower trapezius contract to approximate the scapulae. The torso is thus lifted out from the corner. The elbows and feet stay in the same place. The degree of resistance involved in the exercise is controlled by the distance of the feet from the corner.

can use the ball to treat trigger points near the lateral border of the scapula (in the infraspinatus, teres major and minor, and anterior serratus muscles) by lying partly on the side with the ball under the trigger points. If the joint or muscle area is too tender for the use of a firm ball, a roll of socks or a hackey sack can be used initially.

TREATMENT PROTOCOL

The following protocol summarizes the elements that may need to be addressed to successfully and quickly treat frozen shoulder and shoulder dysfunction:

NOTE: The examiner should evaluate for other conditions that may have a similar presentation, including cervical radiculopathy, slipped bicipital tendon, and torn rotator cuff muscles. The protocol proposed is for treating a frozen shoulder or shoulder dysfunction without these other confounding conditions.

Also, the protocol is not intended to present a cookbook approach. The myofascial dysfunctions listed below are those most commonly encountered as part of the functional unit. The joint dysfunctions listed below are those that most commonly accompany the myofascial dysfunction. It is generally most efficient to treat the muscles that affect structural relationships first, and then to adjust or mobilize the restricted joint areas. It is also important to perform bilateral myofascial release, because latent trigger points on the opposite side of the body may perpetuate the postural patterns involved in frozen shoulder. How much time the clinician spends addressing the nonpainful side in the positions described (seated, side-lying, prone, and supine) will be determined by the degree of muscle and joint dysfunction encountered in each patient.

1. a. Perform myofascial release of the neck muscles, especially the levator scapula, scalene, splenius, and upper trapezius.

   b. Adjust or mobilize the subluxations of the cervical spine, which generally involve a lack of extension and lateral flexion toward the injured shoulder, at the C7, T1 level. Anterior or extension subluxation may accompany the scalene disorder and usually involve the C4, C5, C6 levels.

2. a. Release particularly the anterior border of the upper trapezius, which attaches to the clavicle.

   b. Assess and treat any remaining clavicular subluxation. (Usually the myofascial release will be sufficient to restore normal joint mechanics.)

3. a. Release the pectoralis and subclavicular muscles, particularly the band that forms the anterior border of the axilla, and the short fibers just medial to the anterior deltoid, which tend to pull the humerus too close to the clavicle. Also release the pectoralis minor, which tends to pull the head of the humerus forward and downward (inferior or caudad.) Also release the supraspinatus, if it is involved, because it also can hold the humerus too close to the clavicle.

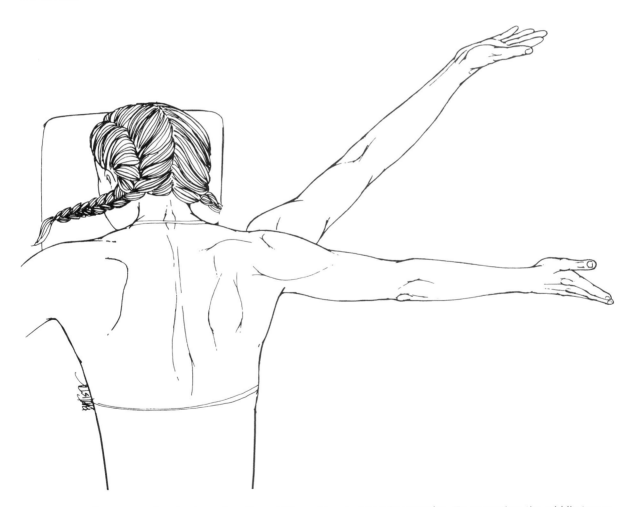

FIGURE 4-13. **Prone exercises to strengthen the middle and lower trapezius muscles.** To strengthen the middle trapezius, the arm is abducted to 90° and then lifted and lowered (toward the ceiling and toward the floor) 20°–30°. The thumb remains pointing toward the ceiling, to supinate the forearm and retract the humerus and scapula, so that the exercise will be localized to the middle trapezius to the extent possible. Then, with the thumb still pointing toward the ceiling, the arm is further abducted another 45°. Then the arm is lifted and lowered (toward the ceiling and toward the floor) 20°–30°. This position will engage the lower trapezius muscle. If the patient's neck muscles tend to tighten during this exercise, the head position can be lowered so that the upper trapezius and paraspinal muscles are placed on partial stretch.

b. Assess and manipulate or mobilize the humerus relative to the glenoid fossa. Also mobilize the humerus away from the clavicle, if there is restriction in this area. Anterior rib subluxations may need to be treated as well.

4. a. Release the subscapularis and anterior serratus, while stretching the humerus away from the scapula and also while stretching the scapula toward the spine and away from the humerus. (The abnormally shortened subscapularis tendon is usually prominent in the axilla with the arm raised.)

b. Mobilize the scapula toward the spine and flatten it against the rib cage.

5. a. Release the teres, triceps, and posterior deltoid to free up normal rotation of the humerus relative to the scapula.

b. Mobilize the humerus and the scapula, restoring a fold between the two when the humerus is in external rotation. (This muscle release and mobilization are critical to restoring the cocking-back movement involved in throwing a ball overhand.)

6. a. Release paraspinal muscles and other muscles medial to the shoulder blade.

b. Manipulate or mobilize the rib–thoracic subluxations and the flexion subluxations of the spine, thereby restoring flexibility to the rib cage. These subluxations are usually interscapular but also can be at levels below the scapula.

7. Evaluate and treat those muscles that contribute to shoulder pain via referred pain from trigger points: infraspinatus, serratus posterior superior, supraspinatus, biceps. These muscles are not as important in controlling structural relationships, but it is important that they be addressed.

8. Have the patient perform stretch retraining at home with all of the muscles involved in the myofascial pain syndrome. Stretches should be modified so that the patient *only stretches within a pain-free range* (not the traditional "no pain, no gain" approach often used with frozen shoulder patients). Also, the involved arm should be supported and extended during sleep, when side-lying on the opposite shoulder.

9. As structural relationships are restored, evaluate the strength of specific shoulder muscles, particularly the rhomboid and the middle and lower trapezius. If these muscles do not resume their normal functions, the shoulder will have a con-tinuing tendency to pull upward and forward. When prescribing exercise, avoid re-triggering the active trigger points that have been treated. This is accomplished by having the patient perform lengthening contractions, or having the patient perform mid-range shortening contractions with stretches of the same muscles before and after the contractions.

THORACIC OUTLET SYNDROME

by Robert Gerwin, MD

Thoracic outlet syndrome (TOS) is a painful condition of the shoulder, arm, and hand, caused by compression of the neurovascular bundle that is made up of the brachial plexus and the subclavian artery. The condition can occur primarily, though infrequently, as a vascular syndrome with features of claudication or embolization to the digits, or of venous congestion. More commonly TOS causes neurologic symptoms of pain in the shoulder and arm, numbness and tingling, usually in the ulnar nerve distribution in the hand, and weakness. The accepted type of TOS, well-defined and unambiguous, is termed true neurologic TOS. A disputed type of TOS, which is the subject of much debate, has been called nonspecific TOS (31,32). Nonspecific TOS is herein renamed myopathic TOS to emphasize the contribution of the myofascial trigger point to its development and persistence (Box 4.1).

The condition is of interest for two reasons. First, the elements of the brachial plexus may become compressed as a result of myofascial trigger points in the scalene muscles, narrowing the interscalene compartment or elevating the first rib toward the clavicle. The latter site of compression is the result of shortening of the scalene muscles by myofascial taut bands, which pull the first rib upward. Anomalous fibrous bands may be present, associated with a cervical rib or with a long C7 transverse process. The cervical rib or fibrous band can compress the brachial plexus. The brachial plexus also can be entrapped under the pectoralis minor muscle by trigger point taut bands, causing the so-called hyperabduction syndrome. Thus, it is possible that TOS, whether neurologic or myopathic, can be caused by myofascial trigger points that lead to nerve entrapment (Fig. 4-14).

Second, myofascial trigger points in the anterior and medial scalene muscles, the infraspinatus muscle, the latissimus dorsi, teres major and minor muscles, and the subscapularis muscle, can refer pain into the shoulder, down the arm, and into the hand. Myofascial pain syndrome (MPS) thus can mimic neurologic TOS in the absence of compression of elements of the brachial plexus. Although evaluation and treatment of shoulder dysfunction as described earlier in this chapter may be of benefit in the treatment of TOS, specific myofascial evaluation and treatment is predicated on an understanding of the locations of possible brachial plexus compression as well as the ability to

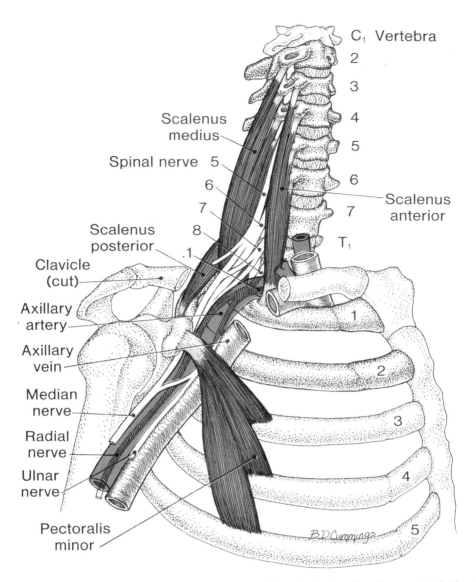

C₁ Vertebra
2
3
4
5
6
7
T₁

Scalenus medius
Spinal nerve 5
6
7
8
.1
Scalenus posterior
Clavicle (cut)
Axillary artery
Axillary vein
Median nerve
Radial nerve
Ulnar nerve
Pectoralis minor
Scalenus anterior

1
2
3
4
5

B.D.Cummings

FIGURE 4-14. Two sites of possible compression of the brachial plexus by trigger points in the scalene muscle. The upper or rostral site is the interscalene compartment, where shortening of the medial and anterior scalene muscles increase scalene muscle diameter and compress the interscalene compartment and its contents. The lower or more caudal site is the costoclavicular space between the clavicle and first rib, where the anterior and medial scalene muscles elevate the first rib and narrow the costoclavicular opening. The clavicle is cut away to show the compressed neurovascular bundle. Reprinted with permission from Simons DG, Travell JG, Simons LS: Travell & Simons' Myofascial Pain and Dysfunction: The Trigger Point Manual, vol 1: Upper Half of Body, 2nd Ed. Baltimore: Lippincott Williams & Wilkins, 1999, fig. 20.9 (p. 517).

BOX 4-1

Types of Thoracic Outlet Syndrome

A. True neurogenic thoracic outlet syndrome

   1. Occurrence: uncommon

   2. Etiology: focal neurologic impairment of lower trunk of brachial plexus function

   3. Symptoms and signs

     a. Paresthesias and sensory loss

     b. Weakness and muscle atrophy

     c. Pain

   4. Diagnostic study: electrodiagnostic studies show lowered ulnar nerve sensory amplitudes and lowered median nerve motor amplitudes

   5. Treatment: surgical

B. Vascular thoracic outlet syndrome

   1. Occurrence: rare

   2. Etiology: compression of the subclavian artery

   3. Symptoms and signs: emboli to the fingers and upper limb claudication

   4. Diagnostic test: angiography (e.g., magnetic resonance angiography)

   5. Treatment: surgical

C. Myopathic (formerly non-neurogenic or disputed) thoracic outlet syndrome

   1. Occurrence: common

   2. Etiology: in dispute (possibly mild or intermittent compression of brachial plexus; referred pain from myofascial trigger points in shoulder muscles)

   3. Symptoms and signs:

     a. Pain and paresthesias

     b. No neurologic impairment

     c. No vascular compression

     d. Myofascial trigger points that

       1) Refer pain to the shoulder, arm and hand, and

       2) Shorten muscles to compress brachial plexus elements

   4. Diagnostic test: clinical examination, including palpation of muscle for myofascial trigger points

   5. Electrodiagnostic studies and angiograms are normal

   6. Treatment: manual therapy directed to shoulder and neck muscles

---

identify and elicit patterns of referred pain from myofascial trigger points that contribute to the symptoms.

The nerve entrapment signs and symptoms of TOS, as well as the vascular manifestations, are well accepted when they are caused by a cervical rib or a demonstrated ligamentous band between the transverse process of C7 and the first rib. Malunion of a clavicular fracture with exuberant callus formation can produce the same findings by compressing the neurovascular bundle. The symptoms of pain and neurologic impairment in the case of brachial plexus nerve compression, and of vascular claudication and thrombotic embolization associated with subclavian stenosis (often with associated aneurysmal dilation), are well described. Results of electrodiagnostic tests often are abnormal in the cases with brachial plexus compression. These conditions may be associated with the development of symptomatic myofascial trigger points in shoulder region muscles. In fact, scapular dyskinesia, and the accompanying shoulder dysfunction with a posture of forward shoulders and head, often accompanies both neurologic and myopathic TOS.

Treatment that is directed toward correcting the anatomic cause is often surgical. The diagnosis is much less certain and is debatable when there is no demonstrated anatomic abnormality such as a cervical rib, and no electrodiagnostic abnormality. In circumstances in which the patient complains of shoulder and neck pain, and arm and hand pain, paresthesias, or numbness, especially in the ulnar and median nerve distributions, other sources of nerve compression, such as cubital and carpal tunnel syndromes, should be considered, and alternative causes of the symptoms should be sought. Myofascial trigger points may produce the anatomic basis for neurovascular compression as described above. Results of electrodiagnostic tests often are normal in these situations, perhaps because compression is intermittent. The two conditions, compression of the neural or vascular bundle and referred pain and sensory symptoms, can occur together. The diagnosis is made by physical examination, at which time the neck and shoulder region muscles are examined for myofascial trigger points. The treatment is directed toward relieving the underlying MPS.

TOS, or its simulated look-alike MPS, can be caused by any of the conditions that results in medial and anterior scalene muscle trigger points. In particular, it has been reported to occur after motor vehicle accidents (a whiplash-associated disorder)(33,34). In the group of 32 patients presented by Mailis et al. (33), the diagnosis was based on clinical findings, exclusion of conditions that could mimic TOS, and "positive objective data (if existent)." Eleven subjects had radiographic abnormalities associated with "droopy shoulders," including long C7 transverse processes. None had electrodiagnostic study abnormalities.

Brachial Plexus Anatomy

The ventral rami of C5 to T1 form three trunks (superior, medial, and inferior) that divide into ventral and dorsal divisions and form three cords. The three dorsal divisions form the posterior cord. The ventral divisions form the lateral and medial cords. The posterior cord gives rise to the radial nerve, the thoracodorsal nerve to the latissimus dorsi muscle, and the nerves to the subscapularis muscle and to the deltoid muscle. The lateral cord of the brachial plexus forms the musculocutaneous nerve and contributes to the median nerve, along with a contribution from the medial cord. The medial cord forms the medial brachial cutaneous nerve and the ulnar nerve.

Symptoms

Thoracic outlet syndrome is an entrapment or compression disorder of the brachial plexus as the nerves traverse the scalene compartment, pass between the clavicle and first rib along with the subclavian artery, and then pass between the pectoralis minor muscle and the coracoid process before entering the arm. Symptoms are pain in the shoulder, often involving the scapular region, radiating down the arm to the hand, particularly in the distribution of C8 and T1. Paresthesias, numbness, and weakness of the arm and the hand may occur, especially in the ulnar nerve distribution, but the C8 component also gives rise to the median nerve, so muscle weakness and atrophy in the muscles of the thenar eminence can result. Pain is generally increased when the arm is elevated above the head, as it is in cubital tunnel syndrome. Bending the elbow greater than 90° increases the symptoms of cubital tunnel syndrome but does not worsen TOS. The subclavian artery and vein also can be compressed in the thoracic outlet.

True TOS can present with either neurologic or vascular symptoms, or with symptoms of compression of the entire neurovascular bundle. Symptoms are increased by any activity that increases tension on the brachial plexus or that increases compression of the brachial plexus at a point of entrapment. The diagnosis is more certain when the full symptom complex is present, including pain, paresthesias, sensory loss, and weakness. The diagnosis is often made with only the complaints of pain and paresthesias. Complaints such as hemicranial headaches and anginal-like chest pains have been attributed to TOS. These nonspecific complaints broaden the differential diagnosis to include a wide spectrum of neck and shoulder problems.

Myofascial Thoracic Outlet Syndrome.

Perhaps more common than actual compression of brachial plexus elements is a myofascial syndrome that mimics TOS and is sometimes called pseudo-thoracic outlet syndrome, but which we prefer to call myogenic TOS. This may account for many of the cases that are classified as disputed TOS. No data are available on the incidence of this condition, nor any that compare the relative frequency of the myofascial TOS with that of true TOS. Macnab and McCulloch (35) state that "thoracic outlet syndromes may be assuming their rightful place as true but uncommon sources of pain in the arm." They mean that such conditions have been fashionable diagnoses, but much overdiagnosed, and that many of the conditions diagnosed as TOS were actually something else.

In myogenic TOS, referred pain from trigger points in the anterior and medial scalene muscles, the infraspinatus muscle, the subscapularis muscle, the posterior serratus superior muscle, and especially the latissimus dorsi muscle gives rise to pain in the shoulder region and down the arm in a pattern that mimics the pain of neurologic TOS. A referral pattern that looks like pain caused by compression of the lower nerve roots that make up the brachial plexus, or like compression of the medial cord of the brachial plexus that gives rise to the ulnar nerve, is seen in particular with trigger points in the latissimus dorsi muscle. Trigger points in the infraspinatus muscle more commonly mimic the pain pattern of the dorsal divisions of the three trunks of the plexus, which make up the posterior cord and the radial nerve.

Weakness that results from trigger points is related to motor inhibition of the muscle that has the trigger point or of a muscle in its functional unit. However, trigger points can develop in muscles within the referred pain zone, and they also may be inhibited and weak. Atrophy and neurologic impairment do not occur in trigger point–related weakness. Paresthesias develop in the pain referral zone, but actual sensory loss is unusual. Weakness in neurologic TOS is a result of nerve entrapment in the ulnar and median nerve distributions and is often associated with muscle atrophy. Sensory loss and paresthesias are often features of neurologic TOS. The following case history serves to illustrate the identification and treatment of myogenic TOS.

Etiology

An understanding of the nature of the problem is gained through insight into the mechanics of neuromuscular injury of the upper body quadrant. Thoracic outlet symptoms develop as a result of direct injury to the structures of the neck and shoulder region, or a combination of anatomic predisposition and overuse. A functional disturbance in the clavicular–first rib inlet to the chest as a result of static work that

CASE 4-4

Myogenic TOS

History

Ms. L.B. is a 38-year-old competitive long distance swimmer who was injured in a rear-end collision in an automobile, suffering a whiplash injury. She complained of neck and left shoulder pain. She reported numbness and tingling along the ulnar or medial aspect of her arm from above the elbow to the ring and fifth finger. Use of her arm and hand increased her arm and shoulder pain. Elevation (abduction and flexion) of her arm increased pain and tingling in the arm.

Examination

Neurologic examination showed sensory loss in the ulnar nerve distribution to the elbow without splitting the ring finger. Motor examination and deep tendon reflexes were normal. She was tender in the supraclavicular fossa. Electrodiagnostic studies were normal. There was no cervical rib. Myofascial trigger points in the scalene muscles, the infraspinatus muscle, the subscapularis muscle, and the latissimus dorsi muscle reproduced the pain and paresthesias reported by Ms. L.B.

Treatment

Treatment was directed toward the elimination of the trigger points through manual therapy directed toward the inactivation of trigger points and the restoration of pain-free range of motion, and through the use of trigger point injections. She continued to work throughout treatment. After 8 weeks of twice-weekly therapy, she was able to resume training in the pool. With continued therapy, reduced to once weekly, her arm pain decreased, and sensory symptoms subsided. She continued with self-stretching, occasional trigger point injections, and resumed training.

Follow-up

Nine months after the injury, she was first in her age-group in a 5-mile open water competitive swim, and she had no further symptoms suggestive of thoracic outlet syndrome.

---

stresses the upper limbs has been cited as a cause of TOS (36). The history and physical examination give insight into the mechanics of injury. Trauma to the neck and shoulder often involves a component of stretch. Whiplash is a common type of trauma in which the symptoms of TOS can occur (37,38). Postural dysfunction, especially rounded shoulders with head-forward posture associated with shortening of the scalene muscles, can lead to brachial plexus compression. People with long necks and sloping shoulders are anatomically predisposed to compression of the brachial plexus and the development of TOS symptoms. In such cases, the development of symptoms is usually indolent and may be associated with periods of unusual physical effort, giving rise to intermittent symptoms. History-taking should assess work and recreational habits for potential postural stresses.

The initial complaint often is pain that can precede other symptoms by as long as years. Paresthesias, dysesthesias, and finally weakness develop over time.

Inspection

The initial physical evaluation of the patient with pain in the shoulder radiating down the arm to the 4th and 5th digits, and with complaints of paresthesias in these digits, is assessment of the neck and shoulders. Patients should be assessed for long, slender necks and sloping shoulders. No literature is available that supports an increased incidence of cervical rib or ligamentous band from the transverse process of C7 to the first rib in such patients, but depressed shoulders seem to be associated with symptoms of TOS. Callus formation at the site of a clavicular fracture is readily visualized. Restricted movement of the neck occurs in cervical radiculopathy as well as in MPS. Restricted range of motion of the shoulder at the glenohumeral joint in internal or external rotation occurs in both MPS and articular disorders of the shoulder. Venous prominence in the arm and shoulder, and distal duskiness in the arm and hand, indicate vascular compression by TOS. Ulcerations of the tips of the fingers and splinter hemorrhages under the nails suggest embolism from a region of arterial stenosis at the thoracic outlet.

Physical Examination (Clinical Evaluation)

The usual tests for TOS are provocative tests that either increase the compression of the neurovascular bundle or stretch the nerves. The traditional tests are the Adson's maneuver, the military brace position, and the disputed abduction, external rotation, and exercise test. A positive response in each of these tests is the reproduction of the subject's symptoms of paresthesias, numbness, or pain. A drop in the radial pulse alone is not sufficient to call the test positive. In the Adson's maneuver, the affected arm is brought behind the body, the head is turned to the opposite side, and the patient is instructed to hold a deep breath. In the military brace position, the shoulders are thrown back with the shoulders in extension, forearms supinated, and the wrists extended with downward and backward traction on the shoulders to further compress the costoclavicular space.

The abduction, external rotation, and exercise test is performed by having the patient abduct the arms to shoulder level, flex the elbows to 90°, externally rotate the arm, and then repeatedly open and close the hands for 3 minutes. The appearance of tingling or pain in the hands or the arm is interpreted as a sign of TOS. However, the interpretation of the test is debated, because it is said to be abnormal in carpal tunnel syndrome as well. A "neurodynamic test" described by Butler and David (39) stresses the ulnar nerve by placing the wrist in extension, the forearm in pronation, the elbow in flexion, and the shoulder in lateral (external) rotation and abduction. To further stress the ulnar nerve, the head is bent laterally to the contralateral side. There are variations on this technique, and Butler and David advise the therapist to take into account the position or activity that brings about symptoms, and to modify the procedure in light of those provocative activities.

Examination of the motor system starts with inspection for atrophy. The most useful motor sign for TOS is atrophy of the ulnar innervated muscles; that is, the intrinsic muscles of the hand, particularly atrophy of the first dorsal interosseous muscle. Atrophy is not specific, in that other conditions such as cubital tunnel syndrome can cause this to occur, nor is the sign sensitive, in that sensory loss is more common and motor signs are not necessarily present. Pain and sensory abnormalities are commonly the early signs that precede motor changes, whereas atrophy of the dorsal interossei is seen in advanced cases. Deep tendon reflexes are generally normal, but the triceps and finger reflexes can be diminished or absent on the affected side.

Examination of the sensory system can show sensory loss in the distribution of the 8th cervical nerve and the 1st thoracic nerve, on the ulnar or medial side of the arm. There is no splitting of sensation of the ring finger as is typical of cubital tunnel syndrome, which occurs only in lesions of the more distal ulnar and median nerves rather than the proximal roots, trunks, and cords of the brachial plexus. Sensory loss in TOS is found in the fifth digit and extends a variable distance up the medial or ulnar aspect of the arm to the elbow or above to the inner aspect of the upper arm, in the C8–T1 dermatome distribution consistent with involvement of the lower trunk of the brachial plexus.

Diagnostic Studies

X-rays of the neck may show a cervical rib. Computed tomography (CT) or magnetic resonance imaging (MRI) scans of the neck can show hypertrophy of the scalene muscles and compression of the interscalene compartment. MRI imaging of the brachial plexus may show compression or distortion of the brachial plexus at the costoclavicular space. Cervical ribs also will be visible on MRI scans, and ligamentous bands from C7 to the first rib can be visualized.

Electrodiagnostic studies are notoriously insensitive to brachial plexus dysfunction in TOS, a source of controversy that has led to the questioning of the concept of TOS, but probably reflecting the mix of true neurogenic and nonspe-

cific myogenic TOS. A reduction in the amplitude of the ulnar sensory and median motor nerve responses are the most useful signs, especially the medial antebrachial cutaneous sensory nerve action potential (40). Results of motor nerve conduction studies and the electromyogram of affected muscles are abnormal in neurogenic TOS, but are unreliable in myogenic TOS and serve at best to identify other abnormalities that are relevant to the differential diagnosis, such as cervical radiculopathy or carpal tunnel syndrome. Attempts to refine the electrodiagnostic identification of TOS, such as using somatosensory evoked potentials, have been mixed and largely unsuccessful when compared with the standard electrodiagnostic tests. The diagnosis of TOS largely remains a clinical diagnosis, with electrodiagnostic confirmation most consistent in true neurologic TOS.

Differential Diagnosis

The differential diagnosis includes any lesion of the brachial plexus that is insidious or traumatic. Acute brachial plexus lesions, such as the Parsonage-Turner syndrome, are not likely to be confused with TOS. However, cervical spondylosis with radiculopathy can be confused with TOS, especially if multiple lower roots are involved. Pancoast's tumor causes pain and sensorimotor loss, and can be symptomatic for as long as months or years before the diagnosis is made by imaging the chest. Postradiation brachial plexitis occurs between 6 and 36 months after the completion of radiation.

Shoulder injuries such as rotator cuff tears can simulate the local pain of TOS. Myofascial pain syndrome can mimic true TOS insofar as it produces a referred pain pattern that can be similar to the distribution of pain in true TOS. Sensory loss and muscular atrophy are not seen in the referred pain syndrome of myofascial trigger point pain unless they occur as a consequence of nerve compression.

Carpal tunnel syndrome (CTS) is most important in the differential diagnosis of TOS, because thenar wasting in the lateral (radial) side of the hand is seen in both neurogenic TOS and in the median nerve entrapment syndrome of CTS. The sensory distribution is different in the two conditions, however. Moreover, the full sensorimotor expression of the two conditions is different because ulnar nerve distribution sensory loss and motor impairment is not seen in CTS, but is seen in TOS.

Conventional Treatment

If there is definite vascular impairment, particularly if there are symptoms of vascular claudication when the arm or hand are used, or if there is thrombosis or embolization to the arm, hand, or fingers, surgical treatment is required. Conventional treatment for neurologic TOS includes the assessment of emotional stress, depression, and sleep disturbance, which is part of the treatment plan for all chronic pain syndromes.

The initial specific treatment of TOS is physical therapy. Physical therapy, including the development of a self-directed treatment program followed by the patient, is directed toward increasing the thoracic aperture through normalizing the relationship between the first rib and the clavicle, and restoring normal motion to the cervical spine. This approach addresses postural dysfunction, relaxation of "tight" muscles, strengthening of the shoulder muscles, sleep positions that may enhance brachial plexus entrapment or compression, and ergonomic or work-related mechanical stresses. A forward-shoulder posture or cervicodorsal kyphosis associated with weakness of the trapezius muscles results in a narrowing of the costoclavicular space. Opening this space by strengthening the trapezius muscles, lengthening the pectoral muscles, and reducing the head-forward position associated with kyphosis is a primary goal of physical therapy.

Recommended treatment protocols currently found in the literature include a set of exercises that involve: 1) bringing the shoulders backwards and up; 2) flexing the thoracic spine and dropping the shoulders forwards and down; and 3) straightening the back and bringing the shoulders backwards again. These maneuvers are supposed to mobilize the shoulder and stretch the pectoral muscles and the middle trapezius and rhomboid muscles. Other exercises include: 4) a chin tuck with the neck straight that is supposed to normalize upper cervical spine movement, to improve scalene muscle function; 5) activating the scalene muscles by isometric contraction of the medial, anterior, and posterior scalene muscles in sequence is intended to restore normal function of the first ribs and the costoclavicular space through which the brachial plexus passes; 6) Stretching exercises for the scalene and levator scapulae muscles completes the treatment (41). Another possible initial treatment is directed toward strengthening shoulder muscles and injecting the trigger points (42).

If physical therapy fails to relieve symptoms, surgery is often recommended. The surgical procedures currently used are resection of the first rib to open the costoclavicular space, and sectioning the anterior scalene muscle (scalenotomy) to relieve compression in the interscalene compartment and assist in the dropping of the first rib. Ligamentous bands and cervical ribs are sectioned or removed when found. The outcome depends on the strictness of the criteria used for surgical selection. When a cervical rib is identified or a ligamentous band is seen on MRI, or the brachial plexus is seen to be deformed on the MRI scan, the surgical outcomes are better than when surgery is performed without objective neurologic signs or the above-mentioned structural causes of plexus compression. Controversy has arisen over the large numbers of surgical procedures done for putative TOS without objective neurologic signs, particularly because there is potential injury to the brachial plexus or the subclavian artery during surgery.

The diagnosis of neurovascular compression may be suspected from symptoms suggesting claudication but is quite firm when there is ulceration or gangrene of the fingers or pallor or duskiness of the hand or fingers. Angiography will confirm the diagnosis of vascular compression, precompression or post-compression aneurysmal dilatation, or stenosis, including that caused by clot. Surgery is definitely indicated when there is unequivocal evidence of vascular involvement.

Myofascial Treatment

Initial treatment for neurologic TOS is appropriately non-operative, unless signs of advanced neurologic impairment with muscle weakness or wasting are present. Nonoperative treatment is certainly indicated for disputed TOS, and for TOS with vague and imprecise symptoms that do not clearly implicate specific neural involvement. This also applies to the diagnosis of myogenic TOS made on the basis of pain and perhaps paresthesias, where myofascial trigger points are involved in the genesis of the symptoms.

TOS is best treated by manual therapy and trigger point injections or dry needling when myofascial trigger points are a major component of the presentation. Trigger points can be central to the development of TOS through the aforementioned compression of the interscalene compartment by scalene muscle trigger points, by elevation of the first rib by shortening of the scalene muscles, by compressing the neurovascular bundle under the coracoid process by trigger points in the pectoralis minor muscle, or because trigger points can cause symptoms that mimic the pain of true neurologic TOS.

The specific manual therapy of the trigger points that are directly or indirectly related to TOS or a TOS-like syndrome includes inactivation of the trigger point by compression and local stretch, then a therapeutic stretch, and instruction in a self-directed program of stretching. In addition, attention always must be directed toward the identification and correction of mechanical perpetuating factors such as ergonomic or postural stresses. Specific therapeutic approaches are described for five key muscles.

Scalene Muscles

1. Trigger point compression. The patient lies supine. The clinician sits at the head of the patient, facing the patient's feet. The clinician's one hand stabilizes the patient's head. The other hand palpates the medial scalene to locate the trigger point. Once found, the trigger point is compressed with the tip of one or two fingers, using moderate pressure. The medial scalene muscle is found ventral to the upper part of the levator scapula muscle. The anterior scalene muscle is located ventral to the medial scalene, under the lateral edge of the sternocleidomastoid muscle. The clinician can confirm the location of each of these muscles by using the "sniff test," by feeling the accessory respiratory scalene muscles contract when the patient performs a short series of vigorous sniffs. Pain may be elicited initially, but it should begin to subside within 15 to 20 seconds. The head is now tilted laterally approximately 20° to the opposite side, and then slowly brought back to the midline for approximately 2 to 5 seconds. This lateral head movement is repeated approximately 5 or 6 times.

2. Local stretch. The clinician's index and middle fingers move together along the scalene muscle trigger point taut band in a rostral to caudal direction for a distance of approximately 1 to 2 inches, providing local tissue stretching. Massage oil or cream will facilitate this movement.

3. Myofascial release. The clinician strokes the side of the neck, including the scalene muscle, using the palm of the hand or the back of the fingers, moving in a rostral to caudal direction.

4a. Therapeutic stretch. The patient lies supine. The clinician stands at the patient's head and bends the neck laterally to the contralateral side with the one hand, while the other hand depresses the first rib ipsilateral to the side being treated (deep to the clavicle, at the anterior base of the neck.) This provides a stretch of the medial scalene muscle and lowers the first rib when it is elevated. The anterior scalene muscle is stretched by bending the head laterally to the opposite side while extending the head, tilting the chin upward while rotating the face slightly to the side being stretched (see Fig. 1-9). Stretch may be enhanced by using the postisometric contraction–relaxation technique described by Lewit (43), or the intermittent vapo-coolant spray and stretch technique.

4b. Mobilization of the ribs. The patient lies supine. The clinician supports the ipsilateral upper arm in 50° of flexion and 30° of abduction, to reduce pectoral muscle tension. The clinician uses the other hand to release muscle tension between the clavicle and the 2nd and 3rd ribs, attempting to make a space. The pressure starts medially, next to the sternum, and continues to the end of the clavicle. During these releases, the patient is encouraged to breathe deeply and exhale fully. With each exhalation, the clinician presses down (caudally) away from the clavicle to further mobilize the ribs.

5. Self-stretch. The patient sits or stands. The patient's head faces forward. The head is passively allowed to fall to the contralateral side, bringing the contralateral ear to the shoulder, to stretch the medial scalene muscle. To self-stretch the anterior scalene, the head is brought into the same lateral bend as in stretching the medial scalene and then extended and the chin elevated. The contralateral arm may be brought over the head, the back of the hand used to gently guide, but not force, the head into the stretch position. The stretch is held for 15 to 30 seconds as tolerated.

Latissimus Dorsi Muscle

1. Trigger point compression. The patient lies supine, the arm on the side to be treated is abducted 90°, the elbow flexed 90° and externally rotated. The clinician sits or stands at the patient's side, facing the patient. The clinician firmly compresses the myofascial trigger point taut band in a pincer group with the fingers and thumb of one hand. The other hand guides the patient in a slow, active (not passive) internal rotation of the arm through a short arc of 5° to 10° and back again to the starting point. This is repeated 5 to 6 times, until the tenderness diminishes.

2. Local stretch. The therapist grasps the trigger point taut band between the fingers and thumb of one hand and moves along the band from the insertion at the humerus toward the thorax, or in a superior to inferior direction. Massage oil or cream will facilitate this movement.

3. Myofascial release. The clinician moves the palm of the hand or the back of the fingers downward along the belly of the muscle from the arm to the thorax, using massage oil or cream to facilitate the movement. This is repeated several times.

4. Therapeutic stretch. The patient lies in the lateral decubitus position; the side to be treated is superior. A pillow or rolled towel is placed under the inferior flank to raise the patient above the waist. The arm is abducted over the head. The superior leg is dropped behind the inferior leg to lower the superior pelvic brim. The clinician stands at the side of the patient and places one hand on the humerus distal to the shoulder, and one hand on the pelvic brim. The therapist then pulls the humerus through abduction toward the side or back of the head and simultaneously pushes the pelvic brim downward (Fig. 4-15). Postisometric contraction–relaxation will facilitate the stretch. Intermittent vapo-coolant spray and stretch can be performed, applying the cold stimulus with one hand, while pulling the abducted arm craniad with the other hand.

5. Self-stretch. The patient sits with a $1\frac{1}{2}$- to 2-inch lift under the contralateral ischial tuberosity to tip the pelvis. The arm on the side to be stretched is abducted over the head and is grasped at the wrist by the other hand. The arm is then pulled upward, across and over the head, as the patient leans to the contralateral side. The tilted pelvis facilitates the self-stretch. The stretch is held for 15 to 30 seconds.

Pectoralis Minor Muscle

1. Trigger point compression. The patient lies in the supine position, with the arm slightly abducted. The clinician sits or stands at the patient's side. One hand stabilizes the shoulder, while the treating hand palpates the pectoralis minor under the pectoralis major muscle. In people of moderate or slight build, the muscle can be palpated through the pectoralis major muscle. In either case, the muscle is located between the superior attachment to the coracoid process and the inferior attachment to the third through fifth ribs. The index and middle fingers compress the trigger point taut band while

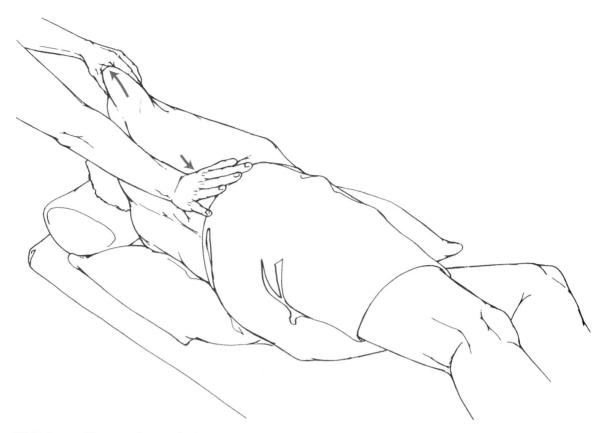

FIGURE 4-15. **Therapeutic stretch of the latissimus dorsi muscle.** The patient is side-lying; the side to be treated is superior. The clinician stands at the side of the table at the patient's back, at the patient's shoulder. To stretch the right latissimus dorsi muscle, the clinician uses the left hand to hold the patient's arm between the shoulder and the elbow. The latissimus dorsi muscle inserts on the humerus below the shoulder. Therefore, the clinician must apply force to the humerus, and not the scapula. The clinician's right hand is placed on the patient's hip. The latissimus dorsi muscle inserts on the pelvic brim, so that the pelvic brim must be moved away from the shoulder. A pillow is placed under the patient's waist to provide more stretch to the long, slack muscle. The direction of force is downward (caudally directed) at the waist and upward (rostrally directed) at the arm. This stretch also stretches the subscapularis and teres major muscles.

the patient slowly moves the shoulder slightly upwards, holds for 2 seconds, and then returns to the starting position. This is repeated 5 to 6 times.

2. Local stretch. The patient and clinician remain in the same position as in the trigger point compression procedure. The index and long fingers move along the trigger point taut band from the coracoid process towards the insertion on the ribs. This is repeated 5 to 6 times.

3. Myofascial release. The patient and clinician remain in the same position as before. The therapist runs the palm of the hand or the back of the fingers down the lateral chest from the coracoid process toward the insertion on the ribs. Massage oil or cream facilitates the movement.

4. Therapeutic stretch. The patient remains in the supine position. A rolled towel is placed under the back to elevate the shoulder above the table. The clinician stands at the side of the patient, facing the patient's head. One

hand holds the patient's elbow, and lifts it approximately 45° above the table and uses the humerus to push the scapula upward, while the other hand pushes the shoulder posteriorly (Fig 4-16).

5. Self-stretch. There are several ways to stretch the pectoralis minor muscle. One way is to stand in a doorway, the arm elevated above the shoulder, and slightly extended, the hand holding the door jamb. The patient then turns with the feet away from the door jamb extending the arm farther to bring the scapula into posterior retraction.

Infraspinatus Muscle

1. Trigger point compression. The patient lies in the lateral decubitus position, the affected side superior. The patient's head, arm, and knees are supported by pillows. The affected arm is flexed to 90° at the elbow. The cli-

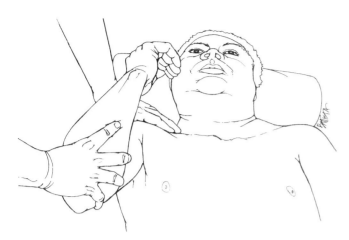

FIGURE 4-16. **Therapeutic stretch of the pectoralis minor muscle.** The patient is supine. The clinician stands at the patient's side. To stretch the right side, the right arm is flexed at the elbow. A pillow is placed under the patient's back, allowing the shoulders to fall backward to the table. The clinician's right hand holds the patient's elbow. The left hand is placed on the patient's right shoulder, contacting the coracoid process and acromion. The patient's arm is angled approximately 45° above the horizontal. The direction of force applied to the elbow by the right hand is toward the shoulder. The direction of force applied to the shoulder with the left hand is downward, to depress the shoulder. The effect is to elevate and retract the scapula.

nician sits behind the patient at the shoulder level. One hand stabilizes the shoulder while the treating hand compresses the trigger point taut band against the scapula with the index and middle fingers. The patient is instructed to raise the forearm while keeping the elbow against the side, thereby externally (laterally) rotating the arm at the shoulder. The forearm is then slowly brought back to the starting position. This is repeated slowly after a 2-second pause for about 5 to 6 repetitions.

2. Local stretch. The clinician moves the thumb or index and middle fingers firmly along the taut band from the inferior and lateral border of the scapular to the shoulder joint. Massage oil or cream will facilitate this procedure.

3. Myofascial release. The palm of the hand or the back of the hand and fingers moves across the skin over the scapula from the lower border of the scapula to the shoulder. Massage cream or oil will facilitate the treatment.

4. Therapeutic stretch. The patient sits with the clinician standing behind the patient. A pillow may be placed between the patient and the clinician to avoid direct body contact. The clinician anchors the scapula by firmly grasping it by the lateral border, and stabilizes the patient by placing the other hand on the contralateral shoulder. The patient brings the affected arm across the chest. The opposite hand grasps the humerus from be-

low and pulls the arm across the chest. The clinician counters the effect of this movement to bring the scapula into protraction by holding the scapula in retraction (Fig. 4-17).

5. Self-stretch. The self- stretch is the same for the patient as the therapeutic stretch, but without the stabilization of the scapula by the clinician.

Subscapularis Muscle

1. Trigger point compression. The patient lies supine, the arm on the affected side abducted and externally rotated. The clinician sits or stands at the patient's side. The trigger point taut band is compressed against the undersurface of the scapula with the long and middle fingers of the treating hand. The other hand guides the abducted and flexed arm as it actively moves slowly in internal and external rotation at the elbow through an arc of 5° to 10°, 5 to 6 times.

2. Local stretch. The clinician's index and middle fingers move along the trigger point taut band in an inferior to superior direction for a distance of 1 to 2 inches, repeated 5 to 6 times.

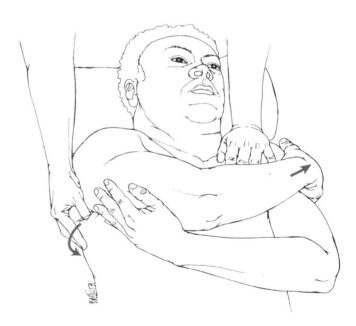

FIGURE 4-17. **Therapeutic stretch of the infraspinatus muscle.** The patient is supine. The clinician stands by the head of the patient on the side to be treated, facing the patient. To stretch the right side, the clinician places the right hand against the patient's right scapula, using the heel of the hand to stabilize the scapula. The clinician's left hand holds the patient's left shoulder to stabilize the patient. The patient holds the right arm to be stretched, above the elbow with the left hand, and pulls the right arm across the chest. The clinician resists the lateral movement of the scapula with the right hand during the stretch.

3. Myofascial release. The patient is in a side-lying position with the arm at the side. The clinician uses cream
or oil and lifts the arm slightly to insert the thumb
between the lateral border of the scapula and the rib
cage and then lowers the arm. The clinician contacts the
subscapularis taut bands high up in the posterior axilla,
and slides the hand along the anterior surface of the
scapula, as far medially as possible, from anterior to
inferior.

4. Therapeutic stretch. The patient is again in supine position with the arm to be treated held in abduction at
the shoulder, flexed 90° at the elbow, and externally
rotated. The clinician stands at the side of the patient
below the abducted arm. One hand is place on the
humerus just above the elbow. The elbow of that arm
is placed on the shoulder to stabilize it and prevent excessive motion at the shoulder. The other hand grasps
the patient's arm at the wrist and moves the arm into
external rotation. The patient alternately isometrically
meets the downward force of the clinician's hand, and
then relaxes as the clinician moves the arm in external
rotation (post-isometric relaxation technique). This
continues until the full tolerable external rotation is
reached (Fig 4-18).

5. Self-stretch. The patient sits and raises the arm to be
treated above the head. The arm is grasped at the wrist

by the other hand and brought over the head to the contralateral side.

CONCLUSION

The treatment model described in this chapter is designed
to address the particular pattern of myofascial involvement
and joint dysfunction commonly seen in patients with
shoulder dysfunction and frozen shoulder. The performance of these procedures generally results in marked and
relatively rapid gains in comfortable range of motion, with
relatively little pain. The success of this treatment approach—even for patients who have long-standing problems including arthritis and joint replacement—suggests
that the central pathologic condition of frozen shoulder is
typically muscle and joint dysfunction, rather than adhesions or fibrosis and shrinking of the capsule.

As summarized earlier in Technique 4-2, the different
types of TOS require different methods of evaluation and
treatment. Because myopathic TOS is the most common of
these conditions, recognition of the role of the myofascial
disorder and appropriate specific myofascial treatment
methods can bring resolution even in patients who have had
chronic problems and previous treatment failures.

References

1. Weber M, Prim J, Bugglin R. Long-term follow up of patients with
frozen shoulder after mobilization under anesthesia, with special reference to the rotator cuff. Clin Rheum 1995; 14:686–691.
2. Ott JW, Clancy WG, Wilk KE. Soft tissue injuries in the shoulder. In:
Andrews JR, Wilk KE, eds. The Athlete's Shoulder. New York:
Churchill-Livingstone, 1994:250–254.
3. Murnaghan JP. Adhesive capsulitis of the shoulder: current concepts
and treatment. Orthopedics 1988;11:153–158.
4. Wiley AM. Arthroscopic appearance of frozen shoulder. Arthroscopy
1991;7:138–143.
5. Noel E. Treatment of calcific tendinitis and adhesive capsulitis of the
shoulder. Rev Rheum [Eng] 1997;64(11):619–628.
6. Nevaiser RJ, Nevaiser TJ. The frozen shoulder: diagnosis and management. Clin Orthop Rel Res 1987;223:59–64.
7. Anton HA. Frozen shoulder. Can Fam Physician 1993;39:
1773–1778.
8. Biundo J Jr. Frozen shoulder. Bull Rheum Dis 1995; 43(8):1–3.
9. Post M, ed. The Shoulder: Surgical and Nonsurgical Management.
Philadelphia: Lea & Febiger, 1988:338–342.
10. Shaffer B, Tibone JE, Kerlan RK. Frozen shoulder: a long-term follow
up. J Bone Joint Surg Am 1992;74:738–746.
11. Rizk TE, Gavant ML, Pinals RS. Treatment of adhesive capsulitis
(frozen shoulder) with arthrographic capsular distension and rupture.
Arch Phys Med Rehabil 1994;75:803–807.
12. Ozaki J, Nakagawa Y, Sakurai G. Recalcitrant chronic adhesive capsulitis of the shoulder. J Bone Joint Surg Am 1989;71:1511–1515.
13. Uitvlugt G, Detrisac D, Johnson LL, et al. Arthroscopic observations
before and after manipulation of frozen shoulder. J Arthroscop Rel
Surg 1993;9:181–185.
14. Bunker TD. Frozen shoulder: unraveling the enigma. Ann R Coll Surg
Engl 1997;79(3):210–213.
15. Bunker TD, Anthony PP. The pathology of frozen shoulder: a
Dupuytren-like disease. J Bone Joint Surg Br 1995;77:677–683.
16. Hulstyn MJ, Weiss APC. Adhesive capsulitis of the shoulder. Orthop
Rev 1993;22:425–433.
17. Wadsworth CT. Frozen shoulder. Phys Ther 1986;66:1878–1883.

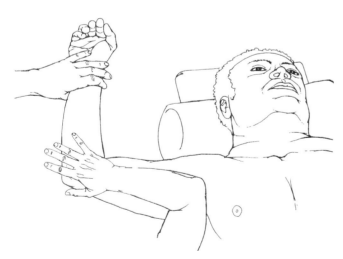

FIGURE 4-18. Therapeutic stretch of the subscapularis muscle.
The patient is supine. The clinician stands at the side of the patient, facing the patient's head. To stretch the right side, the patient's arm is abducted 90°, level with the shoulder. The arm is
bent at the elbow to bring the right hand above the shoulder. The
clinician holds the right arm just above the elbow to stabilize it,
and uses the forearm to press down on the shoulder and stabilize
it, preventing torsion of the shoulder capsule, while the left hand
is placed on the volar surface of the patient's forearm, just above
the wrist. The direction of force is downward, applied to the forearm and wrist, to produce external rotation of the arm.

18. Rizk TE, Christopher RP, Pinals RS. Adhesive capsulitis (frozen shoulder): a new approach to its management. Arch Phys Med Rehabil 1983;64:29–33.

19. Miller MD, Wirth MA, Rockwood CA Jr. Thawing the frozen shoulder: the "patient" patient. Orthopedics 1996;19:849–853.

20. Mao CY, Jaw WC, Cheng HC. Frozen shoulder: correlation between the response to physical therapy and follow-up arthrography. Arch Phys Med Rehabil 1997;78:857–859.

21. Souza TJ, ed. Frozen shoulder. In: Sports Injuries of the Shoulder. New York: Churchill Livingstone, 1994:441–455.

22. Hill JJ Jr, Bogumill H. Manipulation in the treatment of frozen shoulder. Orthopedics 1988;11:1255–1260.

23. Bunker TD. Time for a new name for "frozen shoulder." Br Med J 1985;290:1233–1234.

24. Warner JJP, Allen A, Marks PH. Arthroscopic release for chronic refractory adhesive capsulitis of the shoulder. J Bone Joint Surg Am 1996;78(12):1808–1816.

25. Simons DG, Travell JG, Simons LS. Myofascial Pain and Dysfunction: The Trigger Point Manual, vol 1, 2nd Ed. Baltimore: Williams & Wilkins; 1999:596–611.

26. Calliet R. Shoulder Pain. Philadelphia: F.A. Davis, 1991:1–50.

27. Simons DG, Travell JG, Simons LS. Myofascial Pain and Dysfunction: The Trigger Point Manual, vol 1, 2nd Ed. Baltimore: Williams & Wilkins; 1999:94–177.

28. Simons DG, Travell JG, Simons LS. Myofascial Pain and Dysfunction: The Trigger Point Manual, vol 1, 2nd Ed. Baltimore: Williams & Wilkins, 1999:538–551.

29. Walther DS. Applied Kinesiology, vol 1. Pueblo, CO: Systems DC, 1981.

30. Thie JF. Touch for Health. Pasadena, CA: TH Enterprises, 1987: 11.

31. Roos DB, Wilbourn AJ. Thoracic outlet syndrome (issues and opinions), Muscle and Nerve 1999:126–138.

32. Dawson DM, Hallett M, Wilbourn AJ, eds. Entrapment Neuropathies, 3rd Ed. Philadelphia: Lippincott–Raven, 1999:227–250.

33. Mailis A, Papagapiou M, Vanderlinden R, et al. Thoracic outlet syndrome after motor vehicle accidents in a Canadian pain clinic population. Clin J Pain 1995;11:316–324.

34. Sanders RJ. Etiology. In: Sanders RJ, Haug CE, eds. Thoracic Outlet Syndrome. A Common Sequela of Neck Injuries. Philadelphia: Lippincott, 1991:21–31.

35. Macnab I, McCulloch J. Neck Ache and Shoulder Pain. Baltimore: Williams & Wilkins, 1994:446.

36. Lindgren K-A, Manninen H, Rytkönen H. Thoracic outlet syndrome: a functional disturbance of the thoracic upper aperture? Muscle & Nerve 1995;18:526–530.

37. Capistrant TD. Thoracic outlet syndrome in whiplash injury. Ann Surg 1977;185:175–178.

38. Hong CZ, Simons DG. Response to treatment for pectoralis minor myofascial pain syndrome after whiplash. J Musculoskel Pain 1993;1:89–129.

39. Butler DS. The Sensitive Nervous System. Noigroup Publications, Unley DC, 5061 Australia 2000:332–336.

40. Maggiano H, Levin KH, Wilbourn AJ. Relationship between medial antebrachial cutaneous sensory and median motor response in brachial plexopathy. Muscle Nerve 1993;16:113.

41. Lindgren K-A. Conservative treatment of thoracic outlet syndrome: a two year follow-up. Arch Phys Med Rehabil 1997;78:373–378.

42. Moseley LH, Kalafut RM, Levinson PD, et al. Cumulative trauma disorders and compression neuropathies of the upper extremities. In: Kasdan ML, ed. Occupational Hand & Upper Extremity Injuries and Diseases. Philadelphia: Hanley & Belfus, Inc., 1991:359–362.

43. Lewit K. Manipulative Therapy in Rehabilitation of the Locomotor System, 2nd Ed. Oxford: Butterworth-Heinemann, 1991:190–192.

44. Loeser JD. Pain after amputations, phantom limb and stump pain. In: Bonica JJ, ed. The management of pain, 2nd ed. Baltimore: Williams & Wilkins, 1990:244–56.

5 *Tennis Elbow*

Michael Schneider, DC

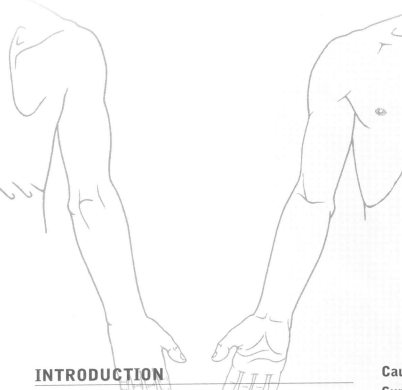

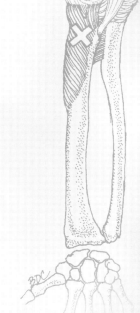

INTRODUCTION

The generic term, tennis elbow (TE), is frequently used by the general public to describe any condition in which pain and tenderness are found in the area around the lateral (radial) aspect of the elbow. The term probably came into popular use because the condition is common among amateur tennis players, and people saw an apparent cause-and-effect relationship. However, clinicians see just as many cases of lateral elbow pain resulting from other causes, and these could be labeled "cashier's elbow," "keyboard elbow," "writer's elbow," "carpenter's elbow," "dentist's elbow," "chiropractor's elbow," and so on. As Travell and Simons note, "the symptoms of tennis elbow appear in the literature as a confusing polyglot of conditions ascribed chiefly to overstrain of the hand extensors at the wrist" (1).

The use of the computer, keyboard, and mouse continues to proliferate in daily life, with the associated problem of pain from repetitive strain of the tissues of the forearm, wrist, and elbow. The term cumulative trauma disorder (CTD) is used to describe any painful condition that has developed as the result of prolonged overuse or repetitive strain. It is becoming commonplace for clinicians to see patients with overuse syndromes involving the muscles of the hand, wrist, and forearms. These CTDs are quickly catching up with lower back pain as the most common "injuries" reported in worker's compensation claims.

Physicians prefer to use the term lateral epicondylitis (LE) instead of tennis elbow, supposedly because it is a more "tissue-specific" diagnosis. This term probably originated with the clinical observation that patients had very localized pain from palpation or percussion directly over the bony prominence of the lateral epicondyle. However, on closer inspection, it is clear the term *epicondylitis* is a misnomer. It is highly unlikely that the epicondyle itself is inflamed. If the epicondyle were truly inflamed, a more appropriate diagnosis would be *periostitis*. The term *epicondylalgia* is gradually emerging in the literature, which is clearly a more accurate and tissue-specific diagnosis.

Most clinicians would concur with the opinion that the pain of LE is generated from injury to, or overuse of, the soft tissues that attach to the lateral epicondyle of the humerus. This chapter focuses on the specific soft tissues that are thought to be responsible for lateral elbow pain.

TENNIS ELBOW: BACKGROUND

The Problem of Diagnosis

Cyriax outlined a very simple and logical diagnostic sequence for determining which type of soft tissues are involved with any case of musculoskeletal pain (2,3). He suggested that the clinician divide all of the soft tissues surrounding a joint into two basic categories: inert tissues and contractile tissues. His method of differential diagnosis between inert and contractile tissues relies on the basic mechanism of *selective tension* applied by manual resistance examination methods.

The inert tissues are examined by applying vectors of force designed to purposefully strain ligaments, joint capsules, or nerves. If the patient feels pain on passive end-range strain, this implicates these inert structures as the pain generators. The anterior drawer test, or Lachman's test, for determining the integrity of the anterior cruciate ligament is an example of passive tension applied to inert structures of the knee. The clinically relevant inert structures in the vicinity of the lateral epicondyle are the joint capsule and ligaments. To determine whether these structures are painful, it is necessary to perform various passive testing maneuvers designed to put stress on these tissues; for example, valgus stress at the end range of an elbow extension tests the ulnar collateral ligament. As a general rule, inert structures around the elbow are not the typical pain generators in cases of LE. Other texts more completely describe testing procedures regarding joint play and ligament and capsular injuries (4,5).

Contractile tissues are the muscles and their associated tendons, which are almost without exception the major pain-generating tissues found to be the cause of LE. They may be functionally examined by manual muscle testing procedures, using the principle of selective tension. By having the patient isometrically contract individual muscles, the clinician expects that lesions within these contractile tissues would be aggravated and evoke a painful response during contraction.

Diagnosis and Clinical Features

The diagnosis of LE is usually made easily from information derived from history taking and physical examination, not from diagnostic imaging. The patient history is straightforward: persistent pain over the radial aspect of the forearm and elbow, usually localized to an area approximately 2 cm in diameter around the lateral epicondyle. There is typically an association between the gradual onset of symptoms and some type of cumulative trauma involving repetitive use of the hand, wrist, or forearm muscles.

Various methods of manual resistance testing can quickly ascertain that LE pain is being generated from contractile tissues. These tests are summarized in Box 5-1. Standard manual muscle testing, as outlined by Kendall and McCreary (6), also can be used by the clinician in an effort to make a more muscle-specific diagnosis.

Examining every muscle of the forearm for trigger points or adhesions would be very time consuming. Therefore, the clinician should start by examining the muscles most commonly known to cause pain in the region of the lateral epicondyle. Simons et al. (7) state that the three most common muscles implicated in the pain of LE, in order of frequency, are the supinator, the brachioradialis (BR), and the extensor carpi radialis longus (ECRL). The extensor carpi radialis brevis (ECRB) lies underneath and is a close companion to the ECRL, and for all effective purposes, is treated along

Manual Diagnostic Selective Tension Tests

Cozen's Test (5)
Positive test is indicated when patient feels sharp pain over lateral epicondyle during the combination movements of making a fist, pronating the forearm, and radially deviating the wrist.

Mill's Method (5)
Positive test when sharp lateral epicondyle pain is elicited during passive extension of the elbow while the forearm is pronated and wrist flexed.

Tennis Elbow Test (5)
Positive test is reproduction of lateral epicondyle pain on manual resistance to extension of the third finger.

Handgrip Test (1)
Positive test is reproduction of proximal forearm or lateral epicondyle pain on performing a firm handshake with the wrist in ulnar deviation.

Compression Test (1)
Same as Handgrip Test, except examiner puts manual pressure over the proximal forearm extensor muscle mass. Positive test is indicated by patient feeling relief of symptoms with compression during firm handshake.

Specific Manual Muscle Tests (6)
Individual muscles can be tested by manual resistance, looking for reproduction of forearm or lateral epicondyle pain on vigorous contraction.

with the ECRL when manual soft tissue techniques are used.

The extensor digitorum and triceps muscles are also frequently involved with cases of LE; the extensor digitorum because of its origin from the common extensor tendon, and the medial head of the triceps because of its attachment site on the distal lateral humerus near the lateral epicondyle. Both of these muscles are known to cause referred pain in the region of the lateral epicondyle. The small and variable anconeus muscle runs between the lateral epicondyle and the olecranon process, and appears as an extension of the triceps. Its referred pain pattern is locally over the lateral epicondyle. Other muscles that are less commonly involved, but also cause referred pain over the lateral elbow region, are the supraspinatus, biceps, and brachialis.

Although muscle testing is useful in the clinic to quickly determine which contractile tissues are the pain

generators, it does not determine the precise location of the myofascial lesion within those tissues. This is where skillful manual palpation of the muscles for taut bands, hypertonic fibers, trigger points, and adhesions plays a role in the examination process. The experienced soft tissue practitioner palpates any muscle that is known to refer to the area of the "sore spot" even if it appears to be remote from the area of complaint. The phenomenon of referred myofascial pain can confuse the unwary clinician into examining only the tissues around the "sore spot" as described by the patient.

The principle of *scanning palpation* is simple in theory, involving the use of light touch to ascertain the amount of tissue tension, shortness, and nodularity of the myofascial tissues. Travell and Simons suggest cross-fiber palpation "across the grain" as the first step in determining the presence of taut bands of muscle tissue. Once a taut band has been identified, they suggest palpating "with the grain," or longitudinally along the muscle fibers, until coming to a "lumpy nodule" known as a trigger point. Other authors have outlined various manual muscle palpation methods in detail (8–13). By using both selective tension tests to determine the specific muscle(s) involved, and scanning palpation techniques to find the localized trigger point within that muscle, the clinician is ready to apply various manual soft tissue procedures to eliminate the cause of the patient's pain.

Conventional Treatment Approaches

Although the standard medical treatment of LE varies somewhat, essentially it is based on the premise that LE is an inflammatory disorder of the common extensor tendon. Therefore, the treatment approach is to use anti-inflammatory medications and modalities in an effort to quiet the inflammation. Bracing and rest are also used to decrease stress and strain on the purportedly inflamed tendon.

A typical case of LE would be managed with nonsteroidal anti-inflammatory drugs (NSAIDs) and a tennis elbow support brace for 3 to 4 weeks. If the patient shows no improvement, physical therapy modalities such as ultrasound, electrical muscle stimulation, or exercises for the forearm extensors would be recommended for 4 to 6 weeks. Steroid medications are commonly driven into the tissues around the epicondyle with ultrasound (phonophoresis) or electrical currents (iontophoresis), and occasionally an oral steroid dose pack is prescribed. In very resistant cases, a steroid injection is performed directly into the soft tissues around the lateral epicondyle. As a last resort, the common extensor tendon can be surgically débrided and released by tenotomy.

This typical clinical management scenario is based on the premise that the condition is merely caused by an inflamed common extensor tendon. Recent research is beginning to shed doubt on this simplistic view of the cause of LE as an inflammatory process only. A recent histopathologic study of 1,000 cases of chronic tendon disorders concluded that the condition termed *tendinitis* is characterized by variable histology, from pure inflammation and acute hemorrhage in acute tendon trauma to calcification and *tendinosis* changes in chronic conditions (14). In fact, during biopsy and histopathologic examination of chronic tendinitis patients, no inflammatory cellular responses were seen in the tendon itself, which has led to the current theory that *most cases of tendinitis are in fact cases of tendinosis* (14).

Tendinosis versus tendinitis is similar to the distinction between osteoarthrosis and osteoarthritis; the tendon or joint surface is degenerated and therefore more susceptible to mild stresses and strains, which may eventually lead to inflammation. This subject is covered in detail later in this chapter. However, clinicians must look beyond simple irritation of the common extensor tendon when considering the alternative myofascial approach to LE.

A MYOFASCIAL APPROACH TO THE DIAGNOSIS AND TREATMENT OF TENNIS ELBOW

Both tendons and muscles are contractile tissues, and they are interdependent from a functional point of view. Therefore, any overuse syndrome could conceivably affect either or both tissues. Those who practice myofascial techniques would argue that tendinitis is often an end-stage manifestation of myofascial dysfunction. Common examples of this scenario are Achilles tendinitis in runners and patellar tendinitis (jumper's knee) in track athletes. Prolonged and excessive contraction of the gastrocsoleus and quadriceps muscles are implicated in the causes of those conditions, respectively. With respect to LE, it is thought that trigger point activity or hypertonicity within the forearm extensor muscles causes prolonged tension along the course of the muscles, and especially in the common extensor tendon. Treatment therefore would be aimed at restoring normal function to the muscles by releasing any trigger points or adhesions by manual methods.

It is also possible that the pain overlying the lateral epicondyle is not arising directly from the tendon, but may be referred pain or tenderness from remote myofascial tissues. Travell and Simons (1) outline at least six muscles around the elbow whose characteristic referred pain patterns encompass the lateral epicondyle region.

Pain around the elbow can be referred from other areas, such as the cervical spine and shoulder. A thorough evaluation of any patient with peripheral upper-extremity complaints should include examination of the major joints and muscles proximal to the painful area. The area of skin overlying the lateral epicondyle region lies within the zone of the C6 and C7 dermatomes. The astute clinician will perform provocative orthopaedic tests of the cervical spine to determine whether pain can be reproduced in the elbow with certain neck movements. Likewise, several muscles in and around the neck and shoulder are known to cause referred pain in the area of the lateral epicondyle: the scalenes, pec-

torals (usually more *medial* epicondyle pain), subscapularis, supraspinatus, and infraspinatus.

The clinician's viewpoint about which tissue is causing the pain and symptoms of LE often determines the type of treatment. Because the medical model has traditionally seen LE as an inflammatory condition, the treatment has been an anti-inflammatory approach. The myofascial viewpoint looks at LE as a problem with muscle–tendon function, with the possibility of inflammation as an associated, but not necessarily causal, factor.

The soft tissue practitioner will attempt to determine which specific muscle, or group of muscles, has become shortened and loaded with trigger points. Such dysfunctional muscles will inevitably cause abnormal stress and strain on the common extensor muscle, causing increased tension on the lateral epicondyle insertion point. In addition, the trigger points within the abnormal muscles may cause referred pain into the lateral elbow, which presents itself as lateral epicondyle pain or tenderness. The myofascial approach rests on the premise of using manual techniques to release these trigger points and restore normal length and function to the affected muscle(s), thereby releasing abnormal tension on the common extensor tendon and eliminating any referred pain.

An Overview of Tennis Elbow

Pain in and around the lateral epicondyle region typically emanates from several of the extensor muscles on the dorsal forearm and the associated common extensor tendon. Cumulative trauma can lead to trigger point or adhesion formation in the muscles, or to inflammation with adhesion formation in the common extensor tendon. Diagnostic testing procedures cannot image these soft tissue lesions; they can only be found on careful and skillful palpation methods.

Trigger points and adhesions within the soft tissues around the elbow may cause dysfunction of the muscles and joints, as well as possible entrapment of peripheral nerves. Manual soft tissue techniques are used by the clinician to release trigger points and adhesions from the myofascial tissues, to restore normal muscle function and blood flow to tendons. Transverse friction massage and various physiotherapy modalities can be applied directly over the common extensor tendon to increase circulation and potentially stimulate the "stalled" healing process within the tendon. Muscle and tendon function are so closely interrelated that both tissues should be addressed by the clinician. In addition to using these manual methods to physically release trigger points and adhesions, clinicians should educate their patients about the chronic and recurrent nature of these CTDs. Patients need to understand how and why myofascitis and tendinitis develop slowly over time from cumulative trauma. They also need to learn simple concepts about the ergonomic design of their workstations, the postures in which they place themselves during daily activities, and especially simple exercises they can readily use to self-treat little aches and pains. The long-term prognosis for many cases of LE and other CTDs may indeed lie in this arena of patient management, in the discovery and elimination of what Travell and Simons so aptly term *perpetuating factors* (1).

Causes

As stated previously, most cases of lateral epicondylitis (LE) occur as an end result of cumulative trauma, by people who repetitiously use their forearm extensor muscles. This leads to hypertonicity and shortening of the myofascial tissues, with eventual formation of trigger points or adhesions. Once this muscle dysfunction has occurred, there may be associated changes within the common extensor tendon.

Tendons are white, chiefly because they are relatively avascular. The blood supply to tendons comes primarily from muscles, where small capillaries pass from the musculotendinous junction along the outer layers of the tendon (paratenon) toward the tenoperiosteal junction. The blood supply to tendons is therefore quite superficial and is susceptible to being compromised by compression, torsion, or friction of the outer layer of the tendon, or by excessive muscular contraction (15).

Because the chief blood supply of tendons comes from the associated muscles, keeping these muscles healthy and free of hypertonicity or trigger points is important. Protracted hypertonicity and shortening of muscle fibers could hamper the circulation to tendons, thereby contributing to further degenerative changes.

When a tendon is overused, it may become fatigued and lose its basal reparative ability. Repetitive microtraumatic processes weaken collagen fibers and vascular elements of the tendon. Cumulative trauma may damage the vasculature enough to cause local hypoxia, and decreased metabolism and nutrition to tendon cells, leading to degenerative changes. This theory of cumulative tendon degeneration is

---

CASE 5-1

Patient History

Mrs. M.R., age 48, complained of left radial forearm and thumb web pain, which was previously diagnosed by an orthopedist as DeQuervain's syndrome. She was employed as an accounting clerk at a large department store, and her job required the frequent use of her left hand on a calculator. Her orthopedist had performed two cortisone injections of the tendons in the region of her distal radius, and then placed the left forearm and wrist in a hard fiberglass cast for 4 weeks. While in the cast, the patient had almost no pain, but all of her forearm and thumb web pain returned on removal of the cast.

Symptoms

On initial examination, Mrs. M.R. complained of pain in the distal radius, thumb web, radial aspect of the forearm, and lateral epicondyle. The pain was most severe over the distal radius, and she did not complain of any pain in the neck, shoulder, or upper arm.

Examination Findings

Examination of the cervical spine, shoulder joint, and proximal muscles of the upper extremity and shoulder did not indicate any abnormalities. Manual palpation detected severe tenderness over the tendons in the vicinity of the distal radius, and Trigger point activity in the left brachioradialis (BR), and the ECRB and ECRL. The trigger points in her BR elicited referred pain down into the distal radius, and during the palpatory examination the patient exclaimed, "That's it; that's exactly my pain." Finkelstein's test (ulnar deviation of wrist with thumb clenched in fist) was positive, eliciting pain over the distal radius. Resistance muscle testing elicited pain in the lateral elbow only when she attempted to flex the elbow against resistance with her forearm in the pronated position, which places strain on the BR muscle. Resisted wrist extension caused some "tightness" in the forearm extensors, but no actual "pain."

Treatment

Mrs. M.R. was treated with manual myofascial release techniques and ischemic compression, chiefly to the BR, ECRB, and ECRL. Adjunctive therapy included interferential electrical stimulation applied through the dorsal forearm muscle mass. No supports or braces were used, because the patient had just been taken out of a rigid cast. Treatments were performed twice weekly for 3 weeks, then once weekly for 2 more weeks. After each visit she reported relief, and after 8 visits, she was essentially pain-free.

Follow-up

Mrs. M.R. was not seen again for 6 months, at which time she returned with a similar complaint, although not nearly as severe. She explained that her company had performed its yearly inventory, and that she had had to work 12-hour days for a week. Her left BR and ECRL were again involved with trigger points, and a similar treatment plan was established. This time, she required only two visits before her forearm pain had quieted down, and she was released to an as-needed basis. She has remained asymptomatic for at least 6 months, and has not returned for treatment.

CASE 5-2

Patient History

Mr. J.S., age 63, complained of point tenderness over the left medial epicondyle. This problem began shortly after he started a course of home exercises, including the use of dumbbell weights, to strengthen his upper-extremity muscles. Specifically, he was performing biceps and triceps curls, as well as forearm curls, by doing wrist flexion and extension exercises.

Symptoms

He reported trouble with grip strength and felt a sharp pinch in the left elbow with certain movements of his left arm and wrist. He had no complaints of neck or shoulder pain, and no symptoms suggesting paresthesia in either upper extremity.

Examination Findings

Physical examination indicated pinpoint tenderness over the medial epicondyle, at the common insertion of the forearm flexor muscles. Orthopaedic tests of the cervical spine and shoulder were negative for the reproduction of elbow or forearm pain. Resistance muscle testing of wrist flexion elicited some moderate pain in the proximal forearm flexor muscles but was negative for reproduction of epicondyle pain. Percussion over the medial epicondyle produced only mild tenderness; no sharp pain was elicited. Passive and active range-of-motion testing indicated that extension of the left wrist and elbow were moderately reduced, probably because of shortening or hypertonicity of the forearm flexor muscle mass.

Treatment

Mr. J.S. was treated with manual myofascial release techniques and ischemic compression four times over the course of 3 weeks. He was advised to cease his dumbbell exercises and to avoid any repetitive use of the hands, such as gardening and yard work. No adjunctive modalities or bracing were used with this patient.

Follow-up

Mr. J.S.'s elbow and forearm pain was completely gone by his fourth visit, and he remained symptom-free for 2 months after his four visits. After 9 months, he still reported having no trouble with his elbow.

CASE 5-3

Patient History

Mr. D.B., age 48, complained of right elbow and forearm pain, which had been present for approximately 3 to 4 months. He blamed the condition on his occupation as a township park maintenance man, which during the summer months meant hours of raking, shoveling, pruning, and other activities requiring frequent repetitive tasks involving his hands. Six months before his initial visit, he had a spontaneous rupture of the right biceps tendon, which on magnetic resonance imaging (MRI) was shown to be severely degenerated and torn. After a consultation and examination with an orthopedic surgeon, he elected not to have it surgically repaired.

Symptoms

Mr. D.B. had very localized pain in the region of the right lateral epicondyle. He did not have any complaints of neck or shoulder pain, and kept pointing to his lateral elbow as the source of his pain. He was losing strength in his right arm at work, and therefore sought treatment out of desperation.

Examination Findings

Physical examination indicated classic signs and symptoms of a localized lateral epicondylitis. Cervical and shoulder joint ranges of motion were within normal limits and pain-free. The patient complained of sharp, severe pain directly over the right lateral epicondyle with any movements involving contraction of the right forearm muscles. Percussion with a reflex hammer, or even light tapping with the index finger, over the lateral epicondyle caused him to wince in pain. Resistance muscle testing of the right forearm extensors by wrist extension or a firm handshake immediately reproduced sharp pinpoint pain over the right lateral epicondyle. Muscle palpation detected numerous trigger points in the ECRB and ECRL, as well as the BR, which caused referred pain into the lateral elbow and forearm regions.

Treatment

Treatment was initiated with deep ischemic compression and myofascial release techniques, using a combination of manual tension over the trigger points while

(continued)

CASE 5-3 *(continued)*

the forearm extensor muscles were stretched either passively by the clinician or actively by the patient. Adjunctive modalities used were continuous ultrasound and microcurrent stimulation applied over the trigger points in the forearm extensors. The patient was also fitted with a tennis elbow support brace and told to wear it only while working, to reduce the strain on his forearm extensors.

After four weekly visits, the patient was about 50% improved with respect to pain and function. However, his sharp lateral epicondyle pain was still present whenever he used his hands. Because his occupation required heavy and continuous manual labor, this was a daily occurrence. Mr. D.B. continued with myofascial therapies and modalities for another 6 weeks at one visit per week, and remained approximately 50% improved. He had a lapse in treatment for about 2 months, then returned again with the same complaint of right elbow pain. The same treatment program was implemented, but after 6 weeks, his pain level would not drop below the 50% im-

provement level. At this point, the patient had been suffering with right lateral epicondyle pain for almost 9 months, and therefore a decision was made to refer him for a steroid injection.

Follow-up

Mr. D.B. was referred to an orthopaedic surgeon, who placed him on a 6-day prednisone dose pack, which reduced the patient's epicondyle pain another 25% from the previous 50% improvement level. He then injected the soft tissues overlying the right epicondyle, and the patient had immediate reduction of all right elbow pain (100% relief). At a 4-week follow-up post-injection point, the patient no longer had any pinpoint epicondyle pain and was released from active care. The patient was seen 1 year later, for treatment of a low-back problem, at which time he reported that his elbow had not bothered him since the injection.

---

very similar to the Simons "energy crisis" model regarding the cause of trigger point formation in muscle tissue (15,19).

Kannus and Jozsa (20) performed histopathological analysis of tendon tissues taken by biopsy from 891 patients who had surgical correction of spontaneously ruptured tendons. They also examined 445 sex- and age-matched tendon specimens from cadavers of healthy individuals who died of accidents and compared the microscopic examinations of the healthy tendon samples with those taken from the ruptured tendons. None of the spontaneously ruptured tendons showed a healthy tissue structure, yet two thirds of the control tendons showed a healthy cellular structure. Some 97% of the ruptured tendons showed various types of degenerative changes, including hypoxic tendinopathy, mucoid degeneration, lipomatosis, and calcification. Most of these surgical patients had no symptoms at all before the onset of their spontaneous tendon ruptures, which tends to discredit the theory that inflammation of the tendon *always* precedes rupture.

One of the new theories about the success of surgical treatment of chronic tendon pain is that the healing process has somehow become "stalled" (14). Surgical debridement of the degenerated tendon tissue is thought to reactivate the healing process by creating a new "surgical wound." This acceleration of wound healing also may explain the therapeutic effects of manual myofascial techniques, transverse friction massage, low-level ultrasound, microcurrent stimulation, and acupuncture, all of which may cause reflex vasodilation or increased local metabolism.

The authors of the previously noted histologic study came to the following conclusion about the cause of painful disorders of tendons:

Tendon inflammation and degeneration may be coexisting, independent phenomena, without a true causal relationship from inflammation to degeneration or vice versa. We suggest that myofibroblasts maintain a prolonged contracted status in their surroundings and thus influence the development of crippling contracture around the tendon. This may lead to constriction of vascular lumina and decreased circulation (18).

Cautions

The use of steroids is one of the greatest advances in suppressing inflammation made in the twentieth century. Hench won the Nobel Prize in medicine in 1950 for reporting the beneficial effects of steroid hormones on the rheumatoid joint (22). This exciting development was quickly dampened a few years later when negative reports began to be published about the adverse effects of steroids, including rapidly progressive degenerative arthritis and decreased synthesis of articular cartilage.

The accepted current viewpoint is that the injection of steroids directly into the belly of a tendon is absolutely contraindicated, because of the undesirable side effects of focal tissue degeneration and necrosis. Intratendinous injection of steroids results in tendon necrosis, reduction of collagen synthesis, and decreased tensile strength of tendons. These effects have led many clinicians to suggest that steroid injections directly into tendons may actually accelerate tendon degeneration and lead to spontaneous rupture.

Despite the large number of steroid injections administered by members of the medical profession, a recent review of the world literature by Assendelft found only 12 randomized clinical trials regarding steroid injections for tendinitis (23). He concluded that the evidence for the clinical effectiveness of steroid injections is not conclusive, but that they appear to be safe and effective in the short term, that is, 2 to 6 weeks. Fredberg recently published a review of the literature and proposed some guidelines regarding corticosteroid injection for sports injuries (36). He states:

It is questionable whether there is a cause–effect relationship between steroid injection and tendon rupture. Rupture may merely be a final manifestation of the disease for which steroids were applied. Peritendinous injection (injection around the tendon, not the tendon itself) may be quite beneficial. It does not seem reasonable to condemn *peritendinous* injection by invoking a direct deleterious effect on the tendon itself. If a local injection does not work the first time, it may be reasonable to repeat it once, for the first one may not have been placed accurately. If injection fails a second time, it is not wise to repeat it (35).

The controversy surrounding steroid injections for treating tennis elbow and other tendinitis conditions is likely to continue until more randomized clinical trials are performed. Most patients will respond quite favorably to manual myofascial techniques and other conservative measures without the need for steroid injection, which should be reserved as a last resort in the myofascial treatment approach.

Note the long-term relief that the patient in Case 5-3 experienced after a single injection; it may be tempting to ask, Why not inject every patient with LE symptoms on the first visit? As mentioned previously, LE is often a chronic and recurring condition, as in the case of this specific patient. The patient probably had some tendinosis, tendinitis, and myofascial trigger points co-existing, which collectively contributed to the symptom cluster he reported as "tennis elbow." The myofascial techniques did relieve his pain by approximately 50%, which most likely eliminated the myofascial dysfunction and trigger point portion of his symptom complex. This may have set the stage for long-term relief, because the injection eliminated the residual inflammation, and the tendon did not become reirritated because normal muscle function had been restored.

In summary, steroid injection probably has a place in the conservative management of LE, but only at a later stage in the treatment process. Patients should first attempt a clinical trial of conservative care for 3 to 4 weeks, expecting noticeable relief of symptoms. If manual techniques and other modalities do not yield favorable results after 4 weeks, more aggressive methods can be used, including forearm braces, complete rest from certain forearm motions, and alteration of daily work duties. Lateral epicondyle pain that is not at least 50% improved after 8 weeks of conservative care may

be the type of case that warrants consideration for steroid injection.

Symptom/Pain Presentation

Patients with LE pain typically have a history of weeks or months of gradually worsening pain, which begin slowly and insidiously. Rarely does a patient with lateral epicondyle or forearm pain state that he or she remembers a specific injury that triggered the pain cycle. The pain is usually associated with cumulative trauma to the forearm extensor muscles, caused by the patient's occupation or hobbies.

Typical LE patients have pain localized to the dorsal aspect of the proximal forearm and lateral elbow, which is provoked by any vigorous contraction of the forearm extensor muscles, such as a firm handshake. With associated tendinitis of the common extensor tendon, the lateral epicondyle itself becomes tender to palpation or percussion. Sometimes this lateral epicondyle insertion point of the inflamed common extensor tendon is so exquisitely tender to even the slightest touch that some patients report feeling pain when they roll over in bed and lean against the mattress.

In the later stages of the process of myofascial pain and tendon inflammation, patients report difficulty holding onto pens and pencils, lifting coffee mugs, sewing, playing musical instruments, and opening jars. They begin to notice definite weakness in their grip strength only when these daily activities are adversely affected. Many people attempt to self-treat the painful forearm and elbow with ice or heat packs, various liniments or ointments, and tennis elbow support braces. These self-help remedies are usually not effective, which prompts these patients to seek professional help.

Myofascial Entrapments

The three most common peripheral nerve entrapments that occur in the upper extremity, in order of frequency of clinical presentation, are the median nerve, ulnar nerve, and radial nerve (37). Each of these peripheral nerves may be entrapped at multiple sites between their origin in the cervical region and their termination in the distal hand. The most common sites where these three peripheral nerves may become entrapped between osseous and myofascial tissues near the elbow and wrist are summarized in Box 5-2. Other entrapment sites also exist but are beyond the scope of discussion of this chapter.

With respect to the forearm extensor muscles, the radial nerve may become entrapped within these soft tissues. Because radial nerve entrapments are the least common of the three upper-extremity entrapment syndromes, they may not be seen in the average private clinic except on rare occasions, or in association with traumatic lesions such as fracture or dislocation.

The radial nerve follows the course of the radial groove in the humerus, until it separates into two branches near the radial head and lateral epicondyle. At this point, the radial

Peripheral Nerve Entrapment Sites (37)

Median Nerve

Frequency—Most common entrapment of upper extremity.

Symptoms—Numbness/paresthesia in digits 1, 2, and 3 of hand. Weakness of thumb muscles with possible atrophy of thenar eminence.

Osseous entrapment—Occurs within the carpal tunnel; a fibro-osseous canal between the carpal bones and the transverse carpal ligament.

Myofascial entrapment—Occurs in the proximal forearm, between the two heads of the pronator teres muscle.

Ulnar Nerve

Frequency—Second most common entrapment of upper extremity.

Symptoms—Numbness/paresthesia of digits 4, 5 of hand. Motor weakness of small intrinsic hand muscles/finger flexors. Possible atrophy of hypothenar eminence.

Osseous entrapments—Two possible osseous sites of entrapment are proximally at the olecranon groove ("cubital tunnel syndrome") and distally at the Tunnel of Guyon ("handlebar palsy").

Myofascial entrapment—Occurs within a triangular myofascial tunnel through the flexor carpi ulnaris muscle, near its attachment at the medial epicondyle.

Radial Nerve

Frequency—Least common of the upper extremity entrapment syndromes

Symptoms—Numbness and paresthesia over the thumb web and dorsal hand. Weakness of the wrist and finger extensors

Osseous entrapments—Rare except with associated fractures of the head of the radius and humerus (spiral groove)

Myofascial entrapments—Two muscles are responsible for radial nerve entrapments; The supinator may entrap the deep branch of the radial nerve (motor only), causing weakness but no paresthesia. The ECRB may entrap either the deep (motor) or superficial (sensory) branches of the radial nerve, causing weakness or paresthesia.

nerve divides into deep and superficial branches. The deep branch of the radial nerve (also known as the posterior interosseous nerve) is a motor nerve only; it innervates most of the finger and wrist extensor muscles except for the ECRB and ECRL. This deep branch passes through openings in both the supinator and the ECRB, and therefore is susceptible to myofascial entrapment by either of these muscles. The superficial branch of the radial nerve may be entrapped where it passes through an opening in the ECRB.

Isolated entrapment of the deep (motor) branch of the radial nerve will cause a painless weakening of the finger and wrist extensors, whereas isolated entrapment of the superficial branch will cause a sensation of numbness and tingling over the dorsum of the hand and thumb web without weakness. However, in clinical practice, it is rare to see such "pure" entrapments without also seeing associated myofascial referred pain patterns. For these entrapments to occur, the ECRB or supinator would have to be hypertonic or shortened, with many trigger points. In that case, the muscles would likely be causing referred pain around the region of the lateral epicondyle and elbow, which the patient would describe as a "deep tenderness and ache."

Treatment
Manual Myofascial Techniques

Many different manual techniques are used to treat soft tissue lesions, some with "brand" names usually associated with an entrepreneurial developer, and others with "generic" names based on anatomic or physiologic descriptions. Three generic manual myofascial techniques are discussed that are used regularly in this author's clinic. A brief discussion about the use of another soft tissue technique, transverse friction massage (TFM), then follows. In the author's clinic, TFM is applied directly over tendons or myotendinous junctions but is not used as a myofascial technique per se. Also, the rationale for the use of TFM is different from the reasons to use myofascial techniques.

Many other soft tissue techniques and methods exist, which may very well give equally effective clinical results; however, for purposes of brevity, only the four methods noted are discussed in this chapter.

The first manual myofascial technique is firm, steady pressure applied directly over trigger points, which has been commonly referred to as *ischemic compression*. With this method, the clinician applies deep, firm manual pressure directly over the trigger point and holds this pressure steady for approximately 5 to 10 seconds. No rubbing, stroking, or stripping movements are used with this method. In chiropractic circles, this generic method is commonly known as *Nimmo technique*, named for the chiropractic pioneer who first developed the procedure, Dr. Raymond Nimmo (24). Massage therapists, physical therapists, and other body workers may call variations of this method *myotherapy* (25) or *neuromuscular therapy* (26,27). Technique 5-1 outlines the basic fundamentals of this method.

TECHNIQUE 5-1

Trigger Point Pressure Release (trigger point PR, ischemic compression)

This technique begins with scanning palpation, performed in a gentle manner across the fibers, to locate taut bands. Once a taut band has been located, the clinician palpates longitudinally along the muscle fibers to locate trigger points, while asking the patient to report any areas of referred pain. Immediately on palpating a trigger point that reproduces the patient's complaint, the clinician applies steady manual pressure directly over the trigger point. In the methodology advocated by Nimmo and others, previously termed ischemic compression, the manual pressure is rather deep and held for approximately 7 to 10 seconds, then released. This deep pressure is applied 3 to 4 times during the course of one session (11,12,13,24–27). In the current methodology advocated by Simons, Travell, and Simons, termed trigger point pressure release (trigger point PR), the amount of manual pressure used is gentler than ischemic compression (7). In trigger point PR, the clinician applies firm pressure directly over the trigger point, with the intent of engaging a barrier of resistance. The pressure is held steady until some release of the barrier is felt, at which time the clinician applies more pressure, following the tissues to a new barrier. This process is repeated approximately 3 to 4 times during one session.

Common reasons for failure with this technique:

- Clinician is too aggressive with the amount of pressure applied or repeats too many applications of pressure during one visit. This may lead to bruising or damage to the muscle tissues, causing the formation of new trigger points or muscle problems.

- Certain patients may not be good candidates for this method, such as frail or elderly patients, or those on anticoagulant or steroid medications. Never apply deep pressure directly over hematomas, acute muscle strains, or other areas of trauma.

The term *ischemic compression* probably developed as a result of the clinical observation of skin blanching during the application of this deep-pressure technique, followed immediately by a red response, in which the tissues become red and hyperemic. It has been generally assumed that this hyperemic response brings in fresh blood supply to the muscle tissue, "washing out" biochemical exudates and thereby relieving pain, but no research has emerged to support this concept. However, Simons has downplayed this "ischemia theory," and proposed alternate theories about the possible mechanisms of action of deep manual pressure applied to trigger points, including mechanical disruption of the locked actin-myosin cross-links in the trigger point nodule (15,19). Simons and Travell now suggest that the term ischemic compression no longer be used, proposing the use of a new term, trigger point pressure release (trigger point PR) (7). Actually, on closer inspection, these two methods are not quite exactly the same, with some major differences in manual application.

The method of trigger point PR involves the use of lighter pressure than ischemic compression methods, with the intent of *avoiding ischemia*. Before applying any manual pressure, the muscle is slightly lengthened to put the fibers in slight tension. Manual pressure is then applied over the trigger point or area of taut muscle tissue until a *barrier of resistance* is felt by the clinician. This pressure is held long enough to feel some release of the barrier, at which time the clinician applies additional pressure until another barrier is engaged. This technique may be augmented by having the patient perform muscular contraction of the antagonist muscle during the procedure, which combines reciprocal inhibition, stretching, and manual pressure. In some ways, trigger point PR as described by Simons is similar to certain aspects of myofascial release techniques as described by Leahy and Mock, which are discussed later.

The second commonly used manual soft tissue technique is post-isometric relaxation (PIR), which is best described by Lewit (28) and more recently by Liebenson (29). In this method, the clinician has the patient very gently contract the affected muscle against light resistance (10%–25% of maximal effort) for approximately 3 to 10 seconds. Immediately after this isometric contraction, the patient is instructed to "let go" and allow the muscle to be passively or actively stretched and lengthened. The line of stretch must pass along the fiber orientation of the muscle being treated; otherwise, other muscles may inadvertently be stretched instead. The therapeutic effect of this method seems to be predicated on the patient being able to completely relax during the procedure, thereby allowing for elongation and release of the hypertonic muscle fibers. There may be somewhat of a "biofeedback effect" with this method, in which the patient learns some self-control of his own muscle tension.

This technique is thought to work on the principle of the *refractory inhibition*, the phase immediately following a muscle contraction during which muscle fibers are temporarily inhibited and more easily stretched. When the patient actively contracts the antagonist muscle to stretch the painfully tight muscle, *reciprocal inhibition* comes into play. In either case, PIR is based on the premise that spinal motor inhibition facilitates the therapeutic stretch of hypertonic and painful muscle tissue. Technique 5-2 describes the major steps in performing post-isometric stretches.

The third soft tissue technique to be discussed is generically known as myofascial release techniques (MRT) as described by Leahy and Mock (30). Leahy (31) has developed his own proprietary version of this method known as *Active*

Release Techniques® (ART), whereas Mock (32) has continued to publish using the generic term MRT. This particular method of soft tissue therapy blends some degree of manual pressure with active or passive stretch of the affected muscle tissue. To a casual observer, it would appear that this technique is nothing more than trigger point PR, applied while the patient or clinician applies an active or passive stretch. However, MRT is more related to the family of stretching procedures than to deep-pressure procedures, such as trigger point PR or ischemic compression.

Tension and stretch, rather than pure compression, are the key ingredients in the method of MRT. Leahy and Mock describe the soft tissue lesion which they are attempting to treat as an *adhesion*, whereas ischemic compression or trigger point PR is attempting to treat *myofascial trigger points,* and PIR technique is designed to treat *hypertonic or shortened muscles.*

Although the original intent and design of MRT was to treat adhesions and not trigger points, this method also may be quite useful for myofascial lesions as well. In this author's clinic, MRT-type procedures are successfully used to treat myofascial trigger points and taut bands. Although it is possible to feel differences in tissue texture over what seems to be a trigger point versus an adhesion, it is speculative for clinicians to state that they can clearly distinguish trigger points from adhesions by palpation alone, when neither of these clinical entities can be absolutely verified by any objective diagnostic test. Mock has stated that he notices distinct palpatory differences between trigger points and adhesions, and that he first releases trigger points before using MRT to release adhesions (personal communication, 30.)

Leahy and Mock describe four levels of MRT. Levels 1 and 2 are variations of muscle stripping, in which the clinician applies longitudinal manual pressure "along the grain" with the muscle in a neutral position (level 1) or with the muscle pre-positioned in a position of passive stretch (level 2). MRT Levels 3 and 4 involve passive and active movements of the muscle to be treated, respectively. MRT levels 3 and 4 both use a broad, flat-finger contact just distal to the muscular lesion while the muscle is passively stretched by the clinician in level 3, or actively stretched by antagonist muscle contraction in level 4. Technique 5-3 summarizes the four different levels of MRT.

Several mechanisms of action may explain the clinical results of MRT. First, the longitudinal nature of the muscular stretch and stripping actions may pull apart contracted actin–myosin filaments found in trigger points, or abnormal scar formations or adhesions as proposed by Leahy and Mock. Second, the active and passive stretching may inhibit hypertonic muscle fibers and taut bands by virtue of mechanically altering muscle spindle activity so that intrafusal fiber activity more closely "matches" extrafusal resting tonus, thereby restoring better muscle organization and function. Third, in MRT level 4, the principle of reciprocal inhibition is combined with specific stretching.

The next section reviews the most commonly affected muscles involved in the development of LE. The anatomy of these muscles is reviewed, along with the typical referred pain patterns. Techniques then are described for the treatment of soft tissue lesions within these muscles.

Treating Specific Muscles

Supinator. The supinator is often overlooked as a cause of lateral elbow pain, yet it is the most common cause of lateral epicondyle pain, according to Travell and Simons. Supination of the forearm occurs mainly from contraction of the supinator and biceps brachii muscles. The biceps is a

---

TECHNIQUE 5-2

Post-Isometric Relaxation (PIR)

The clinician begins by visualizing the origin and insertion of the muscle to be stretched, which assumes a good working knowledge of anatomy. Manual contacts are taken on the patient, applying a mild stretch to draw up tissue slack over the muscle fibers. This creates a pre-tension "along the grain" of the muscle fibers, and the clinician stops stretching once a barrier of resistance is felt in the muscle. While the clinician holds this mild pre-tension stretch position at the barrier of resistance, the patient is instructed to isometrically contract the muscle, using up to 25% of maximal strength. *This is not a tug of war.* The idea is for the patient to hold a submaximal isometric contraction for 3 to 10 seconds, then stop contracting and "let go" of all tension. On release of the isometric contraction, the clinician gently stretches the muscle further, until a new barrier of resistance is felt. While holding the muscle at this new barrier, the patient is again instructed to perform another 3- to 10-second isometric contraction. This process is repeated approximately 3 to 4 times in one session (9,10,28,29).

Common reasons for failure with this technique:

- Clinician applies aggressive stretching rather than gentle relaxation, which may cause micro-tears in the skeletal muscles. Also, the patient may perform an intense isometric contraction rather than a mild (10%–25% of maximal effort) contraction, which may cause reactive muscle cramping that is counterproductive to the technique.

- Stretching methods should be avoided across unstable or swollen joints, through muscles which have been acutely strained, or over inflamed nerves. For example, it is not wise to stretch the hamstrings in a patient with sciatica, nor to stretch the pectoralis major in a patient with an unstable shoulder that has been previously dislocated.

Myofascial Release Techniques (MRT)

Myofascial release techniques (MRT) is a procedure that combines manual pressure over a specific part of a muscle, while simultaneously applying some type of stretching procedure. The method is described in detail by Leahy and Mock (30–32). There are four levels of this procedure, beginning with level 1, in which the patient is passive, *no stretch or pre-tension is applied*. The clinician uses a longitudinal gliding pressure along the grain of the muscle fibers, passing through the Trigger point or adhesion. With level 2 MRT, the patient is still passive, but positioned in such a manner that muscle to be treated is *pre-tensioned in a state of mild stretch*. The same gliding pressure or stripping-like action is applied as in level 1. MRT levels 1 and 2 appear to be similar in application to a light version of generic *stripping massage*. MRT levels 3 and 4 use manual gliding tension-pressure through the adhesion or trigger point, while simultaneously stretching the tissues under the manual contact. The clinician should visualize pulling the muscle fibers in one direction with the stretching action, while the manual gliding pressure longitudinally stretches a specific portion of the soft tissue in the opposite direction. With MRT level 3, the clinician *passively stretches the muscle*, whereas in MRT level 4, the *patient actively contracts the antagonist muscle*. The major difference between MRT levels 3 and 4 is the *passive stretch* applied by the clinician in the former, and the *active antagonist contraction* by the patient in the latter. MRT level 4 combines manual gliding pressure, active stretching of the muscle to be treated, and *reciprocal inhibition* because of the antagonist contraction.

Common reasons for failure with this technique:

- Clinician applies overly aggressive and deep stripping pressure (MRT levels 1 and 2) for too long or too many applications in one visit, which may cause muscle bruising. This is similar to the contraindications in the use of trigger point PR and ischemic compression.

- With MRT levels 3 and 4, clinician may inadvertently use deep pressure and stripping-type manual pressure, instead of *tissue tension*. The patient may not be able to tolerate the intensity of the pressure and often will ask the clinician to stop.

- Just as with the PIR and trigger point pressure release, the clinician should avoid deep pressure with elderly or frail patients who bruise easily and those patients taking steroids or anticoagulant medications. Applying stretching methods across unstable joints or inflamed nerve roots is also contraindicated.

much more powerful supinator of the forearm, but only when the elbow is somewhat flexed. When the elbow is in complete extension, the biceps can act to produce flexion of the elbow if there is a load, but the only muscle capable of significant action to supinate the forearm is the supinator muscle itself. Many movements tend to overload the supinator muscle, such as quick contraction as in the backhand stroke of tennis, or prolonged forearm supination while the elbow is flexed as in chiropractors performing manipulation, hairdressers cutting and brushing hair, walking a dog on a leash, carrying a heavy box from underneath, and so on. Figure 5-1 shows the anatomy of the supinator. Notice that the supinator has an origin on the dorsal aspect of the ulna, then wraps around the radial head to attach on the volar aspect of the radius. The insertion on the proximal radius is just distal to the crease of the elbow near the lateral epicondyle. This muscle is placed at tension and stretched by pronation of the forearm, which winds the supinator muscle around the radial head. As the supinator contracts, the attachment on the radius is pulled laterally, and the forearm is brought into supination. As noted previously, the supinator contracts most intensely when the elbow is locked in complete extension, a position that inhibits contraction of the biceps brachii.

The primary referred pain pattern of the supinator is focused around the region of the lateral epicondyle, on both the volar and the dorsal aspects of the elbow. Another area of referred pain or paresthesia associated with supinator trigger points is the dorsal thumb web. This area is supplied by the radial nerve, which can be entrapped by hypertonic supinator fibers as the nerve passes through its belly or the Y-shaped opening (Arcade of Frohse) near the origin of the muscle. Figure 5-2 illustrates these referred pain patterns, and Figure 5-3 reviews radial nerve anatomy in the region of the elbow and proximal forearm.

To palpate the supinator for myofascial trigger points, the clinician must be sure not to mistake it for the nearby brachioradialis and/or pronator teres. The supinator is easily palpated in the space between the biceps tendon, pronator teres, and brachioradialis, with manual pressure on the supinator against the underlying radius. The clinician should verify the palpation location by having the patient perform an isometric supination while simultaneously holding the palpating finger over the supinator. During this maneuver, with correct placement, the clinician should feel the supinator muscle "pop up" into the palpating finger.

Manual treatment of the supinator muscle with trigger point PR is typically performed with the clinician's thumb directly over the trigger point locations. Clinicians with small fingers should consider using a double-thumb contact, placing one thumb directly over the other thumb, and applying deep pressure to the supinator. This deep pressure is held for approximately 7 to 10 seconds, then released. Application of the deep muscle compression is repeated approximately 3 to 4 times during the treatment session.

To perform post-isometric relaxation, the patient should first be positioned properly, with the elbow in complete ex-

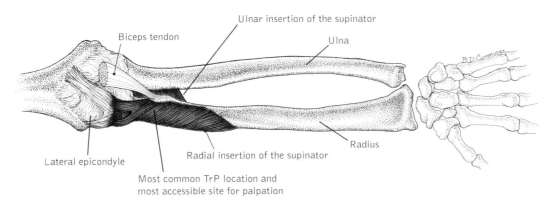

FIGURE 5-1. **Anatomy of the supinator (right forearm).** Reprinted with permission from Simons DG, Travell JG, Simons LS: Travell & Simons' Myofascial Pain and Dysfunction: The Trigger Point Manual, vol 1: Upper Half of Body. 2nd Ed. Baltimore: Lippincott Williams & Wilkins, 1999, fig. 36.2A (p. 730).

tension and the forearm in a pronated position. The clinician can hold the patient's hand, as if to perform a handshake. The clinician then asks the patient to perform an isometric contraction of forearm supination while resisting the clinician, to a level of approximately 10% to 25% of maximal contraction, for approximately 3 to 10 seconds. After this contraction, the clinician passively rotates the forearm further into pronation, which places a specific stretch on

the supinator muscle. This process is repeated 3 to 4 times during the course of one office visit.

When using myofascial release techniques, longitudinal tension is applied along the fibers of the supinator, while stretching the muscle by pronation of the forearm. This stretch can be performed either actively by the patient or passively by the clinician. Two contact points are possible for applying the manual tension/pressure: the dorsal aspect

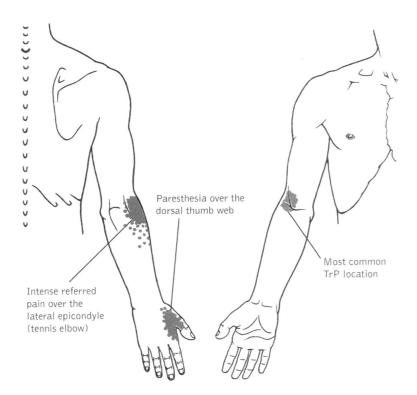

FIGURE 5-2. **Referred pain patterns of the supinator.** Note that the paresthesia over the dorsal thumb web is indicative of radial nerve entrapment between the fibers of the supinator. Reprinted with permission from Simons DG, Travell JG, Simons LS: Travell & Simons' Myofascial Pain and Dysfunction: The Trigger Point Manual, vol 1: Upper Half of Body. 2nd Ed. Baltimore: Lippincott Williams & Wilkins, 1999, fig. 36.1 (p. 729).

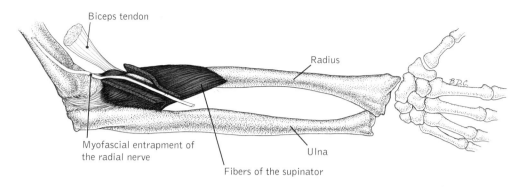

FIGURE 5-3. **Radial nerve entrapment at the supinator.** This view shows the potential site for my-ofascial entrapment of the radial nerve between fibers of the supinator. Notice that the forearm is shown in the position of mid-pronation, to view the dorsal aspect of the muscle. Reprinted with permission from Simons DG, Travell JG, Simons LS: Travell & Simons' Myofascial Pain and Dysfunction: The Trigger Point Manual, vol 1: Upper Half of Body. 2nd Ed. Baltimore: Lippincott Williams & Wilkins, 1999, fig. 36.2C (p. 730).

of the forearm, deep to the extensor muscle mass, or the volar aspect of the forearm, between the biceps tendon and brachioradialis. As the forearm is stretched into pronation, the "tissue pull" being applied by the clinician's fingers should follow and augment the line of stretch.

Brachioradialis. The brachioradialis (BR) is the second most common myofascial cause of lateral epicondyle pain (1). The action of this muscle is chiefly elbow flexion, especially when the forearm is pronated. As noted previously, the biceps and brachialis muscles are the prime elbow flexors when the forearm is supinated. Because the brachioradialis does not cross the wrist, it does not play a role in wrist extension. Holding objects in the hands with the palms facing down, while the elbow is partly flexed, can overload this muscle and cause the development of myofascial trigger points.

The BR originates from the supracondylar ridge of the distal humerus, crosses the elbow joint, and inserts via a tendon on the styloid process of the radius. There are some anatomic variations in which the tendon inserts onto the navicular, scaphoid, or third metacarpal, in which case this muscle could assist in radial deviation of the wrist. Note that the brachioradialis does not have an origin from the common extensor tendon and, therefore, cannot directly cause a true extensor tendinitis. The referred pain pattern of this muscle is very similar to that of the supinator—intense pain over the lateral epicondyle region, with some light referred pain along the radial aspect of the forearm. The dorsal thumb web also may be affected when the radial nerve is compressed between the brachioradialis and the underlying extensor carpi radialis longus. Figure 5-4 shows the anatomy and referred pain patterns of the brachioradialis.

One interesting observation is that some people diagnosed with DeQuervain's syndrome, who have pain and tenderness over the tendons at the radial styloid process, are relieved of these distal symptoms by treatment directed to the

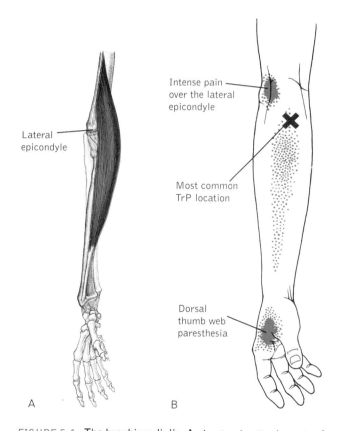

FIGURE 5-4. **The brachioradialis. A.** Anatomic attachments of the muscle, with an origin from the distal humerus and an insertion onto the distal radius. **B.** The myofascial referred pain pattern of the brachioradialis, typical of tennis elbow pain. Note the thumb web paresthesia, which may indicate radial nerve entrapment. Note also the most common trigger point location, the proximal third of the belly. Reprinted with permission from Simons DG, Travell JG, Simons LS: Travell & Simons' Myofascial Pain and Dysfunction: The Trigger Point Manual, vol 1: Upper Half of Body. 2nd Ed. Baltimore: Lippincott Williams & Wilkins, 1999, fig. 34.4 (p. 696), fig. 34.2 (p. 693).

belly of the brachioradialis. Case 5-3, described earlier, is an example. This woman had very severe and apparently local symptoms over the distal radius, which was unresponsive to a hard cast and steroid injections. She was completely relieved of her pain by application of myofascial techniques to the proximal bellies of the brachioradialis and ECRB/ECRL.

Trigger point PR is readily applied to the BR by using a broad thumb contact on trigger points found within the belly of the muscle. Deep pressure is held over each palpable trigger point for approximately 7 to 10 seconds. Trigger points may be found in the portion of the muscle near its attachment on the distal humerus or in the belly of the muscle as it courses along the proximal half of the radius. Because this muscle is very superficial, it is not difficult to palpate or treat with manual pressure techniques.

Post-isometric relaxation as a treatment for brachioradialis hypertonicity or trigger point activity starts with the forearm in mid-pronation and the elbow at slight flexion. The patient is asked to mildly pull the forearm toward the shoulder, against the clinician's resistance, attempting to flex the elbow. The resistance is held for roughly 3 to 10 seconds, after which the patient is told to "let go," and the clinician passively stretches the muscle by extending the elbow and slightly pulling the wrist into ulnar deviation.

Myofascial release techniques involve a combination of manual tension along the grain of the muscle fibers and the stretching position described above for post-isometric relaxation. The clinician first finds the trigger point or adhesion by flat palpation then takes a tissue pull longitudinally along the course of the muscle fibers. While holding this contact firm, the clinician passively stretches the muscle by extending the elbow, or has the patient actively perform elbow extension by contraction of the antagonist triceps.

Extensor carpi radialis longus and brevis. The third most common muscle group involved with the pain of lateral epicondylitis is the extensor carpi radialis longus (ECRL) and brevis (ECRB). These two muscles are so closely connected functionally and anatomically that they can effectively be considered one muscle group. For purposes of manual palpation, it is almost impossible to distinguish a separation between the muscle bellies of the ECRL and ECRB. Figure 5-5 shows the anatomy of the dorsal forearm muscles, with special attention to the ECRL and ECRB.

There are, however, some important distinctions in anatomy, function, and referred pain patterns between the ECRL and ECRB worthy of discussion. The ECRL closely follows alongside the brachioradialis and has an origin on the distal humerus, *not* the lateral epicondyle or common extensor tendon. Therefore, like the BR, the ECRL cannot directly contribute to common extensor tendinitis by mechanical "pulling overload."

Although the ECRL does not attach directly to the common extensor tendon, it does contribute to the pain and symptoms of lateral epicondyle pain by the mechanism of referred pain. The referred pain pattern of the ECRL is

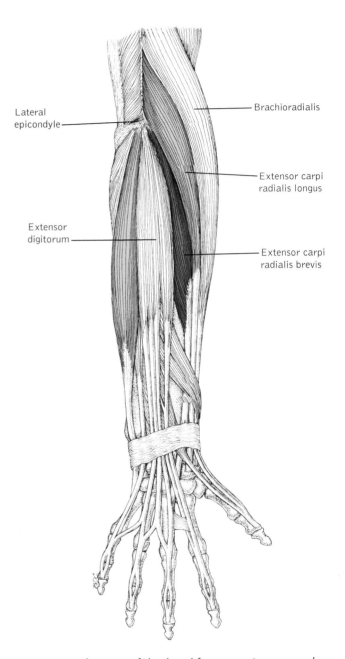

FIGURE 5-5. Anatomy of the dorsal forearm extensor muscles. The extensor carpi radialis longus (ECRL) attaches to the supracondylar ridge of the humerus, and runs alongside and underneath the brachioradialis. The ECRL does *not* attach to the common extensor tendon. The extensor carpi radialis brevis (ECRB) *does* have an origin from the common extensor tendon and the underlying radius. The ECRB runs alongside and underneath the ECRL. Reprinted with permission from Simons DG, Travell JG, Simons LS: Travell & Simons' Myofascial Pain and Dysfunction: The Trigger Point Manual, vol 1: Upper Half of Body. 2nd Ed. Baltimore: Lippincott Williams & Wilkins, 1999, fig. 34.3A (p. 694).

chiefly around the area of the lateral epicondyle, with some radiation down the forearm and over the dorsal wrist and hand (Fig. 5-6). The ECRL inserts onto the second metacarpal, and, therefore, crosses two joints (the elbow and wrist). It flexes the forearm and is also a true wrist extensor, unlike the brachioradialis, which only flexes the forearm. A strong contraction of the ECRL will extend the wrist and pull it into radial deviation.

The ECRB does take its origin from the common extensor tendon and inserts distally to the base of the third metatarsal. The referred pain pattern of the ECRB is *not* over the lateral epicondyle, but distally over the dorsal wrist and hand (see Fig. 5-6). The ECRB therefore may contribute directly to common extensor tendinitis, rather than causing referred pain over the lateral elbow. Also, the ECRB only crosses one joint (the wrist) and therefore is involved in wrist extension but not flexion of the forearm at the elbow. The thickest portion of the belly of the ECRL is near the level of the lateral epicondyle, whereas the belly of the ECRB is at its thickest at about one-third the distance from the elbow to the wrist. As noted earlier, the distinctions between the ECRB and ECRL are somewhat academic, because they are so functionally related that clinically they can be considered one functional muscle unit.

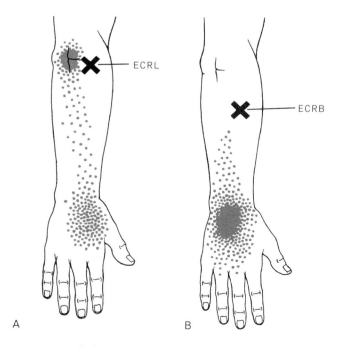

FIGURE 5-6. **Referred pain patterns of the extensor muscles of the forearm.** Note that the ECRL exhibits an intense referred pain pattern directly over the lateral epicondyle region, whereas the ECRB only refers pain distally over the dorsal hand and not over the lateral epicondyle. Reprinted with permission from Simons DG, Travell JG, Simons LS: Travell & Simons' Myofascial Pain and Dysfunction: The Trigger Point Manual, vol 1: Upper Half of Body. 2nd Ed. Baltimore: Lippincott Williams & Wilkins, 1999, fig. 34.1 (p. 692).

Any repetitive use of the forearm extensor muscles, such as typing, playing musical instruments, holding or grasping tools, and so on, may lead to overuse syndromes of this muscle group. The ECRL, ECRB, and other forearm extensor muscles are essential to maintaining a "power grip" on any hand-held tool. When these muscles develop hypertonicity and trigger point activity, patients commonly notice a pronounced loss of grip strength and have difficulty holding objects and performing fine motor tasks. Elderly patients who do gardening, sewing, or other manual crafts may be especially prone to overuse syndromes, because their soft tissues may have lost elasticity and are more susceptible to injury. Many of these patients may be given the simplistic diagnosis of "arthritis," when in fact they have a myofascial pain syndrome.

Trigger point PR is readily applied to these muscles using a single- or double-thumb contact. Most trigger points are located within the thickest portions of the muscle bellies. In the ECRL, trigger points are located in the proximal portion of the muscle, in an area near the lateral epicondyle and brachioradialis. The best location to palpate and explore for ECRB trigger points is right in the center of the extensor muscle mass, in the proximal third of the dorsal forearm. Applying cross-fiber palpation to these trigger points often evokes a local twitch response (LTR), in which the fingers extend by reflex reaction. Very often, after successful manual treatment of the ECRB and ECRL, this LTR will no longer be present.

Post-isometric relaxation of the ECRL first requires the patient to contract the muscle, with extension and radial deviation of the wrist. It is also useful to pull the elbow into slight flexion as well. After the patient relaxes and "lets go," the clinician gently stretches the ECRL by extending the elbow, and by pushing the wrist down into palmar flexion and slight ulnar deviation. The patient also can be taught to perform this PIR at home as a self-stretch. Remember that although the ECRB does not cross the elbow joint, it will simultaneously be stretched along with the ECRL positioning. Again, these muscles are considered a functional unit and should be stretched together.

Myofascial release techniques (MRT) levels 1 and 2 also use a thumb contact; however, a form of gliding pressure is applied along the grain of the fibers of the ECRL and ECRB. The clinician needs to be careful not to apply excessive pressure directly over the lateral epicondyle. With MRT levels 3 and 4, the clinician applies a manual tension-type tissue pull directly over the trigger point or adhesion, then either passively stretches the muscle (level 3) or has the patient contract the antagonist muscle (level 4). The stretching action of the ECRL is accomplished by elbow extension, ulnar deviation of the wrist, and palmar flexion of the wrist and hand. The ECRB is stretched by the movements of flexion and ulnar deviation of the wrist, but elbow extension is not required. The difference in the use of elbow extension as part of the stretching technique relates to anatomy: the ECRL crosses both the elbow and wrist joints, the ECRB only crosses the wrist joint.

Extensor digitorum and triceps. As noted previously, other muscles that commonly cause referred pain and tenderness over the lateral elbow region include the extensor digitorum and triceps. The extensor digitorum has its origin from the lateral epicondyle and the common extensor tendon and inserts into the phalanges. Trigger points in the extensor digitorum are usually found in the proximal one-third of the muscle, in the midline of the dorsal forearm. Having the patient perform resisted extension of the ring or middle finger will cause visible contraction of the muscle fibers. Because this muscle extends both the wrist and fingers, post-isometric relaxation and MRT levels 3 and 4 methods both require that the wrist and fingers be moved into *flexion* to create a specific stretch of the fibers. Elbow extension is not required during stretching techniques, because this muscle does not cross the elbow joint. Trigger point PR or MRT levels 1 and 2 are easily applied to trigger points or adhesions in the belly of the extensor digitorum, because it is a superficial and readily palpable muscle.

The medial head of the triceps is the usual culprit involved with lateral elbow pain, because it tends to refer pain directly over the lateral epicondyle. A simple procedure to scan for a shortened triceps is to have the patient reach toward the ceiling, extending the elbow, and bringing the arm up against the ear. A shortened triceps (especially the long head) will not allow for full elbow extension or full elevation of the arm. The region just above the lateral epicondyle, in the distal and lateral portion of the medial head of the triceps, is where most trigger points can be located by palpation. Trigger point PR or MRT levels 1 and 2 can easily be applied to any trigger points or adhesions found in this region of the muscle. This can be followed by, or combined with, some post-isometric stretches in which the patient actively flexes the elbow, engaging the principle of reciprocal inhibition.

Stretching the medial and lateral heads of the triceps only requires elbow flexion, because these heads do not cross the glenohumeral joint. The long head does cross the shoulder joint and, therefore, requires both elbow and upper arm flexion for an effective stretch.

Transverse Friction Massage (TFM)

Two reasons for primarily treating the forearm extensor muscles, rather than the common extensor tendon itself, are 1) the neurologic phenomenon of referred myofascial pain to the lateral epicondyle, and 2) the biomechanical phenomenon of "pulling action" by hypertonic muscle fibers on the common extensor tendon.

Yet there is one more manual soft tissue technique that deserves some discussion, the method of transverse friction massage (TFM). TFM was first introduced into the literature by the orthopaedic surgeons Mennell (33) and Cyriax (2,3) and popularized within the chiropractic profession by Hammer (5).

This technique is different from the myofascial techniques in several ways. First, TFM is *applied across the grain*

of tissues and involves vigorous rubbing. Second, TFM is typically *applied directly to a tendon or ligament*, not usually over muscle tissue, except for myotendinous junctions or adhesions between fibers of muscles. Third, TFM is applied to the tissues for a much longer period than any myofascial method, anywhere from 10 to 20 minutes according to Cyriax and Cyriax (2). However, in reality, it is rare to apply TFM for longer than 10 minutes, and many clinicians stop the application of TFM once an analgesic effect has been produced.

Typically, TFM is used in cases of LE in which the clinician suspects that the actual pain is coming directly from the common extensor tendon (tendinitis or tendinosis), rather than from trigger points within the forearm extensor muscles. One major clue to this clinical possibility would be the lack of favorable response after a short course of myofascial therapy applied to the forearm extensor muscles. Clinically, the patient with acute tendinitis would be distinguishable from the myofascial referred pain patient by showing a very circumscribed pain directly over the lateral epicondyle with resisted wrist extension. The lateral epicondyle would be exquisitely painful to even light percussion or palpation.

The rationale and theoretical mechanism of action of TFM is based on the resultant intense hyperemia that occurs after the application of this technique, which is thought to stimulate blood flow and increase healing. Cyriax believed that transverse friction applied at right angles to the tissues would not injure the normally healing tissues, but would break down abnormal scar tissue that had been laid down in a disorganized matrix within the tendon after acute inflammation or injury (2,3).

Cyriax's theory is probably not too far off the mark, based on recent basic scientific studies about tendon injury and repair (18,20). Earlier we discussed the recent evidence that most cases of tendinitis appear more likely to be cases of tendinosis. Abundant histologic evidence indicates that tendons go through a degenerative process, which is usually quite advanced before some form of trauma or repetitive strain injures those weakened tissues and acute inflammation sets in. Based on these recent data, TFM may mechanically accelerate the "stalled" healing process, much like the purported mechanism of action for surgical debridement of chronically "inflamed" tendons discussed earlier.

Technique 5-4 summarizes the salient features of the clinical application of TFM as described by Cyriax and Cyriax (2). Hammer has an excellent chapter on friction massage in his text, including illustrations of specific manual procedures (5).

Bracing and Adjunctive Modalities

The widespread use of tennis elbow braces and various physiotherapy modalities as adjunctive aides in the treatment of lateral epicondylitis (LE) deserve some mention. Numerous types of tennis elbow supports are on the market, which claim to effectively take stress off the common

TECHNIQUE 5-4

Transverse Friction Massage (TFM)

The clinician first localizes the ligament, tendon, or myotendinous junction to be treated by the use of manual resistance tests (selective tension). In the case of lateral epicondylitis, the tissue to be treated is usually the common extensor tendon. The clinician positions the patient such that the tissue being treated is under some amount of mild tension. Deep manual pressure is applied *across the grain* of the fibers, at a right angle to the orientation of the tissue being treated. Transverse friction, not mere pressure, is what is thought to make this treatment effective. TFM is applied to the tissues for 10 to 20 minutes, or until anesthesia has occurred (2,3,5,34). TFM should not be confused with another technique known as *strumming*, which is essentially a cross-fiber version of trigger point PR and stripping massage, described by Simons et al. (7).

Common reasons for failure with this technique:

- Clinician uses overly aggressive pressure during the friction massage, or applies the method for too much time during an office visit. Typically, the TFM should be applied only until the patient begins to experience an analgesic effect from the procedure, usually approximately 5 to 10 minutes.

- Application of TFM over an acutely inflamed tendon or soft tissue may aggravate the condition and lead to increased swelling. Also, TFM should not be used directly over areas of acutely traumatized soft tissues.

extensor tendon. The presumption is that by applying a force over the bellies of the forearm extensor muscles, that an alternate "insertion point" is created proximal to the lateral epicondyle. This is also the basis for the compression test described in Box 5-1, in which manual pressure applied to the extensor muscle mass relieves LE pain during resisted wrist extension.

Two specific tennis elbow support braces are recommended: the Aircast® tennis elbow brace (Aircast Inc., Summit, NJ) and the Epi-Lok® tennis elbow brace (CMO Inc., Barberton, OH). The Aircast® brace has a plastic "bubble" integrated into a wide forearm band, which can be placed directly over the most painful trigger points in the proximal forearm. This bubble tends to concentrate force in a more localized area, compared with standard forearm braces, which are merely wide straps. One preliminary study using 10 normal subjects showed that the Aircast® support significantly reduced EMG activity of the extensor digitorum and ECRB muscles, whereas usual tennis elbow braces did not (35).

The Epi-Lok® tennis elbow support also incorporates a novel design; it uses a padded bar about 10 cm long with two forearm straps. The padded bar is designed to be placed longitudinally "along the grain" of the ECRB, ECRL, or extensor digitorum muscles, using the two straps around the forearm to hold it in place. The bar exerts pressure along a greater surface area of the muscle, thereby bracing much more of the muscle tissue than a standard tennis elbow support.

Physiotherapy modalities have been used in the treatment of LE and tennis elbow for many years. It is beyond the scope of this text to provide a comprehensive discussion of all the various types of adjunctive therapies used. However, some of the more popular modalities used in clinical practice are ultrasound (38), microcurrent stimulation (MENS) (39), transcutaneous electrical nerve stimulation (TENS), acupuncture (both needle and laser), interferential stimulation, iontophoresis, and phonophoresis.

A review of the modality literature can be unsettling, because various studies both support and refute the clinical usefulness of most adjunctive therapies. For example, one randomized study of patients with LE treated with either placebo or pulsed ultrasound showed no statistical differences between the groups (41). However, another randomized study of LE patients with similar research design (placebo versus pulsed ultrasound groups) concluded that there was a highly statistical difference between the treatment groups, with 63% of the pulsed ultrasound group improving, compared with only 29% of the placebo group (40).

Another confounding variable in the research of modalities is that they are rarely used as stand-alone therapies in the treatment of LE. Typically these modalities are used in conjunction with manual techniques, forearm bracing, medications, and rehabilitative exercise. However, considering the fact that there is very little, if any, evidence that these adjunctive modalities cause severe iatrogenic side effects, their use in the clinical setting is likely to continue. Clearly, more definitive studies are needed to clarify the role that adjunctive modalities should play in the treatment of soft tissue lesions.

Patient Exercise and Home Care

The patient with a chronic case of soft tissue pain surrounding the lateral epicondylar region will require some self-care tips and suggestions to prevent recurrence. The patient should understand that this condition is almost always related to some type of cumulative trauma to the common extensor tendon (which is typically somewhat degenerated) by repetitive use or overactivity of the forearm extensor muscles. It should be emphasized that the condition is not *caused* by weak extensor muscles, as many patients presume is the case. Rather, the associated muscle weakness occurs as a secondary problem from disuse caused by avoidance of activity because of pain.

In the very acute phase of the condition, resting the swollen tissues is the first course of action. No vigorous stretching or strengthening exercises are recommended while the patient is in the acute phase. Patients should avoid any home activities that are potential aggravating or perpetuating factors, such as prolonged grasping of garden tools, screwdrivers, hammers, paintbrushes, and the like. If the patient's occupation requires prolonged use of the forearm muscles, such as carpentry, the judicious use of a tennis elbow support brace during working hours is warranted. Patients who play racquetball, squash, or tennis should be encouraged to use such a brace prophylactically during games and practices, especially if they have a tendency to develop lateral elbow pain during or after exercise.

Very gentle stretching exercises can be incorporated into the clinical management of LE from the first visit, unless the patient reports that such stretching aggravates the condition. The clinician can passively stretch the muscles for the patient, using PIR or other stretching methods. Once the patient sees and experiences the positioning and degree of tension involved with the stretches, he may be able to perform self-stretching techniques. The simplest way to self-stretch most of the forearm extensor muscles is to have the patient pronate the forearm, flex the wrist and fingers with the elbow in complete extension, then extend the upper arm at the shoulder. Ten to twelve repetitions of this stretch should be performed approximately twice daily. The patient could easily perform these stretches while at work or home, whenever the tissues feel tight.

Strengthening exercises are often used adjunctively in the management of LE pain, but it is important that they be used properly, *after the acute pain has subsided*. As a rule of thumb, before starting any strengthening program, there should be little or no sharp epicondyle pain on resistance testing of wrist extension. Many patients attempt to perform vigorous wrist extension exercises with Thera-Bands or hand weights during the acute phase of their condition, which exacerbates the problem. If the common extensor tendon is truly swollen and inflamed, attempts at strengthening are doomed to failure, because the increased tension generated during the exercises will irritate the already inflamed tissues. Therefore, the timing element of when to begin strength training is critical to the success of such exercise.

Once the acute pain has subsided and the patient is ready to begin strengthening the forearm extensors, such a regimen is relatively easy and straightforward. The patient can be given a Thera-Band or small dumbbell and instructed to perform wrist extensions against resistance, with the forearm lying flat on a table, the arm of a chair, or the patient's lap. Handgrips, resistance-type putty, or small balls can be used to perform hand squeezes against resistance. These handgrip exercises will stimulate muscles of the forearm extensors and flexors, as well as the intrinsic hand muscles.

The supinator muscle can be strengthened, but to isolate it from the synergistic biceps brachii, the patient must have the elbow in complete extension. With even mild elbow flexion, the biceps brachii muscle becomes a powerful supinator of the forearm and will overshadow the supinator

during any strengthening exercise. The patient can lock the elbow in complete extension by using the other hand to support the underside of the elbow, pushing up on the olecranon and holding the elbow in extension. While in this position, the patient can perform 10 to 12 repetitions of supination against resistance by using Thera-Bands or small dumbbell weights.

CONCLUSION

The diagnosis of lateral epicondylitis (or more appropriately, *epicondylalgia*) is relatively simple when the patient's symptoms can be reproduced by resistance testing and palpation over the soft tissues in the area of the lateral elbow. Some cases are more complicated and may involve referred pain patterns from trigger points in the neck, shoulder or chest muscles—most commonly the scalenes, pectoralis major and minor, the infraspinatus, and the subscapularis. Pain may be referred into the elbow from inflammatory lesions within the glenohumeral joint, such as chronic dislocation with instability, arthritis, or other conditions.

The cervical spine is also a potential source of referred pain to the shoulder and elbow by the mechanisms of sclerotogenous pain from degenerative facet joints, or nerve root entrapments from cervical disc lesions. Note that the character of sclerotogenous referred pain from the shoulder or cervical facet joints is "deep and toothache-like," whereas the patient with cervical nerve root or brachial plexus irritation will complain of "numbness, tingling, warm or cold feelings." In either case, orthopaedic tests that place stress on the shoulder and cervical facet joints should reproduce the elbow symptoms.

To manage patients with LE pain, the clinician must understand how to diagnose and treat the various soft tissues of the forearm and upper extremity. Knowledge of the muscular origins and insertions, joint mechanics, referred pain patterns, and muscle action is very important to clinical success when implementing conservative manual techniques. If the clinician is well versed in the anatomy and biomechanical function of these soft tissues, then manual myofascial treatment techniques can be applied easily in an appropriate manner.

The role of patient self-care cannot be underestimated. Patients must be educated about the cause of this cumulative trauma disorder and the role of tendon degeneration that is often associated with the condition. They must be willing to take time and care to rest their swollen tissues and modify their lifestyle accordingly. Good compliance with a forearm brace may help enough that some patients can perform their normal duties without much job modification. Other patients may require substantial changes in work duties to adequately rest the muscles and tendon from functional overload. Managing patients with respect to alterations in lifestyle and eliminated perpetuating factors may present the greatest challenge to the soft tissue practitioner.

Algorithm for treatment of Tennis Elbow Pain

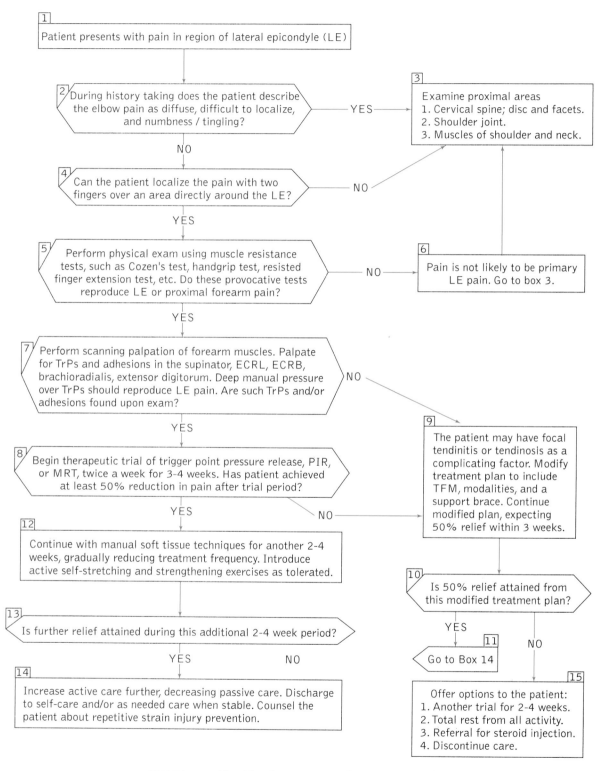

FIGURE 5-7. Algorithm for treatment of tennis elbow pain.

Most myofascial techniques, when applied properly, result in very rapid relief of symptoms, many times after just a few office visits. These techniques should be applied about twice weekly, to allow the tissues some time to heal in between treatment sessions; otherwise, it is possible to cause iatrogenic muscle damage. If the patient is not at least 50% improved within 3 to 4 weeks, the clinician should reexamine the patient and consider other treatment methods. Also, it is important to look at the shoulder and neck for other potential causes of the presenting pain syndrome. The reader is advised to review the treatment protocol section in this chapter and the algorithm for clinical management of tennis elbow pain (Fig. 5-7) for a game plan by which to treat and clinically manage patients with lateral elbow pain.

Clinicians who understand the concepts presented in this chapter will be able to appropriately diagnose and successfully treat most cases of LE with conservative manual techniques. They will also understand when it is appropriate to refer patients for more aggressive diagnostic testing or treatment.

TREATMENT PROTOCOL

1. Perform a physical examination by using muscle resistance tests such as Cozen's test, the handgrip test, and resisted wrist extension, and observe whether the patient has pain reproduction around the lateral epicondyle or proximal forearm extensors.

2. If the patient does not localize the pain to the lateral epicondyle or forearm extensors with provocative muscle resistance tests, consider the possibility of a primary cervical or shoulder joint or muscle dysfunction with referred pain to the forearm. Also consider that the patient may simultaneously have multiple areas of dysfunction, including both soft tissues and joint dysfunction in the elbow, shoulder, or cervical spine.

3. Check for joint play and other signs of dysfunction in the various joints of the elbow, especially the radial head in its articulation with the ulna (proximal radio-ulnar joint). The ulno-humeral and radio-humeral joints also should be assessed for joint dysfunction. Standard manipulation and mobilization techniques can be used by qualified clinicians to correct these joint dysfunctions.

4. If the patient does localize the pain to the lateral epicondyle or forearm extensors with provocative muscle resistance tests, perform scanning palpation of the forearm extensor muscles. Palpate for taut bands in the supinator, ECRB, ECRL, and brachioradialis. Search within these taut bands for trigger point knots or nodules that reproduce the patient's pain. Also scan the triceps and extensor digitorum for potential trigger points and taut bands.

5. If scanning palpation fails to detect trigger point nodules that reproduce the pain pattern, yet lateral elbow pain is clearly reproduced with muscle resistance tests, consider the possibility of tendinosis or tendinitis of the common extensor tendon as a complicating factor. Modify the treatment plan to incorporate direct treatment of this tendon, using modalities such as ultrasound, interferential stimulation, and TFM. Avoid vigorous stretching techniques, so as not to aggravate the tendinitis.

6. If trigger point nodules and taut bands are detected on scanning palpation, proceed to treat them with one or more of the manual myofascial techniques discussed in this chapter: Trigger point PR (ischemic compression), post-isometric relaxation (PIR), or myofascial release techniques (MRT).

7. The initial treatment program should be twice per week for 3 to 4 weeks. The patient should be expected to have at least 50% reduction in all symptoms and comparable increase in function after this time frame.

8. If the patient does not respond with at least 50% improvement after 4 weeks of myofascial treatment, further treatment is highly unlikely to be helpful. Some complicating factor probably is present, such as common extensor tendinitis or tendinosis. Again, remember the possibility of cervical spine or shoulder dysfunction that may refer pain down to the lateral elbow region.

9. If the patient is at least 50% improved after 3 to 4 weeks of myofascial treatment, it is reasonable to continue treatment for an additional 2 to 4 weeks, expecting complete resolution within this extended time frame. Treatment frequency should be gradually reduced during this time, with active self-stretching and strengthening exercises introduced as tolerated by the patient.

10. Before discharging the patient, review the principles regarding the mechanism of injury that occurs with all cumulative trauma disorders. The patient must understand how to avoid repetitive strain of the forearm extensor muscles by modification of activities. A review of self-stretching and strengthening exercises is also in order.

11. The algorithm outlined in Figure 5-7 is provided as a general outline for the clinical management of tennis elbow pain. It can serve as a quick guide to the clinical decision-making steps along the pathway of diagnosis and treatment options for this condition.

References

1. Simons DG, Travell JG, Simons LS. Myofascial Pain and Dysfunction: The Trigger Point Manual, vol 1, 2nd Ed. Baltimore: Williams and Wilkins, 1999.

2. Cyriax JH, Cyriax PJ. Illustrated Manual of Orthopaedic Medicine. Butterworths. London, UK: 1983.

3. Cyriax JH. Textbook of Orthopaedic Medicine, vol 1 and 2. Philadelphia: Balliere Tindall,1984.

4. Laslett M. Mechanical Diagnosis and Therapy: The Upper Limb. Self published; available from OPTP, Minneapolis, MN. 1996.

5. Hammer WI. Functional Soft Tissue Examination and Treatment by Manual Methods. Gaithersburg, MD, Aspen, 1991.

6. Kendall FP, McCreary EK. Muscles: Testing and Function, 4th Ed. Baltimore: Williams and Wilkins, 1993.

7. Simons DG, Travell JG, Simons LS. Myofascial Pain and Dysfunction: The Trigger Point Manual, vol 1, 2nd Ed. Baltimore: Williams and Wilkins, 1999.

8. Greenman PE. Principles of Manual Medicine. Baltimore: Williams and Wilkins, 1989.

9. Lewit K. Manipulative Therapy in Rehabilitation of the Motor System. London: Butterworths, 1987.

10. Lewit K, Simons DG. Myofascial pain: relief by post-isometric relaxation. Arch Phys Med Rehabil 1984;65:452–456.

11. Schneider MJ. Principles of Manual Trigger Point Therapy. Self published, 1720 Wash. Rd., Suite 201, Pittsburgh, PA 15241, 1994.

12. Schneider MJ. Chiropractic management of myofascial and muscular disorders. In: Advances in Chiropractic, vol 3. St Louis: Mosby, 1996:55–88.

13. Schneider MJ, Cohen JH. Nimmo receptor tonus technique: a chiropractic approach to trigger point therapy. In: Sweere JJ, ed. Chiropractic Family Practice Manual. Gaithersburg, MD: Aspen, 1992: 3–3–1–18. Chapter 3, Section 3, 1–18.

14. Jarvinsen M, Jozsa L, Kannus P, et al. Histopathological findings in chronic tendon disorders. Scand J Med Sci Sports. 1997;7:86–95.

15. Simons DG. Clinical and etiological update of myofascial pain from trigger points. J Musculoskel Pain. 1996;4(1/2): 93–121.

16. Hoppenfeld S. Physical Examination of the Spine and Extremities. New York: Appleton-Century-Crofts, 1976.

17. Magee DJ. Orthopedic Physical Assessment. Philadelphia: Saunders, 1987.

18. O'Brien M. Structure and metabolism of tendon. Scand J Med Sci Sports. 1997;7:55–61.

19. Simons DG. Myofascial pain syndrome due to trigger points. Chapter 45. In Goodgold J, ed. Rehabilitation Medicine. St Louis: Mosby, 1988:686–723.

20. Kannus P, Jozsa L. Histopathological changes preceding spontaneous rupture of a tendon: a controlled study of 891 patients. J Bone Joint Surg Am 1991;73:1507–1525.

21. Sandmeier R, Renstrom PA. Diagnosis and treatment of chronic tendon disorders in sport. Scand J Med Sci Sports 1997;7:96–106.

22. Hench PS, Kendall FC. The effect of adrenal cortex of pituitary adrenocorticosterone hormone on RA: Preliminary report. Proceedings of the staff meeting of the Mayo Clinic, 1949 (abstract).

23. Assendelft WJ, Hay EM, Adshead R, et al. Corticosteroid injections for lateral epicondylitis: a systematic overview. Br J Gen Pract. 1996;46:209–216.

24. Nimmo RL, Vannerson JF. The Receptor: A 7 part series of monographs self-published by Nimmo from 1958–1980. Reprints available from MJ Schneider, 1720 Wash. Rd. Suite 201, Pittsburgh, PA 15241.

25. Prudden B. Pain Erasure. New York: Ballantine Books, 1980.

26. Chaitow L. Soft Tissue Manipulation. Wellborough, Northamptonshire, UK: Thorsons Publishing Group, 1987. [First published in 1980 under the title: Neuro-Muscular Technique]

27. St. John Neuromuscular Seminars. 10710 Seminole Blvd, Suite 1, Largo, FL.

28. Lewit K. Post-isometric relaxation in combination with other methods of muscular facilitation and inhibition. Manual Medicine 1986;101–104.

29. Liebenson C. Active muscular relaxation techniques, Parts 1 & 2. J.M.P.T. 1989;12:446–454 and 1990;13:2–6.

30. Leahy PM, Mock LE. Myofascial release technique and mechanical compromise of peripheral nerves of the upper extremity. Chiro Sports Med 1992;6:139–150.

31. Leahy PM. Manual and videotapes published by Active Release Techniques, LLP. Copyright 1996. 10. N. Meade Ave, Colorado Springs, CO, 80909.

32. Mock LE. Myofascial release treatment of specific muscles of the upper extremity (Levels 3 & 4). Part 1; Clin Bull Myofasc Ther, 1997;2:5–23. Part 2; Clin Bull Myofasc Ther, 1997;2:5–22. Part 3; Clin Bull Myofasc Ther, 1997;2:51–69. Part 4; Clin Bull Myofasc Ther, 1998;3:71–93.

33. Mennell JB. Physical Treatment by Movement: Manipulation and Massage, 5th Ed. Boston: Blakiston, 1947.

34. Chamberlain GJ. Cyriax's friction massage: a review. J Ortho Sports Phys Ther. 1982;4:16–22.

35. Snyder-Mackler L, Epler M. Effect of standard and Aircast tennis elbow bands on integrated electromyography of forearm extensor musculature proximal to bands. Am J Sports Med 1989;17:278–281.

36. Fredberg U. Local corticosteroid injection in sport: review of literature and guidelines for treatment. Scand J Med Sci Sports. 1997;7:131–139.

37. Nakano KK. Peripheral nerve entrapments, repetitive strain disorder, occupation related syndromes, bursitis, and tendonitis. Curr Opin Rheum 1991;3:226–239.

38. Frieder S, Weisberg J, Fleming B, et al. A pilot study: the therapeutic effect of ultrasound following partial rupture of Achilles tendons in male rats. JOSPT 1988;10(2):39–46.

39. Cheng N, Van Hoof H, Bockx E, et al. The effects of electric currents on ATP generation, protein synthesis, and membrane transport in rat skin. Clin Orthop Rel Res 1982;171:264–272.

40. Haker E, Lundeberg T. Pulsed ultrasound in lateral epicondylalgia. Scand J Rehabil Med 1991;23:115–118.

41. Binder A, Hodge G, Greenwood AM, et al. Is therapeutic ultrasound effective in treating soft tissue lesions? Br Med J (Clin Res Ed) 1985;290:512–514.

6 _Carpal Tunnel Syndrome_

Lewis Mock, DC

INTRODUCTION

Carpal tunnel syndrome (CTS) is one of the most common mono-neuropathies (a disorder involving only a single nerve), and it is the most common peripheral nerve entrapment in the arm (1–3). CTS is one of several peripheral nerve entrapment syndromes and **cumulative trauma disorders** (CTDs) that have a significant impact on Americans in the workplace (4–9). The condition occurs most often in persons with jobs requiring repetitive motion activities, including keyboarding, carpentry, using vibrating tools, or operating heavy machinery. In occupational carpal tunnel syndrome (OCTS), the symptoms and signs are work-related.

Traditional medical treatments have not produced adequate results in many cases. This chapter presents an approach based on the diagnosis and treatment of CTS as an entrapment neuropathy. This treatment approach is based on the concept of **nerve excursion** and the identification and treatment of restrictions of nerve excursion by using myofascial release techniques. This approach is promising because even after failed surgery, 6 to 10 treatments over the course of 3 to 5 weeks typically result in patients returning to work. Comparing the expense of eight myofascial release treatments with the overall cost of a traditional medical approach clearly shows the economic benefits of this myofascial approach as well.

CARPAL TUNNEL SYNDROME: BACKGROUND

In recent years, the general public has come to use the term *carpal tunnel syndrome* to describe any symptom experienced in the upper extremities. According to the U.S. Bureau of Labor Statistics, CTDs have accounted for more than 60% of all occupational illnesses since 1991 (4). Employers and health care professionals also have become more aware of these disorders, because the associated costs are between $60 and $100 billion annually. Cumulative trauma disorders are thought to affect the very survival of certain industries (4).

CTS is a type of peripheral nerve entrapment involving the median nerve and its entrapment at the carpal tunnel. The terms *peripheral nerve entrapment* and *compression neuropathy* are conventionally used interchangeably to describe the idea that a nerve is entrapped or compressed somewhere along its course from origin to termination.

- **Compression neuropathy** is the result of damage to a peripheral nerve by pressure. This pressure may occur anywhere along the course of a nerve, and at multiple sites. Certain sites along the nerve tract are more vulnerable than others, and the carpal tunnel is one of them.

- **Peripheral entrapment neuropathy** is a specific type of compression neuropathy, in which a nerve is compressed by some other anatomic structure (10). This usually occurs where a nerve passes through a muscle or fibro-osseous passageway and, therefore, is more susceptible to compression (11). To cause nerve injury, these structural restrictions usually must be combined with external pressure, positioning, or other factors. Repetitive movements seem to play a role, in combination with these other factors (4,12).

In compression neuropathies the different sites of entrapment name the diagnosis. For example, cubital tunnel syndrome is entrapment of the ulnar nerve at the cubital tunnel; thoracic outlet syndrome is entrapment of the neural or vascular structures at the thoracic outlet. It is also possible for the nerves to be entrapped at several different areas at the same time.

The median nerve is extremely vulnerable to compression and injury in the region of the wrist and palm, where it is bounded by the carpal bones and the **flexor retinaculum** (FR). The most common site of compression is at the proximal edge of the FR (near the crease of the wrist).

Although CTS may have other causes such as pregnancy, acromegaly, myxedema, osteoarthritis of the carpal bones, contraceptive pills, hemodialysis, infiltration of the transverse carpal ligament in amyloidosis, and rheumatoid arthritis (RA) (3), the literature reports an occupational cause in more than 47% of the reported cases (8).

Diagnosis and Clinical Features

CTS diagnosis involves several considerations. The condition occurs more often in women than men, is more often unilateral (although it may be bilateral), and is rarely seen in children. It occurs most often in people with occupations requiring constant, repetitive motions over long periods, peculiar postures, exposure to high-frequency vibration, and direct trauma.

In certain instances, CTS is caused by some known disorder involving increased pressure within the carpal tunnel. Such situations include a displaced fracture of the distal radius, a lunar or perilunar dislocation, and swelling of the common flexor tendon sheath. Other conditions such as myxedema and RA may have CTS as an attendant condition. In rare cases of CTS, the carpal tunnel may be congenitally small, the tunnel may be compromised by the ganglion, or anomalous tendons and muscles may be present (3).

The differential diagnosis should include C6 or C7 nerve root involvement and discogenic disease. Multiple sclerosis also should be considered if the physical findings do not support the subjective complaints.

The myofascial treatment recommended in this chapter is mainly useful for CTS related to work or cumulative trauma. However, it is also useful for releasing postsurgical adhesions and in alleviating symptoms of some of the abovementioned conditions, once the primary pathologic situation has been addressed.

As described by Travell and Simons (13), trigger points in the upper torso can refer patterns of pain and paresthesias that mimic the neurologic symptoms of compression and entrapment neuropathies into the hand, fingers, and distal extremities. Trigger points and their referral patterns must be considered for a thorough differential diagnosis. In patients with upper-extremity complaints, identifying trigger points may be part of the complete diagnosis. Myofascial pain syndromes are common in patients whose jobs require working at computers, desks, or other types of workstations for long periods. The head-forward posture used in these positions also may lead to rolled-in shoulders, which may result in scalene or thoracic outlet problems, leading to nerve entrapment syndromes.

Initial Diagnosis

Initial diagnosis of CTS always begins with history taking and physical examination, which establish the foundation for subsequent diagnostic and therapeutic procedures.

History. History taking should address the occupational situation. Activities requiring continual use of the hands, or repetitive motions using force, may result in OCTS. Such motions include prolonged flexion or extension of the wrists, gripping, pressure over the palm, trauma, fractures, and vibration. Typists, data-entry workers, supermarket cashiers, meat cutters, assemblers, and instrumental musicians all perform these activities.

Symptoms. The onset of symptoms is usually insidious. Symptoms usually occur at night or in the early hours of the morning and awaken the patient with paresthesia or burning of the hand. The pain involves the distal median nerve distribution into the first three or four digits of the hand, mainly on the palmar side. Pain also may be felt in the hand, wrist, forearm, elbow, or shoulder. Proximal pain is not uncommon.

The distribution of the sensory symptoms of the median nerve may vary considerably. Before passing through the carpal tunnel, the median nerve gives off a sensory branch above the wrist, which innervates the skin of the palm. CTS will not affect the median sensory distribution in the palm but will result in altered sensation in the fingers (14). Although the nerve only goes to the thumb (1st digit), the index finger (2nd digit), the long finger (3rd digit), and half of the ring finger (4th digit), patients may report numbness, tingling, or burning in any or all of the fingers of the entire hand.

Symptoms are usually relieved temporarily by shaking the hands, immersing them in hot water, or simply by a period of rest. Diminished sensation may bring on clumsiness, which may be accompanied by decreased grip strength and a history of dropping things. Cyanosis may be noted as well. Subjective complaints of actual weakness are rare.

Physical Examination. Physical examination should include observation and inspection. Watching the patient attempt fine finger movements such as handling buttons or other fasteners, may provide clues about the extent of involvement. Examination for thenar atrophy should be per-

formed, although atrophy usually occurs only in chronic or severe cases. Initial objective findings consist of impaired sensation of pinprick over the median nerve distribution area; usually the index and middle fingers are involved, the thumb less frequently. Sensory splitting of the ring finger (fourth digit) only occurs in peripheral involvement of the median and ulnar nerves and distinguishes CTS from proximal lesions such as cervical radiculopathy. Loss of temperature, light touch, and position sense are uncommon.

Atrophy of the thenar eminence in the short abductor of the thumb may appear when the condition is severe or prolonged. The typical motor deficit resulting from median nerve entrapment is the wasting of the thenar eminence and loss of thumb abduction—the so-called simian hand, in which the thumb is restricted to the plane of the palm and lies extended next to the index finger, preventing oppositional movement. Weakness of the abductor pollicis brevis (APB) is the most sensitive motor sign of CTS, because the thenar muscle is the muscle least likely to receive anomalous ulnar innervation. It is best to examine the APB in relative isolation by ensuring that the thumb is held parallel to the index finger while testing the abduction up from the plane of the palm (3).

Weakness of opposition of the thumb and 5th digit suggests median nerve involvement. The median nerve enables opposition of the thumb to the index and middle fingers and is essential for precision grip. Opposition should be tested with the wrist supinated, pronated, and with flexion and extension added to each of the above wrist positions. Weakness on resistive testing is not highly reliable as an objective test, partially because of the overlapping or substitution of innervation. However, it can add extra information for a more thorough examination.

Pronator Teres Syndrome

One of the many things to consider in the differential diagnosis of CTS is the variations between **pronator teres syndrome** (PTS) and CTS. PTS involves the entrapment of the median nerve between the two bellies of the pronator teres muscle. This muscle attaches at the common flexor tendon and the medial epicondyle of the humerus. It then passes obliquely across the forearm and ends in a flat tendon that inserts on a rough impression midway along the lateral surface of the body of the radius. Because the movement of pronation is very repetitive in keyboarders and other types of assembly line workers, the pronator teres is a common location for entrapment of the median nerve.

PTS is often misdiagnosed as CTS because both conditions involve the median nerve. The pattern of sensory loss with CTS spares the palmar surface of the hand and usually involves only the thumb and three and a half digits. In PTS, sensory loss usually involves the entire median nerve field of the hand. However, as mentioned earlier, nerve distribution varies among individuals. Therefore, attempting to treat only the carpal tunnel when the pronator teres may be a contributing factor, or even the primary cause, is inadequate

TABLE 6-1		
Several Common Provocative Tests for Carpal Tunnel Syndrome		
Name of Test	Technique	Positive Signs
Phalen's test	The patient's wrists are flexed and the dorsal surfaces of the hands are pushed together. The position is held for 1 minute.	Symptoms of discomfort, numbness, and tingling paresthesia are reproduced or exaggerated in the hand and digits.
Tinel's sign	With a reflex hammer, the practitioner gently taps over the carpal tunnel at the wrist and over the pronator teres at the proximal forearm and over the nerve course in the forearm.	A transient, often painful tingling sensation is experienced in the distal distribution of the injured nerve (not in the area percussed). This tingling persists for several seconds.
Reverse Phalen's test	Patient holds hands in a ''prayer position'' with the wrists extended and palmar surfaces together. The position is held for 1–2 minutes.	Symptoms of discomfort, numbness, and tingling paresthesia are reproduced or exaggerated in the hand and digits.
Tethered median nerve stress test	The patient supinates the wrist and simultaneously extends the distal interphalangeal joint of the index finger and the wrist. The position is held for 1–2 minutes.	The most common provocative complaint is discomfort characterized as aching and myalgic, which increases the longer the test position is held.

and unwise. Likewise, not treating the carpal tunnel because the patient has pronator teres signs is also inadequate and unwise.

Aggravation of the nerve anywhere along its course, from the spinal cord to the tips of the fingers, makes the nerve vulnerable to compromise elsewhere. The whole nerve becomes involved. Therefore, rather than using the more traditional term **double crush**, which suggests compression at two areas, the term **whole nerve syndrome** is preferred. In cumulative trauma-related CTS, areas other than the carpal tunnel are almost always involved. For example, entrapment of the median nerve at the pronator teres elicits a positive Tinel's sign at the wrist.

Diagnostic Tests

The following tests are useful in the diagnosis of CTS (Table 6.1).

Phalen's Test. A positive Phalen's test is considered a reliable diagnostic sign of CTS, with an 80% specificity (15). In this test, the examiner places the patient's flexed wrists together, dorsal surface to dorsal surface, with the fingers pointing toward the floor, and holds them in this position for 1 minute (Fig. 6-1). A positive sign is indicated by tingling into the thumb, the index finger, and the middle and lateral half of the ring finger, as the flexed wrists place pressure on the median nerve.

Tinel's Sign. Although commonly used as a diagnostic test for CTS when performed at the wrist, Tinel's sign is most reliable when combined with other clinical findings. Although it is considered one of the least sensitive provocative tests, it is considered fairly specific, with only a 6% false-positive rate (15). In this test, the examiner taps digitally or with a

reflex hammer over the carpal tunnel at the wrist. Paresthesia felt distal to the point of pressure is considered a positive sign. This test may indicate the rate of regeneration of the sensory fibers of the median nerve. The most distal point at which the abnormal sensation is felt represents the limit of nerve regeneration (14). Evaluation for contralateral signs is recommended because of the frequency of bilateral involvement.

Reverse Phalen's Test. The reverse Phalen's test is performed with the wrists in extension. The patient assumes a palm-to-palm prayer position with the wrist and fingers

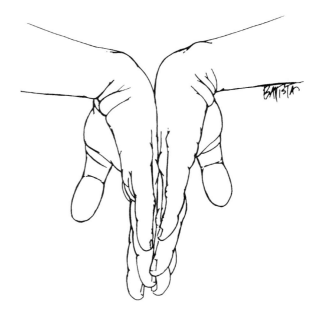

FIGURE 6-1. **The Phalen's test.**

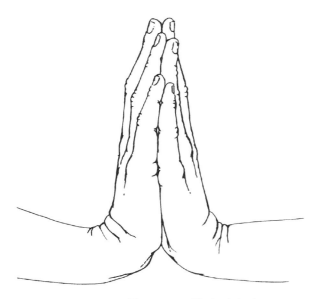

FIGURE 6-2. The reverse Phalen's test.

index finger and, while holding the finger by the distal phalanx, holds the finger in forced extension. This extension provides a significant amount of distal median nerve excursion and combines forced extension and traction on the nerve as in the reverse Phalen's test. This nerve excursion may produce radiation of pain from the tunnel up to the pronator teres. The pain, usually described as aching, increases as the position is maintained. The pain is primarily myalgic, and its intensity is temporally related to the activity that precipitates it.

Characteristically, patients with positive TMNST results show few motor signs of thenar muscle weakness or atrophy and have minimal electromyographic findings. However, their symptoms can be quite severe, particularly at night or with repetitive manipulative activity. Patients with negative TMNST results probably have acute CTS with symptoms that have been present for less than 3 weeks (17).

in full extension (Fig. 6-2) and attempts to maintain this position for 2 minutes. This position causes a steady increase in pressure in the carpal tunnel. This pressure is different from that elicited by the Phalen's test, which tends to plateau after approximately 20 to 30 seconds. In one study, Werner, Bir, and Armstrong state that the pressure at the carpal tunnel during the reverse Phalen's test averaged 34 mm Hg at 1 minute into the test, and 42 mm Hg at 2 minutes, significantly higher than the 4 mm Hg average change during the Phalen's test (16). These results suggest that finger and wrist extension actually may be a more useful test.

Tethered Median Nerve Stress Test. In a chronic, low-grade median nerve compression, in which motor signs are minimal and symptoms are mostly sensory, the tethered median nerve stress test (TMNST) may be useful. Tension on the median nerve is produced by simultaneous extension of the supinated wrist and the distal interphalangeal joint of the index finger (Fig. 6-3). The examiner grasps the patient's

Upper Limb Tension Test. Butler describes several variations of the upper limb tension test (ULTT), also called the straight leg raise test (SLR) of the arm (18). According to Butler, this test is as useful for examining upper limb and neck disorders as the SLR is in assessment of patients with lower limb and spinal disorders. Because this testing method is complex, interested readers are referred to Butler's text for a description of this method.

Palpation for Restriction at Flexor Retinaculum. Sucher discusses the possibility that a "threshold" of mechanical restriction exists in the wrist or carpal canal that, once reached, generates enough pressure within the carpal tunnel to physiologically compromise the median nerve (19). To assess for such restriction, he uses standard range-of-motion procedures and a modified palpatory examination of the wrist. The patient is seated and faces the examiner with the elbows flexed to 90°. Initially, the patient's forearms are supinated, and restriction is best detected by the examiner placing the thumb pads over the ventral aspect of the patient's carpal canal, up against the flexor retinaculum (FR) (Fig. 6-4).

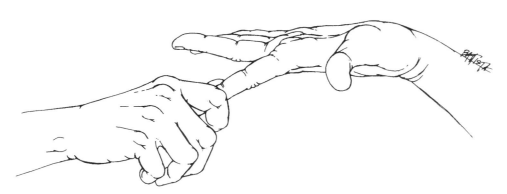

FIGURE 6-3. The tethered median nerve stress test (TMNST). The median nerve is put under tension by extending the elbow, wrist, and index.

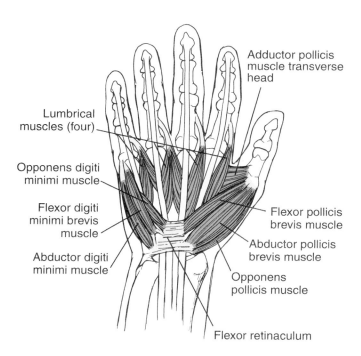

Adductor pollicis muscle transverse head

Lumbrical muscles (four)

Opponens digiti minimi muscle

Flexor digiti minimi brevis muscle

Abductor digiti minimi muscle

Flexor pollicis brevis muscle

Abductor pollicis brevis muscle

Opponens pollicis muscle

Flexor retinaculum

FIGURE 6-4. The flexor retinaculum.
Reprinted with permission from Hendrickson T: Massage for Orthopedic Conditions. Baltimore: Lippincott Williams & Wilkins, 2003, fig. 10.8 (p. 394).

The phases of palpation include palpation of the FR during:

1. Wrist extension and flexion

2. FR extension

3. Thenar radial abduction/extension

4. Radial and ulnar deviation

5. Forearm wrist supination and pronation (which involves placing the thumb pads over the dorsal wrist and palpating the FR with the fingertips)

6. Wrist relaxation (i.e., the wrist in a neutral position)

7. Thenar in abduction with extension and lateral rotation (retroposition)

The primary focus of this examination is on a sense of soft tissue or ligamentous bind.

Electrodiagnostic Tests. Electrodiagnostic tests are the most accepted laboratory procedures for the diagnosis of CTS. The most generally accepted, well-established, and widely used electrodiagnostic procedure is the **nerve conduction velocity** (NCV) **study**, which is used to localize the source of the neurologic symptoms of CTS. An NCV test may not always be positive, and in 3% to 8% of the cases in which a clinical diagnosis of CTS is suspected, results of NCV studies may be normal (20). Grundberg reported an 8% false-negative rate in a group of 32 subjects (21).

The NCV test usually is used in conjunction with electromyography. Nerve conduction velocities can be measured along both sensory and motor nerves, but a requirement for this procedure is that the nerve must be stimulated at two points along its course (12). Nerve conduction studies may detect evidence of demyelination, which usually precedes axonal degeneration in compression neuropathy. Nerve compression will cause a focal conduction block or localized slowing of nerve conduction.

Sensory fibers are usually affected earlier than others in compression neuropathy. Sensory nerve conduction studies can detect a slowing of conduction across the lesion and a decrease in the amplitude of the sensory nerve action potential. Axonal loss is demonstrated on electromyography, usually after the lesion has had time to produce axonal degeneration. Axonal degeneration usually takes 2 to 3 weeks and presents with fibrillations, fasciculation, neurogenic recruitment, and polyphasic units (reinnervation) of the thenar muscles. The NCV study, conversely, will show changes within a week of nerve injury.

Diagnostic Imaging. Diagnostic imaging studies have not played an important role in the evaluation of CTS. Conventional radiographs are of little help if the bony structures are intact. **Computed tomography** (CT) is of limited use because of the similar attenuation values of the contents of the carpal tunnel. When an imaging study is necessary, **magnetic resonance imaging** (MRI) has been shown to be the most helpful.

Four major MRI findings have been described for CTS:

1. Proximal swelling of the median nerve

2. Distal flattening of the median nerve

3. Increase of the median nerve signal intensity

4. Pronounced palmar bowing of the flexor retinaculum at the level of the hook of the hamate (22)

Some authors have suggested dynamic high-resolution sonography as a low-cost alternative, although its definitive role has yet to be established (23).

Laboratory Studies. If the patient's history suggests infection, or metabolic or endocrinologic or arthritic disorders such as rheumatoid arthritis or ankylosing spondylitis, or if the patient has a history of prolonged use of medications such as nonsteroidal anti-inflammatory drugs (NSAIDs), appropriate laboratory tests should be performed for the most thorough diagnosis. As suggested above, many conditions may produce symptoms of CTS.

Conventional Treatment Approaches

Conventional medical treatment of the early stages of CTS includes avoidance of the activity that produces the symptoms, followed by wrist splinting and the use of NSAIDs. If the condition does not respond to these treatments, physical therapy, a cortisone injection into the carpal tunnel, or decompression surgery may be used. Many clinicians who treat CTS conservatively experience frustration about treatment outcomes. Splinting may help for a short time, but long-term splinting can cause atrophy and weakness. Carpal tunnel pressure can increase from 3 to 30 mm Hg when the wrist is placed in extreme positions. Because the splint holds the wrist in a neutral or slightly extended position, its intended use is to relieve pressure on the median nerve.

One of the problems with using splinting to treat CTS is that there is disagreement about the cause of the symptoms. Some authors suggest that the "pins and needles" and numbness in the fingers are a pressure phenomenon (24), whereas others suggest that they are the result of a vascular mechanism (25,26).

Cailliet discusses this mechanism: "Inflating a sphygmomanometer cuff around the arm or manually compressing the radial or ulnar artery at the wrist causes an unpleasant tingling and numbness in the fingers. Release of the pressure results in a 'pins and needles' sensation lasting as long as 5 to 10 seconds... Pressure on the nerve at the wrist causes no dysesthesia; therefore, the mechanism must be considered to be vascular" (25).

Others have suggested a mechanism of nerve stretching or traction resulting from entrapment or **adhesion**, which disrupts action potential propagation, causing impairment of sensory or motor function (11,22,27). This idea has a high correlation with the types of cases seen most often in daily clinical practice. If the nerve does not glide through the tissues freely because of an adhesion, continuous flexion or extension of the wrist puts prolonged traction on it, causing increasing irritability. The reason that splinting is of temporary help is that it prevents movement of the wrist, relieving nerve traction, which allows the symptoms to decrease. This splinting will not, however, fix the problem. The adhesions must be removed from the areas around the nerve to improve gliding and excursion.

NSAIDs may help in certain cases; however, they have serious side effects, including stomach ulceration and digestive disturbances and renal toxicity. By alleviating pain, NSAIDs may simply postpone the inevitable, long-term effects of CTS.

Physical therapy modalities, such as iontophoresis and ultrasound, may help temporarily. However, they have not been shown to have significant results with CTS. Some rapid recovery programs can actually make the patient's condition worse (27).

Although surgery may be offered as the definitive treatment for CTS, it is often only the beginning of a whole new set of problems. Hand surgeon Raoul Tubiana states: "Despite its high incidence and its reputation for simplicity and efficiency, carpal tunnel release [surgery] does not invariably produce good results, and dissatisfied patients are not infrequently encountered" (28). Hand surgeon James M. Hunter states: "Recurrent carpal tunnel syndrome is becoming a real problem in increasing numbers, and numerous complications are also increasing. I am particularly concerned about the number of patients with CTS that do not return to the work force after surgery" (27).

When myofascial release techniques are used to treat hundreds of failed carpal tunnel surgeries, it becomes apparent that surgical failure is often attributable to the fact that the problem is not at the carpal tunnel but higher up at the pronator teres. Failure of efficacy is thus the result not of inadequate decompression, but rather of the misdiagnosis or inadequate diagnosis of the problem. Carpal tunnel release will not correct entrapment at the pronator teres or elsewhere along the course of the median nerve.

NERVE MOBILIZATION USING MYOFASCIAL RELEASE TECHNIQUE

The carpal tunnel is usually visualized as a tiny space that is easily compromised and cannot accommodate the structures inside. However, Hunter says that in over 700 staged tendon surgeries, approximately 200 multiple rods have been placed in the carpal tunnel without one case of compression neuropathy of the median nerve, because the space in the carpal canal is big enough for up to four tendon rods at a time. He also describes easily moving large instruments through the canal during surgery, including three Kelly hemostats at the same time. He concludes that, with the exception of tumors, displacement of carpal bones, or synovitis, there is plenty of room in the bony carpal canal for the nine flexor tendons, their sheaths, and the median nerve. "There must, therefore, be other factors present" (27).

A myofascial approach specifically addresses these other factors, particularly nerve excursion. The concept of excursion is essential to understanding the treatment approach from a myofascial standpoint. A nerve may adhere to other structures along its course from origin to termination (11,18,28,29). To function properly, nerves must be free to move and glide through the tissues and structures of the upper extremities.

The normal anatomy of the hand is one of a splay of the sensory branches of the median nerve in the palm. This splay easily permits the thumb and the fingers to spread without discomfort in the hand. Loss of this splay from fibrous fixation after injury may lead to traction of the median nerve against the carpal bones, like a bow string, allowing no movement whatsoever. Flexor tendon synovial fixation to the epineurium on the dorsal surface of the median nerve disrupts nerve excursion and causes traction with any wrist extension. The result is numbness and weakness from simple use.

Previous injury to the wrist or upper extremity may predispose a person to median nerve and carpal tunnel compromise. If the tissue surrounding the median nerve or the nerve itself is injured, the repair process that follows may gradually cause fibrous changes in the epineural structures of the nerve and surrounding the nerve. These changes may form specific scar fixations or adhesions anywhere along the course of the nerve, affecting its elasticity and its ability to reform as structures around it move and contract.

Hunter's description of a nerve fixation suggests that it is a common underlying problem relating to peripheral nerve conditions (27). A forgotten childhood injury, such as falling from a skateboard; an armed services injury; a sprained wrist that was passed off and forgotten; a car accident many years ago when the hand hyperextended on the dashboard; or a fall on the ice with a fracture are examples of "old" injuries that may cause nerve fixation.

Nerves are not resistant to stretching by sudden, violent trauma, such as the mechanics of injury described above. The adhering of two or more surfaces together restricts a nerve's ability to glide, thereby inhibiting its ability to conduct impulses. Such adhesions can be treated with myofascial release techniques.

The conventional medical approach to treating musculoskeletal conditions addresses only the area of pain or discomfort. If the wrist is painful, the wrist is treated. If the shoulder is painful, the shoulder is treated. Manual medical practitioners have come to understand that treating only the specific area where the patient feels pain often will lead to poor results. The area of pain is often not the primary site of dysfunction but a result of the body's inability to compensate. Removing a trigger point, for example, without addressing the postural, nutritional, lifestyle, and emotional components that led to the formation of the trigger point in the first place, is often ineffective. Travell and Simons call these perpetuating factors (13).

In the myofascial treatment for CTS, it must be understood that the median nerve originates from nerves in the cervical spine and passes through and between tissues all the way to the fingers (Fig. 6-5). The nerve course traverses a considerable distance, and anything that compromises the nerve along its course can compromise the nerve's ability to innervate distal structures.

Another consideration is that the symptoms of nerve irritation usually occur first in the terminal or distal distribution of the nerve. In the case of the median nerve, this location would be in the fingers. Entrapment of the median nerve, whether at the carpal tunnel or the pronator teres, will be indicated by symptoms in the fingers. A positive Tinel's sign at the wrist may be indicative of entrapment at locations other than the wrist, because the same nerve axons are involved. Addressing only the carpal tunnel and leaving out the other areas that may impede median nerve function is addressing only part of the problem.

Myofascial release techniques (MRT) is a collective term for many different types of treatment for soft tissue disorders. Several similar approaches have been described in the literature, all with the basic premise of locating impediments to normal function in and around the myofascial structures and then removing them manually (19,29–37).

The basic goal of the approach presented in this chapter is to locate and eliminate sites of myofascial compromise (adhesions, scar tissue) that interfere with normal biomechanical function. These lesions are evaluated by using static and motion palpation. The clinician palpates along the longitudinal axis of the muscle fibers as they are located along the length of the median nerve, as these tissues are moved passively or actively through their range of motion. Once restriction is located, reduction of the lesion is accomplished by manually placing a broad, flat contact on the tissue, applying traction to it to trap the adhesion, and then drawing it under the contact passively (MRT level 3) or actively (MRT level 4). This releases the adhesion and allows normal function to return. This method stretches and softens fibrous scar tissue, resulting in decreased restriction of circulation, increased range of motion, and increased strength (36,37). The direction of motion used is that which takes the tissue from its shortest to its longest length.

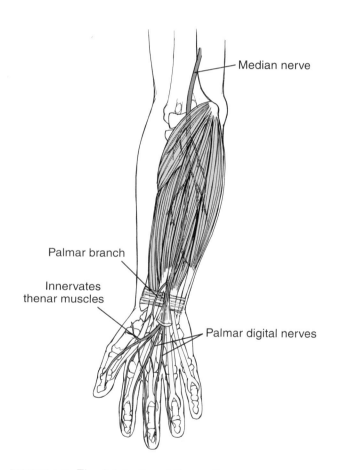

FIGURE 6-5. The distribution of the median nerve. The median nerve arises from C6, C7, C8, and T1 fibers, and forms part of the medial and lateral cords of the brachial plexus that pass between the anterior and middle scalene, between the clavicle and the 1st rib, and under the pectoralis minor muscle. Near the pectoralis minor muscle, portions of the medial and lateral cords separate and form the median nerve that passes through the middle of the anterior surface of the upper arm as shown. It then enters the forearm between the humeral and ulnar heads of the pronator teres muscle, passes under the aponeurotic arch of the flexor digitorum superficialis, and enters the hand under the flexor retinaculum.

Reprinted with permission from Hendrickson T. Massage for Orthopedic Conditions. Baltimore: Lippincott Williams & Wilkins, 2003, fig. 10.3 (p. 382).

CASE 6-1

Patient History

Ms. J. M., age 30, was referred by a local occupational medicine center for evaluation and treatment of her right forearm after all other treatments had failed. She worked as a receptionist for a local company, and her duties included typing and data entry.

Symptoms

Over the previous year, Ms. J. M. had experienced various degrees of pain and paresthesias in her right forearm. She was of normal height and weight, was a non-smoker, and appeared healthy and well hydrated. She described her symptoms as "pins and needles" and "numbness" in her right hand, specifically in the tips of her thumb and first two fingers. Although she did not experience these symptoms in her palm, she did experience aching in her forearm from her wrist to her medial epicondyle. The paresthesias would sometimes awaken her from sleep. At first, she could shake her hands and they would "come around." But after a while, not much seemed to help.

Ms. J. M. had been through a series of NSAIDs combined with wrist splinting. She did notice some relief at first from the splinting, but it did not last. After 4 to 6 weeks, she felt worse.

She stated that her hand felt weak and that she had recently been dropping things, including a carton of milk and her favorite coffee cup. Her husband told her that she should do grip exercises because she was getting weak. She tried using "grippers," but they just made her symptoms worse and her hand hurt.

After the splinting and NSAIDS failed to produce results, Ms. J.M. was sent for physical therapy and spent approximately 6 weeks with hot packs, paraffin baths, and iontophoresis, which "felt good but didn't really change anything." She was given putty to squeeze, which only made her hand hurt. When her symptoms failed to respond positively to any of these procedures, she was referred for a cortisone shot into the carpal tunnel, which "hurt when they did it but didn't make any difference." Because this was a worker's compensation case that included specific cost guidelines from the state, electrodiagnostic studies were not performed. As a last resort before surgery, she was referred for care with a diagnosis of "cumulative trauma disorder, carpal tunnel syndrome."

Examination Findings

The referring physician requested evaluation and, if indicated, MRT level 3 and 4. On examination, the patient had palpable restriction throughout the area of the FR with decreased range of motion at the wrist in extension, in the thenar in retroposition, and with the wrist in neutral. Testing of opposition using the opponens pollicis and opponens digiti minimi showed a 4/5 grade of the opponens pollicis in all phases of wrist motion (flexion, extension, pronation, supination), and her grip strength was poor. A Phalen's test was positive beginning at 30 seconds, and Tinel's sign was positive over the carpal tunnel. Tapping with a reflex hammer gently over the pronator teres also produced a positive Tinel's sign. Palpation over the FR (compression test) produced an increase in her paresthesias, as did palpation along the volar forearm and at the pronator teres. Specific areas of adhesion were palpated just lateral and medial to the FR, and in and around the muscle substance at the pronator teres. She had a decreased sensitivity to pinprick over the distal lateral surface of the index fingertip.

Although CTS was the diagnosis at referral, based on examination findings, CTS was too specific a diagnosis. A more appropriate diagnosis was "whole nerve syndrome of the right median nerve with compromise at the carpal tunnel and pronator teres." This case is typical of what clinicians see on a daily basis.

Treatment

Ms. J. M. was immediately treated with MRT level 3 and 4 (Technique 6-1). Treatment began with level 3, and as treatment progressed, she was able to move her wrist and forearm actively using level 4. The patient was advised that she might feel some post-treatment discomfort that night and possibly the next day. She was also told that she might feel more numbness or tingling for a little while post-treatment. She was scheduled to return for treatment twice per week over the next 3 to 5 weeks. At her second visit, she noticed decreased sensitivity and less tingling. At that visit, she was instructed to perform home care stretching exercises three times every waking hour for 5 to 10 seconds, even while working. By the fourth visit she was working without pain.

It is usually helpful to keep patients working, so that improvement can be demonstrated while they are still performing their routine activities. If patients stop their work activities, they will often feel better simply because they quit doing motions that were aggravating them.

By the sixth visit, Ms. J. M. was essentially symptom-free and was working without pain or discomfort. She

(continues)

CASE 6-1   Continued

TECHNIQUE 6.1

MRT Levels 3 and 4

Four levels of myofascial release have been established to describe the position, tension, and activity of the tissues to be treated as the practitioner applies manual contact. MRT level 1 is the treatment of tissue with no tension involved and the patient passive. The practitioner's contact moves longitudinally along the muscle fibers in a stripping action, distal to proximal, and in the direction of blood flow to the heart. MRT Level 2 places the tissue to be treated in tension, with the patient passive, with the practitioner's contact moving longitudinally along the fibers in a stripping action, distal to proximal, and in the direction of the heart.

MRT Levels 3 and 4 involve motion. The use of motion in MRT produces the most consistent and dramatic results. In both Levels 3 and 4, the muscle is shortened. Then the practitioner places a static contact just distal to the lesion, and the lesion is drawn under the contact by lengthening the tissue, using

passive or active motion. In MRT level 3, the patient is passive but the tissue to be treated is moved through its range of motion from its shortest to its longest length by the practitioner or an assistant. In MRT level 4, the patient actively moves the tissue to be treated through its range of motion from its shortest to its longest length, using either body weight and gravity to provide resistance or a dumbbell, a weight, or surgical tubing to increase the resistance. The patient also may use the opposite hand to add resistance.

With levels 3 and 4, the practitioner tries to keep the contact static. Only the tissue moves. The movement of the myofascial structures through their range of motion from shortest to longest length under a static contact provides a stripping technique that breaks up adhesions and restores function. The motion component of levels 3 and 4 MRT is the main factor that differentiates myofascial release as described in this text from other techniques with the same name.

was no longer waking up at night with the paresthesias. By the eighth treatment, both Phalen's and Tinel's signs were negative.

She was discharged with the stipulation that she continue with her prescribed stretches indefinitely.

Follow-up

At a 3-month follow-up visit, Ms. J. M.'s symptoms had not returned. She was working without pain or discomfort and had continued to perform the prescribed stretches as recommended.

An Overview of Carpal Tunnel Syndrome

To explain the application of MRT level 3 and 4 in the treatment of CTS, the concept of nerve excursion is discussed. The common sites of adhesion or restriction of nerve excursion also are presented.

Causes

Nerve Excursion

Nerve excursion is an aspect of the anatomy of the median and other peripheral nerves of the upper extremities that must be understood by the clinician (11,38–40). When considering any mechanical nerve compromise in the upper body, understanding that the nerves run along an undulating course both grossly and microscopically is essential.

The nerve trunk runs along an undulating course in its bed, as do the funiculi in the epineurium and the nerve fibers inside the funiculi. The length of nerve fibers between any two fixed points is considerably greater than a

straight line between those points. The initial effect of stretching a nerve is to take out the undulations in the nerve trunk. With continued stretch, undulations in the funiculi are removed, and finally those of the nerve fibers. At this last point, the nerve fibers are subject to tension (11).

The brachial plexus and its peripheral nerve trunks are free to move. As the peripheral nerve trunks traverse the upper extremities, they are able to glide several millimeters in a longitudinal fashion, thus protecting the nerve from stretching or kinking. In 1975, McLellan and Swash discovered, as an incidental finding during action potential recordings of the median nerve, that the median nerve trunk slides longitudinally in its bed when the limb is moved (39). They found that with limb movement the tip of the needle electrode that had been inserted in the median nerve would angulate, indicating that the tip had moved relative to its site of entry through the skin. The movement was always in the long axis of the nerve. If the electrode was withdrawn 1 mm and left in the skin, the movement disappeared, indicating that the adjacent soft tissues did not move.

The longest excursion was produced by extension of the wrist and fingers, which in turn produced 7.4 mm of downward excursion and by flexion of the elbow which produced 4.3 mm of upward excursion. Active and passive movements had equal effect. When recordings were made at the wrist in four subjects, 4 to 5 mm of upward displacement occurred when the index finger or middle finger was flexed. Hyperextension of the index or middle finger caused the median nerve to slide downward by an estimated 10 to 15 mm. Median nerve displacement was therefore two to four times greater at the wrist than in the upper arm.

The wrist has an added complication. The retinaculum is carried proximally over the nerve during flexion. Extension of the fingers with flexion of the wrist is therefore the position in which the median nerve is displaced furthest under the retinaculum into the hand. The segment of the nerve distal to the retinaculum is relatively short, providing little room for stretch. The force of the downward traction during finger extension is likely to be much greater than the upward traction, exerted only by the nerves' elasticity, during finger flexion (39).

In 1986, Wilgis and Murphy studied nerve excursions in cadaver specimens (40). They noted during abduction–adduction of the shoulder that the excursion of the brachial plexus measured 15.3 mm. When measured proximal to the elbow, the median nerve excursion was 7.3 mm during full flexion and extension of the elbow. Proximal to the carpal tunnel, the excursion of the same nerve was 14.5 mm, whereas distal to the tunnel, the measurement was 6.8 mm. If the normal sliding of the median nerve is restricted as a result of adhesions or compressive entrapments, nerve stretching or traction can result in temporary or permanent disruption of action potential propagation, causing an impairment of sensory or motor function (11,22).

McLellan and Swash suggest that pathologic changes at one level along the nerve, perhaps by altering the nerve's capacity for stretch, could make other levels more vulnerable to damage during limb movement. To-and-fro sliding across a site of potential entrapment in a person performing repetitive tasks over prolonged periods could cause perineural damage, leading to a restriction of sliding at that point. If sliding were restricted at more than one level, the capacity of the nerve to accommodate limb movement could be reduced (39).

When considering the pathogenesis of stretch–compression neuropathy, the following should be considered. Normal nerve fibers possess a remarkable tolerance for mechanical deformation, but once damaged, they are particularly sensitive to mechanical deformation and ischemia. Nerve fibers subjected to abnormal stretch or compression suffer by sustaining structural damage that is directly attributable to the deforming force, by impaired blood supply, and by constriction from fibrosis developing inside and around the funiculi, and around the entire nerve trunk. According to Sunderland, traction may contribute to the production of a chronic lesion (11). Therefore, adhesions that fix a nerve trunk in its bed or reduce its mobility, and changes in the connective tissue of a nerve that reduce its elasticity, compromise nerve fibers by lowering the threshold at which stretching produces pathologic effects.

Entrapment/Adhesion Affecting the Median Nerve

A nerve is vulnerable when it passes through fascia or fibrotendinous tissue, crosses a fibrotendinous ridge, passes beneath a fibrotendinous arcade, is in contact with an unyielding surface against which it can be compressed, or is so intimately related to another structure that enlargement of the structure could stretch or compress the nerve.

Several areas are more prone than others to entrapment and compression along the course of the median nerve. Entrapment occurs most commonly at the thoracic outlet as the nerve passes through the costoclavicular interval, as it passes in front of the subscapularis in the axilla, as it passes between the heads of the pronator teres and under the anterior interosseus membrane in the forearm, and distally as it passes through the carpal tunnel at the wrist. Although these are the most common areas, the nerve may be entrapped anywhere along its course.

Treatment

Palpation of Adhesion Tissue Restrictions

The best way to make a patient with muscle or other soft tissue dysfunction tighten up and draw away from the examiner is to poke into the tissues with the tips of the fingers. To get optimal information regarding the restriction of nerve excursion from static and motion palpation of the tissues, the practitioner must retrain himself to palpate with the broad, flat palmar surfaces of the fingers or thumb and thenar muscle area. With practice, the examiner will find that this form of contact is the most effective. The patient can relax with the gentle laying of the flat surface of the fingers or thumb against the area to be palpated, allowing the clinician to better evaluate the tissues involved. Slowly sliding the fingers or thumb along the longitudinal orientation of the fibers, without having to lift the fingers and replace them all the time, gives the practitioner much better coverage of the tissues. It is also helpful to passively move the area (motion palpation) from its shortest to its longest length with the noncontact hand while feeling for restriction to range of motion and changes in tissue texture with the palpating hand. Palpation is an art, and just like other manual procedures, it requires time, patience, and practice.

Injuries involving myofascial structures may have several different textures. They may feel fibrous. They may feel "ropey" or have a "leathery" feel. New injuries tend to feel ropey, and the leathery feel comes after the condition has existed for a while. During treatment, the clinician may feel the adhesion break, although this does not always happen. Usually the patient does not feel this. An adhesion may simply involve adherence of two structures together. There may not be a "nodule" or fibrous area. Motion palpation of the muscle structures, and the way they relate to their surrounding tissues, is essential when trying to find a lesion that may not be palpable as a distinct disruption in the texture of the tissue.

Although this chapter addresses the diagnosis and treatment of CTS, these procedures may be applied to any structure on the body. Restrictions can occur anywhere, and adhesions can form anywhere. Applying MRT levels 3 and 4 to shoulder dysfunction or ankle problems, for example, can produce excellent results. Simply follow the same guidelines and apply them to the area in question. As will become clear from this discussion, many of the problems seen in daily practice may respond well to myofascial release. Finding and addressing these problems involves the following three factors:

1. Practitioners must first suspect that the problem exists by understanding the mechanisms involved.

2. They must know the anatomy of the areas involved to properly examine and diagnose the problem.

3. They must continually practice to develop the tactile skills necessary for finding lesions and differentiate them from normal tissues and normal anatomic structures.

General Principles of MRT Levels 3 and 4 Treatment

This treatment has shown good results in the correction of peripheral nerve entrapment, cumulative trauma disorders (CTD), and athletic injuries (26,29,37). The basic principles may be applied to any muscle group in the body, and almost any musculoskeletal injury can benefit from this approach. Several guidelines will insure adequate treatment results:

1. MRT should not be performed if inflammation is present.

2. MRT should not be performed more often than every other day. Ideally the patient is treated twice per week. This gives the tissues time to recover so that they will not be too sensitive when the next treatment is performed.

3. The contact should be soft and as broad and flat as possible. The flat of the thumb is preferred in most areas, with traction and control being provided by the flat of the opposite palm placed on top of the thumb contact. Gripping the area and using the flat ends of the fingers to draw the tissues apart works well in the hands.

4. The tissues should be worked longitudinally, allowing deeper work with less discomfort. Working transversely across the fibers can cause much discomfort and questionable results.

5. When working longitudinally along muscles, the contact should conform to the muscle contour to prevent the muscle from rolling out from under the contact. This can be very uncomfortable for the patient.

6. Lotion may be used to minimize the feeling of the skin being stretched. However, the lotion should not be too greasy. Using lotion makes the tissue slippery and harder to control, requiring more strength on the part of the practitioner. The clinician's tactile sense also may be affected.

7. Passive or active range of motion should be performed as slowly as possible.

8. The practitioner should always work with the contact moving in the direction of the heart to minimize backward pressure on the valves of the veins to prevent bruising the patient.

9. The practitioner should perform 3 to 5 passes over each area at each visit.

10. The practitioner should perform 6 to 10 treatments over the course of 3 to 5 weeks as the standard protocol for most conditions.

MRT does not continue over the course of several months. Results should be rapid, and a considerable change is often noticed after the first treatment. If no change is seen in 4 to 6 treatments, the patient should be reevaluated and the approach changed or different treatment considered. MRT works very well in conjunction with other myofascial techniques, such as trigger point pressure release (formerly ischemic compression). It is wise to remove myofascial trigger points with trigger point pressure release before MRT level 3 or 4. Passively or actively pulling a muscle through its range of motion as is done with MRT, without removing these trigger points, will be less effective.

The practitioner does not apply pressure straight down into the tissues. A tissue pull is taken just distal to the lesion to be treated, with the practitioner applying traction in a proximal direction (Fig. 6-6). The clinician takes up the tissue slack, applying traction proximally toward the lesion, trapping it. This contact is then held static, and the area to be treated is then passively or actively lengthened under the practitioner's static contact. As mentioned above, if using lotion, it must not be too greasy. Slippery tissues can affect the practitioner's ability to traction them properly, and the pressure into the tissues will increase. This will lead to more discomfort for the patient and poor results. Several "dry oils" work exceptionally well for this type of soft tissue treatment.

When passively or actively taking myofascial tissues from their shortest to longest length, the clinician should visualize a line from insertion to origin. The tissue pull and traction of the treating hand contact occurs along that line, giving the best alignment of the fibers of each portion to be treated.

If the patient is too weak to perform the active motion in level 4, the clinician should begin using level 3 for several treatments. This usually will allow level 4 treatment to begin, and the patient will gradually be able to perform the active motion herself.

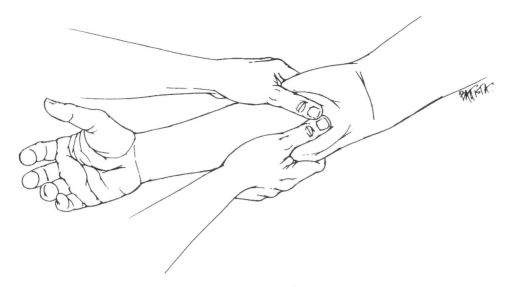

FIGURE 6-6. Tissue pull and tractioning of the tissue.

MRT may be painful to the patient because the practitioner must physically break up the adhesion, and adhesions often involve nerves. To minimize the patient's discomfort, the clinician should work very slowly. Whenever possible, he should have the patient actively move the structure herself and do it as slowly as possible. Using as broad and flat a contact as possible, he must be very sensitive to the patient's tolerance of the contact pressure. The patient often will say, "It hurts, but it feels good." The clinician must always work within patient tolerance.

When using myofascial release to treat peripheral nerve entrapment, the practitioner must discuss possible short-term side effects following treatment. The patient's symptoms may increase for a short time after the treatment. Often the patient will feel the paresthesias increase as the practitioner is working on them. Muscle soreness may follow treatment as well. Both of these symptoms may continue into the next day. This is normal and should be explained. If any symptoms increase and do not resolve in a reasonable amount of time, the clinician should reevaluate the patient.

Specific Application of MRT Levels 3 and 4 to Median Nerve Compromise

The following approach to treating CTS involves evaluating the tract of the median nerve and removing, manually, any restriction that may be involved. Beginning at the hand, the practitioner motion-palpates the tissues in the general vicinity of the median nerve. This motion involves taking the extremity by the wrist with the noncontact hand and gently moving the limb through its different ranges of motion. At the same time, the palpating hand begins at the palm and wrist and slowly, centimeter by centimeter, moves up the forearm following the general tract of the nerve.

For the most part, the practitioner cannot actually palpate the median nerve itself. The idea is to palpate the tissues around the nerve and feel for restriction. The clinician may feel the restriction just as the patient says, "That feels just like it" or "That makes my fingers go numb." As with most orthopaedic tests, the practitioner tries to reproduce the patient's symptoms. He or she should then make a mental note and continue up the forearm. As the practitioner becomes more proficient at palpating adhesions, he or she should treat them as they are identified with the MRT level 3 and 4. The practitioner proceeds up the forearm, keeping in mind the anatomy of the structures that are being palpated and how those structures could be trapping or impeding nerve gliding. Three sites are commonly involved in median nerve entrapment, from distal to proximal:

1. At the carpal tunnel, where the anterior wall is formed by the FR, and the posterior surface of the tunnel is formed by the carpal bones. In cases of displacement of carpal bones, or where there has been swelling because of synovitis, the structures may become compromised.

2. At the anterior interosseus membrane in the anterior/proximal forearm

3. Between the bellies of the pronator teres in the proximal forearm

In resistant cases, another area to consider is the axilla, over the face of the subscapularis (which involves the brachial plexus before the splitting off of the terminal branches). This area is commonly injured from throwing, pushing, and falling on an outstretched arm. The resultant inflammation may cause adhesions that restrict the cords, leading to tractioning or entrapment.

Palpation of the Flexor Retinaculum. The basic idea of motion palpation just described may now be used to describe the palpation of the flexor retinaculum (FR). According to *Gray's Anatomy*, the FR was originally called the transverse carpal ligament (TCL) (41). It is a thick fibrous band that arches over the deep groove on the palmar surface of the carpal bones, forming the anterior surface of the fibro-osseus carpal tunnel through which the long flexor tendons and the median nerve pass. The FR is attached medially to the pisiform and the hamulus of the hamate and laterally to the tuberosity of the scaphoid and the medial part of the palmar surface and the ridge of the trapezium.

Palpation begins with the patient seated and facing the practitioner; the forearm to be palpated is supinated with the elbow flexed. The FR can be located by first finding the pisiform by palpating the ulnar styloid process and moving just distal to it. Radially deviating the wrist moves the triquetrum out from under the ulnar styloid process. Because the triquetrum is beneath the pisiform, manipulation may make the pisiform more prominent for palpation. The pisiform is considered a sesamoid within the tendon of the flexor carpi ulnaris. The tension on the pisiform from the flexor carpi ulnaris helps to keep the transverse carpal ligament taut. From a myofascial standpoint, compromise of the flexor carpi ulnaris may affect the tension in the FR, which also must be addressed when treating CTS.

Once the pisiform is located, the practitioner moves slightly distal and radial to it. Deep palpation should locate the hook of the hamate. At this point, the medial border of the FR has been located. To palpate the lateral border, the practitioner locates the styloid process at the distal radius. By ulnar deviation of the wrist, the scaphoid will slide out from under the styloid process, making it accessible to palpation. Just distal to the scaphoid is the trapezium. The medial and lateral borders of the FR have now been identified.

The practitioner gently palpates the FR and feels for restriction of motion, flattening of the structures, or tightness. He should attempt to reproduce the patient's symptoms by tapping the area or by simply pressing over the medial, lateral, and central surfaces of the structure. Note that the small branches of the median nerve at the base of the thenar eminence may become fixated to the surrounding structures. Once any areas of restriction or compromise have been identified, treatment can proceed.

Flexor Retinaculum Treatment. To treat the FR, the patient should be seated and facing the practitioner, with the elbow flexed and the forearm supinated. Now that the FR has been identified, the forearm should be pronated. The practitioner places both thumbs on the dorsum of the hand and cups the radial and ulnar sides of the retinaculum under the flat surface of the fingertips (Fig. 6-7). Using a gentle pressure, the practitioner slowly applies traction to the retinaculum by drawing the contact fingers away from each other. Three to five passes of slow, gentle tractioning should be sufficient at each treatment.

After applying traction to the FR using MRT level 3, the practitioner then proceeds to level 4 by having the patient cup the hand as tightly as possible, and then positions his hands as described above. The patient should then try to

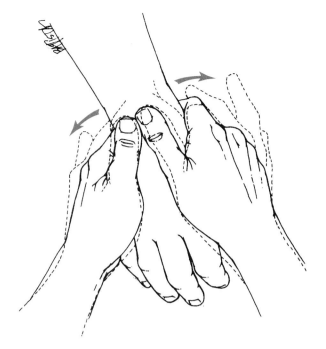

FIGURE 6-7. **Treating the flexor retinaculum.** For MRT3, the thumbs are static on the dorsum of the pronated wrist, while the fingers contact the palmar aspect of the wrist at the ulnar and radial ends of the flexor retinaculum and apply medial to lateral traction, as shown. MRT4 is then performed with the thumbs in the same position, and the fingers static at the ends of the retinaculum, and the patient starts from a position of the hand in a ball and then spreads and extends the fingers and wrist under the clinician's contact.

slowly splay the hand as wide as possible while the practitioner statically holds the FR. This action is used to help the tissues regain their tonus, as well as to release any adhesions within the areas around the median nerve at that level. The patient repeats the active motion 3 to 5 times while the practitioner continues to hold the contact.

Palpation and Treatment of the Thenar Muscles. To address the thenar muscles and the surrounding tissues just distal to the FR, the patient is seated and faces the practitioner with the involved extremity flexed at the elbow to approximately 130°. The hand should be supinated and relaxed. The practitioner pronates the patient's forearm and holds the patient's thenar eminence by placing the practitioner's thenar eminence against the dorsum of the patient's thumb, and cups the substance of the thenar muscles with the flattened surface of the fingertips. The practitioner then places the patient's thumb into adduction by rolling it into the palm. The practitioner should feel for tension and restrictions along the muscles as the thumb is gently flexed and extended. Any restriction or reproduction of the patient's symptoms suggests involvement at that level.

Treatment of the thenar muscles with MRT begins with the patient's thumb in flexion, to shorten the thenar muscles. The practitioner grabs the substance of the thenar eminence

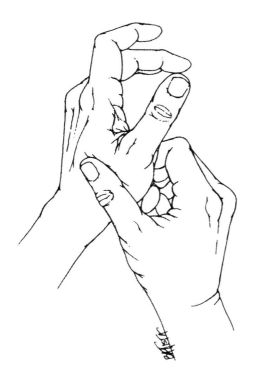

with the flat surfaces of his contact fingers, essentially gripping the substance between his thumb and fingers (Fig. 6-8). The tissues are slowly and gently pulled or lengthened as the practitioner extends the thumb, rolling it out and away from the palm (retroposition). This motion is performed slowly and gently 3 to 5 times. Proceeding to MRT level 4, the patient actively flexes the thumb. The practitioner takes a broad, flat finger contact and holds it as the patient actively extends the thumb, rolling it away from the palm. This is performed 3 to 5 times.

Palpation and Treatment of the Distal Forearm. Palpation of the distal forearm begins at the thenar and hypothenar eminences. It is the continuation of the motion palpation method described above to palpate along the path of the median nerve. The patient is seated, facing the practitioner. The practitioner moves the contact just proximally, to feel the thickened annular band of the antebrachial fascia (also called the superficial part of the FR). This band is attached medially and laterally to the radial and ulnar styloid processes. It merges distally with the FR. The practitioner should palpate the substance of the retinaculum and feel for restrictions.

Performing MRT on the tissues around the median nerve in the distal third of the forearm involves tractioning any restriction in the tissues as the limb is moved through its range of motion. With the patient's wrist flexed, the practitioner places a broad, flat contact across the structures proximal to the volar wrist (Fig. 6-9). The tissues are gently

FIGURE 6-8. **Treating the thenar muscle.** For MRT 3, the clinician grasps the thenar eminence at the base of the thumb as shown, and pulls the patient's thumb into extension and away from the palm. For MRT 4, the patient flexes the thumb, and the clinician grasps the thumb in the same way and maintains a static contact while the patient extends the thumb away from the palm.

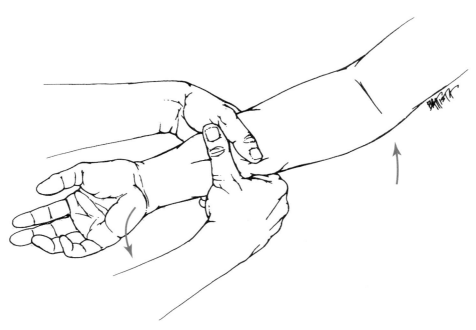

FIGURE 6-9. **Treating the flexor surface of the forearm.** For MRT 3, the clinician contacts the tissues over the course of the median nerve in the volar aspect of the forearm with one hand, while placing the patient's wrist in flexion. The contact is maintained while the clinician takes the wrist into full extension and also extends the elbow. For MRT 4, the clinician uses both hands as contacts on the volar forearm, and the patient takes the hand actively from wrist flexion to full wrist and elbow extension, as shown. MRT 3 and 4 are repeated every few centimeters up the forearm, treating each location of restriction of the median nerve in the surrounding tissues.

pulled in a proximal direction. With the noncontact hand, the practitioner slowly moves the patient's wrist from full flexion to full extension. As the wrist is extended, the elbow should also slowly move into full extension. The wrist and elbow movement should be one smooth motion. This should be performed 3 to 5 times. After the level 3 procedure, the patient actively performs the motion as the practitioner supports the contact. MRT level 4 is performed 3 to 5 times. Each time the passes are completed, the practitioner moves the contact up the forearm a few centimeters and repositions the contact at the proximal end of the tissue that was just treated. The procedure then starts from that point and continues from there.

The practitioner treats the entire area of the volar forearm where the median nerve passes through. By using trapping, traction, and motion, the practitioner removes adhesions and restrictions in and around the tissues and frees up the median nerve to improve its ability to glide. As the practitioner proceeds up the forearm, he or she will reach the pronator teres muscle. This muscle is essential to consider when dealing with median nerve problems.

Palpation and Evaluation of the Pronator Teres Muscle.
The pronator teres has two heads (Fig. 6-10). The origin of the humeral head is from the medial epicondylar ridge and the common flexor tendon. The origin of the ulnar head is from the medial side of the coronoid process of the ulna. Both heads insert on the middle lateral surface of the forearm. The action of the pronator teres is to pronate the forearm and flex the elbow (41).

Although the pronator quadratus is thought to be the prime pronator muscle, the pronator teres is very important because of its common involvement in peripheral nerve entrapment of the median nerve (42). The median nerve passes between the two bellies of the pronator teres and may be entrapped between those surfaces, causing symptoms of CTS distal to the entrapment. For example, the pronator teres is subjected to constant repetitive motion during keyboarding work. As a result, inflammation, infiltration, and fibrous adhesions may form in the tissues. The proximity of the median nerve to this area of constant trauma places it in a position of extreme compromise. The nerve may adhere to the surrounding tissues, and a neurodesis may form. In this case, the median nerve becomes fixed between the bellies of the pronator teres.

Constant tugging distal to the nerve fixation by day-to-day wrist and arm movement then may lead to irritation of the nerve. Because the symptoms usually begin in the destination of the nerve at the fingertips, this may lead to a possible misdiagnosis of CTS. The pronator teres is the most common area of median nerve entrapment in the upper extremities, and symptoms at the carpal tunnel may be attributable to entrapment higher up at the level of the pronator teres (29).

To examine the pronator teres, the attachments and the muscle bellies must first be located and identified. The ori-

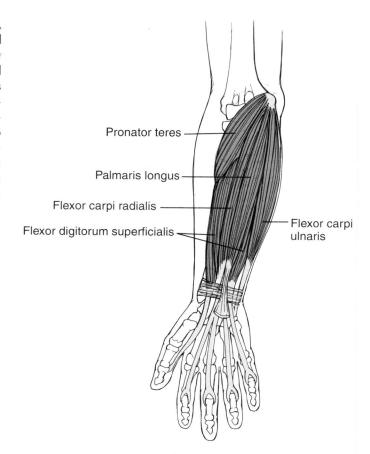

FIGURE 6-10. **The pronator teres muscle.**
Reprinted with permission from Hendrickson T. Massage for Orthopedic Conditions. Baltimore: Lippincott Williams & Wilkins, 2003, fig. 10.5 (p. 384).

gins of the humeral head of the muscle are just proximal to the medial epicondyle on the humerus, and from the common flexor tendon. It passes obliquely across the forearm, where it becomes a flat tendon, and inserts at the middle of the lateral surface of the body of the radius.

To find the insertion of the pronator teres, the practitioner holds the pronated forearm of the patient at the wrist and asks the patient to try and resist as he or she tries to supinate the forearm. This resistance will tighten the pronator teres and make it easier to palpate. The practitioner finds the proximal insertion and follows it diagonally to its distal portion and insertion. Palpating the pronator teres may reproduce the patient's symptoms. This is a good indication that the practitioner has found an area of entrapment.

If the patient is in a job that requires repetitive motion, this area may be tender. As the practitioner palpates the pronator teres, many patients will say, "That's it" or "That's where it's coming from." Patients also may ask why the elbow would have anything to do with their hand hurting or being numb and tingly. The practitioner must explain that the nerves are like a long cable, traveling from the neck to the hand. Once they understand it is the same nerve at the elbow that is traveling to the hand, the treatment makes much more sense.

Once the muscle and its attachments have been located, the patient must relax the forearm. Palpation of the muscle begins with a broad, flat, gentle contact. The forearm is moved very slowly back and forth from pronation to supination by the practitioner's noncontact hand. As the motion is performed, the practitioner's contact glides from distal to proximal along the muscle fibers, all the way up to the common flexor tendon. Once the muscle is identified, the practitioner may want to test the pronator teres for strength. When peripheral nerve entrapment of the median nerve is involved, the pronator teres may test at a 3/5 or 4/5 grade when using standard muscle testing procedures.

The resistive test for the pronator teres places the patient supine with the forearm in pronation, the elbow held to the side of the body and flexed to 60°. The practitioner stabilizes the patient's elbow at the side of the torso with the noncontact hand to prevent shoulder abduction and then uses the contact hand to grasp the wrist and apply force to the forearm in a direction of supination. The patient should try to resist. The patient should not be overpowered. This test is simply to provide some additional information.

Treatment of the Pronator Teres Muscle. Any areas of adhesion or restriction at the pronator teres should be treated as they are found. The patient should completely pronate the forearm. The practitioner places a broad, flat contact distal to the lesion, tractions the tissues, and then draws the lesion under the contact by passively (level 3) moving the muscle from pronation to supination 3 to 5 times. The practitioner then proceeds to MRT level 4 (Fig. 6-11). The contact should be held while the patient actively moves the muscle from its shortest to its longest length. This procedure using the active motion is performed 3 to 5 times.

Other Areas of Entrapment. Essentially, the median nerve may be entrapped anywhere along its course. Symptoms may occur from entrapment of portions of the brachial plexus over the subscapularis muscle in the axilla, under the pectoralis minor, or at the divisions of the scalene muscles. These other areas must always be considered to achieve the most complete results.

One area that is rarely involved in median nerve entrapment is at the ligament of Struthers. This ligament occurs only in 1% of the population (14,33), and when it is involved, the condition is usually referred to as a humerus supracondylar process syndrome. The ligament attaches on an anomalous spur on the humerus called the humeral supracondylar process (visible on a radiograph). It then passes over the median nerve and sometimes the brachial artery, and attaches on the medial epicondyle of the humerus. This is an area of potential entrapment.

Patient Exercise and Home Care

The standard protocol involves 6 to 10 treatments over 3 to 5 weeks. The patient is seen twice weekly for MRT and is

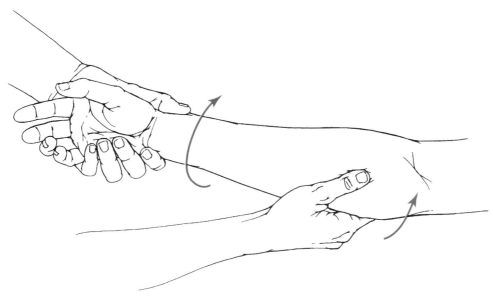

FIGURE 6-11. **Treating the pronator teres muscle.** For MRT 3, the clinician contacts the pronator teres over the median nerve with the thumb while the arm is fully pronated, and then maintains the contact while using the other hand to take the patient's forearm into full supination (as well as extension at the elbow) as shown. For MRT 4, both of the clinician's hands can be used to contact portions of the pronator teres muscle while the patient takes the forearm actively from full pronation to full supination, with extension of the elbow.

prescribed home care stretching exercises within the first few treatments. The first treatment may be uncomfortable for the patient, and waiting until the next visit to prescribe the home care is recommended.

The patient is advised not to rub or massage the areas that are being treated between visits because the tissues need time to recover. Massaging the areas will prolong their recovery period. Patients also must understand that sometimes their symptoms will increase at first, because the treatment is being performed over areas that are already irritated.

Usually the patient's condition will begin to improve within four treatments. Improvement includes a decrease in symptoms, fewer problems working, and improved strength. Waking up at night with paresthesia-type symptoms decreases. This treatment works very well when the patient follows the recommendations. The patient must understand that the stretching exercises are part of the treatment. The combination of MRT and home care exercises produces the best results. The continuation of home care after the patient is discharged also will maintain results and help prevent future injuries.

The practitioner prescribes specific stretching exercises, to be performed hourly at first, then gradually decreased. These stretching exercises should be started immediately after treatment begins, and the procedure must be carefully explained. Patients should only be required to perform a few simple stretching exercises. Patients who are overwhelmed with too many stretches will simply not do them. Patients should demonstrate the stretching exercises to the practitioner at each subsequent visit, to ensure that they have not changed the procedure in any way.

Because this approach assumes a different perception of this condition and a different way of treating CTS and related conditions, the rationale for home care also must be considered differently. The prescribed exercises are not as much about stretching the muscles as they are about drawing the nerve through the tissues and facilitating the nerve's gliding properties. For example, after the nerve has been freed from adhesions and restrictions, the patient moves the limb through specific ranges of motion to facilitate nerve gliding. These actions are performed every waking hour, three times, for 5 to 10 seconds each time.

Two specific stretches for the forearm will cover most conditions. The first stretch is for the pronator and flexor groups in the forearm (Figure 6-12). The affected arm is relaxed at the patient's side with the elbow flexed to 90° and the palm supinated. The shoulder must be relaxed throughout the motion and must not rise up during the stretch. The purpose of the stretch is to extend the elbow and extend the wrist. The palmar surface of the fingers of the treating or opposite hand is placed over the palm on the side to be stretched. The elbow is then slowly extended while the opposite hand gently guides the affected hand into extension. The final position is: the arm outstretched, the wrist and elbow in extension, and the oppo-

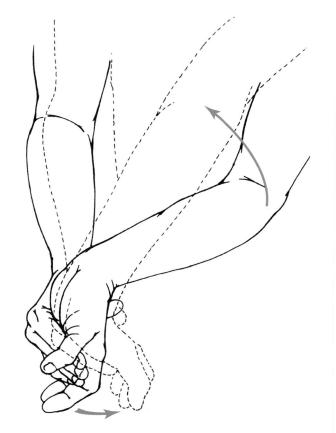

FIGURE 6-12. **Stretching exercises for the flexor and pronator group.** Starting position: with the elbow flexed to 90° and the palm up. Ending position: upper arm flexes at the shoulder to 90°, elbow fully extends, wrist and fingers extend as shown, and forearm is fully supinated until the fingers rotate medially as far as possible.

site hand gently extending and rotating the involved hand until the extended fingers are brought toward the midline of the body (maximal supination.) This position is held for 5 to 10 seconds, and then the forearm is relaxed and lightly shaken. This is repeated three times.

The second stretch is for the extensor group and involves the patient relaxing the shoulder and letting the arm hang at the side (Fig. 6-13). The dorsal surface of the hand faces anteriorly and the palmar surface posteriorly. The patient is instructed to point the fingers back and up. This places the wrist into flexion with the fingers flexed as well. This stretch is held for 5 to 10 seconds, and then the arm is relaxed and lightly shaken out. This stretch is performed three times also, every waking hour.

Patients should understand that the stretching exercises should not be forced through pain. They should be essentially easy and not uncomfortable. Patients must be made aware that they do not have to feel anything for the exercises to be working. This is not a "no pain, no gain" activity. They are simply drawing the nerves through the adjacent tissues regularly to keep the nerves free to glide. Patients may stop

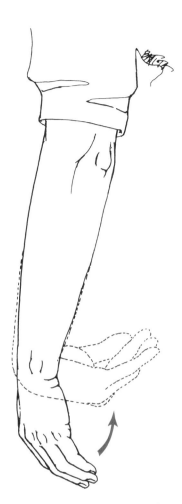

FIGURE 6-13. **Stretching exercises for the extensor group.** Starting position: with the arm relaxed at the side. Ending position, with the wrist flexed and the fingers curled, and the forearm rotated into maximum pronation.

performing the stretching exercises because they cannot feel anything. Therefore, it is essential that they understand the underlying principles.

Patients who perform repetitive motion tasks must be advised to continue the stretches indefinitely to prevent future entrapment. The typical case that recurs is the patient who did not continue with the stretching exercises because the symptoms abated. Clinical experience indicates that the person who experiences CTS once may experience it again if proper exercise is not maintained. Without the exercises to draw the nerves through the tissues and keep them moving freely, after several days of heavy repetitive motion followed by sleep, new adhesions can form and entrap the nerves again. In occupations with a high risk of CTS, the importance of prevention and maintenance cannot be overstated.

Once a full range of motion, without pain, has been restored, the patient may add some strengthening exercises using surgical tubing. Tubing provides resistance in the motions of wrist flexion, extension, pronation, and supination (Fig. 6-14). The resistance should be fairly light, and the exercises should not be over-performed. Tubing exercises should be preceded and followed by stretching exercises.

Patients generally seek this treatment approach after other treatments have failed. Many have been in wrist splints for months or even years. Their forearms and whole upper extremities are often weak, and there is significant atrophy. The patient must be weaned away from the splints as soon as possible. MRT will help restore the tonus in the tissues as circulation increases and the nerve entrapment is released. Once the nerve entrapment has been removed, patients do not need splints to prevent movement of the extremity. The extremity must move to keep the nerves gliding and prevent adhesions from reforming. Often when patients first present, they are in so much pain that they need some support. The practitioner should tell them to use the splints when performing certain activities (such as driving), and then remove them.

Other activities involving repetitive motion must be minimized. Vibration and vibrating tools must be avoided. If the condition is not extreme, most patients will continue to work. Continued work helps determine that the treatment is working, that improvement is not the result of ceasing the aggravating activity. Most patients on this program continue to work, and most handle it well.

Ergonomic factors at the workstation, as well as other perpetuating factors, must be addressed. For keyboard workers, the positioning of the shoulders is of utmost importance. The shoulders must be relaxed when seated at the keyboard. Although the position of the wrists has been considered the primary factor, if the shoulders are relaxed, the rest of the upper extremity will follow suit. To assess correct posture, the practitioner should instruct the patient to sit at the workstation with a coworker standing who places hands on the patient's shoulders as the patient types. If the coworker feels the patient's shoulders rise up at all, the chair, desk, or keyboard must be adjusted. If the patient sits with shoulders relaxed, elbows bent, with the forearm at approximately 90° to the upper arm, and with the wrists straight or slightly flexed, where the hands "fall" is where the keyboard should be located. If the patient has to raise, lower, or move the hands forward to reach the keyboard at all, then the shoulders and arms cannot stay relaxed. An obese patient's hands will "fall" wide of a standard keyboard, and only a split keyboard will prevent the recurrence of CTS in such a case. In fact, a split keyboard is inexpensive and would reduce the muscular tension for all CTD sufferers. Having a coworker take photographs of the patient at the workstation also can be helpful.

At the end of the treatment period, patients should be ready to be discharged. As stated above, they should continue with the home care exercises indefinitely. At this point most will be symptom-free, but some will still have occasional symptoms. Continued home exercises should continue to decrease their symptoms.

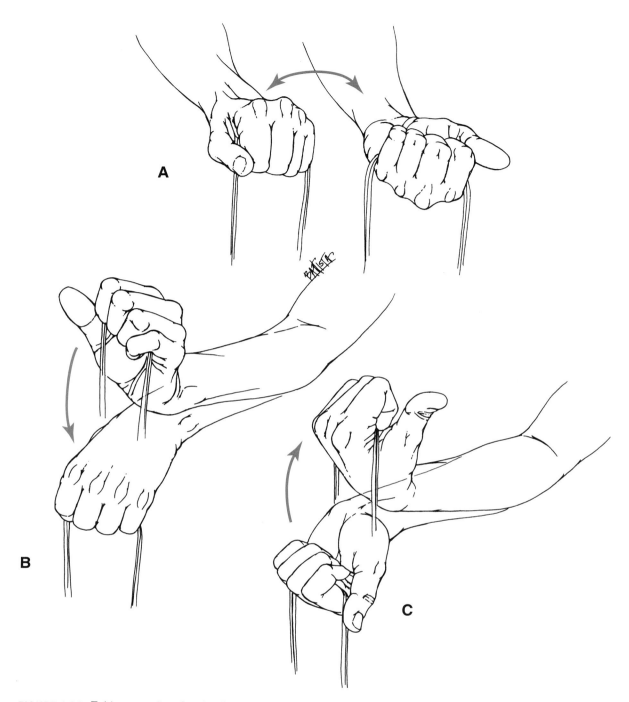

FIGURE 6-14. Tubing exercises for the flexor, extensor, pronator, and supinator groups. Exercises are performed by taking the wrist through the ranges of motion, with the stretch tubing providing resistance. Initially, the repeated contractions can be performed within the mid-range of the range of motion. As muscles strengthen and symptoms subside, strengthening can be performed with the wrist taken through the full range of motion against resistance. Stretches (Figures 6-12 and 6-13) can be performed after the strengthening exercises, to avoid redeveloping trigger points and tension on the median nerve.

CONCLUSION

Even though CTS has been a well-known, common affliction for many years, conventional treatment approaches have not been entirely effective. Conservative medical care and surgical care leave many patients in continual distress and disability. In worker's compensation cases, the procedure has been to place patients at maximal medical improvement (MMI) and discharge them regardless of whether their condition has improved. It is hard to fault a caregiver who honestly believes that all useful treatments have been given and does not know what else to do.

The myofascial release approach has been used to treat thousands of cases of occupational OCTS and other cumulative trauma disorders since 1991. MRT has enabled workers to stay at their jobs and provide for their families when all other forms of treatment, including surgery, were not successful. Even among patients whose symptoms were not completely resolved, most had improvement, at the very least. Unless this approach has been tried, all bases have not been covered.

TREATMENT PROTOCOL

1. **Begin myofascial release at the thenar muscles. With the patient seated and facing you, with the involved limb flexed at the elbow to 130°, perform 3 to 5 passes of MRT level 3 followed by MRT level 4.**

2. **Move proximally up the forearm to treat the flexor retinaculum and the substance of the distal third of the forearm. Perform 3 to 5 passes of MRT level 3 followed by MRT level 4.**

3. **Move proximally into the wrist flexors, and perform 3 to 5 passes of MRT level 3 followed by MRT level 4.**

4. **Palpate and treat the pronator teres muscle, performing 3 to 5 passes of MRT level 3 followed by MRT level 4.**

5. **Follow the tract of the median nerve along the medial upper arm. Treat any areas of involvement with 3 to 5 passes of MRT level 3 and 4.**

6. **Consider other areas that may be involved, including the cervical spine, thoracic outlet, or axilla, and treat them accordingly.**

7. **Prescribe home care, including hourly stretching exercises and an increase in water intake.**

8. **Evaluate the patient's workstation for aggravating factors.**

9. **If needed, prescribe strengthening exercises using surgical tubing.**

References

1. Phalen G. The carpal-tunnel syndrome: seventeen years' experience in diagnosis and treatment of six hundred fifty-four hands. J Bone Joint Surg Am 1996;48:211–228.
2. Diamond MR. Carpal tunnel syndrome: a review. Chiropractic Sports Medicine 1989;3:46–53.
3. Anto C, Aradhya P. Clinical diagnosis of peripheral nerve compression in the upper extremity. Orthop Clin North Am 1996;27:227–237.
4. Millender L, Conlon M. An approach to work-related disorders of the upper extremity. J Am Acad Orthop Surg 1996;4:134–142.
5. Verdon M. Overuse syndromes in the hand and wrist. Prim Care 1996;23:305–319.
6. Hales T, Bernard B. Epidemiology of work-related musculoskeletal disorders. Orthop Clin North Am.1996;27:679–709.
7. Baker EL, Ehrenberg RL. Preventing the work-related carpal tunnel syndrome: physician reporting and diagnostic criteria. Ann Intern Med 1990;112:317–319.
8. Occupational disease surveillance: carpal tunnel syndrome. MMWR 1989;18:36–44.
9. Gerr F, Letz R, Landrigan PJ. Upper-extremity musculoskeletal disorders of occupational origin. Annu Rev Publ Health 1991;12:543–566.
10. Reddy MP. Peripheral nerve entrapment syndromes. AFP 1983;28:133–143.
11. Sunderland S. Stretch-compression neuropathy. Clin Exp Neurol 1981;18:1–13.
12. de Araujo MP. Electrodiagnosis in compression neuropathies of the upper extremities. Orthop Clin North Am 1996;27:237–245.
13. Simons DG, Travell JG, Simons LS. Myofascial Pain and Dysfunction: The Trigger Point Manual, vol 1, 2nd Ed. Baltimore: Williams and Wilkins, 1999.
14. Magee D. Orthopedic Physical Assessment. Philadelphia: WB Saunders, 1987.
15. Gellman H, Gelberman R, Mae Tan A, et al. Carpal tunnel syndrome: an evaluation of the provocative diagnostic tests. J Bone Joint Surg Am 1986;68:735–737.
16. Werner R, Bir C, Armstrong T. Reverse Phalen's maneuver as an aid in diagnosing carpal tunnel syndrome. Arch Phys Med Rehabil 1994;75:783–786.
17. LaBan M, Mackenzie J, Zemenick G. Anatomic observations in carpal tunnel syndrome as they relate to the tethered median nerve stress test. Arch Phys Med Rehabil 1989;70:44–46.
18. Butler D. Mobilization of the Nervous System. Melbourne. New York: Churchill Livingstone, 1991.
19. Sucher B. Palpatory diagnosis and manipulative management of carpal tunnel syndrome. JAOA 1994;94:647–663.
20. Occupational carpal tunnel syndrome. Colorado Department of Labor and Employment, Division of Worker's Compensation, Physician Accreditation and Treatment Guidelines, 1997; Rule XVII, II-1–II-20.
21. Grundberg AB. Carpal tunnel decompression in spite of normal electromyography. J Hand Surg 1983;8:348–349.
22. Horch R, Allman K, Lauberger J, et al. Median nerve compression can be detected by magnetic resonance imaging of the carpal tunnel. Neurosurgery 1997;41:76–83.
23. Chen P, Maklad N, Redvine M, et al. Dynamic high-resolution sonography of the carpal tunnel. AJR 1997;168:533–537.
24. Kessler R. The wrist. In Kessler R, Hertling D, eds. Management of Common Musculoskeletal Disorders. Philadelphia: Harper & Row, 1983:311–329.

25. Cailliet R. Hand Pain and Impairment. 3rd Ed. Philadelphia: FA Davis, 1982.

26. Nau H, Lange B, Lange S. Prediction of outcome of decompression for carpal tunnel. J Hand Surg Br 1988;13:391–394.

27. Hunter J. Recurrent carpal tunnel syndrome, epineural fibrous fixation, and traction neuropathy. Hand Clin 1991;7:491–504.

28. Tubiana R. Carpal tunnel syndrome: some views on its management. Ann Hand Surg 1990;9:325–330.

29. Leahy M, Mock L. Myofascial release technique and mechanical compromise of peripheral nerves of the upper extremity. Chiro Sports Med 1992; 6:139–150.

30. Mock L. Myofascial release treatment of specific muscles of the upper extremity (levels 3 & 4): Part 1. Clin Bull Myofasc Ther 1997;2:5–23.

31. Mock L. Myofascial release treatment of specific muscles of the upper extremity (levels 3 & 4): Part 2. Clin Bull Myofasc Ther 1997;2:5–22.

32. Mock L. Myofascial release treatment of specific muscles of the upper extremity (levels 3 & 4): Part 3. Clin Bull Myofasc Ther 1997;2:51–69.

33. Mock L. Myofascial release treatment of specific muscles of the upper extremity (levels 3 & 4): Part 4. Clin Bull Myofasc Ther 1998;3:2–10.

34. Sucher B. Myofascial manipulative release of carpal tunnel syndrome: documentation with magnetic resonance imaging. JAOA 1993;93:1273–1280.

35. Sucher B. Myofascial release of carpal tunnel syndrome. JAOA 1993;93:92–101.

36. Leahy M, Mock L. Altered biomechanics of the shoulder and the subscapularis. Chiro Sports Med 1991;5:62–66.

37. Leahy M, Mock L. Synoviochondrometaplasia of the shoulder: A case report. Chiro Sports Med 1992;6:5–9.

38. Totten P, Hunter J. Therapeutic techniques to enhance nerve gliding in thoracic outlet syndrome and carpal tunnel syndrome. Hand Clin 1991;7:505–520.

39. McLellan DL, Swash M: Longitudinal sliding of the median nerve during movements of the upper limb. J Neurol Neurosurg Psychiatry 1976;39:566–570.

40. Wilgis E, Murphy J. The significance of longitudinal excursion in peripheral nerves. Hand Clin North Am 1986;2:761–766.

41. Clemente CD. Gray's anatomy. 30th Ed. Philadelphia: Lea & Febiger, 1985.

42. Hartz CR, Linscheid RL, Framse RR, et al. The pronator teres syndrome: Compressive neuropathy of the median nerve. J Bone Joint Surg Am 1981;63:885–890.

7 Dystonia and Pseudodystonia of the Wrist and Hand: A Myofascial Approach

Nancy Shaw, CMTPT and Robert Gerwin, MD

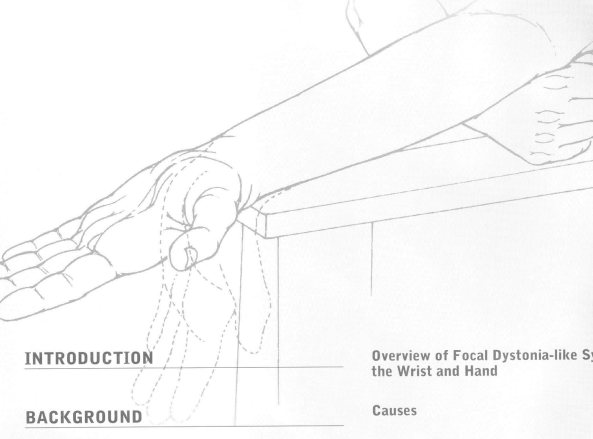

INTRODUCTION

Wrist and hand weakness and pain are common conditions in people who depend on repetitive, small movements or gripping movements, such as musicians, writers, computer operators, artists, tennis players, golfers, among others. This chapter discusses the management of upper extremity dysfunction characterized by **dystonia** and dystonia-like movements. Dystonia is defined as a syndrome of sustained muscle contractions, frequently causing twisting and repetitive movements or abnormal postures (1). Dystonia is increasingly found to be a genetic disorder, with more than 25 different types of primary genetic dystonias described. Sporadic dystonia remains a large percentage of clinical cases and can be secondary to a variety of causes, including trauma, encephalitis, antiphospholipid syndrome, drug-induced, and metabolic (including hypoxia), among other causes. Dystonia may be focal or generalized, but most dystonias start as focal, action-specific movement disorders, even those that become generalized. Electromyographic studies show co-contraction of agonists and antagonists. Changes are seen in cerebral cortex and in the basal ganglia. There is reduced thalamic inhibition by the globus pallidus, resulting in overactivity of frontal and prefrontal cortex, and underactivity of primary motor cortex. The internal globus pallidus shows abnormal firing (2). Dystonia can be action specific (e.g., writing, keyboard use, walking forward), especially in the early phases, although the specificity of action can persist in **focal dystonias**. The important concept is that dystonia is a cerebral disorder, whether primary genetic or secondary. Even secondary dystonias, associated with occupationally related movements such as keyboard use, are associated with changes in the brain (3,4).

Treatment of dystonia depends on whether it is generalized or focal. Focal dystonia is usually treated with botulinum toxin, with generally good success. The injections must be repeated approximately every 3 months. Deep brain stimulation (DBS) is promising as a treatment for severe generalized or unilateral dystonia. Drug therapy other than botulinum toxin remains of very limited benefit. Of interest are two recent reports of local treatment of the affected limb in focal dystonia. Fixation of the normal fingers through splinting with repetitive exercise of the dystonic fingers produced functional improvement in some musicians (5). Conversely, immobilization of the dystonic forearm and hand by splinting resulted in long-term improvement in a small series of patients with occupational focal dystonia (6). Furthermore, sensorimotor training based on the principles of neural adaptation has resulted in clinical motor function and cortical somatosensory response improvement in individuals with focal hand dystonia and a history of repetitive hand use (7).

This chapter focuses on a myofascial approach to the treatment of dystonia and dystonia-like movements of the muscles that control movements of the shoulder girdle, arm, and hand. We have used the term **pseudodystonia** because some movements caused by myofascial trigger points mimic the movement disorder of true dystonia. The subjects described in this chapter have been diagnosed clinically as having dystonia but have not had genetic testing or functional magnetic resonance imaging or positron emission tomography scans. The clinical diagnosis is made on the basis of physical examination, observation, and the exclusion of other conditions. Separating a true dystonia from the dystonic movements associated with myofascial trigger points, or dystonia that is accompanied by coexistent myofascial trigger points, may be clinically impossible. This is especially true for sporadic cases of dystonia that are not inherited. The myofascial approach presented in this chapter treats the underlying musculoskeletal abnormality that leads to dystonic arm and hand dysfunction, or that aggravates a preexisting dystonia. The contribution of proximal shoulder girdle and torso muscles to wrist and hand pain and movement dysfunction is important and is emphasized in discussing the diagnosis and treatment of these conditions.

BACKGROUND

Repetitive strain, repetitive motion, and cumulative trauma injuries are major problems that have been known for more than a century. Sir Charles Bell described writer's cramp in 1833, and Robinson described telegraph operators cramp in 1883. Gowers, in 1888, described writer's cramp as "an occupational neurosis" (8). Workers' compensation claims involving the musculoskeletal system (including low back pain) exceed all other types of claims. According to a survey conducted by *Cumulative Trauma Disorder News*, the rise in wrist and hand pain and dysfunction affects more than 14 million American workers. Many of these cases involve carpal tunnel syndrome, but focal dystonia and repetitive strain–related syndromes also account for a large number of cases (9).

Diagnosis of focal dystonia includes persons who have carpal tunnel syndrome, tennis elbow, golfers' elbow or cramp, psychogenic movement disorders, arthritis, and writers' cramp, even though these conditions are not primarily true dystonias (10–12). Misdiagnosis of dystonia is common because symptoms may be similar to those of other conditions. Seventy-one percent of dystonia patients in one study reported that they had difficulty in obtaining a diagnosis and had to travel an average of 160 miles for treatment (13). They reported decreased social activities and reduced work hours, and 26% reported that they could not work.

Dystonia is an abnormality of muscle tone that presents as a movement disorder. Focal dystonia is a sustained muscle contraction restricted to a particular part of the body, such as the arm and hand. Pseudodystonia refers to a group of muscle dysfunction syndromes in which the symptoms and signs closely resemble those of the true neurologic dystonia, but in which the problem lies in the development of persistent muscle trigger points with contracted taut muscle bands. This distinction may not be possible to make clinically, because true dystonias also can show trigger points, or the persistent contraction of the muscle and dystonic movements may make the examination for trigger points impractical. The term *pseudodystonia* is used in this chapter at times to emphasize the role of the trigger point in cause and in treatment.

Dystonia and pseudodystonia can cause the hand and finger muscles to contract and to exhibit slow or halting movements, uncoordinated movements, and abnormal postures. The disorder is often described as occupational dystonia because of its association with work-related activities (14). It is often triggered by fine motor movements of the hand and fingers, as opposed to gross or bulk movements of the forearm. Musicians and keyboard operators describe movements as uncoordinated. Recovery time is slow, movement is sluggish and muscles are prone to early fatigue. Weakness and pain may travel from the hand and wrist proximally to the forearm and arm. Patients learn "tricks" to dampen the dystonic movements, such as holding an object in the hand. Pseudodystonia, like true neurologic dystonia, can be disabling and devastating. It can lead to loss of ability to work and ruination of career. The characteristics of activity-specific cramps, abnormal postures, dystonic movements, fatigue, and slow and uncoordinated movements can be seen as well in regional myofascial pain syndromes.

Patients with dystonia complain of wrist and hand weakness, altered and uncontrollable movements, and pain. The clinician may initially focus on cervical root compression or median nerve entrapment (carpal tunnel syndrome; see Chapter 6) as causative factors. Electrodiagnostic studies are useful in reaching a diagnosis. No denervation changes or conduction block is found in either true dystonia or pseudodystonia, unless there are associated abnormalities such as nerve entrapments or compression.

A primary cause of pseudodystonia of the wrist and hand are keyboard and similar tasks such as computer use and piano playing or playing other musical instruments. Sign language signers and other professions are at risk, however, including seamstresses, knitters and crocheters, gardeners, writers, carpenters, craftsmen of all sorts, chefs, dentists and surgeons, manual therapists, and others who use their upper extremities in a repetitive manner for prolonged periods.

Conventional Therapy

Identifying the myofascial complications of the dystonias, which can be treated specifically by the means discussed in this chapter, is essential. Moreover, true dystonia also can be helped by these techniques. No published studies exist on this topic. However, this approach is based on clinical experience in treating these conditions.

Nonpharmacologic therapies include:

- Prescribed rest, with cessation of repetitive hand motion

- Elimination or reduction of repetitive motion or the particular offending strenuous activity thought to have initiated or maintained the dystonia or pseudodystonia

- Splinting the forearm or wrist, preventing excessive flexion or extension

- Physical therapy to strengthen forearm extensor muscles and counterbalance flexor muscle overactivity

- Stress management and relaxation training to reduce muscle tension

- Altering work or activity ergonomics to provide better body mechanics

Conservative conventional management is usually tried for a period of months. However, conservative conventional therapy is usually ineffective or may be only partially effective. In cases in which the problem is really pseudodystonia, or is primarily caused by trigger points, the conventional treatment for dystonia will not be very effective. However, botulinum toxin also will work in pseudodystonia caused by myofascial trigger points. Even when botulinum toxin is effective, the outcome is usually less than full restoration of normal movement, and the benefit is often lost by the second or third month. Consequently, a different approach that addresses the dysfunction of the muscle and of related muscles that share control over specific actions is needed.

MYOFASCIAL APPROACH TO THE DIAGNOSIS AND TREATMENT OF PSEUDODYSTONIA

An additional diagnostic paradigm to evaluate and treat wrist and hand weakness, pain, and dysfunction is needed. Muscle trigger points are consequences of muscle overuse. Muscles "learn" shortened functional patterning in response to repetitive activity and overload. The trigger point may persist for months and years if untreated, or if the mechanical stress continues. Flexor muscles tend to be dominant in non–antigravity muscles, resulting in flexion postures at rest. Shoulder and arm muscles also respond to a constant tendency to fold or roll forward. This is seen in the tendency for persons to develop a forward head posture and rounded shoulders. This posture, often accompanied by neck pain and headache, is also associated with shortening of the pectoralis major and minor muscles and chronic stress on the extensor muscles of the neck and shoulders. Likewise, the subscapularis muscle is also shortened and limited in its function in this posture. Symptomatic, active trigger points and asymptomatic, latent trigger points are likely to develop in both the extensor and flexor muscles. The function of these proximal muscles directly affects the function of the more distal muscles of the forearm and hand. For example, full supination of the forearm cannot be achieved in the face of subscapularis shortening.

Myofascial trigger points mimic many other conditions, and can be comorbidities with them. This is true for cervical radiculopathy, and muscle entrapments, including thoracic outlet syndrome, accounting in part for the confusion surrounding this latter condition, especially the form that Wilbourne has called "disputed thoracic outlet syndrome" (15). If the clinician focuses on the site of the complaint, rather than tracing the problem back to its origin, the problem will be sought in the zone of referred pain rather than in the more proximal trigger point origin of the problem. When pain is not the issue, but clumsiness and incoordination is the problem, the origin of the difficulty is even more obscure. A myofascial trigger point syndrome may be misdiagnosed as dystonia in these circumstances. This is an especially critical problem for persons in whom fine motor coordination is essential for performing their activities, such as, for example, musicians.

When a particular group of muscles is overused or repeatedly stressed, as extensor muscles of the forearms may be in keyboard use, whether in computer users or pianists, trigger points also will develop in the muscles of the functional motor unit, that is, in the agonist and antagonist muscles. Therefore, a spread of the muscles involved in the myofascial pain syndrome occurs. Moreover, postural stresses develop because of limitations of movement, and these changes also induce the development of trigger points. Thus, myofascial trigger point pain can spread from an initial focal area to involve a much larger portion of the body (16). This principle, applied to the upper extremity, requires a critical look at those myofascial trigger points that refer pain and dysfunction to the wrist and hand from the torso, shoulder, neck, and arm muscles.

Muscles above the elbow that are relevant to this discussion include the latissimus dorsi, serratus posterior superior and serratus anterior, pectoralis major and pectoralis minor, subscapularis, infraspinatus and supraspinatus, coracobrachialis, subclavius, scaleni, triceps, biceps, and brachialis. Muscles below the elbow that also refer pain from their trigger points to the wrist and hand include the brachioradialis, the extensor carpi radialis and ulnaris, the flexor carpi radialis and ulnaris, the extensor carpi radialis brevis and longus, the extensor indicis, pronator teres, the palmaris longus, and the supinator muscle. Pain and dysfunction in the wrist and hand may direct attention away from the source of the pain in trigger points that are present in more proximal muscles. Tightness and restricted motion in the neck and in the shoulders may be considered "normal" and thus not attract attention as needing treatment.

Once the role of muscle trigger points and local muscle dysfunction is identified as a cause, contribution to, or a comorbidity of focal dystonia, structural abnormalities or mechanical limitations also must be considered as contributing factors to the development of myofascial trigger points or recurrent muscle stress. In particular, biomechanical restrictions of cervical spine function are important, as are nerve impingements and entrapments. These problems also need to be addressed when treating upper extremity dystonias or dystonia-like syndromes.

CASE 7-1

Patient History

Z., a 17-year-old high school junior, was noted to be declining in his musical performance abilities by his piano teacher. The young man had been a piano student since age 8. He also played the French horn and was a drum major in the high school band. His activities, including note taking in class, writing, piano playing, and conducting, all included intensive use of forearm extensor and flexor muscles. He had not been involved in other physical activities such as athletics in or out of school. He had no cross-training activities and no cardiovascular training program. He was taking no medications or drugs. He complained of fatigue, heaviness, weakness, and lack of control in the right forearm, wrist, and third, fourth, and fifth digits, as well as in the left forearm and wrist. He noted a "knotting" in his left forearm. The symptoms were present for approximately 5 months before referral to this clinic. He attributed the symptoms to an intensive 4-hour practice session in which he believed he had used improper technique. He experienced fatigue and weakness for about 3 weeks after this intensive practice session. He felt stiff and a lack of control when playing the piano and when conducting. He experienced pain if he continued either activity. Fatigue and weakness became evident, without pain, even when he was not playing. However, he had not experienced pain or weakness in the upper back, shoulder, or neck muscles. Slight and transient relief was obtained with heat and rest. The diagnosis by his physician was focal dystonia.

Z's eating habits were typical for a teen-ager, emphasizing sugared cereal, pastries, and other foods with a high content of refined sugars, but his diet was deficient in protein.

Examination

Z. had typical myofascial trigger points with painful, tight bands of muscle, local twitch response in affected muscles, decreased range of motion, and pain referred from the forearm muscles to the hand. The affected

CASE 7-1   Continued

muscles included the latissimus dorsi, the infraspinatus, teres major and minor, deltoid, pectoralis minor, triceps, biceps, brachialis, brachioradialis, supinator, and forearm extensor and flexor muscles of both the right and left forearm. The interossei muscles were involved on the right side. Latent trigger points characterized by tender, taut bands that did not reproduce his pain when manually stimulated by applying pressure were found in the posterior cervical muscles, the sternocleidomastoid, triceps, pectoralis major, pronator teres, rectus abdominis, serratus anterior, and serratus posterior superior muscles. There was no limitation of range of motion in torso rotation, flexion, or extension. Internal rotation of the right shoulder was limited to 25 % of normal, and external rotation to 35% of normal. Left shoulder range of motion was slightly better. Cervical rotation was 85% of normal to the right and to the left. Lateral neck bending was 65% of normal. Neck flexion and extension were normal. Elbow extension was limited 25 % on the right and 15% on the left. Wrist flexion was normal. Supination of the forearm was limited by 75% bilaterally. Standing and sitting postures were good, with little to no adaptation to upper back, neck, or shoulder tightness.

Treatment

A program of dietary improvement and physical exercise (cross-training) was undertaken. Symptoms of stiffness, heaviness, and weakness began to subside with this general program even before any manual therapy directed toward the trigger points was begun. Manual therapy consisted of trigger point compression of the trigger points in the upper shoulder and neck muscles, especially of the muscles related to scapular stabilization. The upper arm muscle trigger points were treated similarly, using vapo-coolant spray and stretch techniques. A self-directed stretching program was prescribed, to be done every 1 to 11/2 hours to maintain lengthening of the muscles. This was later reduced to once every 3 hours. The stretching program took approximately 2 minutes to complete and could easily fit into his schedule. Initial treatment was directed at the proximal muscles and not the muscles distal to the elbow.

Z. felt better after the first treatment, and had no sense of weakness, fatigue, or stiffness. He returned for a second treatment to address the forearm muscles in addition to the proximal muscles of the shoulder. The second treatment session again included inactivation of muscle trigger points through trigger point compression and vapo-coolant spray and stretch. Proprioceptive neuromuscular facilitation (PNF) was used for the rotator cuff muscles, and the arm and forearm muscles. The intrinsic muscles of the hand were also treated. The result was the elimination of stiffness and weakness and return of more normal range of motion of the limb. He began to swim several days a week as cross-training and continued to do self-stretching every 2 hours. He was able to return to conducting and to practice the piano 5 hours daily without return of symptoms. There was no return of his symptoms when he was reevaluated 9 months later. He performed his senior recital, and continued to perform in later years.

CASE 7-2

Patient History

E., a 47-year-old professional pianist, came to the clinic when he could no longer practice at the level necessary to perform on stage. He had played the piano since childhood and now performed solo concerts on a regular basis. This required him to practice at an intense level up to 5 to 7 hours a day, often 5 or 6 days per week. He had also been a professional piano tuner for 18 years. This often occupied as many as 6 hours per day. E. worked with free weights several days per week and enjoyed hiking and cycling with his family. A diagnosis of focal dystonia and carpal tunnel had been given, although no magnetic resonance imaging (MRI) nor electromyography (EMG) had been performed. The patient was taking no medications.

Symptoms

E. had begun experiencing a sense of tightness in the forearms and fingers, particularly on the left, some months previous to his office visit. He had also begun to experience occasional burning on top of the right hand. At times, the patient experienced severe muscle spasm in the midthoracic and cervical area with considerable involvement extending into the arms. He noticed a significant reduction in range of motion, stiffness, weakness, and fatigue during this time. There was discomfort when attempting full range of motion in daily movement. He sensed his forearms and hands "jumping around" when he attempted to practice. E. also felt he was losing "perfect pitch" hearing. He sought help after experiencing a burning sensation in the upper back,

(continues)

CASE 7-2   Continued

shoulder, and arm after a 7-hour practice session. Fatigue and a lack of coordination were also of concern. The symptoms were present when practicing and, occasionally, when piano tuning. E. noticed that stiffness and weakness, but not the burning, remained even after cessation of practice. He felt no pain. He was able to find some relief with rest, but the symptoms returned within a few minutes of resuming practicing or tuning. A pain chart and verbal documentation were recorded by the clinician and reviewed by the patient to ensure an accurate understanding of the problem.

Examination Findings

Myofascial examination showed characteristic trigger point involvement, that is, palpable taut bands, decreased range of motion, and referred pain, in the upper trapezius, levator scapulae, latissimus dorsi, pectoralis major and minor, infraspinatus, teres major and minor, biceps, triceps, and forearm flexors muscles. Interossei also were restricted in motion. Latent trigger points were evidenced in the entire functional unit of the torso, neck, and arms.

Range of motion showed restriction of torso rotation and extension. Internal rotation of the left shoulder was limited to 25° and external rotation to 34°, with only slight improvement on the right. Cervical rotation was 45° right and 65° left. Triceps and biceps extension were restricted. Abduction of the arm was limited to 110° on the right and 120° on the left. Wrist flexion was normal. Wrist extension was limited to 15° on both right and left. Forearm supination was negligible both right and left.

E. had a very thick, stocky body build with slight rounding of the upper torso. His standing and sitting postures were good, consistent with the learned posturing of a professional pianist. He did, however, when playing a dynamic portion during a performance, have his right foot on the pedal and actually lifted his body off the piano bench approximately 3 to 4 inches with his left leg/quadriceps. This necessitated tensing the upper torso in a way that would maintain his erect posture without any underlying support.

Perpetuating factor evaluation indicated a slight small hemipelvis/short leg on the left.

Evaluation of eating habits and nutritional intake found E. to be typical of many professional performers. Breakfast consisted of coffee and toast, lunch was often skipped, with dinner being the main meal of meat, pasta/starch, vegetable, and bread. Dinner was often at 9:00 PM or later because of rehearsal or performance schedules. Although his dinners were adequate, there was little nutritional intake, especially protein, during the day or evening, when muscle demand was highest.

Sleep was in a supine position but with slightly too high a pillow. The pillow was also under the shoulders.

Although his schedule did not allow a great deal of time for the cycling, hiking, and free-weight training, they were excellent cross-training for both cardiovascular fitness and muscle use. However, the piano tuning, cycling, and weight training all involve gripping and wrist and finger flexion.

Treatment

Initially, the perpetuating factors of eating and sleeping were addressed. E. was asked to eat every 3 to 4 hours. He was to include some protein each time he ate a meal or snacked (albeit protein was to be a side dish, not necessarily the main entree.) He decreased his caffeine intake and increased fruits and vegetables. Sleep was modified by the use of a lower pillow that allowed his neck to be in a more neutral position. He also removed it from under his shoulders to avoid pushing the shoulders forward and tightening the chest. These changes were addressed before hands-on therapy began.

The short-leg/small hemipelvis discrepancy was alleviated with the insertion of a heel lift in the left shoe. Lift correction must be the entire length of the heel; many lifts on the market begin to taper off immediately from the back of the heel. Use of an ischial lift was important, because he sits with the piano while playing and with tuning. As little as 1/4-inch imbalance at the heel or hip level can mean as much as 1+ inch right-to-left discrepancy at the shoulder level.

E.'s position at the piano was not changed except for bringing him slightly closer to the keyboard. This allowed for increased volume when playing strong segments, because the force exerted by the upper torso, shoulders, and arms was on a more perpendicular line to the keys rather than horizontal.

Hands-on treatment began with the patient in a prone position, arms hanging loosely, and the head in a face-down position. The gluteals, latissimus dorsi, and trapezius were treated with myofascial release technique 4 (MRT4.) (For a fuller discussion of the use of patient movement during myofascial release: MRT3 and MRT4, see Chapter 6.) This consisted of slowly applying pressure parallel to and approximately 2 to 3 inches from the spine. When a taut band or area was found, the pressure was sustained while E. was asked to perform alternate leg lifts for the gluteals, arm forward lifting for the latissimus, and arm abduction for the trapezius. Moving slightly closer to the spine, the technique was repeated, working along the paravertebral muscles. Specific trigger point release using sustained pressure then was performed on the same musculature.

CASE 7-2   Continued

Still in the prone position, the patient's arm was brought into internal rotation with the arm behind the back, winging the scapula. This was extremely difficult for E. to do, the right arm only reaching to the right gluteal area. The rhomboids trigger points were released with sustained pressure, followed by MRT4 with the arm moving from abduction to behind the back. The rotator cuff trigger points then were treated with sustained pressure, the arm resting beside the body. The lateral border of the scapulae was addressed with the patient in a side-lying position and the arm extended overhead. MRT4 and sustained pressure trigger point release were used in treating this area. The pectoralis minor and serratus also were treated in this side-lying position.

In a sitting position, MRT4 was performed on the levator scapulae, upper trapezius, and sternocleidomastoid. The head was rotated right to left as the pressure was held on the various points in the taut bands of muscle fibers.

Specific stretches were given to further the muscle release and to reestablish a new functional range for the treated muscles. Those stretches included a supine bent cross-leg hip and torso rotation, a standing torso rotation, shoulder rotation with the arm in an abducted position, lateral overhead reach, and large arm circles backward. Two repetitions of each stretch were performed every 1 to 2 hours. Patient education is critical, because the patient must understand the importance of doing the stretches frequently, rather than a lot of repetitions once or twice a day. Changing muscle patterning requires the frequency. If the stretches are simple, few, and only two repetitions are required, most patients are compliant.

Before the next session, E. sustained a severe cut on his right hand that required three layers of stitches. Taking pain medications, he forced himself to practice 5 to 6 hours/day in preparation for an upcoming concert. This caused him to use his shoulders and arms in stressed positions to compensate for the hand, resulting in an awareness of a "burning" sensation in the right 4th

finger, in the thumb, and palm. Trigger point release was repeated on the upper back, shoulders, and scapulae to counteract this compensation. With the patient in a prone position, arm abducted at 90°, trigger point release also was performed on the triceps and biceps by using sustained pressure. The concert performance of three very taxing pieces was "superb on one piece, and okay on the other two." Practice then fell to approximately 3 hours per day, which allowed for greater stretch retraining results.

Within a couple of weeks of the concert, when the larger muscles, that is, trapezius, rotator cuff, latissimus dorsi, triceps, biceps, and pectoralis, were maintaining a good range of motion, treatment became focused on the forearms and hands. With the patient in a supine position and the forearm resting on the treatment table, the supinator and pronator were treated with intermittent coolant with stretch. The forearm flexors were treated with sustained pressure combined with MRT4, the patient alternately flexing and extending the wrist while the pressure was held. Stripping release moving from the wrist toward the elbow followed, with the pressure being sustained when particularly taut areas were noted. The forearm extensors were treated in the same manner.

The palm of the hand was treated by using the therapist's thumb in a stripping motion horizontally and at an angle toward the fingers. Pincer sustained pressure using the thumb and first finger was used to address the muscles of the fingers. Direct sustained pressure was used between each joint on the anterior of the fingers, and on the tip of each finger.

E. continued to play throughout the treatment, which prolonged the treatment time, but within 4 to 5 months he was again playing with good coordination, only normal fatigue, and no pain. Occasionally, he experienced a "burning" sensation between the scapulae. This, with E., indicated vertebral fixation and was addressed with chiropractic treatment.

Overview of Focal Dystonia-like Syndromes of the Wrist and Hand

Patients who present with wrist and hand weakness and pain and motor incoordination usually also have some degree of upper body and arm dysfunction. In most patients, the upper back, chest, neck, and shoulder girdle regions are primary sources of pain and dysfunction, affecting hand and forearm use. The more proximal muscles stabilize the arm and forearm, wrist, and hand.

Causes

Wrist and hand dysfunction with dystonic features can develop in situations in which there is trauma to the hand, wrist, or forearm, acute muscle overload or mechanical stress, cumulative muscle overload or stress, prolonged immobilization, prolonged static maintenance of posture, and lack of postoperative rehabilitation that includes restoration of range of motion. The clinician must determine the cause of abnormal functioning. What specific activities produced recurrent muscle shortening? What has led to guarded movements or dysfunctional compensatory movements? The questions are directed toward elucidating the underlying mechanisms that have led to dysfunction, and not just to the nature of the dysfunction itself.

Differential Diagnosis

Atrophy or sensory loss in the upper limb indicates a neurogenic disorder, including entrapment syndromes, that requires further neurologic investigation.

Somatic dysfunction of the first rib at the first thoracic vertebra is a structural disorder, resulting in scalene and serratus muscle dysfunction that can cause hand weakness and pain.

Somatic dysfunction of the lunate bone in the wrist, as a result of hyperextension of the wrist, can cause hand weakness and pain.

Rheumatoid arthritis causes thickening of the transverse carpal ligament, which can compress the median nerve. (Myofascial trigger point therapy is not given during painful acute flare-ups of rheumatoid arthritis.)

Acute gouty arthritis also can cause wrist and hand pain and requires specific treatment by nonsteroidal anti-inflammatory drugs and drugs that lower blood levels of uric acid.

Hypothyroidism can cause thickening of the tissues of the carpal tunnel and also may perpetuate painful myofascial trigger points.

Symptom Presentation

The most common musculoskeletal symptoms of wrist and hand dysfunction are pain, weakness, incoordination, limited range of motion, stiffness, joint clicking, abnormal posturing and dystonic movements, and deformity. Patients also may feel tension and pain in the shoulder and neck. Headache stemming from upper trapezius and sternocleidomastoid muscle trigger points can occur. Weakness and lack of endurance can result from the presence of shortened, taut bands of muscle and associated trigger points. Uncoordinated movements of the fingers and the hands can occur and is especially a problem for musicians and others in whom repetitive, rapid sequences of movements is required. Musicians are especially aware of even mild dysfunctions, because even mild dysfunctions seriously degrade their performance. Stiffness is seen at the beginning of an activity before the patient is "warmed-up" and later in the activity, when fatigue is a factor. Impaired joint mobility and reduced range of motion are factors that affect perceived stiffness. Joint clicking occurs with biceps tendon displacement, degenerative joint disease of the head of the humerus, and temporomandibular joint dysfunction with anterior displacement of the disc. Hand deformities can occur with contractures of the forearm and intrinsic hand muscles.

Nerve entrapments can cause limb dysfunction as a result of compression of neural elements with subsequent motor and sensory symptoms that include weakness, pain, and sensory loss, with clumsiness of fine hand movement.

Entrapments can occur in the interscalene compartment, between the first rib and the clavicle, and beneath the pectoralis minor muscle. The radial nerve can be entrapped by the brachialis muscle, at the supinator muscle, or in the radial tunnel. The median nerve can be entrapped by the pronator teres muscle. Release of muscle trigger points can relieve the nerve compression.

Evaluation

The evaluation begins with the history and proceeds with a mapping of the patient's symptom complex, denoting the location and extent of the dysfunction. (Note: see Tables 7.1–7.8 for information on evaluation of specific regions.) A representation of the pain is drawn on a body diagram. The patient is examined for bodily asymmetries, including scoliosis, swelling, and atrophy. Examination is conducted for abnormal muscle tone and joint mobility (both hypermobility and hypomobility), taut bands, tender nodules, limb temperature and color for evidence of increased or decreased blood flow and sympathetic activity, and joint swelling and tenderness.

Postural assessment is also important. The head-forward, rounded shoulder posture is a common dysfunction that increases in frequency with age, as well as with computer and other keyboard work, including keyboard musicians. In the head-forward, rounded shoulder posture, the sternocleidomastoid and anterior scalene muscles are shortened, and the posterior cervical and upper back extensor muscles are lengthened. Both sets of muscles are vulnerable to developing trigger points, the flexor muscles through chronic shortening and the extensor muscles through persistent contraction required to extend the neck and elevate the eyes to permit forward vision. In addition, the scapulae are protracted and elevated, with shortening of the pectoralis major and minor muscles and lengthening of the latissimus dorsi muscles. Pain referral patterns of the neck, upper back, and shoulder girdle muscle trigger points include the forearms and hands and are important in determining the cause of hand incoordination and fatigue. Scoliosis is an important factor, because it alters neck and shoulder function through asymmetric shortening and lengthening of neck and upper torso muscles. Thus, leg-length inequality, hemipelvis height inequality, and pelvic torsion and sacroiliac joint dysfunctions that cause a scoliosis or pseudo-scoliosis, are important factors in upper limb dysfunction.

Similarly, disordered breathing patterns, namely chest breathing that uses scalene accessory respiratory muscle activity, can affect hand function through activation of scalene muscle trigger points, with all of the consequences that have been mentioned previously.

Range of motion examination is evaluated bilaterally. Active range of motion is evaluated in different positions, sitting, standing and lying down, to increase the ability to detect limitations that may be dependent on joint loading and muscle function. Agonist and antagonist muscles are both assessed for function and limitation of motion around

TABLE 7-1			
Evaluation of the Shoulder			

Normal Range of Motion	Movement	Dysfunction	Notes
180°	Flexion	Restricted movement of the posterior deltoid, teres major, latissimus dorsi, triceps, long head, rhomboid, levator scapulae	Some patients may feel discomfort in the upper trapezius from the added contraction.
	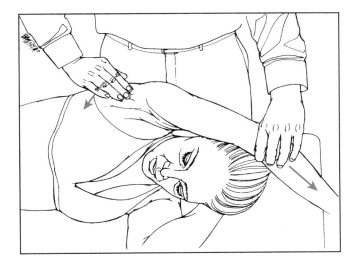		
45°	Extension	Restricted movement of the anterior deltoid, biceps pectoralis major, coracobrachialis	There should be no forward flexion of the hips.
	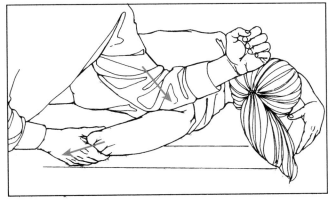		
180°	Abduction	Restricted movement of the latissimus dorsi, triceps, biceps, serratus anterior, pectoralis major & minor, coracobrachialis	Hand in a thumb-down position evaluates the triceps involvement; thumb-up position evaluates the biceps.
	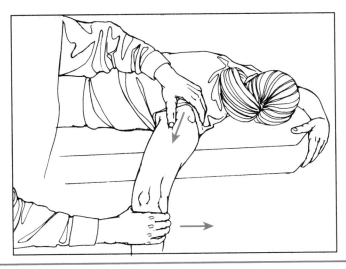		

(continues)

TABLE 7-1

Evaluation of the Shoulder *(Continued)*

Normal Range of Motion	Movement		Dysfunction	Notes
40°	Adduction			Note areas in the arc that are painful on the return.

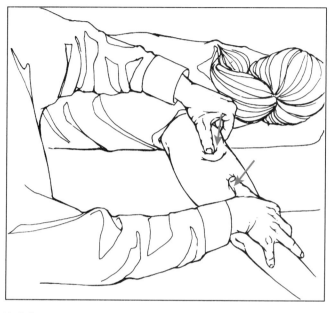

Normal Range of Motion	Movement		Dysfunction	Notes
90°	Medial rotation		Restricted movement in the infraspinatus, teres minor, posterior deltoid.	
90°	Lateral rotation		Restricted movement in anterior deltoid, pectoralis major, subscapularis, teres major, latissimus dorsi.	Note painful arc areas, often on the return movement.

TABLE 7-2

Evaluation of the Elbow

Normal Range of Motion	Movement	Dysfunction	Notes
145°	Flexion	Restricted movement in the triceps and anconeus.	Some patients may feel discomfort in the biceps from the added contraction.
—	Extension	Restricted movement primarily in the biceps, brachialis, brachioradialis.	Some restriction may be present in the forearm flexors.

TABLE 7-3

Evaluation of the Forearm

Normal Range of Motion	Movement	Dysfunction	Notes
85°–90°	Supination	Restricted movement in the brachioradialis, pronator teres, flexor carpi radialis, palmaris longus, pronator quadratus	Support forearm to prevent shoulder rotation
85°–90°	Pronation	Restricted movement in the biceps, brachioradialis, supinator	Support the forearm to prevent shoulder rotation.

TABLE 7-4

Evaluation of the Wrist

Normal	Movement	Dysfunction	Notes
80°–90°	Flexion	Restricted movement in the extensor carpi radialis, longus, brevis, extensor digitorum, extensor carpi ulnaris, extensor pollicis longus	Distinguish between wrist flexion and finger flexion
70–90°	Extension	Restricted movement in the flexor carpi radialis, flexor carpi ulnaris, abductor pollicis longus, palmaris longus, flexor pollicis longus, flexor digitorum supinator, flexor digitorum pronator.	
15°–20°	Radial deviation	Restricted movement in the extensor carpi ulnaris and flexor carpi ulnaris	
30°–45°	Ulnar deviation	Restricted movement in the extensor longus and brevis, abductor. pollicis longus, extensor pollicis brevis, flexor carpi radialis, extensor pollicis longus	

TABLE 7-5

Evaluation of the Fingers

Normal ROM	Movement	Dysfunction	Note
—	Abduction	Restricted movement in the palmaris, int. & adductor pollicis.	Note variances of restriction between different fingers
—	Adduction	Restricted movement in the abductor pollicis longus and brevis, abductor digiti minimus, dorsi int.	

TABLE 7-6

Evaluation of Joint Dysfunction of the Shoulder

Technique	Description
Backward and forward glide of the humerus	The patient sits with her hand and forearm on the clinician's forearm. The clinician stands facing the lateral side of the patient's arm, with his right hand fixating from the ventral side around the patient's scapula and his index finger placed over the acromion. His or her left hand grips around the proximal part of the patient's humerus just lateral to the acromion. The humerus is moved ventrally. For dorsal glide, the same set-up position is used, but with the clinician's left hand fixating the patient's scapula, the index finger over the acromion and the right hand gripping from the medial side around the patient's arm just lateral to the acromion. The humerus moves dorsally.
Lateral distraction of the humerus	The patient sits with her hand resting on the clinician's forearm, the clinician stands facing the patient's lateral side. His or her left hand fixates the patient's shoulder with the thumb dorsally over the scapula and the index finger ventrally over the acromion. The right hand grips from the medial side around the proximal part of the patient's arm, and the arm is moved laterally.
Caudal glide of the humerus (long-arm traction)	The clinician stands facing the patient's lateral side, while the patient sits with her forearm resting on the clinician's forearm. His right hand grips from the medial side around the patient's arm while the left index finger and thumb are placed on the lateral aspect of the humerus just lateral to the acromion. The humerus is moved caudally.

Adapted from Kaltenborn F. Manual Mobilization of the Extremity Joints. Oslo: OPTP, 1989.

TABLE 7-7

Evaluation of Joint Dysfunction of the Elbow and Forearm

Technique	Description
Ulnar deviation of the ulna on the humerus Radial deviation of the radius on the humerus	The clinician stabilizes the patient's elbow by holding her humerus firmly and placing his or her other hand above the patient's wrist, abducting and adducting her forearm. The patient's elbow is straight during the movement, and the end feel should be bone to bone.
Distraction of the olecranon process on the humerus in 90° flexion	The clinician flexes the patient's elbow to 90°. Wrapping both hands around the patient's forearm close to the elbow, he or she then applies a distractive force at the elbow, ensuring that no torque is applied.
Anteroposterior glide of the radius on the humerus	The clinician stabilizes the patient's forearm and holds her arm between his body and arm. He places the thumb of his other hand over the anterior radial head with his index finger over the posterior radial head. The clinician then pushes the radial head posteriorly with the thumb and anteriorly with the index finger.

Adapted from Magee DJ. Orthopedic Physical Assessment. Philadelphia: WB Saunders, 1987.

a specific joint. Limitations of range of motion result from shortening of the lengthening muscles because of the presence of trigger point–associated taut bands, or from pain-induced restriction of contraction of the shortening muscles. Scapular mobility is assessed in the sitting, standing, lateral decubitus, or prone positions. End of range of motion is assessed to determine whether it is pain-free or painful, or whether a "hard-stop" is present, implying a mechanical limitation such as osteoarthritis. Range of motion evaluation helps establish which muscles are harboring trigger points. Taut bands that are associated with both active and latent trigger points will reduce range of motion. Range of motion testing can be indicative of taut bands even when there is little pain and no referred pain. The limitations of latent trigger points that manifest only as taut bands and limited range of motion can be clinically important, because the restrictions result in the development of compensatory move-

ments that can overload muscle and induce or perpetuate other trigger points. Care must be taken to identify those persons, usually women, who apparently have a full range of motion, but in reality are hypermobile and, therefore, should not be treated by stretching. Additionally, limitations of movement caused by tendon or joint disorders (e.g., arthritis or tendonitis) should be identified, because they require specific remedies not addressed in this chapter (Table 7-8). Loss of "joint play" can be a diagnostic feature of limb dysfunction caused by either pain or by muscle shortening, in addition to intrinsic disorders of the joint such as synovial thickening (17). Somatic dysfunctions of the first rib, or of the radius or the ulna at the elbow or the wrist, for example, must be addressed as well as the myofascial component, because the two problems (muscle and joint dysfunction) are intertwined and cannot be effectively separated in management.

TABLE 7-8

Suggested Evaluation of Joint Dysfunction: Wrist

Technique	Description
Long axis extension	The clinician holds the patient's arm with the elbow flexed at a right angle and the forearm in the neutral position. Using the left arm, he or she places the palm of his right hand anteriorly over the condylar region of the humerus at the elbow (no finger grip is used) and grasps the wrist area with his left hand, the thumb being just distal to the radial styloid process, and with his index finger just distal to the ulna styloid process. The clinician takes up the slack at the wrist, stabilizing the forearm with countertraction by applying pressure over the upper arm, and then pulls in the long axis of the patient's forearm.
Anteroposterior glide	The clinician places the crooked knuckle of the proximal interphalangeal joint of his or her index finger over the patient's pisiform bone. Then he places his thumb posteriorly over the lower and of the shaft of the ulna. With the other hand, he or she stabilizes the patient's radius, hand, and other joints of the wrist. Then he or she pinches together the crooked index finger and the thumb and glides the lower end of the ulna forward and, in rebound, backward on the triquetrum, which glides on the meniscus that lies in between.
Side glide	The clinician stands facing the medial side of the patient's hand. His or her right hand grips from the ulnar side around the patient's ulna with the thumb dorsal and index finger palmar. The patient's forearm is stabilized against the clinician's body. His left hand grips from the ulnar side with the thumb dorsal and index finger palmar around the triquetrum and pisiform. The triquetrum is moved in dorsal and palmar directions. Freedom of this joint is necessary for full supination range of motion.

Adapted from Mennell J. Understanding manipulative medicine in general practice. J Manip Physiol Ther 1989;3:12.

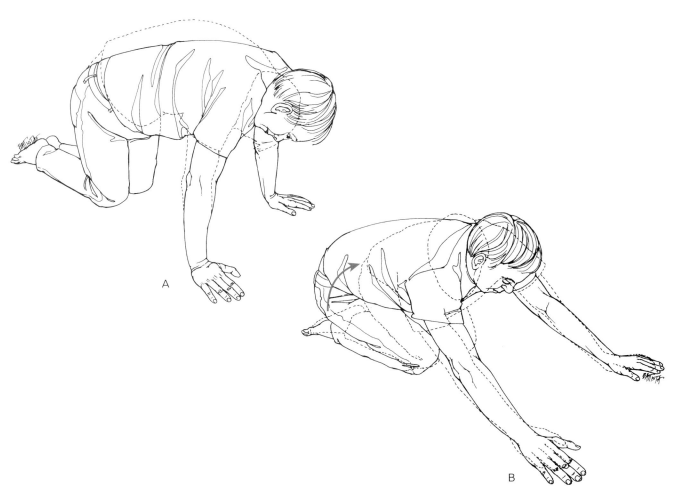

FIGURE 7-1. **Assessment of extension of the shoulder. A.** Head down, arch back upward. **B.** Shift to sitting on heels position.

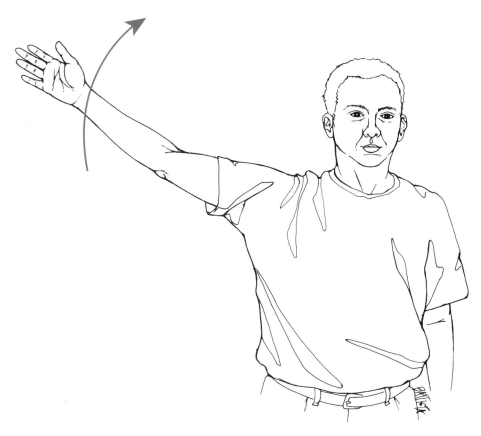

FIGURE 7-2. **Chest muscle stretch to assess shoulder mobility.** Circle the arm backward. Keep arm as straight as possible.

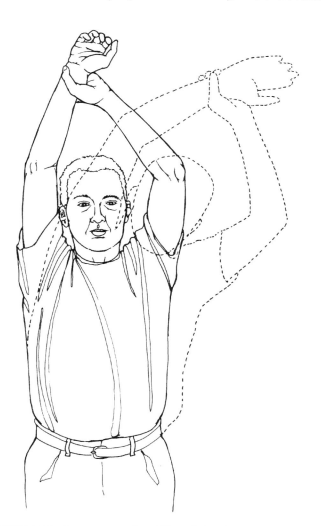

FIGURE 7-3. **Assessment of mobility of the shoulder in abduction.** Grasp arm at wrist. Stretch arm directly up. Maintain pull upward while leaning to side.

Cervical range of motion testing is done in the four cardinal directions of anterior and posterior movement (flexion and extension) and side bending, plus rotation to the right and left. Each direction of movement tests multiple muscles, and each muscle is important in more than one movement. For example, the trapezius muscle is lengthened in neck flexion with regard to its extensor action, in ipsilateral rotation because it is attached to the inion at its origin and to the acromion process at its insertion, and in contralateral side or lateral bending with regard to its ipsilateral side-bending action. The primary muscles that have restrictive trigger points thus can be determined by seeing which directions of movement are limited. Limitation of rotation to the right and side-bending left suggest that the right trapezius, right sternocleidomastoid muscle, and right scalene muscles may be involved. Referred pain from scalene muscle trigger points affects the arm and hand, as well as the upper chest and upper back. The scalene muscle referral pain patterns that extend into the limb, including the hand, mimic cervical radiculopathy, and must be kept in mind

when evaluating a person with arm and hand problems. The infraspinatus and other shoulder area muscles also have referred pain patterns into the arm and hand.

Rotational range of motion testing should be done with the neck in neutral position and also in flexion. Flexing the neck before testing rotation fixes the lower cervical vertebrae and concentrates the rotational motion at the atlas and axis, thereby assessing potential somatic dysfunction at this level. Somatic dysfunction at C1–2 is often associated with suboccipital muscle dysfunction, associated with headache rather than upper limb disorders (see Chapter 1).

Range of motion testing of the arm, wrist, and hand evaluates both primary and satellite trigger points that develop in the region of referred pain. Pronation and supination of the forearm are important and can be limited by proximal muscle shortening such as the limitation of supination by shortening of the subscapularis muscle. Simultaneously, pronation is apparently facilitated (the obverse of supination), again from limitation of stretch of the subscapularis muscle. Wrist extension and flexion are assessed as active movements. Forearm flexor muscles tend to shorten in persons with pain and weakness in the wrist and hand.

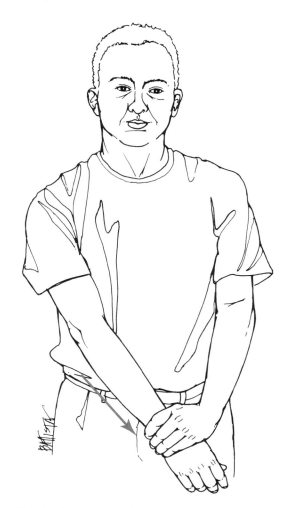

FIGURE 7-4. **Assessment of shoulder flexion.** Pull arm and shoulder down in front of body.

Joint mobility is evaluated for range of motion to identify muscle, internal joint, or capsular components of restriction. A painful arc of movement, such as seen in a shoulder impingement syndrome, may be seen primarily in one movement such as abduction, but it commonly is accompanied by restrictions in other movements as well. In the example of the shoulder impingement syndrome, internal rotation of the shoulder is usually limited, and effort-loaded cross-chest adduction of arm is painful and limited. A capsular pattern of limitation of motion is identified by taking the joint through a passive range of motion. Patients with wrist and hand dysfunction commonly have restrictions in the glenohumeral joint (internal and external rotation and abduction), in the radiohumeral joint (flexion and extension), the radioulnar joint (pronation and supination), and in the wrist (flexion and extension).

Evaluation of joint function is accomplished with the patient comfortable and warm, the limb or part to be examined well supported, and care taken to avoid producing pain. One joint is evaluated at a time, and each movement is assessed separately. The nonmoving part is stabilized, and a mobilizing force is applied to the moving part (Figs. 7-5–7-7).

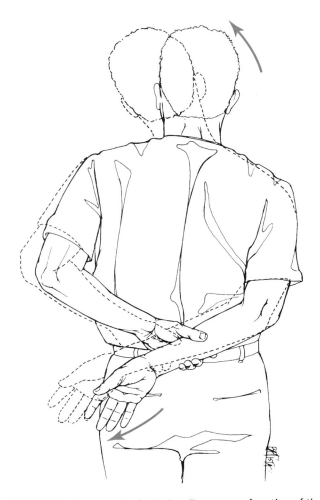

FIGURE 7-6. Assessment of side-bending range of motion of the neck. Grasp arm at wrist, pull arm down and across the back. Lean head to opposite shoulder. Rotate head in varying angles as you continue to lean to shoulder.

Treatment

Treatment is directed to the correction of the underlying causative factors, whether they be a systemic condition such as rheumatoid arthritis, primary joint dysfunction, tendon involvement, soft-tissue myofascial trigger point pain dysfunction, or a combination of these factors. Range of motion increases with treatment, restoring function. Loss of strength caused by muscle shortening and by myofascial trigger points also is alleviated with treatment. Treatment must include addressing the proximal shoulder girdle problems, including those caused by proximal muscle myofascial trigger point syndromes, because of the influence of the pectoral muscles, the serratus anterior, and the subscapularis muscle on forearm and hand function. The pain referral from the pectoralis major muscle includes the hand and the 3rd, 4th, and 5th digits. Body positioning at a keyboard often involves a forward shoulder and head posture, with shortening of the upper, horizontal fibers of the pectoralis major muscles, and potential development and activation of

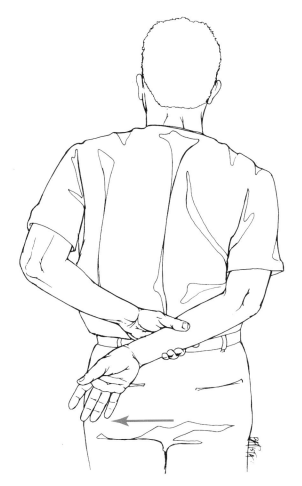

FIGURE 7-5. Assessment of shoulder mobility in extension. Grasp arm at wrist and gently pull across the body at waist level.

consequent trigger point formation in functionally related muscles or satellite trigger points in muscles in the referred pain zones. The proximal muscles are treated with the patient in the prone position for the upper back and shoulder, and in the lateral decubitus position for the scapula and pectoral muscles. The scapula can be mobilized in this position. The patient is instructed in self-stretching techniques for these proximal muscles to maintain the improved range of motion and thereby to encourage restoration of more normal range of motion and function in the distal limb (Figs 7-8–7-9). Inactivation of the trigger points of cervical

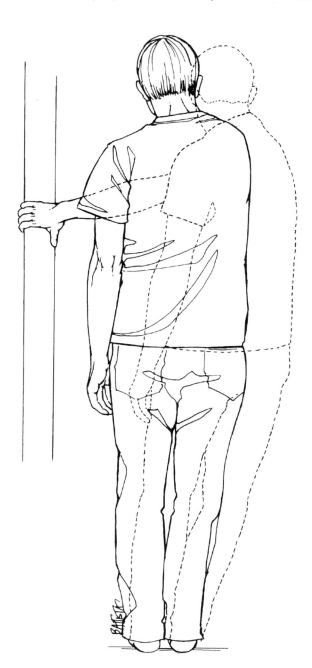

FIGURE 7-7. **Assessment of shoulder and scapula mobility.** Reach across body and grasp door frame in thumb-down position. Lean outward.

trigger points. Therefore, treatment must include addressing the trigger points and the shortening of the pectoralis major and other shoulder girdle muscles, and correcting the postural dysfunction.

Treatment begins with the proximal muscles. This often means treating the neck, upper torso, and shoulder muscles first. These muscles are postural muscles that have secondary effects on the more distal muscles by virtue of causing distal movement limitations as discussed earlier, or by producing referred pain into the more distal limb, often with

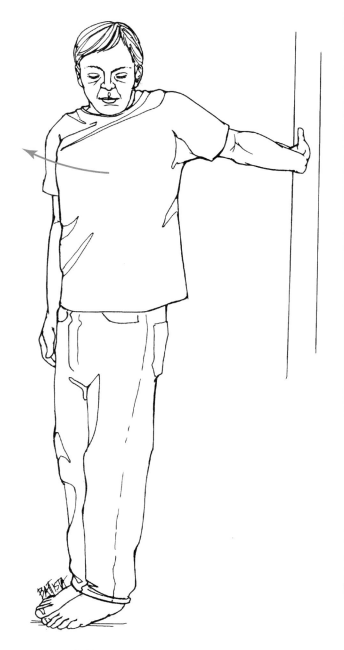

FIGURE 7-8. **Self-stretch of the pectoral muscles.** Place hand on wall in thumb-up position; turn torso away.

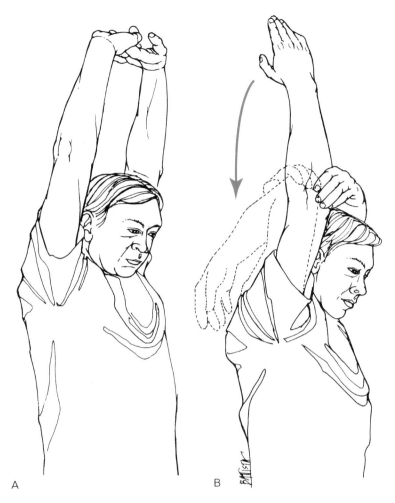

A   B

FIGURE 7-9. **Self-stretch of the shoulder adductors and triceps. A.** Shoulder adductors (subscapularis and latissimus dorsi muscles): Lace fingers. Reach arms forward and upward to overhead position. **B.** Triceps muscle: Reach arm straight overhead with the palm facing backward. Bend at elbow and place hand on shoulder. Keep elbow in close to the side of the head. With the opposite hand, pull the elbow backward.

and upper torso muscles (that also relate to the control of the shoulder) is necessary before achieving long-lasting improvement in distal limb function. The forearm, wrist, and hand are approached after the more proximal muscles and joint dysfunction are approached(Figs 7-10–7-13). The patient also must understand this progression of treatment to avoid anxiety that can occur when the area of concern is seemingly not addressed immediately. The patient must know that an interplay occurs between the proximal and distal muscles in the upper limb and shoulder, and that the hand functionally starts at the neck and shoulder level.

Finally, the ergonomic and biomechanical factors that either precipitated or perpetuated the dysfunction, identified in the initial evaluation, must be corrected to the extent possible. One pianist had a severe problem with the arm, but the real problem was a forceful bending and twisting of the trunk and postural abnormalities of the arm and hand that was partly technique and partly related to a bad seat that was unstable. The problem was compounded by joint hypermobility and marked physical deconditioning resulting

in rapid fatiguing of muscle and the development of muscle overload or stress that led to and maintained widespread trunk and limb trigger points. Part of the treatment had to include the replacement of the piano bench as a mechanical factor in the development of a widespread disorder.

The psychological aspect of the patient's pain syndrome is addressed in treatment. Some persons, particularly musicians and athletes who have a great deal of personal investment in performance, will intensify their practice sessions in the belief that their pain and limitations in movement are the result of under-training or lack of conditioning or practice. They become more aggressive in their training or practice and can aggravate the myofascial syndrome and the movement disorder. Attention to the need to excel and to maintain skills is critical. Teaching the patient pacing and alternative forms of practice or maintaining physical or mental conditioning, such as cross-training for athletes, is useful. Understanding the patient's motives in pursuing a career or an activity is also important. One patient had an action-induced inability to write or to play her instrument,

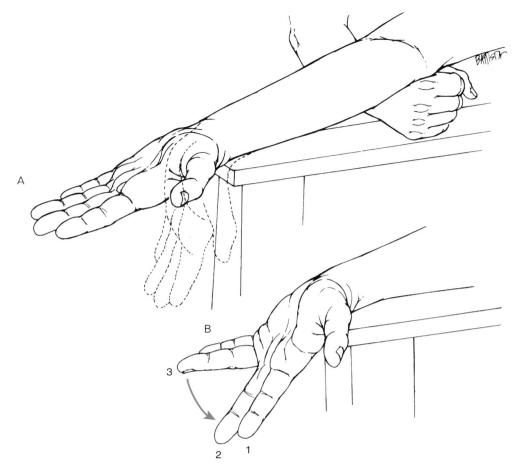

FIGURE 7-10. **Self-stretch of the forearm flexor muscles and flexor digitorum. A.** Forearm flexor muscles: Support the arm with the elbow straight. Palm up, bend the hand downward at the wrist. **B.** Flexor digitorum: Repeat, bending each finger down separately.

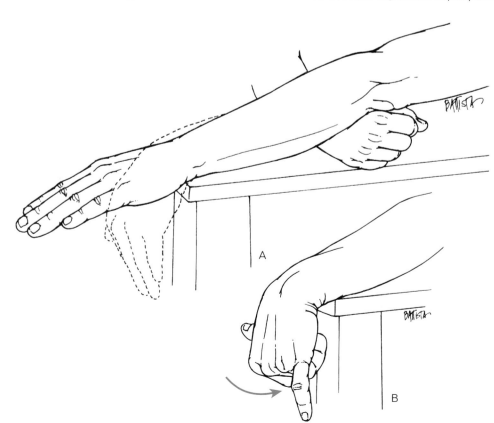

FIGURE 7-11. **Stretch and mobilization of the wrist extensor muscles and wrist and the extensor digitorum. A.** Wrist extensor muscles and wrist: Support the arm with the elbow straight. Palm down, bend the hand downward at the wrist. **B.** Extensor digitorum: Repeat while tucking the middle finger into the palm, then bending the wrist downward.

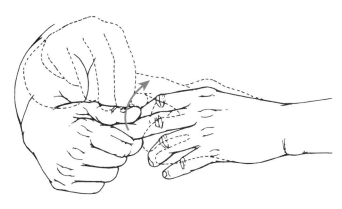

FIGURE 7-12. **Finger rotation/twist.** Rotate and twist each finger separately.

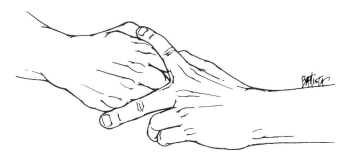

FIGURE 7-13. **Finger spread.** Stretch in all combinations (e.g., 1–5, 2–5, 3–5, 4–5; 2–4, 3–4, etc.).

associated with upper limb pain and abnormal forearm and hand posture. The underlying problem was not physical but rather was an unacknowledged desire not to pursue a concert career but to work in a nonperforming aspect of the arts. When this conflict was brought into the open and accepted by the performer and her family, the limb pain and movement disorder ceased.

CONCLUSION

Forearm, wrist, and hand incoordination, stemming from myofascial trigger point development in the upper limb, as proximal as the neck and upper torso muscles, can produce clumsiness, fatigue, weakness, and loss of fine motor control. These symptoms and loss of function can be devastating to those whose activities rely heavily on the skilled use of the hands and fingers. The clinical picture can sometimes look quite like true dystonia, which is a deep brain disorder. Treatment of the myofascial trigger point syndrome is directed toward release of the trigger points and the associated taut bands, and restoration of normal muscle length, range of motion, and function. Awareness of the contribution of the proximal muscles to the syndrome of upper limb dysfunction is critical to the design of an effective treatment protocol. The treatment of the muscle itself incorporates common techniques that are familiar to all who treat myofascial pain syndrome disorders. Awareness and treatment of joint dysfunction at the neck, shoulder, elbow, and wrist incorporate concepts well known to the chiropractic and osteopathic professions, and increasingly known to the general medical community, the physical therapists, and the myotherapists who treat musculoskeletal pain syndromes. The myofascial syndrome of upper limb disorder is to be differentiated from true dystonia. True dystonia requires a neurologic assessment and generally requires treatment with either botulinum toxin or deep brain stimulation, although two intriguing reports cited in this chapter suggest that local treatment of the limb may have a positive outcome in the management of dystonia.

TREATMENT PROTOCOL

1. Establish a clear idea of the patient's complaint, pain, and dysfunction, including a mapping of the pain.

2. Identify precipitating factors and perpetuating factors, including postural dysfunctions. Include sleep positions and an assessment of breathing patterns as a part of the assessment of biomechanical functioning. Assess for scoliosis and pelvic torsion and asymmetry in the standing and sitting positions.

3. Evaluate range of motion for restrictions and for hypermobility.

4. Evaluate joints for reduced joint play, synovial, or capsular disorders.

5. Evaluate muscles for myofascial trigger points.

6. Evaluate movement patterns, particularly induced by muscle fatigue caused by repetitive movements or prolonged static positioning.

7. Release the shortened torso and proximal muscles, treating the trigger points, the somatic joint dysfunctions, and restoring normal muscle length and function. The muscles of interest include the neck muscles (especially the scalenes), the latissimus dorsi, and the pectoralis major and minor. Upper thoracic spine restrictions also must be released. This may require collaboration with a chiropractor or an osteopathic physician who can manipulate and mobilize the spine.

8. Release the scapula and related muscles, restoring normal scapular glide and movement. The infraspinatus, supraspinatus, rhomboid, and serratus anterior muscles are critical at this point of

treatment, as well as the upper, middle, and lower trapezius, and the levator scapulae. Treatment also is directed to the triceps muscle, the long head of which attaches to the scapula.

9. **Release the deeper shoulder and torso muscles, including the subscapularis and posterior serratus superior. Restore shoulder mobility.**

10. **Treat the trigger points in the arm muscles, including the triceps, biceps, coracobrachialis, and brachialis muscles. Restore normal muscle length and function.**

11. **Treat the forearm musculature. Trigger points in the flexor muscles of the forearm, including the flexor carpi ulnaris and radialis, and the flexor digitorum and palmaris longus muscles. The supinator muscle is always a potential problem, especially when the extensor muscles are involved, and is treated at this point.**

References

1. Fahn S. Concept and classification of dystonia. In: Fahn S, Marsden CD, Calne DB, eds. Dystonia 2. Adv Neurol 1988;50:1–8.
2. Lenz FA, Suarez JI, Metman LV, et al. Pallidal activity during dystonia: somatosensory reorganization and changes with severity. J Neurol Neurosurg Psychiatry 1998;65:767–770.
3. Sanger TD, Pascual-Leone A, Tarsy D, et al. Nonlinear sensory cortex response to simultaneous tactile stimuli in writer's cramp. Mov Disord 2002;17:105–111.
4. Levy LM, Hallett M. Impaired brain GABA in focal dystonia. Ann Neurol 2002;51:93–101.
5. Candia V, Ebert T, Altenmuller E, et al. Constraint-induced movement therapy for focal hand dystonia in musicians. Lancet 1999; 353:42.
6. Priori A, Pesenti A, Cappellari A, et al. Limb immobilization for the treatment of focal occupational dystonia. Neurology 2001:57: 405–409.
7. Byl NN, Nagajaran S, McKenzie AL. Effect of sensory discrimination training on structure and function in patients with focal hand dystonia: a case series. Arch Phys Med Rehabil 2003;84:1505–1515.
8. McClure TA. RSI in Occupational Medicine. San Francisco: Sutter KHS, 1994.
9. Virtual Ergonomics: What is Cumulative Trauma Disorder? Cumulative Trauma Disorder News, www.vergo.com, 1998.
10. Bass T, Gordon MF. Writer's Cramp: A Focal Form of Dystonia. New York: Dystonia Medical Research Foundation, 1988:1–5.
11. Howell TA. Reflections on living with dystonia. US Department of Agriculture, Research, Education, and Economics, Greenbelt, Summer, 1997.
12. Littlejohn G. Key issues in repetitive strain injury. J Musculoskel Pain 3 1995;2:25–27.
13. Frontis E. SD Newsletter, National Spasmodic Dysphonia Association, Chicago, 1998.
14. Office of Scientific and Health Reports. The Dystonias. NIH Publications No.96-717, 1996:3.
15. Wilbourne AJ. The thoracic outlet syndrome is much over diagnosed. Arch Neurol 1990;47:328–330.
16. Simons DG, Travell JG, Simons LS. Myofascial Pain and Dysfunction: The Trigger Point Manual, vol 1, 2nd Ed. Baltimore: Williams and Wilkins, 1999.
17. Mennell J. Understanding Manipulative Medicine in General Practice. J Manipulative Physiol Ther 1989;12:3.

8 _Upper Back Pain_

Gregory M. Berkoff

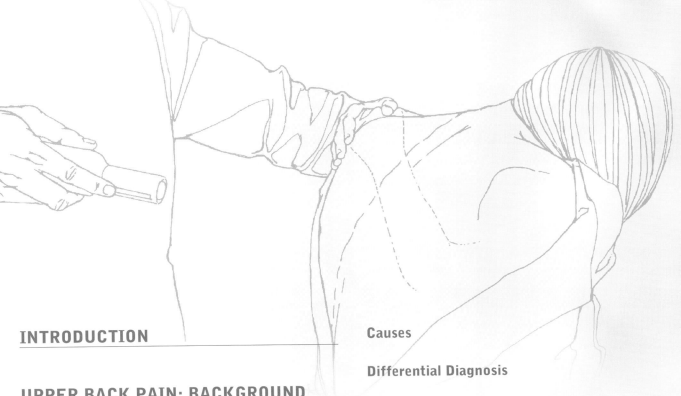

INTRODUCTION

UPPER BACK PAIN: BACKGROUND

The Problem of Diagnosis

Conventional Treatment Approaches

A MYOFASCIAL AND ARTICULAR APPROACH EMPHASIZING THE IMPORTANCE OF SITS IN THE DIAGNOSIS AND TREATMENT OF UPPER BACK PAIN

Case 8-1

Case 8-2

Overview

Causes

Differential Diagnosis

Cautions

Symptom/Pain Presentation

Myofascial Entrapments

Treatment

Box 8-1: Biofeedback and Psychotherapy

Technique 8-1: Treatment Tips for SITS

CONCLUSION

Treatment Protocol

INTRODUCTION

Upper back pain, although not in itself a diagnosis, is a common complaint addressed by clinicians of various disciplines. It may arise from many sources, including muscular trigger points, strain or sprain injury, heart, lung, gallbladder, pancreas, bone, joint, nerve, or disc disease. This chapter focuses on pain caused by muscular trigger points, which is likely the most common (as well as the most commonly overlooked) cause of chronic upper back pain (1). Conventional approaches to diagnosis and treatment are discussed, followed by detailed case histories that demonstrate an approach that derives from a new perspective on the pathophysiology of trigger points in the upper back. Emphases are placed on the limitations of physical modalities and the need to incorporate psychological and emotional considerations into the clinician's approach to patient management.

UPPER BACK PAIN: BACKGROUND

Over a 1-year period (1997–1998) at a family practice medical group in Southern California, 15,120 patients were attended, of whom 221 complained primarily of pain in the upper back, upper back and shoulder, or upper back and neck regions, constituting approximately 1.5% of all new office visits (2). Setting aside infant and childcare visits, well-woman examinations, school and other physical examinations, patients with upper back pain constituted an even higher percentage. In addition, because patients with upper back pain are likely to require more workup and more follow-up visits on average, than, for example, patients with colds, contact dermatitis, seasonal allergies, etc., the percentage of time spent managing these patients in the family practice setting is higher still. Among chiropractic physicians, one large study has shown that in the United States and Canada, from 1985 though 1991, 6.3% of all patients presented with a chief complaint of upper/middle back pain (3). Of the numerous causes of upper back pain, what has been termed "myofascial pain syndrome" is arguably both the most common and the least recognized diagnosis (1).

The Problem of Diagnosis

Visceral diseases of the gallbladder, pancreas, heart and lung, primary bone disease, radiculopathy, and inflammatory arthropathies are relatively uncommon causes of upper back pain. With the exception of Scheuermann's disease, which consists of multiple vertebral body end-plate fractures caused by axial disc herniations (Schmorl's nodes) in the middle and lower thoracic spine, degenerative joint and disc disease in the absence of radiculopathy has been poorly correlated to pain (4–7). When physical and laboratory examination and imaging studies have successfully excluded the presence of visceral, primary bone, radicular, or inflammatory joint diseases, the stakes become lower, and a loss of diagnostic precision can result.

Although acute strain and sprain injury is common, some physical trauma must be identified as a precipitating cause to make the diagnosis. Too commonly, the diagnoses of "strain" or "sprain" are assigned in cases in which no injury has taken place. Patients may be under the impression that childhood falls or motor vehicle accidents from their remote past are suddenly declaring themselves symptomatically, many years later. However, such a belief has no rational basis, and clinicians should avoid the mistake of implanting in the minds of patients the notion of a delayed response (sometimes of years) to traumatic injury. Even when acute over-stretching of muscles (strain) or joints (sprain) does precipitate pain, it is difficult on a pathophysiologic basis to justify the ongoing diagnosis of strain or sprain several weeks, much less several years after injury. Microscopic tears in muscular or ligamentous tissues induced by trauma result in a sterile inflammation that is attended by pain. However, as is true with ankle sprains and brachialis muscle strains (after repeatedly throwing a baseball, for instance), ligaments and muscles do heal with simple measures such as avoidance of re-injury, ice-therapy, NSAIDs, etc., and symptoms typically disappear within days to weeks. This is also true in some cases after strain and sprain injuries to the upper back. Other times, however, pain may persist for months or even years, despite appropriate intervention, including not only avoidance of re-injury, ice therapy, and NSAIDs, but physiotherapy, medicines, and manipulation therapies, stretching, and strength training, as well. The questions we as clinicians should try to answer include:

- Why do some patients with thoracic strain injury recover in days to weeks, whereas others do not?

- What is the pathophysiologic explanation for persistent pain in the scapular region, neck, and shoulder months or years after a 5-mile-per-hour rear-end motor vehicle accident (MVA)? (See Chapter 3.)

In the absence of a pathophysiologic model for chronic upper back pain, many clinicians defer the problem by the use of terms such as "chronic strain." But "chronic strain" is conceptually oxymoronic, as "strain" refers to a specific incident that occurs in a moment when a muscle or tendon is stretched to the point of tissue disruption. Similarly, a sprain refers to an injury whereby a ligament is stretched to the point of tissue disruption. One way to make sense of the discrepancy between the consistently (relatively) brief natural course of strain and sprain injuries to peripheral structures such as ankles and arms, and the wide variation in healing times after upper back (or neck) strain and sprain injuries, is to consider the muscles of the upper back, especially those that connect the spine to the scapulae, not as prime movers, but as preparatory muscles, whose tone is varied by the sympathetic nervous system in response to changes in the environment and fluctuations in emotional stress. The sympathetic nervous system innervates the intrafusal fibers of muscle spindles (8). Muscle spindles are sensory organs found primarily in the bellies of virtually all skeletal muscles (Fig 8-1). They receive efferent connections from both the central nervous system (CNS) and the sympathetic nervous system and feed sensory information via IA and type II afferent neurons back to the CNS at the level of the spinal cord when they are stimulated, such as by mechanical stretch. IA afferent neurons synapse directly on alpha motoneurons in the spinal gray matter, and when the muscle spindle is sufficiently stimulated, the firing of IA afferent neurons triggers the firing of alpha motoneurons, which in turn cause contraction of the extrafusal muscle fibers surrounding the spindle. This monosynaptic sensori-

motor event is encountered in clinical practice when a patient's deep tendon reflex is elicited. Muscle spindles are highly sophisticated sensorimotor organs that set muscle tone by monitoring movement and position and through their ability to contract and cause reflex contraction of surrounding extrafusal muscle fibers (9). Muscle spindles are present in particularly high density in the axial musculature of the neck and upper back (10), the function of which is to closely monitor and control the tension of the muscles providing scapular stabilization in preparation for taking action with the upper limbs. Needle electromyography (EMG) has shown that trigger points identified in the trapezius muscle

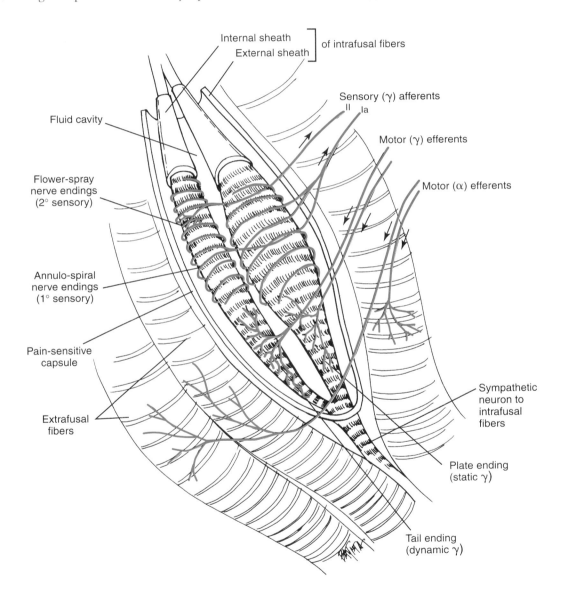

FIGURE 8-1. **The muscle spindle, showing its relationship to extrafusal skeletal muscle fibers.** Gamma and sympathetic motoneurons innervate the poles (contractile ends) of the intrafusal fibers. Various mechanoreceptors supply the equatorial (middle, noncontractile) portions of the nuclear chain and nuclear bag intrafusal fibers and are stimulated by stretch, such as when the entire muscle is lengthened, or when the sympathetic or gamma motoneurons cause contraction at the poles. Adapted with permission from Eriksen K: Upper Cervical Subluxation Complex: A Review of the Chiropractic and Medical Literature. Baltimore: Lippincott Williams & Wilkins, 2003 (fig. 3-4), p. 63.

have a definitive, continuous "spontaneous" electrical activity, whose electromyographic signal is different from normal motor unit action potentials (MUPs). Because this EMG activity is sustained, it cannot be attributed to "insertional activity" (11). Furthermore, studies have shown that this spontaneous EMG activity is of significantly greater amplitude in patients with chronic muscle pain than in asymptomatic subjects with "latent" trigger points; it can be significantly lowered with infusion of sympathetic blocking agents (11); and it fluctuates in direct relationship to psychological stress (12).

Patients with work-related or MVA-related injuries commonly develop chronic upper back, scapular, neck, and shoulder pain. In the worker's compensation and personal injury settings, physical injuries are commonly accompanied by psychological and emotional stress factors peculiar to those settings. Getting the car repaired, obtaining a rental car, sorting out issues of insurance coverage, battling over liability, hassling with claims adjusters, and obtaining legal representation are just a few of the common issues that influence the emotional experience of a patient's life post-MVA. Work-related injuries may become complicated by pressure (real or perceived) from employers, supervisors, or co-workers for patients to downplay their pain and return to work as quickly as possible. The pressures and hassles that attend work-related and MVA-related strain and sprain injuries to the upper back, neck, and scapular areas are real, and recent evidence supports a new perspective that the muscles of the upper back are "wired" by sympathetic innervation of muscle spindles to respond to certain stress conditions and stimuli by tensing as a means of preparing the upper limbs (and jaws, since the muscles of mastication commonly tense as well) for fight.

Unlike other animals, however, humans generally conduct their lives in the context of a psychosocial environment in which the physical act of fighting (as well as that of running away) is typically characterized as inappropriate, and such behavior can carry significant social and legal risk. A conflict between that aspect of normal physiology designed to prepare the human animal to protect and defend himself and the behavioral constraints of society leaves individuals in a state of muscular preparation for an action (fighting, running, falling down and "playing dead") that never occurs. This is especially evident in the context of important, ongoing relationships such as between employees and employers, clients and attorneys, injured subscribers and insurance claims adjusters, where cooperation and adversarial agendas often mingle and the emotional and financial stakes can be high. According to this theory (which will be elaborated in the "Causes" section of this chapter), when stressful condition-stimuli causing sympathetic, fusimotor tension (tension of the intrafusal muscle fibers inside muscle spindles) are not appeased or resolved through action or interaction, but instead are allowed to persist for weeks or months in the forms of strained relationships, financial burdens, discomforting shifts in routine, etc., fatigue and (eventually) pain

develop as a result of unrelieved intrafusal contraction. On palpation, these chronically tensed, sensitized, painful spindles, which are typically found in complex arrangements such that elements are shared between as many as five contiguous spindles (13), would be identified as discretely palpable firm muscle bands that twitch when mechanically stimulated by quick stroking, via the monosynaptic reflex described above. In other words, these chronically facilitated muscle spindles constitute what are known as trigger points and are often the primary source of pain weeks and months after strain injuries.

Given the mounting evidence that chronic muscle pain syndromes may be sympathetically driven or maintained, the author's opinion is that chronic pain in the upper back that is not caused by other identifiable lesions of bone, joint, nerve, or viscera should be approached from the hypothetical perspective described of muscle spindles under chronic sympathetic excitation as a means of preparing the upper limbs for a fight that never comes, than from the more conventional paradigm of "chronic strain." When viewed from this new perspective, the clinical entity known as the "trigger point," a small, localized, firm, tender area of muscle that gives rise to predictable patterns of referred pain, may be conceived of as a cluster of muscle spindles that, because of ongoing or recurrent sympathetic stimulation fueled by emotional stress, has become contracted, fatigued, and painful. On the basis of this understanding, the term "sympathetic intrafusal tension syndrome" (SITS) is proposed to replace "chronic strain," "myofascitis," "myofascial pain syndrome," or "myofascial pain disorder."

Conventional Treatment Approaches

The treatment of chronic upper back pain is extremely variable, both within and across clinical disciplines. Chiropractic doctors have traditionally concentrated on the spine as a source of pain and disease. Little question can exist that the forces exerted by chronic, sympathetically driven muscle tension must have an effect on the joints they support and move. "Fixation," "subluxation," and "misalignment" are some of the terms commonly used to describe the palpatory phenomena of stiffness to gliding forces applied manually by the examiner to spinal joint segments, or prominence over facet or costovertebral articulations, which are typically attended by localized tenderness. Such palpatory findings in the upper and middle thoracic segments are so commonly associated with SITS in the scapular stabilizers (rhomboids, trapezius, levator scapulae, subscapularis, etc.) that failure to uncover evidence of joint dysfunction should lead the clinician to rethink the diagnosis. Typically, spinal manipulative therapy (SMT) is the primary modality in the chiropractic treatment of chronic upper back pain, supported by various physiotherapy modalities such as electrical stimulation and ultrasound in combination, moist heat or ice, trigger point pressure release of trigger points, and spray and stretch of affected muscles. Conventional chiropractic treatment approaches chronic upper back pain from the perspective that the muscle tension, often referred to as "myospasm," is a response to joint dysfunction, the latter being commonly referred to as the "primary lesion."

The physical therapy approach has much overlap with the chiropractic one, using various physiotherapy modalities, especially electrical stimulation and ultrasound, moist heat, or ice. Whereas the conventional chiropractic focus is on joint dysfunction, physical therapists more often focus on limitations in strength and range of motion. An emphasis on function rather than on symptoms has gained popularity, especially with regard to work-related injuries. Spray and stretch is sometimes employed as are various forms of massage and ischemic compression of Trigger points. Strengthening of the affected area, often assessed as "weak," active and passive stretching to increase flexibility, as well as balancing the interplay between antagonistic muscles of the chest and upper back, form the basis of the conventional physical therapy approach to chronic upper back pain. Achieving balanced muscle "tone" by stretching shortened muscles and strengthening weakened muscles may be seen as the primary goal, and the various modalities described above are all tools toward that end. Many physical therapists also perform joint mobilization to address thoracic intersegmental dysfunction. This differs from SMT employed by chiropractors and by some osteopaths in that SMT seeks through the application of quick force to elicit a "pop" or "release" from the affected spinal joints, whereas mobilization employs a slow gliding force to induce movement without taking the affected joints beyond their normal physiologic end range, where an audible "release" would otherwise occur.

The medical approach to SITS (other than referral to physical therapy or chiropractic) has largely consisted of medicines and rest. No surgical treatment exists for this disorder. Instead, the medical or osteopathic physician has at his disposal an ever-increasing arsenal of medicines, including nonsteroidal anti-inflammatories (NSAIDs), antidepressants, and muscle relaxants, which are administered orally, as well as various numbing agents (lidocaine, procaine, bupivacaine, etc.) and steroidal anti-inflammatories (cortisone), which may be injected directly into the affected muscles. The use of tricyclic antidepressants such as amitriptyline hydrochloride for the treatment of chronic upper back pain, though it is not listed as an indication, is quite common and is based on the observation that in low doses, tricyclic medications have an analgesic effect that can be especially useful when NSAIDs have either failed or caused intolerable side effects. Muscle relaxants are chemically similar to tricyclic antidepressants. Cyclobenzaprine hydrochloride, which is one of the most commonly prescribed drugs in this category, is a tricyclic amine salt whose chemical structure (C20H21N-HCl) is almost identical to that of amitriptyline (C20H23N-HCl), differing only by the presence of one double bond in cyclobenzaprine's seven-carbon ring (in amitryptyline the ring is saturated), and the

pharmacologic effects of these drugs are similar. A relatively small number of medical and osteopathic physicians make use of other, nonconventional techniques, such as acupuncture, saline injections of trigger points, and "dry needling," which consists of the insertion of a small-gauge needle (such as an acupuncture needle) directly into the painful nidus of the trigger point.

A MYOFASCIAL AND ARTICULAR APPROACH EMPHASIZING THE IMPORTANCE OF SITS IN THE DIAGNOSIS AND TREATMENT OF UPPER BACK PAIN

A complete evaluation of the patient with chronic upper back pain should include a highly detailed history with a focus on psychologic and emotional factors that might reasonably be expected to increase the sympathetic outflow to the muscles of scapular stabilization. Each patient has his or her own particular set of stress factors, so it is important to get to know each patient as an individual. The clinician should allow sufficient time to hear the patient's full story and gather all necessary information, including a detailed social history, in order to get a sense for whether SITS might be an appropriate diagnosis. The initial contact with the patient is critical in terms of laying the groundwork for gaining the patient's trust. Questions that convey interest in the patient as a person often will elicit a willingness on the part of the patient to discuss ideas and feelings they may be having about their life. During such discussion, the clinician should listen carefully and respectfully, encouraging the patient to speak freely, while making a note of reported feelings (or situations that might lead to feelings) of anger, frustration, irritability, a sense of unfairness or injustice, resentment, or feelings of being trapped, stuck or "caged-in." Patients are often hesitant to discuss the situations that provoke unpleasant emotions, especially when doing so requires that they divulge details of their personal lives. In addition, many patients are unaware of their feelings and often mistakenly conceive of emotions exclusively in terms of either behaviors or cognitions. For example, a patient who is asked whether she feels afraid to be alone when her husband is away on business might reply without much reflection, "I don't let myself get afraid. What good would it do to be afraid?" Such an answer speaks to the common wish to be in control. But the patient in this case mistakes cognition (it would do her no good to be afraid; therefore she chooses not to be afraid) and behavior (by choosing to behave as though she were not afraid, she therefore is not afraid) for her feelings, which are conspicuously excluded from her conception of emotion. In fact, feelings are an essential part of emotion, and they can arise and abate independently of both cognition and behavior. An individual with fear of heights may know intellectually that he is safe in going to the top of a famous skyscraper. He may read and believe that over a million people have gone to the top and none have been injured as a result. He may boldly ride the elevator to the one hundredth floor in strict defiance of his fear of heights (behavior), convinced of his safety (cognition). But neither his knowledge nor his brave behavior will prevent the feelings of panic that will wash through him when he walks out onto the observation deck and looks downward at the city below. Despite both his cognition of safety and his consciously directed behavior, his palms will sweat, his pupils will dilate, his respiratory and heart rates will quicken and he will probably feel nauseated and lightheaded, even to the point of fainting. The patient's feelings (mediated through the unconscious control of the sympathetic nervous system) should be of primary interest to the clinician. Uncovering stressful condition-stimuli and evaluating their potential clinical relevance is vital, regardless of a patient's own understanding of how such stresses may or may not be affecting him. Relaxation and breathing techniques to dampen sympathetic drive, biofeedback therapy, and when necessary, psychotherapy, all may be useful considerations in the treatment of SITS.

For the non-psychologist clinician, leading the patient to make connections between specific condition-stimuli and fluctuations in muscle tension, and between tension and pain, can be challenging. Temporary reduction of trigger point pain with physical medicine procedures should be regarded not only as a means of providing relief, but as an opportunity to bring the patient into a condition of higher awareness with respect to the causes of his muscle tension and pain. "I felt fine when I left here," a patient might say regarding his symptoms since the previous visit, "but then when I got back to work I had another run-in with my supervisor and I could just feel the muscles all tightening up in there." Rather than encouraging patients to ignore or "let go" of the feelings provoked by condition-stimuli, the clinician should lead them to focus on the connections between environment and feelings. They need not understand the detailed physiology of SITS (although in some cases this may be useful), but they must develop an experiential understanding of the connection between stressful situations and muscle tension, and between muscle tension and pain, before they can become motivated to take the necessary action(s) that will ultimately reduce or eliminate the problem(s). For this reason, the combination of the physical medicine clinician and psychologist/biofeedback therapist makes for exceptional patient care. This will be elaborated on as the specific treatment approach to SITS is presented after the Case Histories.

CASE 8-1

Patient History

Ms. KB was a 27-year-old sales representative for a pharmaceutical company, who presented on referral from her family physician, 6 months post-MVA for evaluation and treatment of right scapular, neck, and headache pain. She was the driver of a small car that was struck suddenly and without warning from behind, causing her body to be thrown backward and then forward, causing a typical hyperextension–hyperflexion injury. She stated that although she had headaches before the accident (typically 1–3 per week), their intensity had been minimal and they were typically relieved by ibuprofen. She denied any history of neck or back/scapular pain.

Her car had been only moderately damaged in the rear end. Although this damage had been repaired, she felt the car was not quite right, stating she could hear a grinding sound coming from the wheels when she made sharp turns. She brought her car back to the repair shop, but it was subsequently returned to her 4 days later with the pronouncement that nothing could be found wrong. She had learned to tolerate the noise since that time, stating it would do no good to bring the car back again. When asked whether this made her feel angry, she replied, "Not really, I don't see what good it would do, so I just let it go."

Symptoms

Since the accident, Ms. KB had been experiencing constant headache pain that typically escalated over the course of the day, peaking in the early evening, often on her drive home from work. The headaches were right-sided, temporal, and retro-orbital, without nausea or aura, and seemed to arise out of her right scapula, which was constantly tight and achy. She noticed the headaches seemed to worsen toward the end of the workweek and then improve over the weekends. One exception to this pattern was the weekend before her consultation, when she drove from San Diego to Los Angeles on a Saturday afternoon and then returned the following morning (approximately 2–3 hours' driving each way in moderately heavy traffic). From the time she awoke Saturday morning, until Monday afternoon, she described her upper back and right shoulder as "a brick" and her neck and headache pain as "unbearable." She described her job as very stressful but insisted that, despite this fact, she loved her work as a sales representative, stating, "I see it as a challenge." When asked whether she thought that the stress had any effect on her pain, she answered "No," explaining that she did not really have any unusual stress, just "normal stress." When questioned further, she did concede that while driving she was more "stressed" than she had been before the accident, but stated this was because of having to turn the steering wheel, which was physically demanding on her back and shoulders. She added, "It is not just all mental."

Prior Care

A few days after her accident, she had seen her family physician. She was tried initially on naproxen sodium and carisoprodol, then on cyclobenzaprine. The naproxen sodium caused stomach upset, and the carisoprodol and cyclobenzaprine caused grogginess. None of the medicines substantially mitigated her pain. She was referred to physical therapy, where she was evaluated and found to have a postural imbalance, stemming from a right "short leg," which was causing pelvic unleveling, which in turn caused a left lateral lumbar compensatory lean, followed by a right thoracic compensatory lean, the latter caused by "spasm" in the right paraspinal and trapezius muscles. Treatment consisted of ultrasound and electrical stimulation, stretching of hamstrings, gluteus medius, and upper trapezius muscles, various exercises on a gym ball, especially hyperextension exercises and abdominal strengthening, a heel lift, and weight training of the upper back muscles, including bent-over rows, latissimus pull-downs on a pulley-operated machine, and shoulder shrugs with dumbbells. Ms. KB stated that she attended physical therapy for approximately 8 weeks, during which time she usually felt worse after the treatments and as a result began to miss appointments. She finally discontinued the treatment without discussing it with her physical therapist. She returned to her family physician who referred her for chiropractic evaluation and treatment, but she was hesitant to follow through on the referral because she had "heard horror stories about chiropractors." Approximately 3 months later, the pain, which had not abated, finally spurred her to make an appointment.

Examination Findings

The patient appeared to be a physically fit, 27-year-old woman who during the initial interview was rather agitated. She arrived 15 minutes late for her appointment, and during her time at the office, her pager went off several times. She sat in a kyphotic posture, her shoulders rolled anteriorly and her head markedly anterior with respect to her trunk. As she related her history, her shoulders elevated and descended several times; when the shoulders elevated, she was also observed to clench her hands into fists.

Sensation, muscle strength, and reflexes all were unremarkable. Cranial nerves II–XII were intact. Cervical range of motion was slightly limited in left lateral bending and in right rotation, compared with the opposite sides, because of "pulling" pain in the right scapula and neck. Cervical compression and distraction were unremarkable. Palpation of the right lower, middle, and upper trapezius indicated numerous taut bands with exquisitely tender points that gave rise to referred pain when stimulated with continuous digital pressure, reproducing the shoulder, neck, and head pain complaints. Motion palpation, consisting of gentle gliding movements applied to each vertebral segment, sequentially, showed tenderness and fixation (diminished sense of movement at the joint) at C1/2, C2/3, T2/3, T3/4, T4/5, T5/6, and T6/7. Motion palpation of these joints also reproduced the sensation of stiffness and achiness the patient was experiencing in the midline of the upper/middle back.

Treatment and Follow-up

A treatment plan was formulated based on the following assessment of the historical and examination data:

1. Ms. KB's pain was no longer being caused by the sterile inflammation of acute strain and sprain injuries. She had SITS.

2. Ms. KB was not aware of the connection between stress and emotion, between emotion and muscle tension (MT), or between MT and pain. In fact, she was somewhat hostile toward any suggestion that stress might have an effect on her pain, which she interpreted as implying her condition was "mental" and thus not real.

3. Medicines and conventional physical therapy had both failed.

4. She was suspicious about the qualifications of chiropractors to diagnose and treat her problem.

5. She appeared to be under enormous emotional strain.

6. Several clear-cut stressors seemed to be provoking this emotional strain and fueling the tension in her upper back and neck.

On this basis, it was explained to Ms. KB that her muscles were "in spasm" as a result of the injury, and that they had learned the habit of being that way. In addition, her spinal joints had become stiff and achy as a result of the "spasms." Treatment, therefore, was to try to break the "spasms" and the joint fixations at the same time. A brief overview of biofeedback was explained to her, but she was told there was no need to begin this therapy at the start. Rather, it would be used as a last resort if her treatment was otherwise unsuccessful. She agreed to this plan.

(continues)

CASE 8-1   Continued

Over the next 3 weeks, she was treated 3 times per week with trigger point pressure release of trigger points and spray and stretch of the right lower and middle trapezius and rhomboid muscles, followed by either moist heat or continuous ultrasound to these muscles, and finally, SMT of the cervical and thoracic spine. She was often 10 to 15 minutes late for her 30-minute appointments, usually citing difficulty getting out of meetings or traffic as reasons for her tardiness. After most treatments, she would leave the office feeling dramatically improved, but in the intervening 2 days, the pain and stiffness would gradually return. She was questioned each time as to what factors seemed to be causing the return of pain, but she was generally unable to identify any contributory factors other than driving, which she felt had to do with the action of operating the steering wheel, which was taxing on her upper back muscles. By the end of the second week, she rated herself as 25% improved, overall, since beginning care, with the scapular, neck, and headache pain still constant, but less intense, especially for several hours after each treatment. At the time of her next appointment, Ms. KB presented in a highly distressed state. She related that she'd had some problems at work, on top of which she had also experienced a return of strong pain such that she felt her problem was "right back where we started from." She stated, "This isn't working," and "I never should have gotten involved in all of this. Now it's just more bills I have to pay." She was again asked whether she could identify anything that might have provoked the increase in tension or pain, to which she answered "No." She was then asked whether she thought the problems she was having at work might have caused her muscles to become tense, to which she replied, "No, and I don't see why you keep asking me that over and over again!" The conversation continued as follows:

DOCTOR: Does it upset you when I ask you that question?

MS. KB: Not really, I'm just in a lot of pain right now.

DOCTOR: How *did* it make you feel when I asked you that?

MS. KB: It didn't make me feel anything. I'm just pissed off! I'm sorry.

DOCTOR: What are you sorry about?

MS. KB: I didn't mean to get angry.

DOCTOR: Can you tell me what it feels like when you get angry?

MS. KB: What do you mean, what does it feel like?

DOCTOR: Well, where in your body do you feel it?

MS. KB: Where in my body? I don't know, my hands maybe, my head.

DOCTOR: How do your shoulders feel right now?

MS. KB: Like a brick. Like I just want you to crack it.

DOCTOR: Would that make the angry feeling let go, do you think? If I gave your back an adjustment?

MS. KB: Probably.

DOCTOR: Well, then we should definitely do that today. Tell me though, I'd really like to know, is there anything else you can think of that's been making your back feel like that lately? In the last couple of weeks, maybe?

At this point, Ms. KB began to cry suddenly. She apologized repeatedly for doing so, but was unable to control the tears. She was gently encouraged to talk about her feelings and reminded that anything she said was confidential. In a few minutes, she began to relate a tale that included family issues, a recently failed relationship, work pressures, and a worry that she would soon be past her physical prime and no longer considered desirable. The motor vehicle accident, it turns out, was merely the last straw in a pile of problems that had finally pushed her to an emotional breaking point. She was driving a car that had been pronounced "fixed" but clearly was still having problems caused by the accident. Her claims adjuster had been leaving harassing messages for her at work and at home, insinuating that, so many months later, she could not possibly still be in pain from such a minor accident. In addition, she was having to rush three times per week across town to make her chiropractic appointments because of the relentless pain. She was treated that day with gentle massage and moist heat to the trapezius muscles and SMT to the cervical and thoracic spines. Immediately after the treatment, she felt a significant drop in her tension and pain levels and also reported that her feelings of anger had dissipated. For the first time, she was able to connect her emotions with MT, and the MT with pain. Biofeedback was discussed in greater detail, and she agreed to be referred to a biofeedback therapist 1 day per week, while decreasing her chiropractic treatments to twice per week. The referral was made on the basis that she would learn techniques to get her muscles to relax more, especially because she was having a lot of tension while driving. She was told initially to schedule just one visit, and if she did not like the experience, she did not have to make further appointments, but she was encouraged to keep an open mind and give it a chance.

Ms. KB felt comfortable with the biofeedback therapist, who also happened to be a clinical psychologist. She was given breathing/relaxation exercises and audio tapes to listen to. In addition, surface-EMG electrodes were applied over the tense and painful trapezius muscles in her upper back, and she was given an opportunity

CASE 8-1 Continued

to see how her muscle tension fluctuated in response to the various topics discussed with the biofeedback therapist. She was especially impressed with the fact that discussing her frustrations regarding the unsatisfactory repair of her car, and relating the manner and attitude of the claims adjuster assigned to her case, caused the EMG activity in her trapezius muscles to soar. She continued this combined treatment for approximately 8 more weeks, with biofeedback once per week and chiropractic treatment as outlined above, twice per week, reporting steady improvement in her symptoms. She found another auto repair shop where she was treated respectfully and had her car fixed. She hired an attorney who ordered her claims adjuster to stop contacting her. With the help of the therapist, she took steps toward repairing

a family relationship that had been damaged by a misunderstanding a few years earlier, and worked out an arrangement with her boss to cut down her work hours to 40 per week. She agreed to begin some cardiovascular exercise and immediately felt better about her appearance. She was also sleeping more soundly and waking up more refreshed in the morning. Ms. KB had two follow-up visits, at 2 weeks and then at 6 weeks after the cessation of regular care. At the time of her last visit, she was essentially pain-free and had decided to seek individual psychotherapy. She stated that, in retrospect, she had created an unhealthy lifestyle and that although she suffered quite a bit as a result of the accident, she was also grateful for what she described as the opportunity to make some needed changes in her life.

CASE 8-2

Patient History

Ms. AP was a 30-year-old nurse and single mother, working in a busy family medicine practice, who presented with a complaint of bilateral, left greater than right, upper back pain of approximately 2 years' duration. She stated that as a teenager she had had similar pain for several years, but that it had resolved somewhat mysteriously without any treatment at age 21. Approximately 2 years before her initial presentation to this office, she had begun to notice the insidious return of upper back stiffness and pain. She was unable to recall any specific precipitating trauma to her back but stated that picking up her 18-month-old son and carrying him around sometimes made her arms and her upper back feel "tired." Over the previous 2 years, the problem had seemed to come and go. In the beginning, the pain would typically last a couple of days and then resolve spontaneously or with nonsteroidal anti-inflammatory drugs (NSAIDs) (ibuprofen, nabumetone, or naproxen), and she would be asymptomatic for up to 2 weeks. However, as time went on, the bouts of pain lasted longer, the remissions were shorter, and medicines became progressively less effective.

In the 2 weeks before her initial presentation, her upper back and neck had been constantly stiff and painful, and the pain intensity had twice been so high that she had resorted to taking hydrocodone/acetaminophen, a supply of which she had at home, left over from a tooth extraction surgery 1 year earlier. She denied radiation of pain, weakness, numbness, or **paresthesias**. She felt the pain was typically worse during the week than on weekends, although this was not always true. She also felt that stress seemed to make the pain worse. She cited estrangement

from the father of her child as a source of stress, especially the unpredictable, episodic nature of his involvement with their son, marked by sudden appearances at her home, often after having had no communication from him whatsoever for months. He had been through a rehabilitation program for alcoholism but recently he had called her, obviously drunk, and although she did not believe he was a violent man, his tone was hostile and his words antagonistic. He blamed her for his inability to see his son. The following morning, he called again and apologized. One month before her presentation to the office, he had requested that he be allowed to visit the child more often, and Ms. AP identified significantly increased stress levels since that time. She offered that this might be playing a role in her pain, as she believed that stress can cause pain even if nothing is really wrong physically.

Symptoms

Ms. AP complained of constant, left greater than right, stiffness and ache in the upper back, which was worse during times of stress, and tended to peak in the late afternoon or early evening, when she also experienced neck ache. She denied headaches, upper extremity symptoms, recent illnesses, or infections. She also related poor quality sleep, finding it difficult some nights to fall asleep or stay asleep through the night. She reported having had bad dreams several nights during recent weeks, including one dream in which she was being pursued by a dangerous man; she recalled running as fast as she could while clutching her son, who, in the dream, was an infant, tightly to her chest, and then looking down only to find that her son was gone and that she

(continues)

CASE 8-2   Continued

was carrying a box full of dirty laundry. She awoke from that dream with her jaws painfully clenched. She stated that she had begun wearing her night splint again (provided by her dentist 2 years earlier for bruxing) after having gone several months without needing it.

Examination Findings

Ms. AP appeared her stated age of 30 years. She was moderately obese (5′7″ tall, 180 lbs.) and rather muscular. Her neurologic examination, including reflexes, muscle strength, and sensation, was unremarkable. Range of motion was full in all directions, with left scapular pain at end range of flexion and left rotation, and left upper trapezius "stretching" pain at the end range of right lateral bending. Palpation indicated taut bands with trigger points in the lower, middle, and upper trapezius, bilaterally, with referred pain to the neck and shoulder, the left side more tender than the right. Motion palpation showed C0/1, C1/2, T2/3, T3/4, T4/5, T5/6, and T6/7 fixations, with slight to moderate tenderness, except at T5/6, where there was marked tenderness, prompting the patient to recall that over the previous few weeks she had also begun to have some point pain in the midline over that joint, especially at night. Plain film X-rays were obtained of the thoracic spine (anteroposterior [AP] and lateral views) to rule out primary bone or joint disease. The films were read as normal by a radiologist.

Treatment and Follow-up

The treatment plan in this case was made on the basis of the following assessment of the historical and examination data:

1. There was no significant injury to explain her condition.

2. The patient was able to identify that increased stress levels corresponded to increased pain.

3. The patient described herself as a "tense person" who had difficulty relaxing and "just letting go."

4. The examination was consistent with SITS, including the presence of numerous trigger points in the scapular stabilizing muscles, and spinal joint fixations to motion-palpation, which reproduced a significant portion of her pain (in the absence of trauma).

5. There were clearly identifiable condition-stimuli in the patient's life, which constituted ongoing sources of unresolved conflict and stress.

6. The patient was a health care professional with some understanding of human anatomy and physiology.

On this basis, the patient was educated at length with regard to the physiology of MT (sympathetic intrafusal tension). She was very receptive to the conceptual model that stress (especially frustration, annoyance, or anger-producing stress) activates the sympathetic nervous system to facilitate the scapular stabilizer muscles in preparation for fight, and that if the stress-provoking condition-stimulus is not resolved, this preparatory muscle tension will continue, eventually causing feelings of muscle fatigue, tightness, and pain. She stated that this description seemed to her to be "right on," adding that lately, her whole life seemed to be stressful to her. "If I had to use one word to describe my life right now," she stated, "I'd say, 'trapped.'"

She was given a breathing exercise in which she was to allow her abdomen to expand fully with inhalation while her chest was to remain stationary during the entire breathing cycle. The breaths were not to be deeper than normal breaths, but they were to be slow, with a 2-second pause after each exhalation. This was to be done for five consecutive breaths frequently throughout the day and for 3 continuous minutes at lunchtime and on returning home from work. She was instructed to take hot showers, allowing the water to get her scapular muscles very warm for 5 to 10 minutes at the beginning and end of each day. In addition, she was provided a muscle tension diary and asked to purchase an inexpensive watch with a timer alarm set to go off each hour. In the diary, she was asked to record each waking hour, her levels of MT on a scale of 0 to 10, in which 0 represented no tension and 10 the most tension she had ever experienced. In addition, she was asked to rate her pain levels in the same manner, from 0 to 10. She was also asked to note where she was at the time of each entry, and what she was doing. She was asked to keep the diary faithfully until bedtime and to use simple descriptive words and phrases, such as "at my desk doing paperwork," or "just finished having a conversation with my mother on the phone." She was treated with trigger point pressure release of trigger points, spray and stretch, and continuous ultrasound mixed with galvanic stimulation set to subtetany, to the trapezius and rhomboid muscles and SMT to the cervical and thoracic spine.

Her course of treatment continued in this way for 3 weeks at a frequency of three times per week. During this time, the following observations were noted:

• She generally exhibited a significant rise in MT in the upper back during the last 2 to 3 hours of each work day, when she typically performed her least enjoyable work-related tasks of charting, returning calls to patients, and calling-in prescriptions to pharmacies. She admitted that she avoided this unpleasant work until the end of the day, allowing it to pile up, such that it was common for her to have as many as 30 charts to take care of after her clinical work was complete.

- Although she had had to call the police on one occasion to have her ex-boyfriend (the father of her child) removed from her premises, she had never pressed charges, nor had she sought any legal action against him as she was worried about his record.

- She had exercised daily for several years but had suddenly stopped approximately 3 years earlier when her routine had been interrupted, first by a protracted bronchitis, followed by changes in her work schedule that forced her to stay later at the clinic, and then by her pregnancy. She stated that she had always meant to return to exercising but had become so out of the routine that she had "sort of just let it go." In addition, she related being self-conscious about allowing her body to be viewed by others at the gym, as she had put on approximately 40 lbs as a result of her pregnancy.

Treatments were provided in a very quiet and comfortable setting, with soothing music. At the end of each visit, she was asked to do a minute of abdominal breathing as she lay on the treatment table, supine, beneath a blanket, her head supported by a cervical pillow, in a dimly lit room. She typically felt dramatic improvement after treatments, often leaving the office stating "I just want to go home and take a nap now, I feel so relaxed." At the end of the third week of care, Ms. AP volunteered the following:

"I can see how that stuff is making me get tight up there and causing the pain. But, I mean, I just don't see how I can keep coming three times a week. I think my insurance has like, 20 chiropractic visits a year, but what do I do after that? I mean, if it's all being caused by stress. . ."

This was, in a sense, a breakthrough for her. Clearly, the cure to her problem would not be achieved through therapeutic interventions, no matter how well delivered, if the cause of the MT was not addressed. She still had coverage for 10 additional treatments. A new plan was made to have follow-up visits once per week, and each week she would be given some new task or exercise to be performed outside the office. The first task was to break up her charting work, such that she did approximately 10 charts before taking lunch and then the rest at the end of the day. At her next visit, she was asked to begin using the gym available to employees at her workplace. Specifically, she was asked to head straight to the gym after she had done her morning charting, and to do 15 to 20 minutes of cardiovascular exercise such as treadmill, stationary bicycle, or StairMaster, followed by a hot shower and a light lunch, which she would carry with her to work. Next, she was instructed to schedule a consultation with a lawyer to discuss her legal options for handling the unpredictable actions and volatile nature of her child's father. The following week she was asked to break up her charting duties yet further, so that after her watch alarm went off each hour, instead of recording in her MT diary, she would now spend several minutes doing whatever charting had accumulated up to that point.

Ms. AP was extremely compliant, and over the next 10 weeks, she reported progressive improvement in her MT and pain levels, such that at the time of her last visit she had been pain-free (if not completely tension-free) for almost 3 weeks.

Overview

"Sympathetic intrafusal tension syndrome" (SITS) is probably one of the most common causes of persistent upper back pain, but it is infrequently diagnosed because of a generally poor understanding of the pathophysiology of muscle pain. Psychologists, though highly sensitive to the link between stress and pain, are for the most part prohibited from laying hands on patients. By training, they typically have a comparatively limited understanding of the physical examination and as such are sometimes hesitant to treat back pain. Non-psychologist clinicians, however, often feel ill equipped to venture into the psychological or emotional realms with patients, perhaps for fear of opening "wounds" they are not qualified to attend. The result is that most clinicians who treat patients with chronic upper back and neck pain approach the care of these patients from a predominantly (or exclusively) physical perspective. Because a significant percentage of patients with chronic upper back pain have SITS, physical treatments often provide only temporary relief, resulting in frustration on the part of both clinicians and patients. An integrated approach to patient care that combines increasing the patient's understanding of SITS and emotional self-awareness with muscle-directed treatments is the key to successful treatment of this disorder.

Causes

The cause of SITS may be described as a normal physiologic response to a particular kind of stress, sustained beyond its biologic usefulness to the point of pain. The pain caused by muscle tension increases stress, which enhances and sustains the physiologic response, ultimately creating a self-sustaining loop of stress-tension-pain.

Humans, like other animals, respond to environmental conditions and stimuli in emotional ways. When the silence of a library reading room is suddenly shattered by the sound of a book crashing to the floor, in the moments before cognition can inform our understanding of the intrusive noise, a wide array of physiologic responses, mediated by the sympathetic nervous system, are set in motion, including the tensing of muscles in the upper back and jaws, a slight buckling of the knees, a racy-queasy stomach, **tachycardia**, pupillary dilation, **diaphoresis** of the hands and feet, and **tachypnea**. These are the normal physiologic manifestations of the massive sympathetic discharge associated with the reaction commonly referred to as the "startle response." After the initial startle response, one naturally tries to determine the source of the disturbance, and when the source is found to be innocuous, such as in the example above, this understanding influences not just the intellectual meaning of the incident (the cognition) but subsequent emotional processing as well. The need to be on the alert is assuaged, and the startle response fades. A brief feeling of annoyance or irritation might emerge in reference to the clumsy accidental perpetrator of the emotional startle. What does this annoyed, irritated emotional condition consist of? It is certainly different from the startle response in which nearly the entire body exhibits the effects of generalized sympathetic arousal. With feelings of irritation, annoyance, frustration, the sense of having had one's peace or one's space violated, the sympathetic excitation has a different purpose than that associated with the startle response. A binding feeling between the shoulder blades, a slight clenching of the jaws and a tensing in the stomach are common sensations associated with the more discrete sympathetic facilitation that serves the function of preparing to defend oneself or one's boundaries. Although the sensations attending the startle response are momentarily paralyzing (non-action or ducking down being biologically advantageous under certain sudden, highly threatening conditions), those attending feelings of anger, insult, etc., reflect preparation of the animal for fight. Tensing of the scapular stabilizers and abdominal muscles, a scowling facial appearance, and clenching of the fists and jaws are clearly physiologic precursors to aggression. The fact that the "trespass" (in this case, the sudden intrusion on one's tranquillity) was minor and accidental—the result of some ungainly person's attempt to replace a book on a shelf—changes the real, experiential understanding of the event and with an isolated, nonthreatening condition-stimulus, in which there is no apparent biologic advantage to the perpetuation of "fight mode," the sympathetic outflow to the muscles of the jaws, upper back, and abdomen recedes. One begins to feel more relaxed. The subjective experience of the event passes, and normal resting physiology is quickly restored.

But what if the condition-stimulus is not an isolated, nonthreatening incident, but rather an ongoing theme carrying threatening psychological and emotional undertones (real or perceived), as, for instance, when a conflict arises between co-workers? The emotional response to a condition-stimulus of ongoing interpersonal conflict likely would persist well beyond harsh words exchanged at a company picnic. The individuals involved might ruminate over the scene, replaying the drama in their minds and fantasizing about how they might have acted or spoken differently. They would probably discuss the event with friends and other coworkers, seeking advice or validation. Rumors and innuendo might begin to make their way through the office, with coworkers taking sides. The longer such a situation continues, the harder it becomes to repair the relationship. In such a case, the condition-stimulus, rather than quickly being rendered meaningless, takes on increasing complexity of meaning and the physiologic responses to it; rather than passing away, the responses persist and might even escalate in intensity. Prolonged adversity of this kind could result in ongoing manifestation of muscle tension as preparation for a fight that never comes.

Human emotions tend to occur in clusters rather than singly (14), and furthermore, discrete negative emotions such as fear, anger, frustration, etc. tend to cluster together (as do discreet positive emotions) (15). When the condition-stimulus is persistent or recurrent, complex, and unpredictable in its level of threat, the physiologic responses attending the cluster of emotions can lead to a chronic and self-perpetuating state of MT and pain.

The clinician must bear in mind that emotion is synonymous with neither cognition nor behavior, and that feelings are not subject to rules of logic. Although both cognition and behavior inform an individual's experience of emotion, the various physiologic responses that create feelings (tension in the back and neck, "butterflies" in the stomach, etc.) are an essential component as well. In the clinical setting, where such common ailments as chronic tension-type headache and chronic upper back pain due to SITS are routinely encountered, the "feelings" component of emotion must be addressed. This is a difficult task, because we live and learn in the context of a culture that continues to value emotional stoicism; from early childhood we are taught to subordinate our feelings to the power hierarchies of home, school, and eventually the workplace. Because strong feelings of fear, anger, jealousy, etc., if allowed to result in the biologically determined actions they seem designed to prompt (running away, falling down and playing dead, fighting, etc.), would likely carry grave consequences, the ability to mask one's feelings is advantageous and in many cultures is viewed and taught as a valued skill.

Through cognitively directed effort, we adopt attitudes toward the events of our lives and often frame even our most personal experiences in a context that is consistent with those attitudes. Patients face feelings of rejection, frustration, exclusion, and isolation as a normal part of social intercourse. However, according to the rules of the workplace, home, or of society in general, they often must maintain a controlled, unemotional demeanor. Such feelings have been shown to produce a host of physiologic reactions, including significant increases in tension and blood pressure (16), and conflict between experienced and expressed emotions (emotional dissonance) has been correlated with low job satisfaction (17) and may lead to the amplification and chronicity of negative feelings, in part because individuals who make more effort to maintain and project a "positive attitude" while experiencing negative feelings are typically less likely to seek help for symptoms related to stress, and are less likely to engage in activities that address and alleviate the sources of stress, necessary for mood repair (18). Individuals who suffer from emotional dissonance are particularly predisposed to developing SITS and may be only a 5-mph rear-end MVA away from chronic upper back pain.

SITS is a diagnosis that describes chronic, relatively diffuse pain. The areas most commonly affected are:

- upper back/scapular areas
- neck
- occipital, temporomandibular, and temporal areas of the head
- shoulders and upper arms

The pain of SITS is typically described as an ache, slowly fluctuating in intensity, typically peaking toward the end of the day, or occasionally on first awakening in the morning. Patients with SITS do not report sudden "attacks" of pain, as is common in strain injuries or migraine, for example, but rather a gradual onset. Habitual stretching, rubbing, and self-manipulation of the neck and shoulders is common in patients with SITS, and the clinician typically will observe this during the interview, especially when the patient is asked about stress. Most patients with SITS are aware of this habit and will report that they do it "constantly," to relieve stiffness in the neck or shoulders. On examination, trigger points are palpated in the muscles connecting the spine to the scapulae, and often the scapulohumeral muscles as well; these trigger points give rise to referred pain on sustained digital pressure, reproducing part or the entirety of the pain complaints in the shoulders, neck, head, or arms. Additionally, stiffness or "fixation" occurs with tenderness during gliding palpation of the thoracic and cervical spinal joints. SITS is hypothesized to result from physiologically normal sympathetic facilitation of the muscles of scapular stabilization, prolonged by a persistent or repetitive condition-stimulus. The resultant muscle tension, whose biologic value is the preparation of the individual for fight, when maintained beyond the point of biological usefulness, leads to fatigue and, finally, pain.

A single muscle spindle is on average approximately 5 mm in length and 2 mm in diameter at its thickest point, but most spindles are found in complex arrangements (tandem, parallel, or paired) such that elements are shared between as many as five contiguous spindles (13). The muscle spindle typically contains approximately six specialized muscle fibers (intrafusal muscle fibers), which are subdivided into two categories based on their morphology as follows: nuclear bag fibers, which are longer and thicker, and chain fibers, which are shorter and thinner. Nuclear bag fibers are further divided into dynamic bag 1 fibers and static bag 2 fibers. These specialized intrafusal muscle fibers sub-serve the separate spindle functions of responding to quick changes in muscle length and setting muscle tone.

All intrafusal muscle fibers are contractile at their poles (ends), where they receive both gamma motoneuron and sympathetic nerve innervation. By contrast, the equatorial (middle) region of the spindle is noncontractile and laden with mechanoreceptors highly sensitive to stretch. Spindles are covered by a pain- and pressure-sensitive capsule, inside which is a thick fluid, rich in hyaluronic acid, that bathes the intrafusal muscle fibers. Sympathetic facilitation of spindles cause the poles of intrafusal fibers to contract. This stretches the sensory equatorial region, exciting the mechanoreceptors and provoking **afferentation** at the level of the spinal cord. Afferentation also may occur if the muscle is suddenly stretched, such as during the elicitation of a deep tendon reflex (DTR).

Contraction of the polar regions of the spindle under sympathetic drive places a more gradual, less forceful stretch on the equatorial region than that elicited during a DTR. This relatively slow, sustained stretch stimulates static bag 2 fibers and chain fibers, whereas the sudden tap of the reflex hammer stimulates the dynamic bag 1 fibers. Stimulation of static fibers leads to dorsal horn afferentation designed to set the stage for muscle action, whereas stimulation of dynamic fibers (bag 1) provokes a muscle jerk.

The cause of SITS is theorized to be as follows: certain types of stressful condition-stimuli provoke sympathetic facilitation of spindles in the muscles of scapular (and jaw) stabilization. The biologic function of this facilitation is preparation for fight. If the provocative condition-stimulus is persistent or recurrent, spindle tension can lead to fatigue and pain as well as reflexive, low-grade extrafusal muscle tension. On palpation, chronically tense spindles would be identified as a band of firmness in the belly of the muscle (spindles are linked together in clusters of up to five long) that is extremely tender to mechanical pressure. Quick stroking or plucking across the sensitive spindle cluster would provoke the well-described monosynaptic stretch reflex (referred to by Travell as the "muscle twitch response"). Sustained pressure on the spindle cluster would give rise not only to local, but also to referred pain, because spindle has a pain- and pressure-sensitive capsule, and all encapsulated structures of the body may give rise to referred pain. In other words, this sensitized, fatigued cluster of spindles, driven by persistent or repetitive sympathetic facilitation, is what has traditionally been called a "trigger point," and multiple trigger points in the scapular stabilizers are the primary source of upper back pain in SITS.[1]

---

[1] In contrast to the theory proposed in this chapter that muscle spindles are the cause of trigger points, recent research indicates that abnormal neuromuscular junctions are the cause. See Editor's Note on the Nature of Trigger Points after the Preface for a detailed discussion of this more current hypothesis. Notwithstanding this issue, the clinical evaluation and treatment approach in this chapter remain valid.

Differential Diagnosis

As stated above, upper back pain can derive from many sources. The key in differential diagnosis is to apply an understanding of the pathophysiology of the various conditions under consideration, during the interview and examination. The clinician should begin by settling the issue of which structures or tissues are involved. Upper back pain of a visceral source is uncommon, except for that arising from disease of the pancreas or gallbladder, as described later. The reader is referred to other texts for a detailed discussion of heart and lung disease and their occasional association to upper back pain. Radiculopathy in the thoracic spine may occur but is far less common than in the cervical and lumbar areas, partly because of the relatively small discs and limited range of motion that exists normally in thoracic spinal segments. Thoracic nerve root entrapment may present with pain radiating from the back around the thoracic wall to the chest or breast. The dermatomal pattern of thoracic spinal nerve roots describe narrow, discrete bands of skin that run posterior to anterior, much as the ribs do. In fact, differential diagnosis of thoracic radiculopathy must include rib fracture and costovertebral joint dysfunction, as the symptoms of these conditions are nearly identical. Shingles also may include a prodrome of this same pattern of pain before the outbreak of vesicular lesions. Medical history of herpes zoster should raise the index of suspicion when symptoms of radiating pain from the thoracic spine around the thoracic wall to the chest or breast begin insidiously. The following observations address differential diagnosis with respect to diseases/disorders of muscle, joint, and bone, and, when visceral disease is not in question, may be helpful:

- Spinal joint or bone pain is primarily located in or close to the midline of the body, over the spine, and may be described as a deep bruise or "toothache" type pain (in the case of bone) or as a sharp, stabbing, or "pinching" type pain (in the case of joint).

- Muscle pain is lateral to the spine, usually between the spine and the scapulae, and is typically described as dull and aching.

- Joint disease (because diarthrodial joints are encapsulated) may give rise to referred pain. However, joint pain is usually highly localized to the joint(s) involved, and primary joint disease of the spine, even when accompanied by referred pain, is typically associated with a specific pain area approximately the size of a quarter or half-dollar.

- Muscle pain is diffuse and harder to localize; patients often have to stretch or contract the affected muscle(s) to locate the main area of pain.

- Pain from muscle tension is typically worse in the late afternoon/early evening, or, occasionally, on first waking in the morning.

- Joint pain is typically worse in damp weather.

- Spinal joint pain is made worse by compression, such as when the examiner passively extends the patient's spine, thus compressing the spinal facet joints.

- Application of vibration with a tuning fork to a bone lesion (especially fracture) may significantly increase pain.

In addition, the clinician should keep in mind that muscular trigger points always provoke referred pain when pressed. Active trigger points, by definition, reproduce the pain complaint to some degree. Tenderness in muscle without referred pain, or referred pain that does not at all reproduce the patient's complaint, rules out muscle trigger points as the primary source of the problem.

Cautions

The presence of disease or dysfunction in one structure does not exclude disease or dysfunction in other structures. For example, dysfunction of thoracic spinal facet joints, or articulations between the spine and ribs, are typically associated with muscular trigger points, and vice versa. Muscles crossing affected, painful joints typically will be exposed to mechanical perturbations and will be subject to local spinal reflex arcs, causing facilitation (often referred to as "spasm" or "splinting"). Similarly, with SITS, the repetitive or constant forces exerted by tense muscles on the spine result, over time, in some degree of aberrant joint function, which is usually reported by the patient as middle/upper-thoracic midline stiffness. Finally, visceral disease may coexist with joint and muscle dysfunction, and failure to achieve significant improvement with appropriate treatments directed at somatic (joint and muscle) lesions should raise the clinician's index of suspicion regarding the presence of occult visceral pathology. Whenever thoracic bone or joint disease is suspected, imaging of the affected area should be obtained immediately and pursued until a lesion consistent with both the patient's symptoms and the findings of the physical examination are identified or ruled out. Plain film radiographs, though limited in their diagnostic yield, are still the reasonable first step.

Poor correlation has been seen between spinal degenerative joint disease (DJD) and pain. To the contrary, significant data indicate the absence of a correlation between the radiographic presence or progression of spinal DJD and symptoms (12,13), as well as MRI data indicating a high incidence (35%–54%) of disc bulges and herniations in the asymptomatic adult population (6,7), from which it is clear that the presence of DJD alone on an imaging study probably does not explain back pain. Unless plain films demonstrate advanced, focal DJD at the exact joint the patient identifies as symptomatic and which the examiner identifies through physical examination as the primary source of pain and dysfunction, the clinician should resist a primary diagnosis of DJD.

If spine pain is suspected, the plain films are negative, and manipulative or traction-type therapies do not bring relief, advanced imaging studies should be undertaken. CT is still considered the best technique for the identification of bone disease, although MRI, using STIR technique, is probably close to being as good. The bone scan has little advantage over CT or MRI in identifying spine disease.

A few words about gallbladder and pancreatic disease are appropriate as a final thought here. When distended, referred pain from the gallbladder, a hollow viscus, may be felt in the upper back. Typically, patients describe a quarter-sized burning or aching pain at the inferior pole of the right scapula. As discussed above, muscle pain is not specifically isolated to a small area, and spinal joint and bone pain are typically located toward the midline. However, a muscle strain of the lower trapezius fibers, such as during rowing, or a bone lesion of a rib could cause similar symptoms. The diagnostic pearl is the pain's relation to meals—especially to fatty foods—which exacerbate the symptoms of gallbladder disease, but not muscle, bone, or joint problems. Diagnostic ultrasound will settle the issue of gallbladder disease in most cases. Adenocarcinoma of the pancreas also typically refers to the back, most commonly the lower to midthoracic spine. Depending on the location of the tumor, the pancreatic duct may become occluded, blocking the flow of pancreatic enzymes, resulting in gastritis. The early symptoms of pancreatic cancer are often profuse belching, indigestion, and thoracic pain. Interestingly, depression is extremely common in patients with this disease and often precedes any physical signs or symptoms. Although the cause of the depression is not well understood, it is seen so consistently in patients with adenocarcinoma of the pancreas that symptoms of depression in conjunction with thoracic pain, indigestion or belching in any patient older than 40 years should prompt an investigation for occult disease. CT scanning of the abdomen with the use of contrast medium continues to be the diagnostic procedure of choice for ruling out pancreatic cancer.

Symptom/Pain Presentation

The patient with SITS presents with tightness, or stiffness, and ache in the scapular or interscapular area. Approximately 50% of patients are experiencing, or have experienced in the past, **bruxism**, and many of them have a bite guard or other dental appliance that they make use of from time to time. Sometimes the patient will describe the pain as "soreness," but with careful questioning can differentiate the feeling from the soreness one experiences the day after vigorous exercise, and usually will settle for "ache" instead. The pain fluctuates, usually gradually over several hours, peaking (especially if the patient works) toward the end of the day or early evening. Occasionally the pain is worst on first awakening in the morning. Poor quality sleep is an extremely common associated feature in SITS and may take one or more of the following forms:

- Difficulty falling asleep
- Difficulty staying asleep through the night
- Troubled, anxiety-filled, or frustration-filled dreams
- More than one nightmare per month
- Nonrestorative sleep with the patient typically waking up unrefreshed.

Patients with SITS often have difficulty sitting still, and may want to point to the pain area repeatedly. They usually exhibit unconscious body habits such as rolling the shoulders, deep sighs, stretching the neck from side to side, or self-manipulation of the neck or back, especially when, during the interview, the clinician probes into the personal and stressful areas of the patient's life. Many patients are aware that they manipulate the pain area (though perhaps not of the frequency with which they do so), especially toward the end of the day, when their pain is at its worst, and will explain that they "need" to do it, because it is the only thing that brings relief, albeit temporarily. The astute clinician will make use of these unconscious or conscious mannerisms as clues toward making an accurate diagnosis, keeping in mind that tensing extrafusal muscles (such as hunching the shoulders) unloads the intrafusal fibers (19). Similarly, stretching, rubbing, and tensing the painful muscles all manipulate muscle spindles in some way, and patients intuitively develop these techniques to manage the symptoms of SITS.

Sometimes the patient is highly aware of a relationship between stress and pain; often he is unaware of this connection, but it is always present. The same is true about MT, with some patients fully aware of both the presence of tension and the relationship between MT and pain, and others who are entirely unaware of both. It is up to the clinician to gain insight through the history and physical examination, with respect to the presence or absence of psychological and emotional stress, MT, and trigger points.

When the pain is at its worst, it may be reported as incapacitating, but it is not actually so (patients typically do not leave work, for instance, the way they might during a migraine), and symptoms may spread to one or more of the following areas: neck, head, shoulder/upper arm, hand, and fingers. The referred symptoms are not always categorized as pain but may instead be described as numbness, "tingling," or a "heavy feeling," especially in the upper extremity. Although some patients first state that their pain comes and goes, careful questioning will usually show that there is always some level of pain, stiffness, or discomfort, especially in the neck, though perhaps at times it is ignorable. Patients may recall times in the past when the pain was very bad for several weeks, and other times when they felt much better for several weeks.

If they have a long history of prior treatments, they likely have developed a pharmacologic routine; this typically includes the sparing use of muscle relaxants or narcotic medications (for "really bad days"), as well as the regular use of

NSAIDs. More patients with chronic pain are now using antidepressant medicines. The clinician must obtain a complete and accurate inventory of all medicines, dosages, and usage habits. Narcotic dependency is common among patients with chronic pain, and in many instances, dealing with prescription drug addiction is prerequisite to treating the pain problem. The clinician should also determine where and from whom the patient obtains prescriptions and medications; a careful history will sometimes uncover multiple prescribing sources, and patients may be operating from the misguided belief that several pain medications must be taken in conjunction, one for the headaches and another for upper back pain, for example. Multiple prescribers, difficulty recalling the frequency and dosages of medications, a history of repeated visits to emergency rooms for meperidine injections, as well as defensiveness when questioned directly about their drug usage all may be signs of narcotic dependency. To get control of this problem, the patient must at the outset of care agree to have only one prescriber of pain medicine. An open line of communication must be established between all of the patient's healthcare providers. When narcotic dependency has been established, a drug withdrawal program should be started, and psychological or psychiatric supervision can be extremely helpful at this juncture.

Myofascial Entrapments

No myofascial entrapments are associated with SITS in the upper back. However, as mentioned previously, trigger points can refer pain and paresthesias into the upper extremity, sometimes mimicking neuropathy or radiculopathy. In addition, SITS typically affects not only the upper back/scapular area, but also commonly the muscles of the neck and jaws. When symptoms involve the upper extremity, thoracic outlet syndrome should be ruled out (the pectoralis and scalene groups evaluated), along with radiculopathy. This is true even when manual stimulation of the trigger points in the spino-scapular or scapulohumeral muscles reproduce the upper extremity complaints.

Treatment

As with any condition, effective treatment of SITS begins with an understanding of its pathophysiology. Unlike some medical problems, however, not only the clinician but the patient must develop an understanding of what is happening if SITS is to be successfully treated. Many patients with chronic pain have already formulated an idea regarding the cause of their pain before seeking treatment. Common examples are sleeping on a bad mattress, arthritis, scar tissue or adhesions in muscles (usually from some long-ago injury), inflammation, weakness, bad posture, fluctuations in weather, spinal misalignment, a familial disorder, fibromyalgia, and disc herniation. These ideas may come from prior physicians or therapists, the internet, television, magazines, or books. Some patients have friends with similar symptoms who have been given one of these explanations. When the clinician is sure of the diagnosis of SITS, the first priority is to educate the patient as to the real cause of the pain. Ultimately, patients must learn to gain control of MT, and to do this, they must become partners with the clinician and work together by the light of common understanding. Disabusing patients of previously held false ideas about their problem can be one of the most difficult aspects of treating patients with SITS. This is especially true when they have been shown X-rays by a previous orthopedist or chiropractor showing "arthritis."

The clinician must keep in mind what is at stake when the patient accepts a diagnosis of SITS. That one's problem is "stress-related" carries numerous implications and ramifications, including the fact that the patient is, in a sense, both responsible for the problem and the solution. In a non-confrontational manner and in the simplest terms possible, the clinician should present a clear and systematic explanation as to why the patient's prior diagnosis does not explain the condition and the reasons why SITS does. For example, if the patient believes the problem stems from DJD of the spine, the clinician might compare the patient's pain area to the area of the DJD, demonstrating that they are not the same. A very effective technique is to grasp a trigger point between the thumb and forefinger (the upper trapezius muscle is ideal for this purpose) and, having identified the tissue as muscle, apply pressure to the trigger point, thereby reproducing the patient's pain and demonstrating experientially that the source is muscular. Although needle EMG also can document the intrafusal muscle contraction in the spindle (16), this procedure is not commonly used in clinical practice. It should be emphasized that muscle tension is not "in the head" but, rather, is the normal response of a healthy body to persistent or recurrent stressful condition-stimuli.

Getting patients to make the connection between tension and pain is relatively easy compared with getting them to connect emotion to MT. Most patients are under the misapprehension that emotions are "mental" and are synonymous with thoughts. Others think of emotions as descriptions of behavior. The following represents a common dialogue between a doctor and a SITS patient:

DOCTOR: When was the last time you felt angry?
PATIENT: I don't really get angry.
DOCTOR: How is it that you never feel angry?
PATIENT: I just try to keep a positive attitude.
DOCTOR: How would you know if you did feel angry?
PATIENT: I don't know, I'd be angry.
DOCTOR: And how would that *feel*?
PATIENT: I'd probably start yelling.
DOCTOR: That's how you'd be *acting* angry, but what would it *feel* like? In other words, where in your body would you feel it and what would it actually *feel* like if you were angry?
PATIENT: Where in my body? I don't know, everywhere.

At first, the patient confuses feelings with mental attitude. By keeping "positive," he assumes he never experiences feelings of anger. Later in the dialogue, the patient confuses feelings with action. As long as he does not act angrily, he does not feel angry. In such cases, the clinician should continue to use the word "feel" while gently pursuing the line of inquiry as follows:

"Do you think you could have unpleasant feelings even if you had a positive attitude? For instance, if a person close to you died, and you kept a positive attitude, do you think you might still feel somewhat sad underneath?"

-or-

"I think I understand what you mean, but the thing I'm getting at is the actual *feeling*. You know, feelings are called *feel*-ings because they actually do involve the sensation of feeling something, and I want to know what it is you physically feel."

-or-

"Well, let me ask this in a different way. You know when you have to get up and make a speech, you get a specific kind of feeling in your body, some people call it "butterflies," right here, in the stomach? Clinically we call that feeling "anxiety." What I'm getting at is, what does it feel like, not when you're anxious, but when you feel angry?"

There are endless permutations of this interaction. The goal is to get the patient to begin thinking about emotions as body sensations, rather than as cognitions or behaviors. The clinician should be non-confrontational, and if the patient is resistant after two or three attempts to make the point, it should be dropped and picked up again at a future visit. It is also good to keep in mind that intellectual understanding by itself will not eliminate the sympathetically driven physiologic state of MT. This can only be accomplished through an experiential process of identifying the stressful sources of tension and then taking some action to change them. The clinician should think about himself and the patient as working as a team over time.

One of the most effective tools for leading patients to an experiential understanding of SITS is to provide them with relief. Because of the persistent or recurrent nature of the condition-stimulus, even complete relief from pain will be temporary, but it is the contrast between relaxed, relieved muscles, post-treatment, and tense, aching muscles, that demonstrates to the patient that his pain is coming from MT, which in turn is caused by the stressful condition-stimulus. To this end, trigger point pressure release of trigger points, followed by spray and stretch, followed by moist heat or continuous ultrasound (by itself or mixed with alternating current electrical stimulation set to sub-tetany), and finally, by SMT of the mid-thoracic and cervical segments, is an extremely effective protocol.

As any clinician knows, the effectiveness of treatment relies in part on the skills of the clinician. The key to the physical medicine treatment is to get the patient to relax. In the treatment room, quiet music and slightly dimmed lighting may be helpful. On visits in which relief is the goal, the clinician should not have a lot of verbal interaction with the patient beyond the medically necessary gathering of information before the treatment. The clinician should convey as much as possible a supportive, caring disposition toward the patient, speak directly to him or her in a calm voice, answer any questions simply, and encourage the patient to let go of all concerns while the treatment is taking place. Tense, guarded muscles should not be aggressively stretched, and the clinician should take measures to get the patient relaxed before and during spray and stretch. If the patient is not able to relax his muscles, the spray and stretch should not be undertaken on that day. Any fears the patient may have should be taken seriously and addressed to the patient's satisfaction. The clinician should empower the patient to decline any part(s) of the treatment with which he or she is not comfortable. Inducing relaxation in the tense patient is of primary importance.

Each visit, the patient should be given some homework. The successful treatment of SITS does not take place solely within the treatment room. The first assignment should consist of having the patient discontinue any use of cold packs, self-manipulations, stretching, rubbing, or pressing on sensitive areas. This may be quite difficult for patients, especially because so often these maneuvers are either unconscious or believed to provide some relief, but the patient must be strongly encouraged to break these bad habits. It may be useful to explain this to the patient in the following way: "I know it feels good when you stretch and poke on the trigger points, but it's like scratching a rash; it feels good while you're doing it but it inflames the rash and makes it worse in the long run." In place of these maneuvers, the patient should be instructed to purposely relax the upper back. It is essential to educate the patient that tension-relaxation is not accomplished by slouching, wiggling the neck and shoulders, or by pulling the shoulders down. Rather, tension-relaxation consists of the progressive un-tensing of the muscles in the upper back. It may be helpful to give the patient an image to use, as follows: "Think about your shoulder blades as being like balloons filled with air. The air is like tension and I want you to just let it out like a balloon deflating. Each time you exhale, try to let more air out of the balloons until they are completely relaxed." Moist heat, especially hot showers, should be done twice per day if possible, with the patient allowing the hot water to relax the interscapular muscles. Electric or microwaveable heating pads are to be used sparingly or avoided altogether, because dry heat may cause congestion in the muscles, and patients are prone to overuse of these comfort items, thereby diminishing the time they spend taking stock of the fluctuations in their tension levels. If the patient consumes more than two caffeinated beverages per day, cutting back would be helpful because increased arousal caused by stimulants can result in an increase in negative feelings such as anger (20), which in turn can escalate SITS. If the patient appears hesitant to cut back on caffeine, the issue should not be pushed but should instead be dropped until the patient has made significant symptomatic progress and reports some mood improvement. At this time, the subject may be broached again, but the clinician should do so in a casual manner: "Have you given any further thought to cutting back just a bit on the caffeine?" If he is amenable to decreasing or eliminating caffeine, the patient should be instructed to consume at least six, 8-ounce glasses of water each day in its place. NSAIDs might be a good idea for one week if the patient decides to completely eliminate caffeine, to manage withdrawal headache.

Next, the patient should begin to engage in some form of cardiovascular exercise each day, which will help improve mood (21) and will give the patient a chance to break away from his routine to do something positive and healthy for himself. Again, this should not be pushed too hard on the patient, and he should be allowed to pick whatever form of exercise is most appealing to him. The exercise, if possible, should be sustained at least 15 to 20 minutes, a minimum of 3 days per week (5 is optimal), and it must be cardiovascular in nature.

The next assignment is to purchase a small notebook pad and to record his MT levels (on a scale of 0–10) and pain levels (0–10), as well as the place and time. This should be done every day: in the morning when the patient first wakes up, during the day just before taking lunch, in the evening on leaving work, and at night before bedtime. With more motivated patients, hourly recording prompted by a watch alarm provides even more information.

When the muscle tension diary is explained to the patient, a technique called progressive tension-relaxation (PTR) should be taught to the patient as well. The clinician stands behind the seated patient, the clinician's thumb gently pressing on a trigger point in the lower or middle trapezius muscle, for example. Next, the patient is asked to squeeze the muscle being pressed on without moving the shoulders. This may take some coaching, because often patients have a poor sense of how it feels to be tense but can easily appreciate the sensation of having their shoulders raised up toward the neck. Tensing, it should be explained, does not necessarily involve gross body movements such as raising the shoulders. After approximately 10 seconds of continuous tensing without moving the scapulae, the patient should next be coached to release all of the tension from the muscle(s) in question. After a few relaxed breaths, the patient should next be asked to squeeze the muscle(s) again, this time creating only half the amount of tension as before. The clinician's thumb stays on the trigger point with slight to moderate pressure to monitor both the tension and relaxation phases of the PTR technique. After 10 seconds, the patient once again is coached to drop out the tension completely. Again, after a few relaxed breaths, the patient squeezes one final time, this time with half-again the amount of tension as the previous PTR cycle (one-quarter the amount of the first cycle) and then, after 10 seconds, lets go completely once again. Explain to the patient that he or she probably is holding about the same amount of tension

as the third PTR cycle, on and off, all day long. The patient should be encouraged whenever they check their tension level and record it in their muscle-tension diary (MTD), to also take themselves through one round (the three cycles) of PTR. If there is not enough time for this, the patient should employ the simpler tension-relaxation technique of letting go of the back muscles, as described above. The patient should bring the MTD to each office visit, and the clinician should begin some office visits after that time with an inspection of the MTD, looking specifically for times of day, events, people, or places that seem to correlate with either an escalation or a decrease in MT or pain. When these are identified, the patient should be asked to elaborate on what was going on during those times and why they think their MT changed. The clinician should ask open-ended questions that encourage the patient to talk; for example, if a patient's MTD shows a consistent increase in MT and pain in the late afternoon hours, the clinician might ask, "I can see that your tension seems to escalate almost every afternoon when you're working. What causes that, do you think?" The goal is to continually put the patient in contact with his or her emotional fluctuations and with the condition-stimuli that fuel them. Once again, this should be done gently, and if the patient is resistant to associating a particular condition-stimulus with MT or pain (even if the condition-stimulus takes place just before each recorded escalation in MT), the issue should not be pursued to the point of causing the patient to become defensive. More than likely, the point has been made, and the patient will be more aware next time of the connection. Biofeedback is an excellent tool to help the patient who has difficulty with developing the awareness of the connection between the condition-stimulus, the MT, and the pain (Box 8-1).

Once a time of day, situation, person, or place has been connected to the escalation of MT, the patient should be given a breathing/relaxation technique, in which they are taught to inhale through the nostrils, causing the abdomen to expand, and then exhale through the mouth, causing the abdomen to recede. These should not be deep breaths, but they should be slow breaths. The patient should not pause or hold his breath after inhalation, but he should pause for a slow mental count of three following each exhalation. He should sit in a relaxed position or lie down if possible, and the exercise should be done for approximately 3 to 5 breaths. The patient may use this exercise instead of PTR, immediately after each time they write in their MTD, and for longer periods (up to a minute, continuously) in the morning and before bedtime.

Approximately every third visit, the patient should be encouraged to speak more extensively about his or her experience with the treatment. Each day the MTD will give an index of the symptomatic progress, and this should be averaged each third visit to show the patient the changes in his or her condition over time. The patient should be allowed to ask whatever questions they wish and a brief discussion of the pathophysiology of SITS, using simplistic language,

BOX 8-1

Biofeedback and Psychotherapy

As the clinician gains experience in treating SITS, he or she will undoubtedly become skilled at quickly recognizing those patients who will be highly resistant to a form of care that requires their participation and, especially, which requires them to look closely at their feelings, their lives, and to what extent their condition is a physiologic manifestation of psychological and emotional stress. Poor compliance often may simply reflect an unconscious wish to avoid facing uncomfortable feelings. Losing their Muscle Tension Diaries, failing to "find time" to exercise, "forgetting" to do the breathing/relaxation or PTR exercises, etc., are common forms of avoidance behavior. In such cases, the help of a well-trained psychologist can be extremely valuable.

Biofeedback, which uses (among other things) surface EMG as a tool for teaching awareness of muscle tension and techniques for muscle relaxation, is also extremely helpful because it provides experiential understanding of how muscles can be tense or relaxed while also helping the patient to feel better. A psychologist trained in this form of biofeedback is particularly helpful to the physical medicine clinician, for it is generally far easier to persuade a resistant patient to see a "biofeedback therapist" who happens also to be a psychologist than to simply see a psychologist. When making the biofeedback referral, the clinician should ask the patient for permission to speak with the therapist about the case, and if possible, this line of communication should remain open.

A team effort, in which the physical medicine clinician is able to share the role of leading the patient toward self-awareness with a talented, experienced psychologist, is ideal for both the clinician and the patient. It is unfortunate that insurance restrictions limit the number of patients who can be managed this way. In the post-MVA setting, anxiety while driving is common and is a reasonable cause for referral to biofeedback. Once there, the patient may discover that the therapist has much more to offer than help with just this isolated psychophysiologic symptom.

---

should be regularly undertaken to reinforce the guiding principles of treatment. The patient's own views on the cause of his or her problem should be solicited, and the evidence from his or her own case should be used gently to prod the patient into an awareness of the connections between the condition-stimuli and his or her MT and pain. As the patient begins to make these connections, some practical steps can be discussed for addressing the condition-stimuli. Many patients with SITS are aware that they are under a lot of pressure and that they have developed unhealthy living habits (lack of exercise, poor diet, insufficient sleep, etc.), but they also are convinced that they have no reasonable options for changing their situation. The clinician's job is to lead patients toward understanding in such a manner that they begin to see options that would enable necessary changes to take place. For example, the clinician might offer the following: "I was wondering, do you think your boss would be willing to let you come into work an hour later if you also stayed an hour later? This way you could do a little exercise in the morning and miss both rush hours." Helping patients resolve some of the associated ongoing issues is an extremely important part of the doctor–patient relationship, for it is by taking action that patients gain the experiential understanding that addressing and resolving specific condition-stimuli reduces muscle tension and pain. As always, the clinician must resist the temptation to push the patient, as this may provoke defensiveness and poor compliance. In addition, patients may need to experience success to proceed to further action; therefore, the clinician would be wise to guide the patient at first toward addressing those condition-stimuli that are relatively straightforward and easy to resolve.

Although patients with SITS often have a central issue fueling their tension, several smaller issues may play a role as well. Chronically running late may not be the primary cause of the problem, but it probably contributes to the overall high level of sympathetically induced intrafusal tension. A similar observation can be made of numerous common problems people face repeatedly in their daily lives; driving in rush hour traffic, not getting a pay raise that was promised, having a noisy next-door neighbor, or dealing with an adversarial claims adjuster are a few examples of condition-stimuli that can escalate tension in the preparatory "fight" muscles of the upper back. When the physiological responses to condition-stimuli such as these are superimposed on a muscle strain injury, their effect is amplified. For example, between the pain caused by the muscle strain, insurance issues, having to make doctors' appointments, missed time from work, auto repairs, disruption of routine, financial issues, etc., it is not hard to see why even very low speed rear-impact motor vehicle collisions are a common cause of chronic pain in the neck and upper back (22). Patients who are suffered to endure numerous, repeated frustrations on top of strained, painful, sensitized upper thoracic muscles are likely to develop SITS as they move from the acute strain injury phase to the chronic phase.

If the patient feels overly burdened by the clinician's demands, this will work against the compliance necessary for ultimately undoing this complex problem. To ask a patient to make even small lifestyle changes is asking a lot, and the clinician who appreciates this fact will transmit a sense of supportiveness, whereas approaching this aspect of patient management in a cavalier or impatient manner will garner only resentment from the patient.

As the patient gains awareness of their feelings, the clinician continues to provide treatment focused primarily on the muscles and secondarily on the spinal joints. Each treatment should include identification of the current active trigger points. When the taut bands are found, digital pressure is applied over the most tender nidus provoking referred pain. The clinician should never fail to ask the patient what he or she is feeling and where. It is also helpful if the patient can tell which muscle is being palpated and to this end, the affected muscles being treated should be named each time so that the patient can learn them. By continuing to involve the patient in their own care, the clinician reinforces not only the sense of teamwork, but an understanding of the essential nature of the problem as being that of muscle tension.

Once the patient has begun to get some control of their MT (by breathing/relaxation exercises, PTR, and tension/relaxation techniques, release of tension through cardiovascular exercise, taking action to reduce or eliminate the sources of tension, and by treatments), gentle stretching may begin. Stretching should be done three times per day (in the morning, evening, and before bed). The stretches should be named according to the muscles involved, (lower trapezius, rhomboids, infraspinatus, etc.) and should be done very slowly, very gently, and without any pain whatsoever. Patients must understand that the goal of stretching is not to take shortened, tight muscles and force them to painfully elongate, but to gently coax these muscles into letting go. The clinician should be careful not to institute self-stretching too soon during the treatment program and should keep in mind that according to the pathophysiologic construct of SITS, trigger points are chronically facilitated muscle spindles. Muscle

spindles are stretch receptors that, if stretched too hard or too quickly, will provoke more muscle tension via the monosynaptic stretch reflex. In addition, SITS patients, especially at the beginning of care, usually have a poor sense of body awareness; this, combined with the state of impatient agitation that is common in the postinjury or chronic pain settings, can easily lead to over-stretching, causing, in effect, recurrent strain injuries. Only when the patient begins to develop a sense of control over the muscle tension and an experiential understanding of his or her condition should the clinician feel comfortable giving the patient some gentle home stretches.

At the end of a successful course of care, the patient parts ways with the clinician, having quit the habits of ignoring their feelings and performing unconscious self-manipulations. The patient has learned to like their cardiovascular and gentle stretching routine. He or she has learned to be aware of subtle escalations in MT and has learned to identify the sources of those escalations. The patient also has learned that acting constructively, though not always easy to do, brings rewards in terms of reducing tension and eliminating pain. The patient has learned to view physical medicine treatments as an aid in managing his or her problem and not as a remedy for immediate cure. Not uncommonly, the patients having conquered SITS, will report during the last weeks of care (or at follow-up) that they have done a lot of thinking and have decided to make some significant change in their lives (change jobs, go to college, quit smoking, etc.).

Much has been written on the treatment of trigger points. Spray and stretch, as described by Janet Travell, followed by moist heat or continuous ultrasound (with or without alternating current electrical stimulation set to subtetany) is a reasonable and effective protocol. Modifications for treating trigger points associated with SITS in the upper back, affecting lower trapezius, middle trapezius, or rhomboids are described in Technique 8-1.

TECHNIQUE 8-1

Treatment Tips for SITS

The patient must be coaxed into a relaxed state before attempting spray and stretch. Once relaxed, trigger point pressure release ("ischemic compression") is performed with the patient seated in a slouched position, arm crossed in front, back rounded and relaxed, the scapula abducted (Fig. 8-2). No more than two trigger points should undergo trigger point pressure release during a single treatment, as a certain amount of soreness and slight bruising can sometimes occur the day after treatment. Trigger point pressure release involves the use of the thumb or of a device to apply pressure directly to the extremely tender nidus of the trigger point (Fig. 8-3). The amount of pressure should be enough so the patient reports a strong stimulation of local and referred pain, but the clinician should try to

minimize the risk of bruising. The compression should be held with a constant amount of pressure until the patient reports a reduction in the tenderness/pain of 75% or more. Pressure should not be applied for more than 2 minutes continuously, and if the patient has not reported sufficient reduction of tenderness/pain by that time, trigger point pressure release should be stopped. In most cases, patients experience nearly a complete resolution of the local tenderness/pain after approximately 30 seconds if they are relaxing sufficiently. If significant improvement is not obtained after 30 seconds, the clinician should encourage the patient to relax more, even though there is pain. Use of the breathing/relaxation technique is extremely helpful in this regard.

TECHNIQUE 8-1

Treatment Tips for SITS (*Continued*)

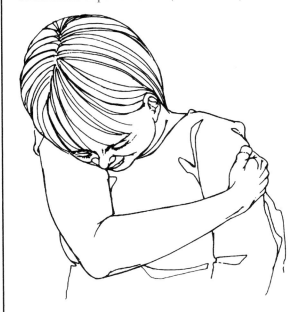

FIGURE 8-2. Relaxed starting position for trigger point pressure release of upper back muscles. The patient sits in a slouched position, with the hand of the side being treated grasping the opposite shoulder at the level of the mid-scapula.

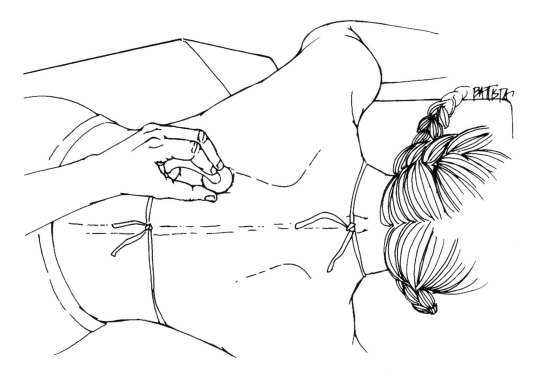

FIGURE 8-3. Use of a hand-held wooden device to apply trigger point pressure. The device can be used with the patient seated, or prone as shown here. The pressure is removed when the patient reports 75% or more reduction in local tenderness.

TECHNIQUE 8-1

Treatment Tips for SITS (*Continued*)

During stretch and spray, lower trapezius and middle trapezius fibers are stretched together by having the patient grasp the opposite shoulder with the hand of the affected side (the side being stretched). The clinician then guides the patient's elbow across the body as sweeps of vapocoolant are applied along the direction of the fibers of the muscle from origin to insertion, followed by three spray applications from the trigger points to the areas of pain referral (Fig. 8-4A). From this position, the patient is encouraged to lean backwards toward the clinician, who simultaneously continues to draw the pa-

tient's elbow to bring the muscles into further stretch and also contacts the inferomedial edge of the patient's scapula, adding slightly more stretch to the muscle. This stretch should be held for approximately 30 seconds to 1 minute, as the patient is continually coaxed to let go of tension and relax into the stretch. Finally, the patient is gently returned to a normal resting position, and the muscle warmed with the clinician's hands.

The second stretch begins with the patient in the same resting position as for the first stretch. The clinician reaches beneath the opposite side arm and takes

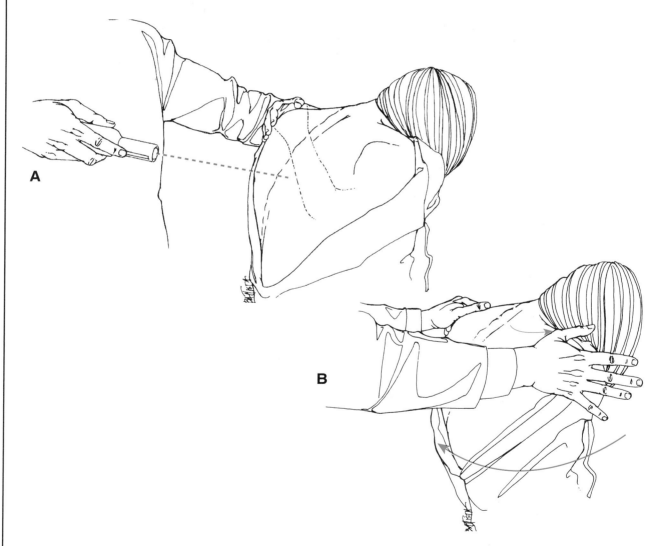

FIGURE 8-4. **Stretch and spray of the lower and middle trapezius. A.** Starting position. The clinician guides the patient's elbow across the body to effect greater spraying from origin to insertion. The clinician holds the patient's hand in place and has the patient lean backwards and relax completely as he gently guides the scapula into further protraction and abduction to increase the stretch. **B.** The clinician completes the stretch by contacting the border between the muscle and the scapula and manually stretching the scapula further from the spine.

TECHNIQUE 8-1

Treatment Tips for SITS (*Continued*)

hold of the elbow on the side that is to be stretched (contact left elbow to stretch the left side, etc.). The patient is encouraged to fall backward against the chest or hip of the clinician and to relax. It may be suggested that the patient pretend to relax back into a big, comfortable chair. As the patient falls progressively backward, the elbow on the side to be stretched is brought straight across the body and beneath the opposite arm, causing scapular abduction and protraction, as sweeps of vapocoolant are applied along the direction of the fibers of the muscle from origin to insertion, followed by three spray applications from the trigger points to the areas of pain referral (the upper neck and the mastoid, the acromion and the suprascapular region, and the medial surface of the scapula.) As in the first stretch, the clinician at this point should put down the vapocoolant and contact the medial edge of the patient's scapula, further abducting and protracting it to slightly further stretch the muscle (Fig. 8-4B). This should be held for approximately 30 seconds to 1

minute as the patient is continually coaxed to let go of tension and relax into the stretch. Finally, the patient is gently returned to a normal resting position and, as before, the muscle is warmed with the clinician's hands. The clinician may do both stretches once, or either of the stretches twice per treatment.

The rhomboids are stretched and sprayed with a slightly different technique that may be done in conjunction with the lower and middle trapezius stretches. The patient makes a fist on the affected side (the side being treated), which is placed firmly on the same side hip. The patient is then told to relax the shoulder while maintaining the fist on the hip. The shoulder should not be pulled forward or back but should simply be allowed to slide on its own. The patient is then asked to slowly begin leaning backward while the clinician holds the elbow gently in place. The result is that the dorsal spine moves backward while the scapula slightly wings and is protracted and abducted as the clinician applies the vapocoolant spray (Fig. 8-5). This should be held for a slow

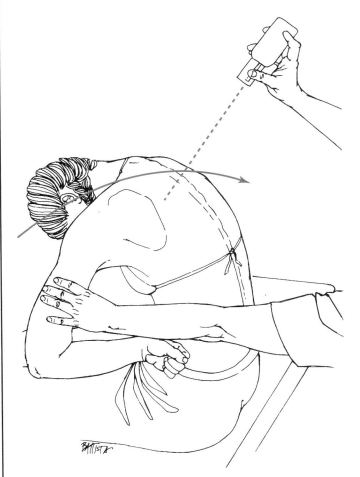

FIGURE 8-5. **Starting position for stretch and spray of the rhomboid muscle.** The patient sits in slouched position, fist of side to be treated placed firmly on the iliac crest. The shoulder is completely relaxed. The clinician stabilizes at the elbow and applies the spray from origin to insertion, while the patient leans back toward the clinician. Once stretched, the clinician warms the muscle with the free hand and gently guides the patient forward to a balanced, seated position.

TECHNIQUE 8-1

Treatment Tips for SITS (*Continued*)

count of 5. Then the clinician lets go of the elbow and uses the free hand to guide the patient gently back to a normal resting position. The muscle is again warmed with the clinician's hands. This procedure may be performed once or twice.

Stretch and spray of the pectoral muscles, infraspinatus, teres major and minor, levator scapulae, latissimus dorsi, and scalenes also may need to be performed. In each case, the first step is patient relaxation, followed by gentle stretch and spray. Warming with the clinician's hand completes the protocol.

Moist heat or continuous ultrasound (with or without alternating current electrical stimulation set to subtetany) should be applied immediately after the completion of stretch and spray, with the patient either seated in a relaxed position or prone on the treatment table with

arms hanging freely so that the scapulae are abducted (for rhomboids, middle and lower trapezius, levator scapulae). For other muscles, the patient should also be positioned such that the treated muscle is placed on a slight stretch and the patient is comfortable and relaxed. Sufficient toweling between the moist hot pack and the patient's skin is important to avoid burns or intolerance, and the heat should be left on for approximately 3 minutes. The patient should be able to report that the heat has penetrated such that the muscle (and not just the skin) has been deeply warmed. If continuous ultrasound is applied instead of moist heat, it is important that the applicator head be moved slowly but constantly to achieve a sedative warming of the muscle without causing burning. Internal appliances, such as a pacemaker, contraindicate the use of both ultrasound and electrical stimulation.

CONCLUSION

SITS is the most common cause of chronic upper back pain. Four hallmarks and four associated features to the disorder are noted, as follows:

Hallmarks:

1. Patients experience constant stiffness/discomfort in the neck.

2. Patients perform frequent stretching, rubbing, tensing, squeezing, or self-manipulation of the pain area.

3. Trigger points are present in the muscles of scapular stabilization that reproduce the pain complaint.

4. Gradual fluctuations in pain are seen, rather than sudden attacks of pain.

Associated Features:

1. Some form of sleep disturbance is present, such as difficulty falling asleep; difficulty remaining asleep through the night; bad dreams; unrefreshing, non-restorative sleep.

2. Bruxism or TMJ pain are common.

3. Pain is worse during times of higher stress.

4. Pain is worse at the end of the day or on first waking in the morning.

The clinical diagnosis of SITS may be made on the presence of at least three hallmarks and one associated feature, or at least two hallmarks and three associated features.

Once the diagnosis of SITS has been established, treatment is organized around the pathophysiology as follows:

1. Patient education

2. Pain relief

3. Providing patients with tools to control their muscle tension

4. Empowering patients to take action to reduce or eliminate stressful condition-stimuli causing MT

Emphasis should be placed on patients gaining an experiential understanding of the connection between stress and MT, and between MT and pain. A team approach with physical medicine clinicians and psychologists is ideal.

TREATMENT PROTOCOL

1. **Begin the process of educating the patient about the pathophysiology of SITS.**

2. **Instruct the patient to discontinue stretching, rubbing, poking the affected area, applying cold packs or topical balms, or self-manipulating the neck or back. Limiting or discontinuing the use of stimulants such as caffeine may be appropriate if the patient is amenable to the suggestion.**

3. **Administer trigger point pressure release (ischemic compression), followed by spray and stretch, followed by moist heat or continuous ultrasound with or without electrical stimulation of the affected muscle areas.**

4. **Perform SMT on the fixated cervical and thoracic spinal segments.**

5. **Instruct the patient to begin regular cardiovascular exercise.**

6. **Educate the patient in the use of progressive tension-relaxation technique (PTR) and in the use of a muscle tension diary, to be consulted at each visit to identify condition-stimuli causing MT, and to help the patient make the connection between changes in MT and pain.**

7. **Instruct the patient in abdominal breathing/relaxation exercise.**

8. **As the patient begins to form a good understanding of the connections between condition-stimuli, fluctuations in muscle tension, and pain, develop a practical plan for taking specific actions to address the problem(s) fueling MT.**

9. **Instruct the patient in gentle home stretches to be done within pain-free limits.**

References

1. Bonica J: The Management of Pain, vol. I, 2nd Ed. Philadelphia: Lea & Febiger, 1990:180–196.
2. Unpublished data, collected by the author at his private practice clinic, La Jolla Village Family Medical Group, in La Jolla, California.
3. Hurwitz EL, Coulter ID, Adams AH, et al. Use of chiropractic services from 1985 through 1991 in the United States and Canada. Am J Public Health, 1998;88:771–776.
4. Gore DR, Sepic SB, Gardner GM. Roentgenographic findings of the cervical spine in asymptomatic people. Spine 1986;11:521–524.
5. Gore DR, Sepic SB, Gardner GM, et al. Neck pain: a long-term follow-up of 205 patients. Spine 1987;11:1-5.
6. Boden S, Davis D, Dina T, et al. Abnormal magnetic resonance scans of lumbar spine in asymptomatic subjects. J Bone Joint Surg Am 1990;72:403–408.
7. Weinreb JC, Wolbarsht LB, Cohen JM, et al. Prevalence of lumbosacral intervertebral disc abnormalities in MR images in pregnant and asymptomatic non-pregnant women. Radiology 1989;170:125–128.
8. Barker D, Banks RW. The muscle spindle. In: Engel A, Banker B. eds. Myology. New York: McGraw-Hill, 1986:309–341.
9. Grassi C, Passatore M. Action of the sympathetic system on skeletal muscle. Ital J Neurol Sci 1988;9:23–28.
10. Voss VH. Zahl und Anordnung den Muskelspindeln in den Oberen Zungnbeinmuskeln, im M. Trapezius und M. Latissimus Dorsi. Anat Anzeiger 1956;103:443–446.
11. Hubbard DR, Berkoff GM. Myofascial trigger points show spontaneous needle EMG activity. Spine 1993;18:1803–1807.
12. McNulty WH, Gevirtz RN, Hubbard DR, et al. Needle electromyographic evaluation of trigger point response to a psychological stressor. Psychophysiology 1994;31:313–316.
13. Boyd IA. The isolated mammalian muscle spindle. TINS November 1980;258–265.
14. Polivy J. On the induction of emotion in the laboratory: discrete moods or multiple affect states? J Pers Soc Psychol 1981;41:803–817.
15. Diener E. Introduction to the special section on the structure of emotion. J Pers Soc Psychol 1999;76:803–804.
16. Stroud LR, Tanofsky-Kraff M, Wilfley DE, et al. Ann Behav Med 2000;22:204–213.
17. Abraham R. The role of job control as a moderator of emotional dissonance and emotional intelligence-outcome relationships. J Psychol 2000;134:169–184.
18. Goldman SL, Kraemer DT, Salovey P. Beliefs about mood moderate the relationship of stress to illness and symptom reporting. J Psychosom Res 1996;41:115–128.
19. Boyd IA, Ward J. Motor control of nuclear bag and nuclear chain intrafusal fibers in isolated lining muscle spindles from the cat. J Physiol 1975;244:83–112.
20. Erdmann G, Janke W. Interaction between physiological and cognitive determinants of emotions: experimental studies on Schachter's theory of emotions. Biol Psychol 1978;6:61–74.
21. Simons CW, Birkimer JC. An exploration of factors predicting the effects of aerobic conditioning on mood state. J Psychosom Res 1988;32:63–75.
22. McConnell WH, Howard RP, Guzman HM, et al. Analysis of human test subject kinematic responses to low velocity rear-end impacts. Society of Automotive Engineers (SAE Technical Paper Series 9308889 1993;21–31.

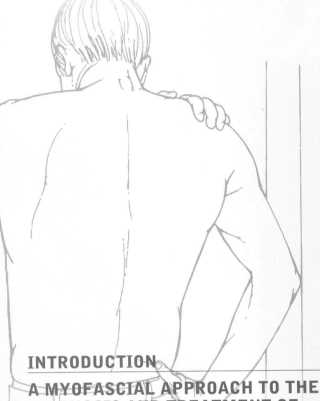

9

Interscapular Pain: A Myofascial Composite Syndrome

Tasso G. Spanos

TABLE 9–1

•••

Right Scapular = Pain	Location of Pain	Muscle	Distinguishing Characteristics that may be Present	% Encountered by Author
	Upper 1/4 of vertebral border	Levator scapula	Pain also at angle of neck, limits rotation to opposite side (often accompanied by 1st rib dysfunction that limits rotation to same side)	30%
	Upper 2/3 of vertebral border	Scalene	Pain in lateral aspect of upper arm; thumb and index finger, 2 finger-like projections over pectoral region almost to nipple level	80%
	Middle 1/2 of vertebral border	Infraspinatus	Deep pain in front of shoulder and down front of upper arm (biceps) Difficult to reach behind the back	20%
	Lower 1/3 of vertebral border (inferior angle) of scapula, fist size	Latissimus dorsi	Light pain in ring and little fingers, triceps	30%
	Lower 1/3 of vertebral border, inferior angle of scapula, 2 thumb digits size	Serratus anterior	Pain anterolaterally at mid-chest level. Sense of air hunger with short panting respiration	20%
	Lower 4/5 of vertebral border, narrow in width.	Lower trapezius	Slight burning pain, not severe	10%
	Medial pain inferior end of scapula and lighter in pain along vertebral border	Iliocostalis thoracis	Pain along inferior medial border of scapula, less intense pain along vertebral border.	10%
	Upper 1/2 of vertebral border and deep pain under scapula	Serratus posterior superior	Pain in entire little finger. Deep pain cannot be reached by patient	5%

TABLE 9–1 *(continued)*

Right Scapular = Pain	Location of Pain	Muscle	Distinguishing Characteristics that may be Present	% Encountered by Author
	Middle 1/2 of vertebral border and toward spine	Multifidi thoracis	Most pain toward the spine	10%
	Middle 1/2 of vertebral border between the scapula and paraspinal	Rhomboid	Complaint is of superficial aching pain at rest, not influenced by ordinary movement	5%

Data from Simons DG, Travell JG, Simons LS. Travell & Simons' Myofascial Pain and Dysfunction: The Trigger Point Manual, vol 1: Upper Half of Body. 2nd Ed. Baltimore: Lippincott Williams & Wilkins, 1999. Presented by Tasso Spanos at the American Academy of Pain Management Meeting in 1999. The table shows a drawing of the right scapula, repeated 10 times. The interscapular pain pattern is shown in red at or close to the border of the scapula. A written description of the location of the pain is followed by the name of the offending muscle. Distinguishing characteristics that may be present help to differentiate similar pain of two or more muscles. The percentage of the time that each muscle contributes to the pain is noted, as encountered by one pain center. Note that the percentages add up to more than 100%, because there are often several offending muscles for each patient with interscapular pain.

INTRODUCTION

The interscapular area can be a location of pain and suffering in many patients. When there is direct injury to this portion of the upper back, the problem usually resolves when the appropriate orthopedic, chiropractic, vascular, neurologic, or physical therapy treatment is focused to the traumatized zone. However, when there has been no trauma to the painful interscapular area and the same treatments yield no improvement, great frustration arises for both the patient and the healthcare practitioner. Practitioners may be unaware that trigger points in a muscle in another part of the body can refer pain to the interscapular area.

A MYOFASCIAL APPROACH TO THE DIAGNOSIS AND TREATMENT OF INTERSCAPULAR PAIN

If one has never been taught that a myofascial pain syndrome exists, then it is simply not part of the diagnostic consideration. The examination of library cards for volume 1 of *Myofascial Pain and Dysfunction, The Trigger Point Manual*, from two dozen medical schools and hospitals, show single-digit withdrawals in a 19-year period (1). Furthermore, myofascial interscapular pain can confuse practitioners, because it can be a composite pain referred from as many as 10 different muscles. Imagine that your house has been continuously burglarized and the police have finally caught the burglar, but the theft continues, because there is another burglar in the house. The second burglar is jailed; however, objects are still disappearing but at a slower rate. A third burglar is apprehended but theft continues. However, another undetected seven burglars remain in the house, and unless they are all put in jail, the theft will not be stopped. Likewise, unless all of the different muscles with active trigger points are separately treated, the patient's interscapular pain will not be resolved. This chapter is more about *when* and *where* to treat these 10 muscles than how to treat them. Simons and Travell have given us their knowledge and techniques for treating these muscles in 10 different chapters of *Myofascial Pain and Dysfunction* (2).

This chapter summarizes some of their information. A table is presented regarding how to successfully treat complex, composite interscapular myofascial pain (Table 9-1). A few pain centers have found that, using the information in this table, most of the time they can remove the patient's interscapular pain in one treatment. The pain may come back because of unresolved perpetuating factors or lack of patient cooperation in doing corrective stretches. Thus, this treatment protocol is not necessarily a permanent fix, but the patient who has not had full pain relief in the past learns that relief is possible. In addition, the clinician and the patient learn which muscles require attention to resolve the pain. One pain center has seen approximately 4,000 patients with myofascial interscapular pain. Most of them never had any history of trauma to this area. Those who did and were successively treated in the interscapular area obviously never came to the attention of a myofascial specialist. However, when the patient with nontraumatic interscapular pain received no relief from an articular adjustment, cortisone injection, electrical stimulation, work hardening, ultrasound, heat, cold, massage, surgery, nerve block, hydrotherapy, ointment, or magnetism, it is likely that there was an undiagnosed and untreated composite myofascial pain syndrome.

CASE 9-1

Patient History and Symptoms

Mr. S.D. had severe multiple pains for 17 years after electrocution during a parachuting accident. He consulted with, and was treated by, more than 100 medical practitioners who unfortunately gave him no help. The prognosis of the practitioners was divided into two main conflicting groups. One group said, "He will never be well." The other group said, "It must be in his head." Investigation revealed other earlier and important accidents: a concussion at age 21 months, four severe wrestling accidents, and one football accident. These proved to be significant creators of multiple trigger points, which were causing the major persistent problems. The electrocution was the "icing on the cake," producing a tremendous precipitating factor. The patient confirmed that during two of the wrestling accidents, his clavicle and shoulders were violently pushed upward toward the neck. The compression of his scalenes produced the interscapular pain, which he had, off and on, until the electrocution occurred. The pain then became constant and was accompanied by typical scalene trigger point referred pain in the hand, chest, and lateral upper arm. The pain in his right hand was primarily in the thumb and index finger.

Examination Findings:

Right lateral flexion was limited to 30° compared with left lateral flexion of 65°. He showed no tenderness of his left chest and lateral upper arm.

Treatment and Follow-up:

Three myofascial trigger point treatment sessions used trigger point pressure release to his right scalene Trigger points completely eliminated all these pains. As recommended by Simons, Travell, and Simons, the nonsymptomatic antagonist left scalenes also were treated (3). Follow-up 2 months later confirmed that Mr. S.D. was still doing his corrective exercises and was still pain free. Before these successful treatments, a host of other clinicians had attempted over 17 years to treat the pain-referred areas rather than the source, the scalene muscles.

CASE 9-2

Patient History and Symptoms:

Ms. B.D., an opera singer from New Zealand, came to the United States for further musical studies and medical help for a debilitating pain in her interscapular area. Trigger points can refer not only pain but also autonomic phenomena to another part of the body, and in this case there was also swelling in the interscapular area. Over the years, a variety of physical therapy modalities and cortisone injections were directed to her painful areas. Many practitioners have heard their patients exclaim, "if I had a knife, I would cut the painful spot out!" A major medical complex obliged her wish by surgically removing a portion of the middle trapezius, but the pain remained.

Examination Findings:

When she took a deep breath to sing, her interscapular pain greatly increased. This finding was puzzling to her medical practitioners. Her lung vital capacity seemed normal, yet upper chest movement was particularly annoying. Pain in her right finger and thumb was attributed to a separate problem, perhaps carpal tunnel.

Treatment and Follow-up:

The sharp interscapular pain was greatly reduced in two sessions of myofascial trigger point therapy consisting of trigger point pressure release directed to the scalenes. Thorough treatment to her scalene minimus (which attaches to the pleura of the lung and rib 1) eliminated the increased interscapular pain when she took a deep breath. The patient returned to New Zealand, where she could not receive any additional trigger point treatments. However, she performed regular muscular retraining stretches, corrected many perpetuating factors, and continued to improve.

CASE 9-3

Patient History and Symptoms

Mr. A.B. exhibited interscapular pain for 3 years. His pain was aggravated when he used a computer at his office job.

Examination and Treatment

His pain was primarily caused by the scalene and infraspinatus muscles. Once the trigger points in these muscles were identified, treated, and deactivated, practically all of the pain was gone. Evaluation of seven additional muscles from this chapter's table (Table 9-1) failed to indicate the origin of the remaining interscapular pain. A review of this patient's history showed a hobby of archery. When a heavy-duty archery bow is pulled back, the rhomboid muscle exerts an enormous pull. Listening carefully as Mr. A.B. moved his scapula, the clinician heard a crunching sound. Treating the trigger points in the rhomboid muscles resolved the remaining pain. The improvements continued when the rhomboid stretch was performed daily, along with the scalene and infraspinatus stretches.

Follow-up:

Correction of a short right hemipelvis with a butt lift, lowering his computer keyboard by 4 inches, and substituting a phone headset eliminated three perpetuating factors at his workplace. He continued to do his scalene, infraspinatus, and rhomboid stretches. One year later, he was still symptom free.

Overview of Myofascial Treatment of Interscapular Pain

To effectively treat myofascial interscapular pain, the clinician needs to select the appropriate muscles that may be responsible for that pain out of a list of 10 likely muscles. These are then evaluated and treated successively until the interscapular pain has been eliminated. Once the muscles responsible for the interscapular pain have been identified and treated, the patient is given specific stretches for these muscles. Attention also is turned to eliminating perpetuating factors that affect these muscles.

Causes

Injuries and occupational stresses that compress a muscle can create trigger points that precipitate interscapular pain. The greatest culprit, the scalene muscles, are particularly susceptible to injury from a violent upward thrust of the upper shoulders toward the neck. This motion can occur when hands are on the steering wheel during an automobile accident, or when the arms are extended to break a fall. Surgical cervical spine fusion disturbs the scalene muscles. Levator scapula, serratus posterior superior, lower trapezius, and rhomboids are irritated by prolonged holding and cradling a telephone receiver between the neck and shoulder. Heavy coughing, rib fracture, or thoracotomy can create serratus anterior trigger points. Repetitive strain syndromes can particularly irritate the latissimus dorsi and infraspinatus muscles.

Cautions

Other conditions can mimic interscapular myofascial pain. Cancer can cause interscapular pain without or with the presence of myofascial trigger points. One clinician saw a patient with unresponsive and migrating lower interscapular pain that was caused by metastatic liver cancer. Another patient had interscapular pain that did respond to myofascial treatment, but kept coming back after treatment. The patient had a tumor in the area of the latissimus dorsi. Myofascial treatment of the latissimus muscle eliminated the lower interscapular pain, but the tumor caused the latissimus dorsi muscle irritability to recur.

Entrapments

Myofascial involvement of the scalene muscles can cause compression of the interscalene compartment, entrap the neurovascular bundle, and create the condition commonly called thoracic outlet syndrome (see Chapter 4 for a fuller discussion.) Is the elevated first rib causing the compression, or are highly contracted unreleased scalenes elevating the first rib? The differential diagnosis can include articular dysfunction, scalenus anticus syndrome, and costoclavicular syndrome.

USE OF SYMPTOM PATTERNS IN THE EVALUATION AND TREATMENT OF MYOFASCIAL INTERSCAPULAR PAIN

To effectively treat interscapular pain, the practitioner needs to know when and where to treat each of the 10 muscles that refer pain to the interscapular area. To assist the practitioner in this process, Table 9-1 is presented.

The 10 muscles are divided into two main groups, those responsible most of the time for the interscapular pain, and those that infrequently contribute. *Note that the five most commonly responsible muscles are not located in the interscapular space.* The presentation order of the five major contributing muscles is by the location of the referred pain, beginning from the superior edge of the medial border and continuing downward to the inferior edge.

The five muscles most often responsible for interscapular pain (but not located where the pain is experienced) are: the levator scapula, scalene, infraspinatus, latissimus dorsi, and serratus anterior muscles.

Levator Scapula: Treatment and Stretch

The levator scapula muscle trigger points refer pain to the upper fourth of the vertebral border. It is the only muscle from the group that also refers pain to the angle of the neck and the posterior shoulder. It is responsible for the "stiff neck" syndrome, and the patient usually wakes up one morning with it because they "slept wrong." Although a severely shortened levator scapula would be expected to limit rotation to the opposite side, in the stiff neck syndrome, the shortened levator scapula is accompanied by a 1st rib joint dysfunction, and there is sharp pain when the head and neck are rotated to the same side. Although the levator scapula does not attach to the ribs, the shortened levator scapula and the 1st rib dysfunction commonly occur together. Luckily, trigger point pressure release applied to the lower levator scapula trigger points often also restores improved mobility to the underlying T1–1st rib joint.

If the patient points only to the top of the scapula and has poor rotation of the head to the same side, the levator scapula is probably causing most of the problem. Janet Travell, M.D. insisted that the levator scapula be treated bilaterally even if the complaint is only on one side. This will help relieve very persistent unilateral levator scapula problems. Care should be taken to seek and treat trigger points in all of the first four cervical attachments, besides those at the scapular attachments. An easy way to find these trigger points is by placing one hand on the cervical area, and the other hand restrains the head while the patient attempts to turn the head toward the affected side. The levator trigger points will pop up into the hand holding the cervical area. The inferior trigger points near the scapular attachment can be palpated through the upper trapezius muscle by having the patient shrug the shoulder.

Simons, Travell, and Simons (4) show a half-twist of the levator scapula muscle just before the four cervical attachments (Fig. 9-1). Most other anatomy books show the levator scapula as a straight line. The stretch for the levator scapula muscle requires the arm and the head to move in the same direction (see Fig. 7-6). The arms are behind the back, and one hand grasps the opposite wrist, to pull arm down and across the back. The head is leaned toward the opposite shoulder and is rotated at varying angles to stretch the different slips of this muscle. This muscle is particularly aggravated by perpetuating factors such as a short hemipelvis, or "crunching" the phone receiver between the head and the shoulder. Holding the phone improperly for 30 minutes can reverse a whole month of daily corrective stretches.

Scalenes: Treatment and Stretch

The scalene muscles are the most important to the myofascial interscapular pain, responsible for at least some of the

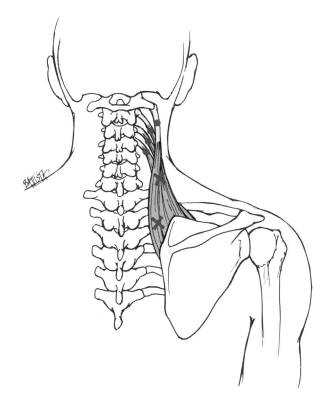

FIGURE 9-1. **Levator scapula trigger points.** Note that the X's indicate the trigger points nearer to the scapula and the O's indicate the upper trigger points near the transverse processes of C1, 2, 3, and 4. Modified with permission from Hendrickson T. Massage for Orthopedic Conditions. Baltimore: Lippincott Williams & Wilkins (fig. 4.29), p. 144.

composite pain in 80% of cases! They refer pain to the upper two-thirds of the vertebral border and slightly into the scapula itself. The referred pain overlaps with levator scapula referred pain in the upper third of the scapula. However, it has unique characteristics, which the levator does not share. It also can cause the following three pain referral patterns: the lateral aspect of the upper arm into the triceps; the whole hand, especially the thumb and index finger; and two finger-like projection patterns below the clavicle into pectoral region. Interscapular referred pain is seen practically all of the time, whereas the other three referred patterns occur at least 50% of the time.

Referred pain from scalene trigger points is so commonly misdiagnosed that many specialists have been led on a wild goose chase. The orthopaedic physician or chiropractor is not looking for the source of the interscapular pain in the anterior neck. The internist or rheumatologist is not looking for the source of the lateral upper arm pain in the anterior neck. The neurologist investigating carpal tunnel is not usually looking for the source of the hand or finger pain in the anterior neck. The cardiologist is not looking for the source of left-sided chest pain in the anterior neck. Nelson Hendler, M.D., suggests that 25% to 75% of misdiagnosed reflex sympathetic dystrophy is really an upper extremity nerve entrapment, often by scalenes and pectoralis minor muscles (5). Unsuspected scalene trigger points can be responsible for so many puzzling pain patterns that it is important to investigate the patient's injury and surgical history. Keep in mind Dr. Travell's dictum, "it is the mystery of the history."

One pain center specializes in the treatment of scalene trigger points. To describe their treatment protocol would require an entire chapter. However, a few of the important treatment highlights are covered. Simons, Travell, and Simons have identified common locations of scalene trigger points (3). In severely affected cases, the practitioner should also seek and treat trigger points in the higher cervical (C2–C4) attachments of the scalene medius and the scalene anterior. Because the thoracic outlet contains many components, isolation of the scalenes can be difficult. The practitioner should place two fingers of the treatment hand into the space anterior to the upper trapezius and posterior to the sternocleidomastoid muscle. The other hand should be placed on the ipsilateral top of the head. The patient is then asked to gently bring the head up laterally against the other restraining hand. This light contraction helps to distinguish

the scalene muscles from the surrounding blood vessels, nerves, and nearby muscles. This same light contraction is performed laterally at three different head angles to isolate the three main scalenes. These investigative angles are the same as the supine stretch angles shown in Figure 9-2. Travell emphasizes that the opposite scalene must be treated. However, in difficult cases, while the "good" side is being stretched, it can annoy the previously stretched "bad" side. Then the "bad" side must be treated and stretched again. Some very difficult cases have required treating and stretching one side and then the other up to 10 times.

The forgotten muscle in this area is the scalene minimus, which inserts into cervical 6, cervical 7, rib 1, and the pleura of the lung. To treat this muscle, the clinician places the patient's head in posterior scalene stretch position and runs one finger down the transverse processes, staying close to the spine. Isolate the scalene minimus with the contraction method described above. Many patients complain of an increasing interscapular pain when they take a deep breath. They have suddenly jerked the pleural attachment of the scalene minimus, overloading the muscle and causing in-

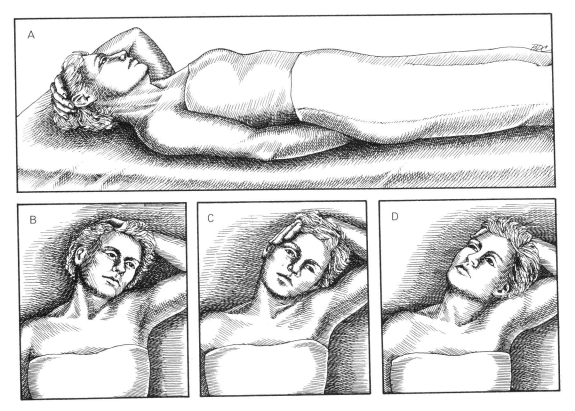

FIGURE 9-2. **Side-bending neck exercise.** This exercise is performed with the patient supine. Each position passively stretches one of the three major scalene muscles. The exercises should always be done bilaterally. **A.** The hand on the side to be stretched is anchored on the buttock. The contralateral hand is placed over the head and assists sidebending away from the muscle with trigger points. **B.** To stretch the scalenus posterior, and minimus, the face is turned away from the involved muscle. **C.** The face looks forward to stretch the scalenus medius. **D.** The face is turned toward the involved muscle to stretch the scalenus anterior.

Reprinted with permission from Simons DG, Travell JG, Simons LS. Travell & Simons' Myofascial Pain and Dysfunction: The Trigger Point Manual, vol 1: Upper Half of Body. 2nd Ed. Baltimore: Lippincott Williams & Wilkins, 1999 (fig. 20.14), p. 531.

creased hypertonicity, with the predictable pain pattern medial to the scapula.

To stretch the scalenes, the shoulder must be anchored by holding onto a chair or sitting on the hand of the affected side. This ensures that the rib attachments of the scalenes do not slip upward, negating a proper stretch. This is the most common mistake of physical therapy facilities in stretching scalenes muscles. The very best stretch for the patient is performed supine, lying with one hand anchored under the buttock. By unloading the spine in this position, it is often easier to perform the stretches. Of course, proper stretching of the scalenes also requires pulling the head laterally to the opposite side at three different angles to localize the stretch to the three different portions of the muscle group. The chin must be tipped down, then straight, and finally up, while the patient is pulling laterally. The scalene minimus is stretched along with the posterior scalene with the chin down.

The scalenes are very susceptible to multiple perpetuating factors. In severe cases, most of the major perpetuating factors must be addressed. It is imperative to review again and again the corrective actions discussed thoroughly by Simons, Travell, and Simons (3). The perpetuating factors that may require attention include paradoxical respiration, body asymmetry, improper lifting, improper pillow height, improper lighting while reading, and numerous other factors.

Infraspinatus: Treatment and Stretch

The infraspinatus is the most overlooked of the first group of muscles. Its predominant referred pain pattern, down the front of the shoulders into the biceps, overshadows its secondary referral to the middle half of the vertebral border. This rare pattern is depicted in Simons, Travell, and Simons (6). This scapular pain pattern has been omitted in the Travell and Simons Trigger Point Flip Charts, Travell and Simons Trigger Point Pain Patterns Wall Chart part I, and the Gebauer spray pattern booklet IRMA—#1 and should be added by the clinician.

The referred pain pattern of the infraspinatus is similar to that of the scalene, and they overlap in the middle of the vertebral border. The distinguishing factor is the patient's inability to place the hand behind the back and reach up the spinal column. Infraspinatus participation in interscapular pain is much rarer (20%) than that of the scalene (80%). However, it often can be the last bit of the interscapular puzzle that needs to be addressed. This trigger point lies caudally, closer to the vertebral border rather than the spine of the scapula.

In the infraspinatus stretch, the patient reaches across the body at opposite elbow height, while holding on to a chair. The body is then turned away from the securing hand (Fig. 9-3).

Latissimus Dorsi: Treatment and Stretch

The latissimus dorsi muscle trigger points refer pain to the lower third of the vertebral border, (inferior angle) of the scapula, about the size of a fist. The distinguishing feature is a light pain in the back of the shoulder and down the

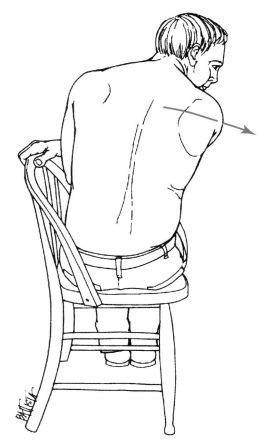

FIGURE 9-3. **Infraspinatus stretch.** The patient holds the back of the chair while seated sideways, and then turns the torso away from the back of the chair. The stretch pulls the scapula away from the spine and then lengthens the infraspinatus fibers between their attachments to the scapula and to the humerus.

medial arm (triceps) and forearm to the ulnar aspect of the hand, including the ring and little finger. The pain can extend across both sides of the middle back if both latissimus dorsi muscles are involved, and the pain pattern can be confused with that of upper rectus abdominis trigger points. The latissimus dorsi referred pain pattern includes the inferior angles of the scapula, whereas the abdominis referred pattern does not. The abdominis can cause nausea and vomiting, whereas the latissimus does not.

All parts of the latissimus dorsi must be stretched for effective release of trigger points, including the lower portion of the muscle that inserts onto the iliac crest near the quadratus lumborum. The arm on the affected side is stretched directly up above the head, while the opposite hand grasps the wrist, maintaining the upward pull while the patient bends at the waist, leaning away from the affected side (see Fig. 7-3). This stretch, when performed while leaning toward the side of quadratus lumborum trigger point involvement, can cause a temporary increase in referred pain to the hip. In fact, quadratus lumborum trigger points often coexist with latissimus dorsi trigger points, so the quadratus lumborum should be examined and

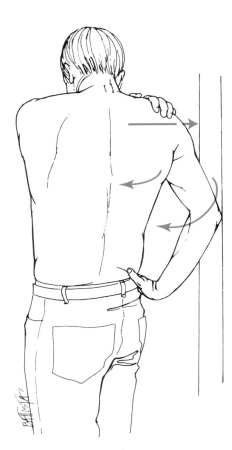

FIGURE 9-4. **Serratus anterior stretch.** The body is turned away from the doorway with the outside of the elbow in contact with the doorway and the hand at the waist. The body leans toward the door frame as the elbow is pushed further behind the back, and the scapula is pressed into further retraction.

treated if necessary in cases of middle back pain. And the latissimus dorsi muscle should be examined and treated when there has been persistent hip pain referred from the quadratus lumborum muscle.

Serratus Anterior: Treatment and Stretch

Trigger points in the serratus anterior muscle also refer pain to the lower third of the vertebral border, including the inferior angle of the scapula, about the size of two thumb digits. Distinguishing features can include a pain anterolaterally at mid-chest level, and sometimes there is a sense of air hunger, with short panting respiration. The size of the referred pain zone, small for the serratus anterior and large for the latissimus, differentiates the two. The intensity of the pain seems to be the same for both. A history of coughing deeply during a bout of bronchitis, pneumonia, or asthma is a clue to serratus anterior involvement. Deep coughing, even years before, irritates the serratus anterior more often than direct trauma to the side of the rib cage. Trigger points can occur on any of the serrations to the upper nine ribs, particularly numbers 3, 4, 5, 6, and 7.

The best stretch is to place one's hand on the hip of the affected side, contact a door frame with the outside of the elbow, and lean toward the door frame (Fig. 9-4). This pushes the elbow behind the back, passively stretching the serratus anterior.

Five muscles infrequently cause interscapular pain, and they are located in the interscapular space. It is clearly a mistake to focus on these muscles that reside in the referred pain zone and not investigate and treat the muscles that contribute but are located elsewhere. However, treatment of trigger points in these muscles may be necessary, once the other muscles have been investigated and treated, to fully eradicate the interscapular pain. The contribution of each muscle to the pain must be removed like layers of an onion, one at a time.

Lower Trapezius: Treatment and Stretch

Trigger points in the lower trapezius muscle refer pain in a narrow pattern, to the upper four-fifths of the vertebral border. Even though it is responsible 10% of the time, the trapezius has the distinction of being the most overworked muscle involved in interscapular pain. Pain practitioners spend 90% of their time treating and retreating this muscle. The most common location of the trigger point is in the superior portion of the lower trapezius muscle, very close to the middle trapezius (Fig. 9-5). When the lower trapezius trigger points cause problems, there is a steady burning quality to the pain rather than a severe ache.

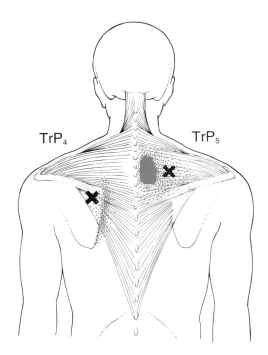

FIGURE 9-5. **Lower and middle trapezius trigger points.** The trigger point in the lower trapezius (left side of figure) is indicated by an X, with the referred pain pattern indicated by the dots.

Reprinted with permission from Simons DG, Travell JG, Simons LS. Travell & Simons' Myofascial Pain and Dysfunction: The Trigger Point Manual, vol 1: Upper Half of Body. 2nd Ed. Baltimore: Lippincott Williams & Wilkins, 1999 (fig 6.3), p. 280.

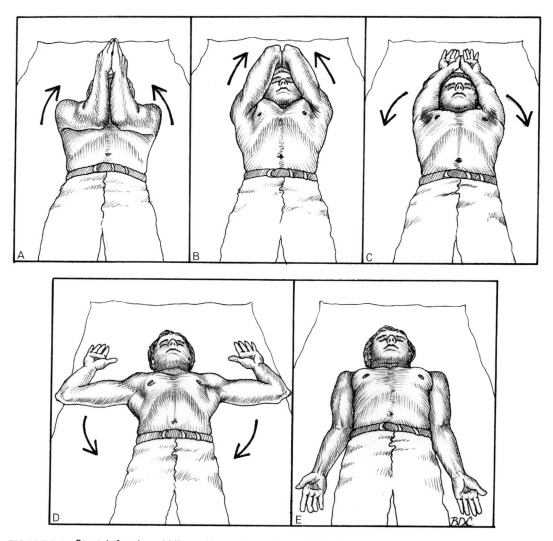

FIGURE 9-6. **Stretch for the middle and lower trapezius and rhomboid muscles.** Movements progress from **A** through **E** with a relaxing deep breath at the end before repeating.

Reprinted with permission from Simons DG, Travell JG, Simons LS. Travell & Simons' Myofascial Pain and Dysfunction: The Trigger Point Manual, vol 1: Upper Half of Body. 2nd Ed. Baltimore: Lippincott Williams & Wilkins, 1999 (fig. 6.15), p. 303.

One stretch is used to address the lower and middle trapezius as well as the rhomboid muscles (Fig. 9-6). This exercise also can be executed while seated. The scapula is fully abducted and rotated by placing the hands and elbows together in front of the upper body, pushing both of them upward above the head. An attempt is made to keep the elbows together until the end of the movement. After the elbows separate, the extension with the hands continues. Then the hands swing gently outward and downward in a graceful arc to the sides of the torso. When completed, the patient pauses and breathes deeply to relax. After relaxation, the sequence is repeated two more times.

Iliocostalis Thoracis: Treatment and Stretch

The iliocostalis thoracis trigger points refer a very light pain along the vertebral border and a medial pain into the inferior end of the scapula. A distinguishing characteristic can be a light pain in the chest below the nipples (Fig. 9-7). The iliocostalis causes problems 10% of the time, but because the pain tends to be slight, it might be overshadowed by more severe pain coming from the more frequently responsible muscles.

Two different exercises help to isolate and stretch the iliocostalis thoracis (Figs. 7-1 and 9-8).

Serratus Posterior Superior: Treatment and Stretch

The serratus posterior superior muscle trigger points refer pain to the upper half of the vertebral border. A unique characteristic of this referred pain is that the patient insists that it is very deep under the scapula (Fig. 9-9). Pain also can be felt intensely over the posterior border of the long head of the triceps, the ulnar side of the forearm, hand, and all of the little finger. The secondary pain patterns are

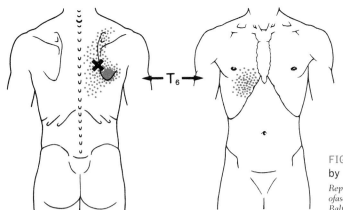

FIGURE 9-7. **Iliocostalis trigger point.** The trigger point is indicated by an X, with referred pain indicated by dots.

Reprinted with permission from Simons DG, Travell JG, Simons LS. Travell & Simons' Myofascial Pain and Dysfunction: The Trigger Point Manual, vol 1: Upper Half of Body. 2nd Ed. Baltimore: Lippincott Williams & Wilkins, 1999 (fig. 48.1A), p. 915.

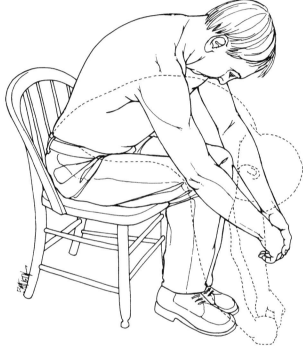

FIGURE 9-8. **Stretch for the iliocostalis thoracis muscle (paraspinal stretch).** The patient starts sitting in a chair and slowly bends over, lowering the shoulders toward the floor. After holding for seconds, the patient returns to the starting position.

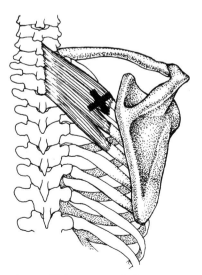

Trigger point palpable

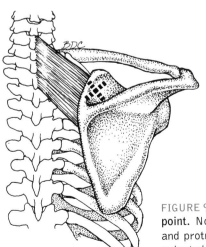

Trigger point not palpable

FIGURE 9-9. **Serratus posterior superior trigger point.** Note that the scapula must be abducted and protracted (left) for the trigger point to be palpated.

Reprinted with permission from Simons DG, Travell JG, Simons LS. Travell & Simons' Myofascial Pain and Dysfunction: The Trigger Point Manual, vol 1: Upper Half of Body. 2nd Ed. Baltimore: Lippincott Williams & Wilkins, 1999 (fig 47.1), p. 901.

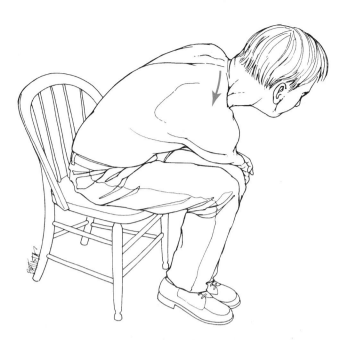

FIGURE 9-10. Treatment position for the serratus posterior superior muscle. The patient leans forward, using gravity to assist in the stretch, with the arm of the affected side drawn across the front of the torso and contacting the outside of the opposite thigh. With the rhomboid fully stretched and the scapula abducted and protracted, the clinician can apply vapo-coolant spray to the posterior serratus posterior and also may apply trigger point pressure release to the trigger points in this muscle that are otherwise hidden under the medial border of the scapula. With the thoracic spine flexed, the clinician increases the stretch by pressing the base of the cervical spine away from the affected side, and asking the patient to exhale. For self-treatment, the patient lies supine and draws the arm across the torso to achieve a similar scapular position, while applying a tennis ball (or, if necessary, a softer ball) to the trigger points in this muscle.

similar to those of the latissimus dorsi muscle. The secondary referred pain from the latissimus is light and not intense. Pain from trigger points in the serratus posterior superior may go untreated for a long time because the source of the pain often is not identified.

Treatment requires careful coordination between patient and clinician. The seated patient rests the arm of the involved side on the outside of the opposite thigh to abduct the scapula. The patient leans forward and drops the head forward slightly so the practitioner can push the base of the neck forward and to the opposite side to stretch the muscle. The scapula must be protracted and abducted to uncover the serratus trigger points beneath the scapula (Fig. 9-10). A similar treatment position can be accomplished by having the patient lean forward and hold onto a chair rung below the chair seat. The serratus posterior superior is palpated through the trapezius and rhomboid muscles. The trigger points often underlie the top quarter of the scapula. In more than 100 affected cases, there was some anatomic and trauma variation, so some trigger points often are found

under the top two-thirds of the scapula. Once the palpable trigger point has been found, the patient flexes the thoracic spine, and exhales deeply (this increases the stretch and makes the chest cavity slightly smaller) while the practitioner performs the trigger point pressure release. Minor changes in the flexion of the thoracic spine, the degree of protraction of the scapula, and the exhalation change the relative tension between the posterior serratus superior and the overlying muscle tissue, so that different trigger points can be palpated and treated. The trigger point pressure release of the trigger point against an underlying rib is often painful and takes the patient's breath away. However, if proper identification and treatment of the trigger point is executed, the patient will immediately experience less pain, more freedom of movement, and less noise in the scapula area.

Thoracic Multifidi: Treatment and Stretch

The thoracic multifidi trigger points refer pain to the middle half of the vertebral border of the scapula. Most of this large referred pain zone is toward the ipsilateral spine, with a slight spillover to the contralateral side. The trigger points in this muscle limit the extension and rotation of the thoracic region, producing weakness. The other nine muscles discussed here do not cause this particular muscle weakness.

The best way to find the offending trigger points is during the corrective stretch (Fig. 9-11). The seated patient

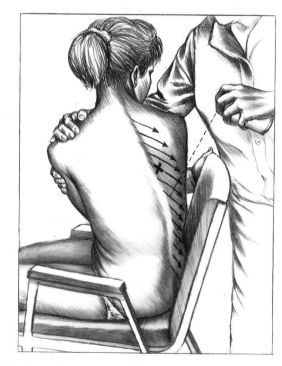

FIGURE 9-11. Treatment and stretch position for the thoracic multifidi. The seated patient's spine is flexed and simultaneously rotated, turning the torso and face to the affected side. The patient may feel more stretch by extending the leg on the affected side.

Reprinted with permission from Simons DG, Travell JG, Simons LS. Travell & Simons' Myofascial Pain and Dysfunction: The Trigger Point Manual, vol 1: Upper Half of Body. 2nd Ed. Baltimore: Lippincott Williams & Wilkins, 1999 (fig. 48.7), p. 928.

flexes forward and rotates the head and torso to look toward the affected side. The leg of the affected side can be extended to increase the stretch on the paraspinal muscles. The clinician's fingers are kept close to the spine, palpating the transverse processes through the superficial paraspinals, seeking trigger point nodules on the multifidi processes.

Rhomboid: Treatment and Stretch

The rhomboid muscle trigger points refer pain to the middle half of the vertebral border between the scapula and the paraspinal muscles. A slight additional pain can extend over the superior spinous area of the scapula. The rhomboids share a similar pain pattern on the vertebral border with the scalene, infraspinatus, middle trapezius, and iliocostalis thoracis. The rhomboid trigger points refer no pain to the upper arm as do the scalenes and infraspinatus muscles. The iliocostalis can refer a light pain into the chest and inferior end of the scapula, whereas the rhomboids do not. At rest, the rhomboids produce a superficial pain that is not influenced by ordinary movements. The steady burning pain referred by the trapezius is affected by movement. However, movements of the rhomboids can produce snapping and crunching noises. Pain is often not identified as originating in this muscle, until trigger points in the neighboring involved muscles, such as the levator scapula and trapezius, have been inactivated. The corrective stretch is the same as that for the middle and lower trapezius.

CONCLUSION

Technique 9-1 shows the application of the investigative process described in this chapter, to treat a very complex case of composite myofascial interscapular pain. Through the use of the approach described, treatment efforts are appropriately focused on the source and most often the multiple sources of the patient's pain. The muscles that are found to have active trigger points that refer pain to the interscapular area are systematically treated, and the pain tends to localize progressively, until the pain has been eliminated. Then the patient is given stretches of those muscles that required treatment to eliminate the pain. Attention is also focused on the perpetuating factors that can affect these same muscles. Thus the clinician has a focused and efficient treatment approach that often produces dramatic and lasting relief in only a few sessions even in those patients who have been suffering with interscapular pain for many years and have unsuccessfully sought care from many other health practitioners.

TECHNIQUE 9-1

Application of Trigger Point Pressure Release: A Diagnostic Sequence

Over the years, a clinician has presented and demonstrated at many public meetings, where volunteers from the audience have been helped with their myofascial problems. A particularly dramatic incident occurred when a volunteer from the audience presented with a far more complex case than anticipated.

Mr. C.F., the volunteer, complained about a stiff neck and a right interscapular pain, pointing to the top of the shoulder. He stated he never had any trauma to the scapular area. He could not turn his head to the affected side as far as he could to the opposite side. This symptom indicated myofascial dysfunction of the levator scapula muscle, which was treated with myofascial trigger point therapy and then stretched. Immediately the head turned normally, and the patient said, "My neck pain is gone, but the scapular pain, though slightly better, is still there."

On questioning, the patient indicated that the pain had moved lower on the scapula, and there was additional pain on the outside of his upper arm. Palpating his right subclavian chest area indicated tenderness that was not present on his left. The right scalene anterior, medius, and minimus were treated with the same therapy and three slightly different scalene stretches. The patient said, "Wow, my arm doesn't hurt and my shoulder blade is much better, but something is still there."

The caudal trigger points of the infraspinatus were treated and stretched. The patient said, "That improved it a bit, but the pain is still there."

The remaining pain was now at the lower end of the vertebral border of the scapula, and was about the size of a fist. Treatment of the right latissimus dorsi trigger points resulted in the patient saying, "Most of the pain is gone, but a little spot is still there".

When the patient was asked to take a deep breath, he indicated that the pain increased. He informed the audience of severe coughing during a bout of pneumonia 2 years ago. The trigger points in his right serratus anterior, particularly around ribs 5 and 6, were treated, and the muscle was stretched. The patient's right hand was placed on his right hip, and his right elbow was abducted (pushed behind his back), stretching the serratus anterior. C.F. said, "I can breathe better, and the pain is all gone". The volunteer's pain pattern was clearly a complex composite caused by multiple trigger points in several muscles. When all of these muscles were investigated and treated, the volunteer experienced total relief.

TREATMENT PROTOCOL

Table 9-1 serves as the protocol for the treatment of interscapular pain.

1. **Find the exact location of the pain on Table 9-1.**

2. **Check the list of distinguishing characteristics to see which apply to the patient and the specific location of the pain. Select the trigger point for treatment.**

3. **Treat the trigger points with trigger point pressure release.**

4. **Perform the corrective stretch specific for that muscle to achieve elongation of taut bands.**

5. **See what pain remains in the interscapular area. Select the next muscle according to the criteria in Table 9-1, and perform the treatment procedure for that muscle.**

6. **Investigate and treat the muscles causing the referred pain, beginning with the most superior and proceeding inferiorly.**

7. **Teach the patient to perform specific corrective stretches for each muscle requiring treatment.**

8. **If pain recurs, investigate and address perpetuating factors that specifically affect the treated muscles.**

References

1. Spanos TG. Informal research in medical school libraries conducted by the author.
2. Simons DG, Travell JG, Simons LS. Myofascial Pain and Dysfunction: The Trigger Point Manual, vol. 1, 2nd Ed. Baltimore: Williams & Wilkins, 1999.
3. Simons DG, Travell JG, Simons LS. Myofascial Pain and Dysfunction: The Trigger Point Manual, vol.1, 2nd Ed. Baltimore: Williams & Wilkins; 1999:504–537.
4. Simons DG, Travell JG, Simons LS. Myofascial Pain and Dysfunction: The Trigger Point Manual, vol 1, 2nd Ed. Baltimore: Williams & Wilkins; 1999:491–503.
5. Hendler NH. The differential diagnosis of complex regional pain syndrome type 1 (RSD). Pan Arab J Neurosurg 2002;6:1–9
6. Simons DG, Travell JG, Simons LS. Myofascial Pain and Dysfunction: The Trigger Point Manual, vol 1, 2nd Ed. Baltimore: Williams & Wilkins; 1999:552–563.

10 *Low Back Pain*

Robert Gerwin, MD, Margaret Royson, DO, Roberta Shapiro, DO, and Lucy Whyte Ferguson, DC, with contributions by Shannon Goossen, AP, CMTPT, and Arnold Graham Smith, MD

INTRODUCTION

Low back pain is a problem of major proportions in the Western world, affecting approximately 70% of the population during a lifetime, and approximately 15% of the population at any one time (1,2). The impact on the workplace is great, as roughly 1% of the adult population in the United States has a back-related permanent disability, and another 1% has a back-related temporary disability. The relapse rate of low back pain is high, approximately 70% to 80%, with roughly 5% of cases developing chronic low back pain lasting 3 months or longer (3). The prevalence of chronic benign pain, which is pain without a link to a specific identifiable cause, is estimated to be 15% (4). No figures accurately describe the prevalence and incidence of low back pain that is primarily muscular, but muscular involvement (i.e., the presence of comorbid myofascial pain syndrome of the low back, abdominal, pelvic, and hip region muscles) appears to be very common in low back pain of all causes. Many chronic benign pain patients or patients with "nonspecific" back pain *may* have myofascial pain syndrome (MPS), because this condition is under-diagnosed.

LOW BACK PAIN: BACKGROUND

The Problem of Diagnosis

Lower back pain can arise from many sources or structures and actually comprises a number of separate and sometimes overlapping conditions, each of which may require a different therapeutic and rehabilitative approach (5). Nachemson and Vingard (6) point out that in common back pain conditions, few patients have a well-defined disorder. After 1 month, only 15% had a definable disease or injury. Although the percentage is higher after 3 months, it is still low. More than 50 different entities have been identified as causing neck and back pain (6). Unfortunately, neither Fordyce nor Nachemson and Vingard recognize referred pain from muscle as a cause of acute or chronic low back pain, ostensibly because MPS has not been proved pathoanatomically (7).

Besides internal organ disorders (intestines, prostate, uterus, and kidneys) that can refer pain into the lower back, a number of pain-generating structures are found in the lower back itself. The lumbar discs can generate pain through pressure on nerve roots, though only when the nerve has been injured and is either inflamed or demyelinated (8,9). Furthermore, pain-sensitive fibers are found in the annulus of each disc, so that injury to the disc and disruption of the annulus can generate pain (10). The lumbar zygapophyseal or facet joints are supplied by nociceptive (pain) sensory fibers (11,12), as is true also of the sacroiliac joints (SIJ) (13). The SIJ have been demonstrated to cause significant chronic pain (14).

The complexity of this picture is increased by the fact that significant disc disorders are frequently identified in asymptomatic individuals in all age groups, including both the young and the older population (15). Moreover, we know from clinical experience that the presence of degenerative joint disease may increase the likelihood of low back injury from lifting and other vigorous activities, but it is not usually the explanation for the chronic cases of low back pain. In other words, the presence and degree of degenerative change does not necessarily correlate with the degree of low back pain. Efforts to treat myofascial involvement and joint dysfunction in patients with significant degenerative joint disease often result in the resolution or improvement of chronic low back pain, although the degenerative arthritis is still present.

Treatment of low back pain is increased by the fact that MPS refers pain into other structures in the lower back. For example, trigger points in the quadratus lumborum, gluteus medius, piriformis, longissimus thoracis, multifidi, and even a muscle as distant as the soleus can refer pain into the sacroiliac joint. The superficial and deep paraspinals, particularly the multifidi, the iliopsoas, and sometimes the abdominals, can refer pain into the lumbar facets, and the gluteus minimus can refer pain into the buttock, thigh, and leg that mimics either an L5 or an S1 radicular distribution (16,17). Furthermore, joint dysfunction or nerve damage in the lumbar facet joints and in the sacroiliac joints can refer pain into other areas of the lower back and into the buttock, thigh, and groin (14). Thus, the presence of pain in a specific location does not clearly indicate the structure that is the source of that pain.

The fact that facet injection (zygapophyseal or facet joint medial branch blocks) can fail to provide clinical relief may indicate that the zygapophyseal joint was not the source of the pain in the first place, that the procedure cannot reliably provide long-term relief (18), or that another comorbid cause of the pain is present, such as a MPS that maintains the pain pattern even when the facet joint source of pain is successfully alleviated. Likewise, most myofascially oriented clinicians have successfully treated patients with "failed low back surgery syndrome." Sometimes it appears that the surgery was performed as an unsuccessful attempt to treat pain that was in fact arising from myofascial and articular dysfunction. In other cases, the surgery did result in successful restoration of reflex function and decreased weakness, but the residual and sometimes very significant pain apparently arose from the presence of untreated MPS and articular dysfunction.

Conventional Treatment Approaches

Continuing advances are occurring in treating disc disorders, facet injuries, nerve injuries, and related disorders. However, the most controversial condition in the field of low back rehabilitation is **nonspecific back pain,** defined as a persistent pain condition in which the source of the pain is not readily identifiable through such studies as radiographs, magnetic resonance imaging (MRI), or electromyography (EMG). Functional restoration has been advocated in the rehabilitation of individuals with nonspecific back pain, and the bed rest approach has been fully discredited. All too often the concept of functional restoration results in prescribing exercises of increasing vigor, while ignoring the patient's complaints of increasing pain. Furthermore, the exercise that is often prescribed uses muscles that have active trigger points or joints that have articular dysfunction, and, therefore, an increase in pain is quite predictable. For example, even though studies have shown that abdominal exercises are very helpful for many patients with lower back pain, they dramatically increase the back pain of patients who have active abdominal and iliopsoas trigger points. The practitioner who fails to find the source of the back pain and has a general prescription for all patients with nonspecific back pain often will overlook readily treatable sources of pain, with disastrous consequences. The myofascially trained practitioner often assesses and treats patients whose problems have been compounded by this neglect.

Psychological factors that lead to low back pain and disability in the person with so-called nonspecific back pain certainly must be considered (19). Job dissatisfaction plays a major role in long-term disability caused by low back pain. However, psychological factors should not be accepted as the cause of low back pain to the exclusion of physical causes. Myofascial syndromes of low back pain should be considered, especially in cases of nonspecific low back pain, because they can be diagnosed by physical examination done by trained examiners, and they can occur in the absence of radiologic abnormalities. MPS may be overlooked by an examiner focused on skeletal abnormalities, neurologic impairments, or psychological issues. In the absence of either orthopaedic or neurologic impairments, low back pain may be termed nonspecific, and psychological factors may be blamed for the chronic pain. In fact, clinicians who are trained in the diagnosis and treatment of myofascial and articular dysfunction and their associated pain syndromes usually find that patients diagnosed with nonspecific back pain have *very specific* sources of pain which, in turn, dictate particular and individualized courses of therapy and rehabilitation. The job of the myofascial practitioner is not complete with the simple relief of pain, unless function has been restored fully, or at least to the extent possible. Functional restoration becomes a part of the overall rehabilitation of individuals in whom every effort has been made to identify and treat the source of their back pain.

A MYOFASCIAL AND ARTICULAR APPROACH TO THE TREATMENT OF LOW BACK PAIN

The physician must evaluate each patient for the cause of pain before starting treatment. Physical examination, laboratory studies, and imaging studies are done to identify causes of low back pain, such as metastatic cancer to the vertebrae or to the pelvic bones in women with a history of breast cancer, for example, or in men with a history of prostate cancer. This assessment must be comprehensive and include conditions that may be co-existent to identify those factors that affect and perpetuate the pain.

Some mechanical conditions necessitating consideration are associated with low back pain. Among these is pelvic torsion, which can be caused by asymmetric shortening of low back, pelvic, and hip region muscles, and sacroiliac joint dysfunction that alters the normal movement of the lower spine, pelvis, and hips and promotes the development of myofascial trigger points. Examination and correction of these conditions is important in the management of low back pain. Evaluation of the role of MPS in the genesis, maintenance, and presentation of these mechanical conditions is also important.

The practitioner beginning to work in the field of myofascial care of lower back pain patients may be frustrated by efforts to relieve back pain when treating the tender knots that are in or near where the pain is experienced. Many myofascial practitioners see patients who have received trigger point injections in tender points in their lower backs and believe that the trigger point injection process has failed because the patients continue to experience characteristic pain. In these cases, the trigger point injections may have been performed in tissues that are in the zones of referred pain but are not the source of the pain; thus, this treatment approach is doomed to failure. Effective trigger point treatment involves awareness of and examination of *all the possible myofascial sources of pain referred into the lower back*, with an attempt to see which trigger points in each of these muscles, when palpated, reproduce the patient's typical pain pattern. When all possible sources of myofascially referred pain are identified, a treatment approach can be developed to address these trigger points and to address the associated articular (somatic) dysfunction or subluxation. The treatment plan also addresses perpetuating factors, including posture, gait, work and sleep positions, as well as other nutritional, biochemical, hormonal, medical, and psychological factors that can affect the rehabilitation process. Articular dysfunction makes its own contribution to low back pain, as well as being associated with chronic myofascial involvement. Therefore, the successful treatment of both myofascial involvement and articular dysfunction or subluxation is essential when addressing mechanical or nonspecific back pain. Furthermore, because both myofascial and joint dysfunction accompany and aggravate other low back pain syndromes, successful treatment of these aspects may bring relief and decrease the need for more invasive and risky treatments. This treatment approach is very individualized; full treatment and functional restoration involve addressing many aspects of daily activity and lifestyle.

The case histories that follow represent a range of types of low back pain patients and demonstrate the complexities involved. The first case shows the relationship between myofascial and joint dysfunction in a patient with a relatively acute and simple back pain disorder, and shows the speed with which such a disorder can be resolved with a combined articular and myofascial treatment approach. The second case presents a more complex and chronic back condition involving traumatic injury, herniated disc with radiculopathy, and lengthy disability. The third case presents a back condition of 15 years' duration, much of it apparently arising from a myofascial disorder of the abdominal muscles, but with other myofascial and articular dysfunctions. The fourth case presents a back and hip pain condition with sciatica of 10 years' duration, with spinal stenosis. The last three cases all involved numerous failed or only partially successful therapeutic interventions.

CASE 10-1

Patient History

Mr. R.H., age 52, presented with a 3-month history of increasing right-sided low back pain. He was unaware of any inciting event, but acknowledged that his pain was at its worst when playing golf. He played three 18-hole games of golf per week and walked the course. He conducted no other exercise and performed no stretches. Past medical and surgical history was noncontributory, and the patient was taking no medication, although he had been taking acetaminophen and ibuprofen for his pain, with minimal relief. A lumbar MRI showed only mild diffuse degenerative joint disease consistent with his age.

Patient Symptoms

The right low back pain was described as a constant dull ache that intensified with twisting and lifting movements. The pain ascended from his lower back to the region he associates with his kidney. During the 2 weeks before being seen, his pain started to radiate to the left groin and buttock, without numbness, tingling, or paresthesia, and he had no bowel or bladder dysfunction. Pain interfered with sleep. Pain intensified when hitting the golf ball with a driver. His most comfortable position was either seated in a reclining position or lying on his back with his legs propped up.

Examination

Mr. R.H., a well-developed man, was in mild distress during movement and transitions. His gait was guarded but otherwise unaffected. The lower right ribs appeared to approximate the right iliac crest when standing, giving the impression of a lumbar scoliosis with convexity to the left. The iliac crests were the same height. There was a positive standing flexion test on the right (Technique 10-1). This suggested a possible restriction of motion of the right ilium on the sacrum, or a tightness of the right quadratus lumborum or left hamstring. The one-legged stork test, a more specific test for iliosacral joint restriction (Technique 10-2), was negative. The seated flexion test, a test specific for sacroiliac joint somatic dysfunction (Technique 10-3), was also negative. Passive range of motion was full in the lower extremities, except for end-range tightness in both hamstrings. The straight-leg raising test was negative bilaterally (Technique 10-4).

Strength was 5/5 throughout both lower extremities as well. Superficial sensation to light touch and vibration was intact, and deep tendon reflexes were 2+, equal, and symmetric. Plantar responses were downgoing bilaterally. There was no apparent leg-length discrepancy. The patient returned 2 weeks later and was pain-free.

The anterior superior iliac spines (ASIS) were symmetric, and the sacrum was in normal anatomic position. L1 through L5 were side-bent right and rotated left, except for L3, which was non-neutral, extended, and side-bent and rotated to the right. There was palpable shortening of the right quadratus lumborum muscle, with numerous tender trigger points that duplicated and intensified the patient's pain, including the referral into the groin and buttock. Significant muscle shortening also was seen, with trigger points in the right lumbar paraspinals, particularly the multifidi and the right iliopsoas muscles.

Diagnosis

The examination did not indicate any neural impairment, but rather a single articular dysfunction involving L3, a group somatic dysfunction of the lumbar spine, and a myofascial disorder, particularly of the right quadratus lumborum, the lumbar paraspinals, and psoas.

Treatment

Muscle energy techniques (Technique 10-5) were performed with complete correction of the lumbar structural dysfunctions, including the central nonneutral segment (Technique 10-6). Myofascial release was performed on all of the muscles listed above. The patient was instructed in an independent stretching protocol to be performed at least twice daily, particularly *before and after* playing golf. He returned 2 weeks later, reporting 75% improvement. On re-examination, there was a recurrence of the quadratus lumborum trigger points and the L3 nonneutral dysfunction. The L3 dysfunction was again treated with a muscle energy technique and the quadratus lumborum trigger points were injected and treated with vapo-coolant spray and stretch according to Janet G. Travell and David S. Simons' protocol (20).

Follow-up

The patient returned 2 weeks later and was pain-free.

CASE 10-1   Continued

TECHNIQUE 10-1

Standing Flexion Test

The patient stands with feet shoulder's width apart, and the examiner is seated behind the patient. The examiner's thumbs are placed under the patient's posterior superior iliac spines (PSIS). The patient is asked to flex forward from the waist (see figure). The examiner follows the motion of each PSIS and determines which of the two moves more toward the patient's head or cephalad. This is the side of the positive standing flexion test, and indicates the side of the iliosacral somatic dysfunction to be treated. (Pelvic landmarks are shown in Fig 10-1.)

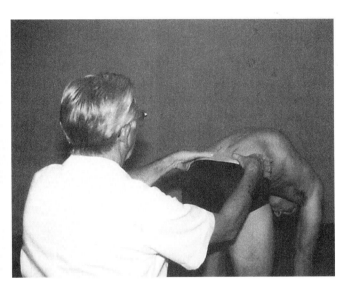

Standing flexion test.

Reprinted with permission from Greenman PE. Principles of Manual Medicine, 3rd Ed. Baltimore: Lippincott Williams & Wilkins, 2003 (fig. 17.6), p. 345.

TECHNIQUE 10-2

One-Legged Stork Test

The patient stands with feet shoulder's width apart. Standing behind the patient, the examiner places one thumb under the PSIS being examined, and the other thumb just medial to that PSIS, on the sacral base. The patient is asked to raise the knee on the side being examined. A normal or negative test result would involve the thumb on the PSIS moving inferior to the thumb on the sacral base as the knee is lifted. A positive or abnormal response would be for the thumb under the PSIS to move cephalad or superior to the thumb on the sacral base, as shown in the figure. The right ilium would be considered hypomobile in its movement on the sacrum.

(continues)

CASE 10-1   Continued

TECHNIQUE 10-2

One-Legged Stork Test   (*Continued*)

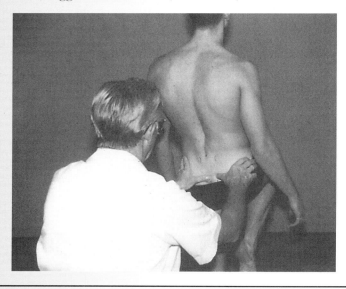

One-legged stork test.

Reprinted with permission from Greenman PE. Principles of Manual Medicine, 3rd Ed. Baltimore: Lippincott Williams & Wilkins, 2003 (fig. 17.12), p. 347.

TECHNIQUE 10-3

Seated Flexion Test

The patient is seated on a stool with both feet on the floor. The examiner kneels behind the patient with thumbs under each PSIS. After the examiner's thumbs are in place, the patient is asked to bend forward (see figure). The examiner observes which of the PSIS moves first and furthest away from the examiner. This is considered the side of the sacral somatic dysfunction.

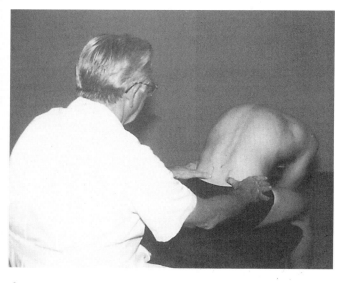

Seated flexion test.

Reprinted with permission from Greenman PE. Principles of Manual Medicine, 3rd Ed. Baltimore: Lippincott Williams & Wilkins, 2003 (fig. 17.17), p. 349.

CASE 10-1 Continued

TECHNIQUE 10-4

Straight-Leg Raising Test

The patient is supine with both legs extended. The examiner elevates the patient's leg on the affected side to 35° to 70° (see figure, shown with solid lines). If pain or tingling is elicited in the elevated leg in the low back, buttock, or along the path of the sciatic nerve, nerve irritation is indicated. If there is a question as to whether the discomfort is related to the hamstring muscle being stretched, the patient's leg is lowered slightly to decrease the pain or pares-thesia, and the patient's foot is dorsiflexed (the Brag-gard test) (shown in dotted lines). If the symptoms reappear, the straight-leg raising test is positive for nerve root irritation as by disc herniation at L4, L5, or S1, because this test places tension along the sciatic nerve and the lumbosacral nerve roots. Hamstring tightness is felt in the posterior thigh, and dorsiflexion of the foot does not cause buttock or back pain.

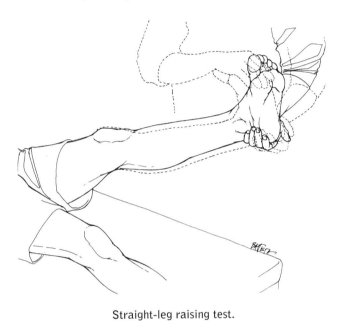

Straight-leg raising test.

TECHNIQUE 10-5

Muscle Energy Technique

This is an "active" technique in which the patient participates in the treatment and a "direct" technique in that the barrier to joint motion is engaged. The joint in question is placed in its position of greatest restriction without causing stress to the patient. The technique is used to restore a joint to its normal physiologic position. The practitioner places the involved joint into a position of greatest restriction and uses an isometric counterforce to resist the patient's efforts to move from that position. Only a slight force is needed to reset the barrier to motion, and the position is held for 3–5 seconds. This procedure is repeated 3-4 times until a full range of motion is restored to the joint. A passive stretch is added at the end of the treatment to relax the muscles attached to the involved joint.

CASE 10-1   Continued

TECHNIQUE 10-6

Specific Muscle Energy Technique for the L3 Single SD and the L1–L 5 Group Somatic Dysfunction

A **somatic dysfunction** (SD) is an impaired or altered function of related components of the somatic (body framework) system: skeletal, arthrodial, and myofascial structures, and related vascular, lymphatic, and neural elements (21). A standardized terminology has been developed by the osteopathic profession to name somatic dysfunctions. The SD is always named for the freedom of motion of the upper vertebrae of the vertebral unit. A vertebral unit consists of two vertebrae and the disc in between. The upper vertebra is off center and stuck in an eccentric position. For example, if L3 is side-bent right and rotated right and fixed in an extended position, the osteopathic diagnosis would be L3 E Sr Rr. This implies that the barrier to motion, or the position that the vertebrae does not go into easily, is L3 in flexion, side-bent to the left and rotated to the left. (Chiropractic nomenclature is somewhat different, but the terms can be translated. For example, the osteopathic point of reference for rotation is the body of the vertebra, but the chiropractic reference is usually the spinous process. When the body rotates right, the spinous process deviates toward the left.) . The clinician first contacts the extended L3 segment and palpates the limits of movement in different

planes. Flexion and extension are assessed by contacting the L3 spinous process and then passively rocking the torso into flexion and extension. The ease of joint play is felt by the examiner, and whether the spinous in question moves readily posterior with flexion and anterior with extension as much as the vertebrae above and below. Lateral flexion is assessed by placing the thumb against the side of the spinous process and determining the lateral to medial and medial to lateral joint play as the torso is rocked into lateral flexion. Rotation is assessed by palpating against the side of the spinous process and assessing how easily it rotates to the left as the spine and torso rotate to the right, and rotates to the right as the spine and torso rotate toward the left.

To apply a muscle energy technique to the L3 E Sr Rr SD, the practitioner places the L3 vertebra in flexion, side-bends and rotates it to the left, until the barriers or endpoints to motion are felt at L3 in all three planes (**A**). The practitioner stabilizes and resists at the L3 segment, and also maintains the torso position, as the patient is then asked to either side-bend or rotate right against the practitioner's resistance. Only one plane of motion, excluding flexion or extension,

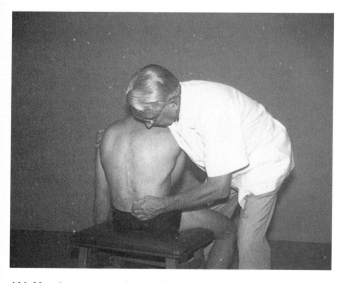

(A) Muscle energy technique for L3 extended, side-bent right, and rotated right (L3 E Sr Rr).

Reprinted with permission from Greenman PE. Principles of Manual Medicine, 3rd Ed. Baltimore: Lippincott Williams & Wilkins, 2003 (fig. 16.5), p. 313.

CASE 10-1   Continued

TECHNIQUE 10-6

Specific Muscle Energy Technique for the L3 Single SD and the L1–L5 Group Somatic Dysfunction   (*Continued*)

needs be engaged to apply muscle energy to a SD. Then the patient relaxes. Next, a new barrier to motion is engaged, as the clinician takes the patient further into flexion, left side-bending, and left rotation. This means that the joint would now move more readily through the previous barriers, because the muscle energy technique had loosened the joint and brought it more toward balance. The technique would be repeated 3–4 times and held for 3–5 seconds with each trial until balance was restored to the joint. The joint would then be in a more neutral position, be more mobile, and returned to its normal physiologic position.

Group somatic dysfunctions for the thoracic and lumbar spine involve side-bending and rotating in opposite directions, so the Group SD treated here involves L1–L5 in neutral position rather than extended or flexed, and they are side-bent right and rotated left.

The Muscle Energy Technique for the L1–L5 N Sr Rl (Ll–L5, neutral, side-bent right and rotated left) group SD requires placing the group curve L1–L5 into

its motion barrier of left side-bending and right rotation with the patient seated. The clinician first contacts the side of the group of vertebrae and palpates the restriction of mobility. Then the clinician places the thumb along the left side of the vertebrae and side-bends the patient's body to the left and rotates the patient's body to the right (**B and C**). While the clinician maintains the body in this position, the patient is asked to attempt either side-bend right or rotate left against resistance. This is repeated 2–3 more times until the barrier to normal physiologic motion has been eliminated. This can be thought of as a slow-velocity, low-amplitude adjustment, rather than high-velocity, low-amplitude (HVLA), because the same motion barriers are engaged in both HVLA and muscle energy techniques but the rate of the adjustment is different.

In Case 1, in which there is a type II SD at L3 in the middle of the L1–L5 type I SD, the L3 SD would be treated first, followed by the treatment of the L1–L5 group SD.

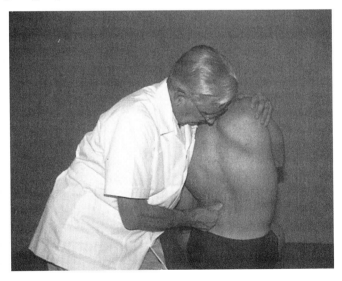

(B) Muscle energy technique to address a group somatic dysfunction L1–L5 neutral, side-bent right, rotated left (L1–L5 N Sr Rl). Back view of the procedure.

Reprinted with permission from Greenman PE. Principles of Manual Medicine, 3rd Ed. Baltimore: Lippincott Williams & Wilkins, 2003 (fig. 16.19), p. 317.

(*continues*)

CASE 10-1   Continued

TECHNIQUE 10-6

Specific Muscle Energy Technique for the L3 Single SD and the L1–L5 Group Somatic Dysfunction   (*Continued*)

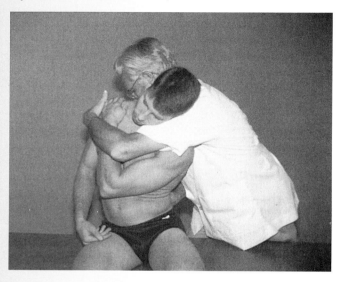

(C) Muscle energy technique to address a group somatic dysfunction L1–L5 neutral, side-bent right, rotated left (L1–L5 N Sr Rl). Front view of the procedure.

Reprinted with permission from Greenman PE. Principles of Manual Medicine, 3rd Ed. Baltimore: Lippincott Williams & Wilkins, 2003 (fig. 16.18), p. 317.

CASE 10-2

Patient History

Ms. A.B., age 42, had a motor vehicle accident 14 months before her examination. Wearing her seatbelt, she was driving through an intersection at approximately 35 miles per hour. Another vehicle struck the left front of her vehicle. Her car spun around approximately 180° and struck a traffic sign on the opposite corner. She denied hitting her head. She was transported to the hospital by emergency personnel because of her complaint of neck pain. X-rays of the cervical spine were negative except for straightening of the normal lordosis. Ms. A.B. was diagnosed with whiplash injury and sent home with acetaminophen with codeine and told to see her primary care physician. Her neck pain worsened over the next several days, and she became aware of severe low back pain as well. A cervical MRI was negative. A lumbar MRI showed a small right paracentral disc herniation at L4–L5. An orthopaedic surgeon prescribed the anti-inflammatory drug oxaprozin, the muscle relaxant cyclobenzaprine, and sent her to physical therapy.

Ms. A.B.'s neck pain gradually resolved with the stretching and modalities in physical therapy. Her low

back pain, however, continued to worsen and seemed to localize to the right, radiating down the right buttock, lateral thigh, leg, and occasionally into the big toe. Her right leg pain was intermittently sharp and shooting and associated with numbness and tingling. She reported performing what seemed to be an extension protocol in physical therapy, but she told the therapist that these maneuvers seemed to intensify her pain. Approximately 10 weeks later, she progressed to a strengthening program consisting of a "back school" and a weight-lifting regimen. She continued to complain of the same pain. She had discontinued use of the cyclobenzaprine on her own because it made her feel "spaced out." She continued use of the oxaprozin, but was unsure whether it helped. She ultimately failed the strengthening program because of persistent pain. She was treated with amitriptyline for depression and told she simply had to exercise and live with the residual pain.

Two other orthopaedic surgeons agreed that she was not a surgical candidate and recommended more physical therapy. She experienced temporary relief this time after the stretching and modalities program in therapy. She also tried three other anti-inflammatory medica-

CASE 10-2   Continued

tions, nabumetone, naproxen sodium, and choline magnesium trisalicylate. Again, she was unsure whether any helped. She was offered, but refused, narcotics. She made no more progress in therapy and could not tolerate a strengthening program.

A repeat lumbar MRI scan showed essentially the same right paracentral L4–L5 disc herniation, without further progression of disc herniation, nor any neural foraminal stenosis, nerve root compression, or effacement of the thecal sac. An electrodiagnostic test was positive for a right L5 radiculopathy.

The patient's medical and surgical history was significant for irritable bowel disease and two cesarean sections. Before the accident, Ms. A.B. had been employed as an accountant, but she was unable to work because of her pain. She was terminated from her place of employment 6 months after the accident and was embroiled in a dispute with her former employer regarding her worker's compensation benefits. She was also in active litigation with the other driver and insurance company.

Ms. A.B.'s MRI films were reviewed in the course of this evaluation. There was effacement of the right L5 nerve root by a disc fragment that was not previously noted. Also not previously noted was significant hypertrophy of the **ligamentum flavum.** There was also an outer annulus tear visualized as a high-intensity zone.

Symptoms

Ms. A.B. had pain with sitting and with walking for any appreciable distance. She complained of numbness and tingling down the right lateral thigh and leg to the big toe. She also complained of right greater than left low back pain and right buttock pain. Her most comfortable position was lying supine with her legs on a pillow. She denied bowel or bladder dysfunction or, as stated above, sleep disorder.

Examination

Ms. A. B. was in obvious discomfort. All movements were guarded and stiff, but her gait was intact. The iliac crests were level. Visible and palpable severe lumbar paraspinal muscle hypertonus on the right, and some on the left, were seen. There was limitation with almost no reversal of the normal lumbar lordosis, on attempted forward flexion. She had a negative standing and seated flexion test that was limited by decreased range in motion. The Stork test was negative. Passive range of motion of the lower extremities was full except for pain radiating into the right posterior thigh at 45° of flexion. Atrophy of the right extensor digitorum brevis was seen. Muscle strength was 5/5 except for the right extensor hallucis longus, which was 4/5. Sensation to light touch

was diminished in the right L5 distribution, and vibration was diminished in the right first and second toes. The deep tendon reflexes were 2+ in both lower extremities, and plantar responses were flexor. The innominate bones were in normal anatomic alignment, and no leg-length discrepancy was present. Significant shortening of the right paraspinal muscles with marked trigger points, including in the multifidi muscles, was found. Palpation of these areas duplicated and intensified her back pain. Trigger points also were identified in the right gluteals, piriformis, and tensor fascia lata muscles.

Diagnosis

The diagnosis for Ms. A.B. was lumbar disc disorder with L5 radiculopathy, complicated by right-on-right forward sacral torsion, and myofascial pain syndrome of the right lumbar paraspinal muscles including the multifidi, the right gluteal, piriformis, and tensor fascia lata muscles, which intensified her lower extremity symptoms.

Treatment

Ms. A.B. initially continued the anti-inflammatory and muscle relaxant medication. She was given a gentle flexion stretching program. Physical therapy included moist heat with electrical stimulation, ultrasound to the right L4–L5 level, myofascial release, stretching, and soft tissue mobilization. She underwent one lumbar epidural block and two selective right L5 nerve root blocks, which alleviated 80% of her peripheral complaints. She was left with a residual decrease in sensation in the right L5 distribution that was not painful. She continued to have localized right low back and buttock pain, as well as mild referred pain in an L5 distribution. She was found to have persistent trigger points in the right gluteus minimus that duplicated and intensified her lateral thigh complaints. She also had a right-on-right forward sacral torsion, which increased her lumbosacral lordosis (Technique 10-7). The latter was corrected with manual techniques (Technique 10-8). Trigger point injections were performed in the involved muscles, with large twitch responses delineated at each location. Vapocoolant spray-and-stretch was performed, and the patient was instructed in a postinjection protocol, as well as in a home program. She continued in physical therapy for an additional 6 weeks and successfully progressed to a strengthening program.

Follow-up

A 3-month follow-up showed continued improvement. Ms. A.B. ultimately returned to work 2 months later, 2 years after her accident.

(continues)

CASE 10-2   Continued

TECHNIQUE 10-7

Right-on-Right Forward Sacral Torsion

This is a right forward sacral torsion in that the *left* sacral base (the widest part of the sacrum that attaches to the lumbar spine) is anterior or rotated to the *right,* giving the left sacral sulcus (the groove between the sacral base and the PSIS) a deeper or more anterior appearance. To compare the depth of the sacral sulci, the examiner places thumb contact on each sul-

cus (**A**), just medial to the PSISs. The inferior lateral angle (ILA) of the sacrum is the point on the lateral surface of the sacrum at the level of the fifth sacral vertebra. The thumbs are placed at each ILA to compare which is most inferior or caudal (**B**). In Case 2, the right ILA is angled more toward the patient's foot. Therefore, the side of a deep sacral sulcus and the side

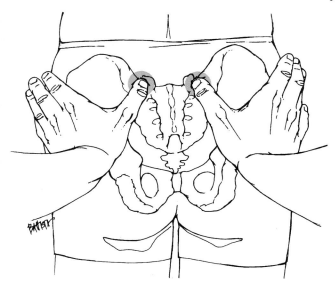

(A) Palpating sacral sulci.

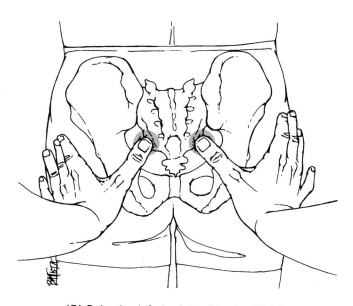

(B) Palpating inferior lateral angles (ILAs).

CASE 10-2   Continued

TECHNIQUE 10-7

Right-on-Right Forward Sacral Torsion   (*Continued*)

of the inferior lateral angle are opposite. In addition, the lumbar spring test (**C**) is negative. This means that there *is* forward motion to the lumbar spine when a

downward force is applied to it. A positive test would find little or no spring in the lumbar spine and is found in a backward sacral torsion.

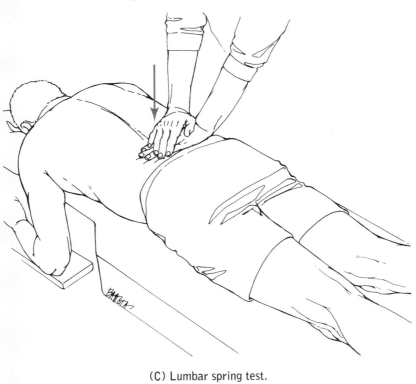

(C) Lumbar spring test.

TECHNIQUE 10-8

Muscle Energy Technique for a Right-on-Right Forward Sacral Torsion

The patient lies prone, with both knees flexed to 90° (Technique 10-8A). The patient's lower body is taken into a twist position with the right hip on the table, and the knees are drawn off the table slightly and the feet are lowered toward the floor. The patient is then instructed to reach for the floor with the left arm to lower the left shoulder closer to the floor. The practitioner supports the patient by leaning into the patient's knees while palpating the lumbosacral junction for motion created by the twist (Technique 10-8B).

The patient is instructed to attempt to lift the ankles against the practitioner's resistance, using 5–10 pounds of force for 3–5 seconds. The practitioner repositions the patient's ankles closer to the floor and

repeats this procedure 2–3 times until the tension in the tissue of the lumbosacral junction is reduced. This technique raises the more inferior right ILA to the level of the left ILA (Technique 10-8C). The patient is then asked to lift the left shoulder toward the ceiling against the practitioner's resistance, using 4–5 pounds of effort for 3–5 seconds. The patient's shoulder is positioned more toward the floor, and this step is repeated 2–3 times and held for 3–5 seconds for each repetition. This maneuver *pops* the left sacral sulcus posteriorly so that it is even with the right sacral sulcus (Technique 10-8D). The sacrum is now balanced, and the surrounding muscles, especially the piriformis muscles, will need to be evaluated and treated for trigger points.

CASE 10-2 Continued

TECHNIQUE 10-8

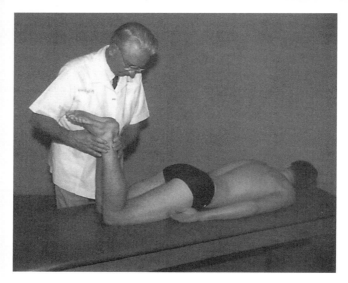

(A) Muscle energy technique for right on right forward sacral torsion.

Reprinted with permission from Greenman PE. Principles of Manual Medicine, 3rd Ed. Baltimore: Lippincott Williams & Wilkins, 2003 (fig. 17.76), p. 377.

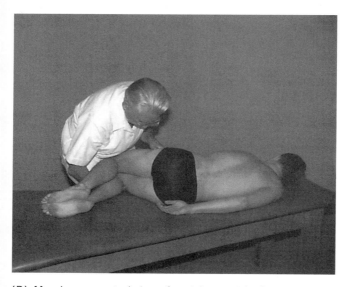

(B) Muscle energy technique for right on right forward sacral torsion.

Reprinted with permission from Greenman PE. Principles of Manual Medicine, 3rd Ed. Baltimore: Lippincott Williams & Wilkins, 2003 (fig. 17.77), p. 377.

CASE 10-2   Continued

TECHNIQUE 10-8

Right-on-Right Forward Sacral Torsion (*Continued*)

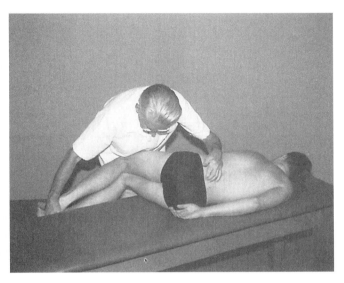

(C) Muscle energy technique for right on right forward sacral torsion.

Reprinted with permission from Greenman PE. Principles of Manual Medicine, 3rd Ed. Baltimore: Lippincott Williams & Wilkins, 2003 (fig. 17.79), p. 378.

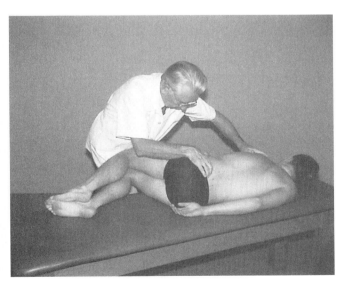

(D) Muscle energy technique for right on right forward sacral torsion.

Reprinted with permission from Greenman PE. Principles of Manual Medicine, 3rd Ed. Baltimore: Lippincott Williams & Wilkins, 2003 (fig. 17.78), p. 377.

(*continues*)

CASE 10-3

Patient History

Ms. F.R., age 48, had chronic back pain for 15 years. She had several falls as a child but could remember no incident or injury associated with the onset of back pain. She previously had a negative neurologic evaluation for pain and numbness radiating down her left leg, which eventually abated. She had a cesarean section for the delivery of twins 15 years previously. A hysterectomy was performed 2 years later. Interstitial cystitis was diagnosed 3 years before evaluation and was fairly well controlled by dietary restriction. She saw several medical doctors for treatment of her back pain, including an orthopaedic surgeon. She engaged in physical therapy, but the exercises bothered her. She saw two chiropractors, one of whom helped a "little bit."

Symptoms

Ms. F.R. had pain in the lumbar area, across her low back. In the 3 months before evaluation, the pain significantly increased with sitting and spread into her midback and around to her chest. For the previous 9 months, she felt pain in her left side, radiating to her left abdomen at the costal margin. She also experienced neck pain and had developed severe headaches, radiating into both temples.

Examination Findings

The right iliac crest was higher and more forward than the left when standing, with the right shoulder lower than the left. Her ears appeared even. There was a slight flattening of the lumbar lordosis, with a fairly acute lumbosacral angle, rounding forward of the shoulders, and forward carriage of the head. All of the lumbar vertebrae were tender to percussion. Heel and toe gait were normal. Thoracolumbar flexion was limited to 75° and caused pain at the lumbosacral and thoracolumbar juncture. Back extension was full but caused pain in the left mid-abdomen. Right and left lateral flexion were normal but caused pain in the left flank. Left rotation caused pain all the way down the spine, from the interscapular area to the sacrum. Rotation to the right caused pain in the same areas, but not as severe. Patellar and Achilles tendon reflexes were equal and active. Valsalva's maneuver (Technique 10-9) caused increased pain at the thoracolumbar juncture. Seated leg extension was not painful, but seated thoracolumbar compression with lateral flexion to either the right or the left caused increased left flank pain. Supine passive straight-leg raising caused left low back pain with lifting of the left leg to 80°. Supine right leg raising to 90° caused pain in the lower back that was less severe than that caused by left leg raising. Dorsiflexion of

the foot to induce sciatic nerve stretch did not accentuate her pain or produce pain with the legs lower than 80° and 90°, respectively. Pain was experienced at the end of internal and external rotation of each femur. The left femur had 15° degrees less internal rotation and increased pain compared with the right. Resistive manual muscle testing showed weakness of the left psoas, adductor, and tensor fascia lata muscles.

Anterior-to-posterior joint glide (femoral head on acetabulum movement) was reduced in the left hip joint. The standing flexion test was positive on the right; the right ilium was superior (cephalad) and rotated forward and resisted mobilization. This signified a right anterior ilium **SD** (Technique boxes 10-10, 10-11, and 10-12). Sacroiliac joint mobility was restricted bilaterally. The seated flexion test was positive on the right, and the upper portion of the sacrum at the sacral base was recessed on the right (rotated left). The lower portion of the sacrum at the inferior lateral angle was posterior and inferior on the left, and a normal Spring test (good spring or anterior motion of the sacral base) signified a left-on-left forward sacral torsion. Tenderness and reduction of normal lumbar spine mobility were found at L5 in extension, on the left. The spinous process deviated to the right and the transverse process prominent and inferior on the left, indicating lateral flexion (side-bending) and rotation of the L5 vertebra to the left (L5 F, Sl Rl). The lumbar and lower thoracic spine deviated toward the left, producing a scoliosis with convexity to the left. There was also tenderness at T11, T12 with restricted joint mobility.

There was significant myofascial involvement of bilateral quadratus lumborum muscles, right paraspinal muscles from T8 to the sacrum, and more severe myofascial involvement of the left paraspinals, from the occiput to the sacrum. The right internal oblique and the left external oblique abdominal muscles were very tender and shortened. There was bilateral myofascial

TECHNIQUE 10-9

Valsalva's Maneuver

This technique is used to increase pressure in the intrathecal space. If there is a herniated disc protruding into the spinal canal, Valsalva's maneuver will enhance the pressure into that space and cause pain. The patient is seated and asked to inhale, hold the breath and bear down as if trying to have a bowel movement. The test is positive if it creates back pain or pain down the leg.

CASE 10-3 Continued

TECHNIQUE 10-10

Dominant Eye Test

Before diagnosing somatic dysfunctions, it is important to know which eye of the examiner is dominant, because this is used in testing structural asymmetries and distortions. The examiner places the index finger and thumb together and makes a circle (as if making the hand signal "OK.") With both eyes open, the examiner looks through the circle at a clock or other stationary object (see figure, part A). The object must be seen equally by both eyes. Then the examiner closes one eye and looks with the open eye, to see whether the object remains within the circle. If it did, the eye that remained open is the dominant eye. (The object would appear nearly identical with the one eye as it did with both eyes in the figure, part A.) Repeat this procedure with the dominant eye closed and the other eye open, and the object should no longer appear within the circle (figure, part B).

In evaluating a patient for a structural asymmetry, such as whether one ilium is more anterior than the other, the dominant eye is placed over the midline of the patient. A left-eye-dominant person would stand on the left side of the supine patient. If the patient were lying prone, a right-eye-dominant person would stand to the left of the patient to have the right eye over the midline of the patient. The left-eye-dominant person would stand to the right of the prone patient.

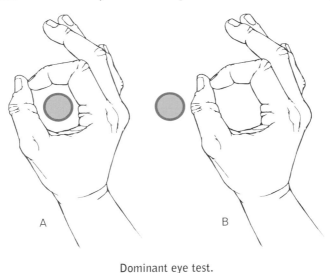

A   B

Dominant eye test.

TECHNIQUE 10-11

Anterior Iliac Dysfunction

An anterior iliac SD is diagnosed by first establishing on which side the standing flexion test is positive. For example, in Case 3, the standing flexion test was positive on the right. This signifies that the right ilium would be evaluated for an anterior (inferior) or posterior (superior) rotation. It was found that the right ilium was anterior and rotated toward the supine patient's right foot. A right-eye-dominant person would stand to the right of a supine patient and place the thumbs on both ASISs; that is, the practitioner's left thumb would be just under the right ASIS. The practitioner's right thumb would be just under the left ASIS. The practitioner, if right eye dominant, would focus the right eye over the midline of the patient. In this case, the right ilium was found to be lower (caudad) or more anterior than the left. In other words, the practitioner's left thumb was lower, more anterior and toward the patient's right foot. This anterior rotation of the right ilium is a somatic dysfunction that can be treated with muscle energy technique.

(continues)

CASE 10-3 Continued

involvement of the iliopsoas muscles, worse on the left, and there was bilateral rectus abdominis muscle myofascial involvement, somewhat in the upper rectus, but with severe bilateral trigger points just above the pubic bone, in the area of the transabdominal incision from the cesarean section. Palpation of the trigger points in the left psoas, rectus abdominis, and quadratus lumborum muscles reproduced her back pain. Palpation of the trigger points in the left external oblique abdominal muscle reproduced the flank and upper abdominal pain just under the ribs. There were no significant trigger points in the gluteal muscles or piriformis muscles.

Cervical flexion caused pain into the left upper back. Extension caused pain into the posterior neck. Both right and left lateral flexion were limited to 60° and produced pain in the left neck and down inside the left shoulder blade. Biceps and triceps reflexes were

equal and active bilaterally. Cervical spine compression produced increased pain in the left neck. There was restriction of normal intersegmental spinal mobility with tenderness at C1, C2, C7, T1, and T5. Tenderness also was found at the left T4 and T5 rib/spinal joints, with restriction of normal joint play. There was myofascial involvement of the left pectoralis and infraspinatus muscles, as well as the left levator scapula, upper trapezius, and sternocleidomastoid muscles. Palpation of the left upper trapezius muscles and sternocleidomastoid muscles reproduced aspects of the patient's headaches.

Diagnoses

Major myofascial disorder of the left paraspinal, neck, shoulder, abdominal, and groin muscles with cervical, thoracic, rib, lumbar and sacroiliac somatic dysfunctions. She also had a left disordered hip complex. (For a

TECHNIQUE 10-12

Muscle Energy Technique for a Right Anterior Iliac Somatic Dysfunction

The patient lies prone with the right hip and knee flexed and suspended off the table.

The clinician stands on the right side of the examination table and supports the patient's knee by holding it in the palm of the right hand as the patient's foot rests against the clinician's left thigh. The clinician's

left hand is placed on the patient's right sacroiliac joint, and the heel of the hand is on the sacrum to fix its position (**A**). The clinician asks the patient to try to straighten the knee by pushing the foot into the clinician's thigh, using 5–10 lbs. of force for 3–5 seconds. The clinician resists this effort. The new motion

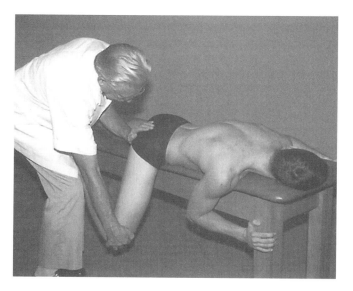

(A) Muscle energy technique for right anterior ilium.

Reprinted with permission from Greenman PE. Principles of Manual Medicine, 3rd Ed. Baltimore: Lippincott Williams & Wilkins, 2003 (fig. 17.67), p. 373.

CASE 10-3   Continued

TECHNIQUE 10-12

Muscle Energy Technique for a Right Anterior Iliac Somatic Dysfunction   *(Continued)*

barrier is engaged, and the same technique is repeated for a total of three efforts. The right ilium is reevaluated for resolution of its dysfunction.

An alternative to this technique is to have the patient in a *supine* position. The clinician asks the patient to bend the right knee and bring it toward the right shoulder. (If there is knee dysfunction, this technique can be modified.) The patient is then asked to position the head on the table so that the chin is tucked and the lower back is flattened against the examination table. The fingers are then interlaced around the right knee **(B)**. The patient breathes out and pushes the right knee into the interlocked hands with 5–10 pounds of force, not allowing the knee to move, while the clinician monitors movement in the right sacroiliac joint. After 3–5 seconds, the patient stops and relaxes. The knee is then repositioned closer to the shoulder (taking up the newly available slack) and the technique is repeated 2–3 more times. This is a muscle energy technique or isometric activity the patient can perform independently for self-care as long as there is no discomfort to the knee or the back.

The anterior ilium is repositioned with these maneuvers and placed in balance with the left ilium. The clinician rechecks both ASIS to assess that they are balanced.

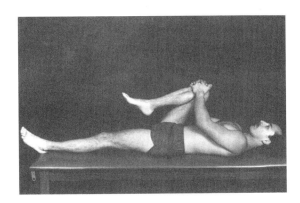

(B) Muscle energy technique for right anterior ilium.
Reprinted with permission from DiGiovanna EL, Schiowitz S. An Osteopathic Approach to Diagnosis and Treatment, 2nd Ed. Philadelphia: Lippincott-Raven, 1997 (fig. 11.30), p. 192.

full discussion of evaluation of the disordered hip complex, see Chapter 11.)

Treatment

Treatment consisted of myofascial release techniques applied to the muscles of the back, groin, and abdomen. Emphasis was placed on rotating the right ilium posteriorly, and pulling the left sacrum and pelvis forward, and then stretching the left lumbar spine away from the pelvis. Particular attention was paid to releasing the portions of the abdominal muscles, the left psoas, and the left quadratus lumborum that had been reproducing the back pain. Myofascial release techniques were also performed on the involved neck, shoulder, and upper back muscles. Moist heat was applied to the muscles after the stretching. The left femoral dysfunction was addressed, and gentle side posture mobilization was used to decrease the sacroiliac and L5 joint restrictions. Anterior to posterior osseous manipulation was used to release the middle and lower thoracic joint restrictions. Gentle osseous manipulation of both the upper and lower cervical spine was performed with rotation corrected in the setup, and a gentle lateral-to-medial thrust was performed that was well-tolerated.

[Note: It is not within the scope of this text to present the details of osseous manipulation, which requires considerable skill and training. Muscle energy techniques for correction of the cervical spine are presented in Chapter 3. The following muscle energy techniques are those that would be applied to this patient, according to the diagnoses stated: Right anterior ilium SD (Technique 10-12); Left on left forward sacral torsion, (Technique 10-13); and L5F, Sl Rl (Technique 10-14). The purpose of the presentation of these techniques is to acquaint the clinician with the importance of articular dysfunction or subluxation, so that appropriate referral can be made of the patient who is not adequately responding to care.]

The patient was initially given a set of gentle stretches to assist in her rehabilitation. More vigorous stretches were given as she improved. She was also encouraged to walk regularly for exercise. She was treated 19 times over an 8-month period. Her symptoms improved markedly. On her second visit, she stated that she had some relief of her back pain, but was still having the left abdominal pain. One week after her initial evaluation and treatment, she stated that she had some good days with little pain. Deeper muscle work was performed to release the abdominal trigger points, and she had

(continues)

CASE 10-3   Continued

TECHNIQUE 10-13

Left-on-Left Forward Sacral Torsion

The same muscle energy technique is used as that which is used for the right-on-right forward sacral torsion except that the patient's lower torso will be rotated so that the *left* hip is on the table. (The positions for these maneuvers are the reverse of those depicted earlier in this chapter (Technique 10-8).) The starting position is prone, with the knees bent at 90°, and then the patient's lower torso is taken into a twist and the knees are drawn off the table slightly and the feet are lowered toward the floor. The patient is instructed to lift the ankles against the practitioner's resistance. Then the patient is asked to lift the shoulder toward the ceiling against the practitioner's resistance.

TECHNIQUE 10-14

Muscle Energy Technique to Correct L5 F Sl Rl SD

The muscle energy technique previously described in Case 1 for the L3E Sr Rr can be applied to this lumbar somatic dysfunction. The exception is that in this SD, L5 moves more easily into flexion, left side-bending, and left rotation. Its barriers to motion are: extension, right side-bending, and right rotation. The barriers to motion constitute the position in which L5 would be placed, to move through its barriers to motion with a muscle energy technique. First the clinician contacts the hypo-mobile L5 and palpates the pattern of movement restriction. Then the spine is moved into extension until the tension is felt at L5. The clinician then takes the patient into right lateral flexion and right rotation (**A**). The patient is asked to either left side bend or left rotate against the clinician's resistance (**B**). After each repetition, the clinician takes the patient further into right lateral flexion and right rotation. The clinician reevaluates the joint mobility at the end of the procedure.

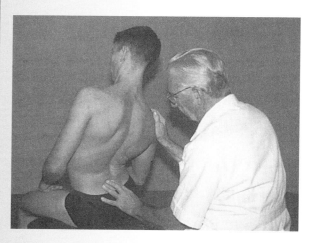

(A) Muscle energy technique for L5 flexed, side-bent left, rotated left (L5 F SI RI).

Reprinted with permission from Greenman PE. Principles of Manual Medicine, 3rd Ed. Baltimore: Lippincott Williams & Wilkins, 2003 (fig. 16.10), p. 315.1

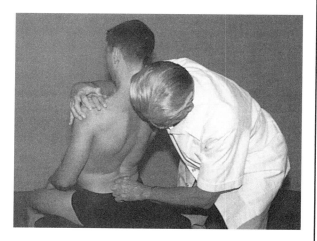

(B) Muscle energy technique for L5 flexed, side-bent left, rotated left (L5 F SI RI).

Reprinted with permission from Greenman PE. Principles of Manual Medicine, 3rd Ed. Baltimore: Lippincott Williams & Wilkins, 2003 (fig. 16.12), p. 315.

CASE 10-3   Continued

increased abdominal pain after that treatment but markedly decreased lower back pain. Gentle techniques were used to continue the abdominal muscle release. An upper respiratory infection then complicated her care, increasing her back pain with coughing and sneezing.

By her seventh visit, pelvic skew was decreasing but was still significant when she was seated, so an ischial lift was tried (a 3/8″-inch-thick magazine was placed under the left ischium.) This balanced the patient's iliac crests while she was seated. By her eighth visit, the patient had good release of lumbar and pelvic somatic dysfunctions. By her ninth visit, it was clear that the left quadratus lumborum was not releasing fully with manual techniques, so this was injected followed by manual care the next day. During the 11th through the 16th visits, her pain shifted mainly to her mid-back and neck. Prolonged sitting still aggravated her low back pain. The use of the ischial lift was discontinued because the articular and myofascial care had balanced the pelvis. Ms. F.R. increased her activity during the last month of this treatment sequence, experiencing some increased pain after vacuuming and cleaning house. She also had reported increased back and left-sided pain after traveling abroad. Examination at that time indicated a recurrence of left femoral dysfunction, which had been stable since it was treated on her first visit. Treatment to address femoral dysfunction and the associated myofascial involvement resulted in a dramatic relief of pain, and the patient's sequence of care was completed on the follow-up visit.

Follow-up

She had numerous episodes of increased back pain over the next year, associated with physical stresses, and requiring further treatment. Then she became mostly pain-free for almost 3 years. She was able to control any minor aggravations with her own exercise regimen. She retired from her job. When she had been in chronic pain, she had stayed at her job because it was a good distraction. She retired and enjoyed her retirement, and then decided to return to a less demanding job working with children. After almost 3 years without significant back pain, some back pain returned 2 to 3 months after her son committed suicide. She found that if she did not control her back pain with her home exercise and efforts to ameliorate her stress, she could not control her pain adequately.

Ms. F.R. received a great deal of care directed to her lower back over a 15-year period, but her condition did not really come under control until the groin and abdominal trigger points were addressed. The cesarean section and the myofascial reaction to it was a major factor in the initial development of her back pain, and to its continuation over the ensuing 15 years. If only the lower back is assessed and treated when there is back pain, patients such as this will fail to find relief.

CASE 10-4

Patient History

Ms. H.H. was 64 when she was first evaluated for her back, hip, and leg problems. She had been having pain problems in her back and both hips and legs for more than 10 years. No traumatic event precipitated her pain. Onset was gradual, starting with bilateral hip pain, right greater than left. Both prolonged walking and sitting increased her pain, and there was pain at night and leg cramping as well.

She took a variety of anti-inflammatory medications over a 10-year period and had physical therapy without substantial benefit. She engaged in a program of home exercise for her back as well. She experienced a significant aggravation of her condition, 3 months before her examination, that started during a car trip between New Mexico and California, when she developed increased back pain and right sciatic pain. After that it became difficult for her to sit in a car for more than 10 minutes. Over the past 6 months, she had four greater trochanteric steroid injections for chronic bursitis without benefit. She had a facet injection and an epidural block with only mild improvement. An MRI scan taken 2 months before examination showed lumbar spondylosis (degeneration of the intervertebral discs) with substantial disc space narrowing at L3–L4, L4–L5, and L5–S1 and stenosis of moderate degree centrally at L4–L5 with bilateral foraminal compromise. There was also a Tarlov's meningeal cyst on the right. Such cysts are most often considered to be non–pain-producing, but her physiatrist suggested that she might be a candidate for meningeal cystectomy.

Symptoms

Ms. H.H. complained of severe, constant low back pain, bilateral hip pain, pain down both legs, worse on the right, and more pain in the front than the back of the legs. The right foot was numb, and use of the right foot while driving was difficult because of increased pain

CASE 10-4   Continued

when using the gas and brake pedals. Nocturnal calf cramps occurred frequently and were made worse by swimming. Both walking and sitting were significantly limited by pain.

Examination

The right iliac crest was significantly higher than the left when standing, and the sacrum also was significantly and visibly displaced forward on the right. A slight decrease in the normal lumbar lordosis was seen. Thoracolumbar range of motion was normal, and pain occurred on back extension bilaterally in the upper sacroiliac area. Patellar and Achilles tendon reflexes were equal and active bilaterally. Valsalva's maneuver did not increase pain. A seated thoracolumbar compression with lateral flexion to either side did not increase pain. Seated leg extension on the right increased right thigh pain. Left lower leg pain and cramping of the left thigh were elicited by left seated leg extension, but there was no increase in back pain with these maneuvers. Supine leg raising was normal, as was Patrick's (Fabere) test for pain on hip motion (Technique 10-15). Weakness of psoas and tensor fascia lata muscles was present bilaterally, as well as weakness of the right posterior tibialis and the left gluteus maximus muscles with resistive manual muscle testing. The iliopsoas muscles were shortened and tender. Numerous tender trigger points were found in the adductor, vastus lateralis, piriformis, gluteus minimus, and tensor fascia lata muscles. The trigger points in the tensor fascia lata and the lateral piriformis reproduced the patient's hip pain. Quadratus lumborum trigger points reproduced her lower back and sacroiliac pain bilaterally. Tender trigger points were also present in bilateral medial calf muscles, including both the soleus and gastrocnemius muscles.

The right ilium was hiked cephalad and rotated forward, with the ASIS low on the right and the PSIS high on the same side. The sacrum was dropped forward on the right and flared posteriorly on the left, and the lower lumbar vertebrae followed this same pattern, but the rotation pattern was not as severe. Lumbar intersegmental spinal mobility was generally reduced, and the lumbar vertebrae deviated somewhat to the left, away from the hiked right hip. Bilateral tenderness and restriction of normal femur mobility in the acetabulum were found, with the femurs palpably in the anterolateral portion of the hip joint. (This mechanical pattern and its implications are addressed in Chapter 11.)

The patient also had very high arches and significant medial pronation of both feet, which were not corrected with her footwear.

Diagnoses

The diagnoses were spinal stenosis, with a severe myofascial disorder of the muscles of the lower back, groin, hips, buttocks, thighs, and calves; also with sacroiliac disorder, bilateral disordered hip complex, and lumbosacral spine hypomobility, complicated by severe foot pronation, and **pes cavus**.

Treatment

Treatment consisted of myofascial release of all of the myofascially involved muscles. The low back muscles were released in seated-forward flexion. The quadratus lumborum then was stretched by placing the patient on her left side with a pillow under her waist, her right arm extended over her head and the right hip and leg dropped posteriorly off the table. In this position, the right ilium was also pulled caudally and posteriorly. The gluteal and piriformis muscles were elongated, with the right thigh pulled both forward and back. The tensor fascia lata was also stretched in this position. While stretching these muscles, pressure on the trigger points was performed to assist in muscle release. With lumbosacral stabilization to prevent excess extension, the iliopsoas and adductor muscles were stretched with the leg straight and drawn into extension, and then into extension with abduction. The knee was then flexed and the stretch was continued, to release the vastus lateralis. Digital pressure to the trigger points also was performed during these and all of the other stretches.

The same or similar procedures were performed with the patient lying on her right side, with her left arm extended and her left hip and leg dropped off the table. In this case, however, she was asked to bring her right hip up onto the pillow, so that it was elevating the hip more than the waist. When the left piriformis was being stretched, the contact was not just to the muscle, but also to the posteriorly flared left sacral base, to mobilize it forward. When releasing the left quadratus lumborum, there was an attempt to lift the left lumbar facets and lower rib cage away from the pelvis, to decrease the functional scoliosis.

Both femurs were then released (see the Wishbone Procedure in Chapter 11). The patient was then placed in a prone position, and her posterior calves were stretched to lengthen the soleus and gastrocnemius. Pressure was used to release the trigger points as well. Moist heat was then provided, with the patient prone. Moist hot packs were placed under the abdomen, groin, and upper inner thigh muscles, over each side of the lower back, each lateral hip, and tucked around to cover the tensor fascia lata and piriformis bilaterally, and also placed on the posteromedial calves. After 10 minutes of

CASE 10-4   Continued

TECHNIQUE 10-15

Patrick's Fabere Test

This test is used to detect pathologic conditions in the sacroiliac joint as well as the hip (see figure). The patient lies supine with the knee and hip flexed, abducted, and externally rotated with the lateral malleolus placed above the patella of the opposite, extended knee. The examiner applies pressure to the patient's bent knee and the iliac crest of the opposite pelvis. If pressure on the patient's knee causes pain, this indicates hip dysfunction. If pressure on the iliac crest causes pain, the patient may have sacroiliac pathology. If both are painful, there may be concurrent hip and sacroiliac dysfunction. Note that the patient may have myofascial trigger points that make end range movement painful in this test, so this factor should be evaluated before a conclusion regarding joint dysfunction or pathology is rendered.

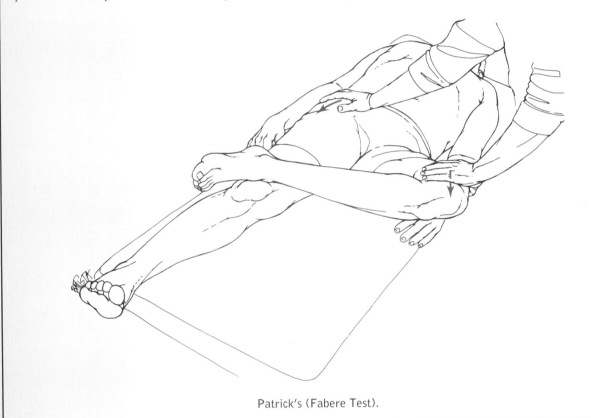

Patrick's (Fabere Test).

moist heat, gentle side posture manipulation of the pelvis was performed, with no impulse. (This maneuver could be considered a mobilization rather than manipulation, but the patient was so relaxed that **cavitation,** a popping sound, was produced.) The right ilium was manipulated to bring it posterior and inferior, and the left sacrum was manipulated to bring it anterior and slightly superior, thus derotating the pelvis. [Note: Muscle energy techniques to address the same restrictions are presented in this chapter, to acquaint the practitioner with the importance of improving restricted articular function.] The patient was then given home stretches to perform and was advised to purchase good supportive shoes and over-the-counter arch supports.

Treatment was tolerated well without excessive soreness after sessions. After three visits, delivered over 7 days, the patient experienced a significant reduction in hip pain and leg cramping. Treatments were given twice per week thereafter, and by the third week of care, Ms. H.H. was sleeping better, with less pain and cramping. Hip pain when walking was reduced, as was her buttock and lower back pain. The femurs were sta-

CASE 10-4   Continued

ble after the first treatment, and the skew of her pelvis was markedly reduced. Her mid-back was unable to accommodate the shift in the functional scoliosis, however, and some pain accompanied restriction of the lower thoracic spine. She had spinal/rib joint tenderness on the left, and left paraspinal tender trigger points.

There was a 2-week hiatus in care because of travel. Although she tolerated the car trip to the airport (over 2 hours) and the flight, she had 2 to 3 nights of increased pain afterwards. She experienced significant pain on the return trip. In the interim, she also performed a cardiac treadmill test, walking fast.

At her next visit, both femurs again showed dysfunctional hip complex and required release, and there had been an increase in myofascial involvement throughout. She again responded well to weekly care, and her hips were stable, the sacroiliac function improved, and the myofascial involvement markedly decreased. By 3.5 months into her care, her main remaining symptom was hip pain that was primarily nocturnal. Ms. H. H. was referred to a neuromuscular massage therapist experienced in specific trigger point release, and then was also referred to a medical doctor for trigger point injection. Trigger point injections were preformed into the piriformis, tensor fascia lata, gluteus minimus and vastus lateralis muscles. With these combined therapies, after 5 months of care, the patient experienced a 60% reduction in the severity of the localized trigger point pain in the hip and lateral thigh.

Although the patient's gait had improved, she was asked to acquire custom-made orthotics. These further assisted her to tolerate walking. She experienced one exacerbation after walking her dog; she did not tolerate the extension of her lumbar spine required to counter the dog's pull on the leash. Walking in deep snow also aggravated her condition a month after the trigger point injections.

She had a second session of trigger point injections and neuromuscular therapy that addressed the fewer and more localized remaining trigger points in the same muscles, and that also included the gemelli and obturator muscles in the lower lateral hips. After 8 months of treatment, Ms. H.H. tolerated a long car trip and walking on hard pavement and hills. Treatment frequency was reduced to once per month. By 9 months into her care, the hip pain had resolved sufficiently that it no longer affected her sleep. By 13.5 months into her care, she tolerated a 3,900-mile car trip and only developed some increased hip pain on the last day of travel. Generally, monthly care has been continued, because increased lifting, gardening, or other changes of activities exacerbate her pain. Pain is easily controlled, however, with a home exercise program and monthly treatments.

Follow-up

With continued monthly care, there has been no recurrence of the hip, back, or buttock pain in the 2 years since completion of rehabilitative treatment.

An Overview of Myofascial and Articular Treatment of Low Back Pain

As already noted, low back pain can arise from many different structures. Treating low back pain requires identifying the specific tissue or tissues involved in the pain (22). Identifying the configuration of myofascial and joint dysfunction that maintains stress on the painful tissues is also necessary. Referred pain arises from both dysfunctional joints and from myofascial trigger points. Therefore, it may take some time and trials of care to identify how much pain arises locally at the site of pain, and how much is referred from other structures. Balancing and stabilizing posture, elongating shortened muscles, and restoring normal patterns of mobility to joints are integral components of managing back pain, no matter which specific tissues are involved in the pain pattern. Identifying perpetuating factors that tend to decrease normal patterns of joint mobility and cause repetitive stress to myofascial structures is also essential in the process of treating low back pain.

For example, if an x-ray shows that a patient has significant disc degeneration in the area of pain, the clinician should not tell the patient that the pain is inevitably the result of arthritis. The lack of normal cushioning in the spine does make it more likely for the back to develop pain, and it also may take longer to get the back out of pain. Also, once the patient feels better, the lack of cushioning may affect the amount the patient can lift or the amount of impact the patient can tolerate without a recurrence of pain. The arthritis is not insignificant, but in the examination, the clinician looks for postural, muscular, and structural factors that are increasing the mechanical stress at the patient's pain area and at the site of the arthritis. If significant mechanical factors are found that increase stress at the site of pain, or that refer pain into the symptomatic region, then the clinician will see whether that pain can be decreased by improving posture, and by decreasing the sources of mechanical irritation, and decreasing the sources of referred pain. Significant mechanical factors and sources of referred pain are almost always present and need to be addressed. Once found, a course of care can be performed to treat these factors.

If pain resolves with treatment, the clinician teaches the patient how to maintain a pain-free state through exercise and self-care activities. If the pain does not change, the clinician reevaluates the patient's condition to discern whether other muscle or joint dysfunctions are present that were not previously identified. The clinician must consider possible missed diagnoses and assess whether treatment methods used to address muscle and joint dysfunctions have been effective. If normal joint or muscle function is not restored with manual techniques, other treatment modalities might be more productive. If the muscle and joint dysfunctions are corrected but recur, then the clinician will investigate perpetuating factors. The ability to simultaneously explore and reevaluate the patient continuously with regard to each of these issues characterizes the effective clinician.

The initial history and examination are only the very beginning of the diagnostic process. That process continues throughout the course of the patient's care. The process becomes easier if the patient can progress from constant pain to intermittent pain, because then the clinician can help the patient identify the perpetuating factors—whether physical, biochemical, or emotional—that may cause the pain to recur. The clinician must not become too strongly wedded to continuing a particular course of care, nor be dogmatic in defending a failing treatment protocol.

For example, if a patient is not making good progress with manual treatment of sciatica, an epidural block can be performed, and then the patient's manual care of the structural factors can resume within a few days. If structural and myofascial factors that are contributing to disc compression are improved, and the factors that are amplifying the pain are decreased, a patient may only require one epidural block to resolve a severe sciatica, whereas a sequence of several blocks might be recommended in the absence of manual care of myofascial and articular dysfunction.

When treating a patient with a major skew of the pelvis, a natural sequence of areas of restriction often will have to be addressed. Consider the patient who has the right hip or ilium pulled up and anterior, the left hip dropped low and posterior (the right ASIS will be lower than the left and the right PSIS will be higher than the left), and the thoracolumbar spine has a functional scoliosis with the spine dropping toward the low left hip. Releasing muscles that are hiking the right hip up and forward, but not sufficiently derotating the left pelvis, will likely result in increased pain in the left lower back or pelvis. If good balance of the pelvis is achieved quickly, the thoracolumbar scoliosis will rapidly come back toward center, with a significant increase in tension in the left paraspinal muscles and the iliolumbar portion of the quadratus lumborum muscle. The patient often will develop increased pain in the thoracolumbar region, around T10 or higher into the middle back. If the clinician can anticipate this sequence, treatment can address the factors necessary to avoid pain moving to a new location. If this is unavoidable, the patient often is reassured when the clinician explains the sequence to them and instructs the patient in what can be done for self-help and to continue the process of treatment.

The myofascial and articular relationships have to be addressed in tandem. The clinician needs to assess the shifts in the patient's pattern of dysfunction and pain to assist the patient throughout the course of care. The patterns of restriction are actually quite fluid. Although there are exceptions, the clinician should not need to perform the same procedures repeatedly when they are not successful. The successfully executed process of treating structural restrictions continually shifts the areas of greatest mechanical stress, and the process of investigating perpetuating factors helps eliminate sources of repetitive stress.

Causes

Taking an adequate history and identifying the circumstances and the time frame of the initial onset of pain are very important. The patient may not be forthcoming with this information. When asked how long they have had pain, patients will often respond "forever," or they may indicate that it has been there for their entire adult life. The clinician should ask patients to recall when they did not have pain and try to recall the circumstances involved in the first episode of pain. The triggering incident may have been a car accident, a fall from a swing, a football injury, a skiing accident, a surgery on the abdomen, a lifting incident, grabbing something to keep from falling, and so on. This aspect of the history taking is key to the focus of the physical examination as well as other evaluations such as x-rays or MRI. The clinician also should try to identify the circumstances that surround the patient's repeated episodes of pain or repeated injuries. Such episodes typically come about when the patient is under stress, even if only a minor lifting incident specifically triggers the onset of pain or a significant increase in pain. The clinician should determine whether the patient spends long periods of each work day sitting, standing, or walking, and how these factors affect the pain. Does the pain interfere with sleep, or is sleep disturbed for some other reason, that, in turn, causes the return of pain?

Acute episodes of pain often occur at times of increased stress. Some clinicians have focused on the idea of repressed feelings, particularly anger, as a contributor to back pain (23). Acute episodes of back pain, or marked worsening of chronic back pain, can occur at times when the patient's "foundation" has been shaken by a wide variety of experiences, including being in a near-accident that is frightening, being close to someone who is dying or has just died, losing one's job or feeling that there is a threat of losing one's job, making a major career move, or moving one's home, even if this is a desirable event. Identifying the role that fear, anger, grief, and depression can play in pain does not mean that structural, muscle, and joint factors are not present that also need be addressed to help to relieve the pain. The task of healing and preventing further painful episodes entails treating both the physical components of the pain and the psychological stresses together (24).

Cautions

The clinician must be careful to assess whether another disorder aside from muscle and joint factors is the primary cause of the patient's back pain, such as cancer, infection, abdominal aneurysm, digestive disorder, inflammatory arthropathies, and ankylosing spondylitis, among other causes. If nerve compromise is present, most often affecting the sciatic nerve, the status of the neural impairment must be monitored so that the patient can be referred for surgical intervention if appropriate, as when there is loss of muscle strength, or of bowel or bladder control.

Viscerosomatic Pain Syndromes and Low Back Region Myofascial Pain Syndromes

Visceral pain syndromes cause coexistent regional MPS, and a regional MPS can both mimic and aggravate visceral pain syndromes (25,26). Ureteral stones cause flank and low back pain. Irritable bowel syndrome and irritable bladder syndrome both result in local muscle wall pain. The pain syndromes result from segmental hypersensitization of the spinal cord. The muscles that typically are involved include the pelvic floor muscles, particularly the levator ani muscle, and the gluteal muscles and the quadratus lumborum in the extensor group, and the psoas and abdominal muscles in the flexor group. Adductor muscles are also frequently involved. Both the visceral component and the somatic component must be treated for a successful outcome.

Symptoms

The patient is asked to describe both the nature of the symptoms and their distribution. The pain may be sharp or dull, or it may be aching, shooting, boring, burning, cramping, or tingling. Pain may be very localized, or it may extend in a longitudinal pattern in the lumbar paraspinals, as can be seen from trigger points in the psoas muscle. A horizontal line across the back is often caused by referred pain from trigger points in the abdominal muscle. Pain or numbness may be present that radiates into the buttock, the groin, or down the leg. The pain can be diffuse and difficult to localize, as is typical of all somatic pain (as opposed to the precisely located pain of cutaneous stimulation), or it may be more distinct in a linear manner, resembling a radicular pattern. Limb weakness or bowel and bladder symptoms also may be present. The patient's primary complaint may be about low back pain. Therefore, the patient may forget to mention abdominal or groin pain because of such oversights.

Myofascial Entrapments

Piriformis Muscle and Sciatic Nerve Entrapment

The sciatic nerve passes ventrally and inferiorly to the piriformis muscle as they pass together through the greater sciatic foramen. A piriformis muscle that is shortened by contracted myofascial trigger point taut bands will of necessity have a greater cross-sectional diameter. In other words, it will be a shorter, bulkier muscle. Under these conditions, the sciatic nerve may be compressed against the edge of the greater sciatic foramen and may thereby be entrapped. One or both divisions of the sciatic nerve may pass through the piriformis muscle as an anatomic variant in approximately 10% of individuals. Theoretically this also could lead to an entrapment syndrome within the shortened, contracted piriformis muscle. The diagnosis of a sciatic entrapment syndrome is made clinically when the symptoms and signs of nerve impairment extend beyond the distribution of a single nerve root—for example, including the dermatomal distribution of both the L5 and S1 nerve roots—when there is no imaging evidence of root compression in the lumbosacral spine, and when pain is felt in the buttock and distally, but not in the low back.

Confirmation of a suspected piriformis entrapment of the sciatic nerve is obtained by a reversal of symptoms when treatment is specifically directed to release piriformis trigger points. A rapid way of confirming the suspected diagnosis is by injecting or needling the proximal and distal regions of the piriformis muscle to inactivate the trigger points and relax the muscle, and then assessing the degree of relief of the radiating pain down the leg and to the foot. (The central portion of the piriformis is not injected, to avoid trauma to the sciatic nerve.) Rapid relief that outlasts any local anesthetic effect is often achieved, thereby pointing to a role of piriformis shortening and compression of the sciatic nerve as a cause of pain. The problem is more complicated when there is both a lumbosacral radiculopathy and a piriformis muscle entrapment of the sciatic nerve.

Psoas Entrapment of the Lumbar Plexus

Another entrapment syndrome is that of the lumbar plexus by the psoas muscle, discussed in Chapter 11.

Myofascial Disorders that Mimic Entrapments

Two myofascial pain syndromes mimic sciatica and are a source of much treatment confusion. These pain syndromes may persist after a disc herniation or other pathologic condition is dealt with, or they may have been the original source of pain, and invasive procedures may have been performed to no avail because of an incorrect diagnosis.

Gluteus Minimus Trigger Points and Sciatic-Like Pain. Trigger points in the gluteus minimus muscle can present as pain radiating down the lateral or posterior aspects of the leg in the same distribution as L5 and S1 radiculopathy. Pain may present in the hip region, with referred pain, similar to lumbosacral radiculopathies. The diagnosis is made by identifying tenderness over taut or hard bands in the lateral hip region above the greater trochanter. Maintaining pressure for 5 to 10 seconds will result in pain referred down the leg. Inactivation of trigger points is accomplished by either manual methods (trigger point compression, stretching) or by intramuscular stimulation through needling with or without injection of local anesthetic. Eliminating the referred pain and the local pain by inactivating trigger points confirms the diagnosis. Attention must be given to precipitating and perpetuating factors, such as pelvic tilt from hemi-pelvis asymmetry and leg-length discrepancy, as well as faulty foot mechanics, to minimize recurrences.

Medial Hamstring Myofascial Pain Syndrome and the Inability to Sit. A recently described syndrome is the inability to sit because of pain located very precisely over the ischial tuberosity (27). The onset most often is insidious, although it can be abrupt and dramatic, as in one gentleman who developed pain while driving for 2 hours, but who had no prior symptoms. The problem is frequently seen in people with more widespread MPS, but it may occur as an isolated regional pain syndrome as well. In some cases, the initial pain syndrome was a pelvic regional pain syndrome (as discussed previously).

The history is that of an individual who cannot sit for more than a limited period. The limitation can be severe, as reported by one patient who said she could sit for only 7 minutes total through the day. In others, the limitation varied from 10 minutes to 20 minutes of sitting at one time. The pain is usually acute at the time of sitting, although in one individual the pain was delayed for 10 minutes after he stood up, after sitting for 10 minutes or longer. He knew that he could sit for no more than 10 minutes without developing the delayed pain.

The physical examination always identifies an upper medial hamstring trigger point that refers pain to the ischial tuberosity. The adductor magnus muscle is frequently, but not always, involved. The piriformis muscle also can be involved, but less frequently. The diagnosis is confirmed when inactivation of the trigger point results in an immediate increase in the time that sitting is possible. Needling or injecting the trigger points is the fastest way to inactivate the trigger points, albeit transiently, but long enough to confirm the diagnosis. Treatment is inactivating the relevant trigger points and treating of the regional and systemic factors that have contributed to the persistence of the symptoms.

Treatment
Evaluation and Treatment of Muscles

The evaluation of muscles starts with postural evaluation. If one hip is higher than the other while standing, usually the quadratus lumborum, the oblique abdominals, or the psoas muscles will be shortened on the side of the high or "hiked" hip. The paraspinal muscles and all three portions of the quadratus lumborum will be shortened on the concave side of a lumbar scoliotic spine. Weak abdominal muscles may be seen when there is excessive lumbar lordosis. Bilaterally shortened iliopsoas muscles may increase the forward tilt of the pelvis, like a bowl that is tipped forward to spill its contents. This posture in the pelvis will necessitate an acute lumbosacral angle and a lordosis localized at the base of the lumbar spine for the patient to stand up "straight." Such localized stress at the base of the spine can accentuate facet- and disc-related pain. Other individuals may have a loss of the normal lumbar lordosis, which is typically attributable to a shortening of the paraspinal muscles. Even when the more superficial portions of the paraspinals have been released, deep paraspinals such as the multifidus can pull the spinal joints together in a way that does not allow for the normal curve or normal mobility of the lumbar spine.

It is too simple to assume that everyone with back pain needs to learn to extend the spine, or to flex the spine. The clinician analyzes what combination of joint and muscle factors are restricting either flexion or extension and plans the appropriate intervention to restore the patient's normal patterns of mobility.

Assessment of standing posture, range of motion of the back while standing, heel and toe tandem walking, and balance is made to assess postural effects of weight bearing and the upright position. When the standing patient bends forward and the spine pulls to one side, the paraspinal muscles on that side are shortened. The clinician assesses relative tension in the quadratus lumborum muscles during side-bending to each side. Sacroiliac joint mobility while standing on one leg and raising the other also is evaluated. The clinician also observes the patient's gait while wearing customary shoes, including orthotics if they are used.

Paraspinal muscle tension also is assessed in the seated patient as the patient leans forward. Pelvic balance is assessed in the seated patient, because this will indicate the areas of joint and muscle dysfunction. The clinician performs other seated tests, such as deep tendon reflex testing, Valsalva's maneuver, and seated leg extension. The sitting position is also an excellent position for assessing the motion of individual joints. With the patient's arms crossed across the chest, the clinician rocks the spine into extension, flexion, lateral flexion, and rotation, and with the other hand palpates the extent to which each segment of the spine can glide freely into each of these positions. Even the gliding movement of the pelvis into extension at the sacroiliac joints can be evaluated in this way.

The patient is examined in side-lying position with a pillow under the waist, the upper arm raised over the head, and the upper leg dropped anteriorly and then posteriorly off the table, to allow access to the quadratus lumborum. In this position the clinician also can assess the degree of tenderness and trigger point activity in the paraspinal muscles. The clinician also evaluates the portions of the quadratus lumborum that are shortened with the hip and leg pulled forward and backward. If the hip is hiked on the side that is examined, the clinician determines which muscles are at their limit of stretch when the hip is stretched away from the rib cage. If the quadratus lumborum comes to tension first, then it is the primary hip hiker. If the hip is pulled up and forward and the abdominal muscles come to tension first, then the internal oblique is the most shortened muscle involved in elevating the hip.

With the patient in this side-lying position, the clinician assesses the various portions of the gluteal muscles and the piriformis. The straightened leg is extended to assess the shortening of the psoas muscle. If a bent leg is more restricted in extension than a straight leg, then the rectus femoris is significantly shortened. In this position, by pulling the arm back as well as up, and by pulling the leg back as well as down, the abdominal muscles can be palpated while they are partially stretched. The rectus is palpated with a cross-wise palpation, along vertical taut bands. The abdominal oblique muscles are palpated by strumming across the fibers perpendicular to their orientation, or by deep pincer palpation, grabbing the muscles from the front and the back of the flank. A mistake can be made by not pinching deeply enough to palpate the oblique muscles, and important trigger points can be missed. The clinician searches for taut bands and tender nodules or trigger points in taut bands during the examination of each of the muscles. As each tender trigger point is palpated, the patient is instructed to indicate where pain is felt and whether it is local or referred elsewhere, and to identify whether any of the trigger points palpated elicit a pain that the patient recognizes as the primary back pain complaint. The deeper layers of paraspinal muscles are often difficult to palpate because discreet tender nodules and taut bands are not discernible. However, the paraspinal muscles will have portions that feel thicker and denser, and these often will correspond to the locations of spinal joint restriction.

In a supine position, the abdominal muscles and the psoas can again be palpated. The psoas muscle starts just under the diaphragm. Abdominal muscle trigger points involved in low back pain are often very near the insertion on the pubic bone. The clinician should pay particular attention to areas where there are scars from past surgeries, because these areas are often sites of persistent trigger points in the musculature and fascia. The patient may discount the tenderness and say, "Oh, that's my appendix, [or hernia or hysterectomy] scar," but it may be a key feature in persistent back pain. The shortened iliacus muscle that contributes to forward pulling of the ilium can also be appreciated. In fact, the clinician can attempt to rock the ilium back slightly and assess the tension in the muscles between the ilium and the leg (iliacus, sartorius, and rectus femoris). The clinician also can palpate and compare tension in different parts of the paraspinals by reaching under the patient's torso and attempting to rock or lift individual spinal segments and feel the muscular restriction that limits this small movement. The tautness of the hamstring muscles can be assessed in this position also, along with the usual tests of nerve involvement, such as straight-leg raising.

It is also recommended that the evaluation of hip function as described in Chapter 11 be conducted as well. The disordered hip complex often accompanies chronic low back pain and is very common in patients with sciatica or disc disorders.

With the patient prone, the clinician can palpate the paraspinal and gluteal muscles. This is also a good position for palpating and assessing trigger points in the psoas and the abdominal muscles. (See the discussion of prone palpation of the psoas in Chapter 11).

Once the significant trigger points have been identified, they are treated by trigger point pressure release, percussion, localized stretch over the trigger point, injection, or other technique, and the muscle is stretched to restore its length. Trigger points are most readily identified when the muscle is on a slight stretch, so it is beneficial to examine and treat the same muscles in a number of body positions and stretches. Different trigger points often will be addressed in different positions. Thus, the psoas muscle, for example, may be treated with the patient side-lying, prone, and supine.

It is also worthwhile to have assessed the locations of joint restriction during the examination, so that joint mobilization can be conducted simultaneously with trigger point release and muscle elongation. For example, to treat the patient with a left posterior sacral flare who also has active left piriformis trigger points, the patient lies on the right side. The clinician stands facing the patient. The clinician rocks the patient's left pelvis forward, toward the clinician's body, and applies pressure first to the wing or ala of the sacrum, and then to the piriformis as it emerges lateral to the sacrum. Pressure is also directed to the insertion of the piriformis at the trochanter, continuing to derotate the pelvis while completing the treatment of the muscle. The trigger points and the joint restrictions are closely and integrally related. Therefore, the most effective treatment combines the release of both the muscle and joint restrictions. It is not necessary to ask whether the joint problem is causing the muscle problem or whether the muscle problem is causing the joint problem. Normal joint function usually cannot be restored and maintained if there is major asymmetric myofascial involvement affecting the joint function; likewise, good myofascial release cannot be effected and maintained if there is significant irritation from dysfunctional joints in the same vicinity.

When treating a patient with an acute episode of back pain, it is usually not productive to attempt to stretch the paraspinal muscles while the patient is seated and bending over because of pain. The clinician focuses on paraspinal elongation when stretching the patient's paraspinal muscles in side-lying position. The clinician can lean the flat of one elbow on the patient's hip and the other elbow on the patient's scapula. Exerting gentle traction by separating the elbows, the clinician can stretch large portions of the paraspinals and the quadratus lumborum simultaneously. The elbows can guide the hip or the shoulder forward or backward to focus the direction of the traction on the tautest portions of these muscles. To localize the stretch further, the clinician can apply compression and traction by placing the hands several inches apart, with one hand at the proximal end of a taut muscle band and one hand at the distal end. Post-isometric relaxation or a contract–relax stretch technique can be used to engage the patient in the treatment process, and to achieve greater elongation of the muscles, as described in Chapter 11.

It is often critical to release the psoas muscle during an acute episode of back pain (as well as to address the disordered hip complex). This muscle can be stretched in lateral decubitus position as well. The clinician must stabilize the lumbosacral spine during the psoas stretch, to prevent excessive or painful extension. This is done in part by flexing the opposite hip and knee, to keep the pelvis in anterior rotation, and the clinician also can contact the lumbosacral spine in such a way that extension is blocked. While the clinician uses one hand to draw the patient's thigh into extension, the other hand can palpate taut bands and press on trigger points in the psoas muscle.

It is imperative to treat only within the range in which the patient's body is able to allow release when treating the patient in acute distress, rather than trying to force more vigorous release than is readily possible. The clinician should address bilateral hypertonic muscles, even if one side is much worse than the other. Vapo-coolant spray-and-stretch release is advantageous when treating patients who are so acute that they have difficulty tolerating much manual handling of the muscles.

Several patterns of myofascial dysfunction have been noted in conjunction with patterns of joint dysfunction. For example, iliopsoas trigger points increase lumbar lordosis by approximating the lumbar spine segments at its origin to its insertion at the proximal medial thigh, thereby anteriorly rotating the pelvis. When the iliopsoas is shortened bilaterally, the pelvis will be tilted with both ilia rotated somewhat forward. Increased lumbar lordosis will be necessary if the patient is to stand erect rather than stooped forward. The lumbar lordosis is often focused at L4, L5, S1, causing a significant increase in pressure on the facet joints. Often a loss of curvature in the upper lumbar segments accompanies localized increased lordosis at the lower lumbar segments.

This problem is compounded by various factors. The stooped-forward posture is often part of an acute lumbosacral strain or sprain and often is a feature in chronic back and buttock pain. At the same time, most people focus on stretching their low back muscles and hamstring muscles because this is where they can feel their tightness and discomfort. Iliopsoas muscle trigger points refer pain and discomfort into the lower back and pelvis, yet few people realize the paramount need to include stretch of the psoas as well. It is rare to see a low back sprain or strain or a chronic low back problem without major psoas involvement. In fact, in acute or chronic low back or buttock pain problem, examination is focused on determining which muscles are most severely myofascially involved and on discerning the pattern of joint and myofascial "wind-up" so that we can unwind the pattern of dysfunction. Myofascial involvement of the quadratus lumborum, iliocostalis lumborum, longissimus thoracis, lumbar multifidi, and iliopsoas is common in any acute or chronic back problem. Abdominal myofascial involvement, including both the obliques and the rectus, and myofascial involvement of buttock muscles, hamstring, and adductor muscles are also very frequent in patients with both acute and chronic low back pain.

Shortened paraspinal and hamstring muscles limit lumbosacral flexion. Paradoxically, whereas shortened abdominal muscles can limit extension, shortened paraspinal muscles clearly also play a role in limiting extension, because they approximate the facet joints so severely that they cannot comfortably glide into extension. Anterior rotation of the ilium often is accompanied by shortened abdominal oblique muscles, shortened iliopsoas, and sometimes sartorius. In fact, when the iliacus muscle stays shortened, it is very difficult to correct an anteriorly rotated ilium. Shortened hamstring and buttock muscles can be involved when there is a posteriorly rotated ilium.

Also, again paradoxically, if the shortened psoas is more prominent than the shortened iliacus, the ilium may be maintained in posterior rotation. A shortened and myofascially involved piriformis muscle will make it very difficult to restore normal alignment to the sacrum. By the same token, the joint dysfunction involving the sacrum often appears to make it more difficult to obtain good and lasting release of the piriformis muscle. Whether the shortened muscles "cause" the joint dysfunction, or the joint dysfunction "causes" the myofascial dysfunction, is unclear. Both features are almost always present from the outset, soon after an acute back injury.

Evaluation and Treatment of Joint Dysfunction

Evaluation is performed by simple observation and by putting the patient through certain maneuvers designed to assess function of specific muscles and joints. Some patients respond better to muscle energy release techniques used by osteopathic physicians, and others are appropriate candidates for and respond better to specific high-velocity but low-amplitude spinal adjustments typically performed by chiropractors, or flexion distraction or other treatment techniques used by chiropractors. In fact, research evidence supports the effectiveness of the high-velocity, low-amplitude chiropractic spinal manipulation in patients with both acute and chronic low back pain (28–31). Besides the change in joint function that results from spinal manipulation, generally significant reflexive decrease in local muscle hypertonicity that accompanies the audible (popping) sound is present. When myofascially shortened muscles are released first, spinal manipulation can be performed with very little impulse or force. Osteopathic maneuvers such as muscle energy techniques are explained here, because they are easier to learn and less likely to have a harmful effect if not performed properly. The primary goal in this discussion is to provide the broad range of health practitioners with some understanding of the relationship between joint and muscle dysfunction. If the practitioner can recognize the presence of joint dysfunction, and can learn the benefits to be derived by improving the joint function, then appropriate referrals can be made for the patient who is not responding adequately to care.

Normal Mechanics of the Pelvis and Lumbar Spine. One must have an understanding of normal mechanics of the pelvis to best understand the treatment of pelvic joint dysfunction or subluxation. The ilia rotate anteriorly and posteriorly in normal gait. The right ilium rotates posteriorly as the right leg is lifted, with the right anterior superior iliac spine (ASIS) moving upward or cephalad and the posterior superior iliac spine (PSIS) moving downward or caudally (Fig 10-1). The lower right extremity initiates the swing phase of the gait cycle. The opposite motion occurs at heel strike, when weight transfers into the right leg; the right ilium rotates anteriorly, moving the ASIS down or more caudal, and the right PSIS moves up or more cephalad. The left ilium does just the opposite. When the weight is transferred into the right leg, the left ilium rotates posteriorly as the left leg is raised. This briefly describes the swing and stance phases of the normal gait cycle.

The ilia are neutral when standing on both legs, or when not bearing weight, as when lying supine on an examining table; the ilia are level rather than rotated either anteriorly or posteriorly. When rotation of the ilia is maintained even in a neutral position, there is a restriction of normal joint mobility at the sacroiliac joint, with one sacroiliac joint being generally more restricted than the other. There are various ways of evaluating which sacroiliac joint is the most restricted, and many of them were described in the case histories (see pp. 230–250). There can be an apparent short leg on the side where the ilium is rotated posteriorly, elevating one ASIS and lowering the ipsilateral PSIS. Conversely, an apparent long leg may be

noted where the ilium is rotated anteriorly, with the ASIS lowered and the ipsilateral PSIS elevated; anterior rotation of the ilium lowers the ipsilateral acetabulum, resulting in an apparent lengthening of that leg.

The sacroiliac joints are complex and are considered arthrodial joints with a joint space, an articular capsule, cartilage, and strong ligamentous support. The movements of the sacroiliac joints are small but significant. Although the actual amount of movement at the sacroiliac joint has been a source of controversy, up to 4° of rotation and 1.6 mm of translation can occur in young adults (32). Investigational studies of sacroiliac movement have shown that symptomatic patients have more rotation and translation than nonsymptomatic patients (33,34). Each joint is crescent-shaped, with an upper and lower axis of rotation, and has complex surfaces that are convex at the upper surface and concave at the lower surface where the sacrum and ilium meet. Because the exact configuration of these convex and concave surfaces varies from one individual to the next, there are different limits to sacroiliac joint mobility in each individual. In addition to identifying which sacroiliac joint is most restricted when there is a dysfunction, one also can determine whether the restriction is more pronounced in the upper or lower portion of the sacroiliac joint.

The sacrum plays a major role in normal and abnormal sacroiliac joint function and mechanics. When weight is transferred onto the right leg and the ilium rotates anteriorly, the right side of the sacrum also moves anteriorly; this movement is called *forward torsion.* A normal locking function takes place as the weight is borne through the right leg

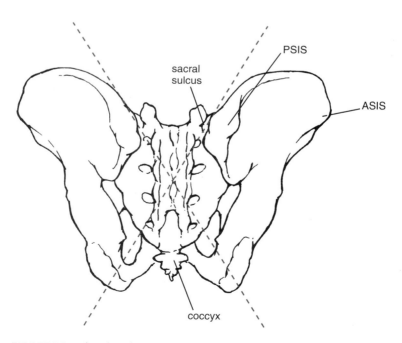

FIGURE 10-1. Landmarks in the pelvis. The pelvis is shown opened at the pubic symphysis and viewed from the back, to depict the ASIS on the front of each ilium.

and the sacroiliac joint, when the sacrum, L5, and the ilium engage. Then, when the right leg is lifted and the ilium rotates posteriorly, the sacrum also rotates posteriorly (*backward torsion*); simultaneously the left sacroiliac joint is engaged, with both the left sacrum and the left ilium moving anteriorly. The sacrum rotates about an oblique axis that runs from one upper sacroiliac joint to the opposite inferior lateral angle (ILA) (see Fig. 10-1).

Assessment of Abnormal Function of the Pelvis and Lumbar Spine. Dysfunction is present when the ilia remain in the normal relationship that they would be in during gait (e.g., one ilia rotated anteriorly and the other posteriorly), even when the patient is in a neutral position. Assessment of ilial rotation was presented in case 3 (see Technique 10-11). Varying degrees of sacral dysfunction can be found that involve the sacrum not following the iliac movement smoothly. For example, the sacrum may be in a torqued position while the ilia are relatively balanced. Sacroiliac joint dysfunction in which the ilium is rotated anteriorly but the sacrum on the same side is in backward torsion is probably the most painful and most difficult dysfunction to resolve. In this instance, it is as though the sacrum and the ilium are gears that are failing to mesh properly. If the clinician corrects the anterior iliac rotation by helping to rotate it posteriorly but does not recognize the concomitant posterior flare of the sacrum, this can aggravate the patient's condition. By the same token, if the clinician corrects the posterior flare or backward torsion of the sacrum by bringing it anterior, but does not recognize the concomitant anterior rotation of the ilium, this can also aggravate the patient's condition. Correcting both sacral and iliac dysfunction to allow them to mesh properly again can be difficult, but when they do, usually a marked decrease in pain occurs.

Sacral dysfunction is assessed in a variety of ways. The tests most used are the seated flexion test and the static evaluation of the sacral sulci and ILAs (see illustrations in Technique boxes 10-3 and 10-7). **Motion palpation** is another assessment technique and can be performed standing, seated, or prone. Motion palpation with the patient supine is performed as follows: the examiner slides one hand under the supine patient and positions it under the sacral base, with the fingers bent or cupped while the back of the hand rests on the examining table. Palpation can be performed unilaterally or bilaterally, whichever gives the clearest information. A gentle posterior-to-anterior rocking motion is introduced by pressing the fingers upward, and the clinician notes the difference in mobility between the right and left sides of the sacral base. Because two axes of rotation exist in the sacroiliac joint, the mobility in the lower portion of the joint can be examined and compared in a similar fashion.

Hip height can be observed while the patient is standing, to see whether one side is higher than the other. Restrictions of mobility that can be responsible for an unbalanced position of the pelvis are evaluated. For example, if the right hip is lowered by lengthening the quadratus lum-

borum muscle, inevitable changes will occur in the dynamics of the joint restriction. Assessment of leg-length discrepancy is unreliable in the presence of a shortened quadratus lumborum or psoas muscle that causes the hip to be elevated, or in the presence of a significant sacroiliac joint dysfunction. The apparent longer leg may no longer appear to be so when an ipsilateral anteriorly rotated iliac bone is corrected. Likewise, when a posteriorly rotated ilium is corrected, the leg that appeared shorter on that side may no longer appear shorter. Leg-length differences are a normal part of the mechanics of gait. It is best to correct myofascial involvement and joint restrictions before assessing leg-length discrepancy.

Often the corrections are performed over several sessions before the clinician decides that an underlying leg-length discrepancy may be present and prescribes the use of a heel lift. The heel lift helps to bring the pelvis and thence the body into balance around a central axis. Because this is a dynamic process, the patient's body may respond to the use of the heel lift and come into balance and no longer need the device days, weeks, or months after it was initially prescribed. The patient must be evaluated and reevaluated frequently throughout the course of care. The use of orthotics to stabilize the foot and improve gait also can result in apparent shifts in leg length, so reassessments also should be made when new orthotics are introduced into the treatment.

One more pelvic joint, the pubic symphysis, must be considered. The symphysis must accommodate the rotational movements of the ilia, which have some upward (cephalad) and downward (caudad) directional components. Restricted mobility can develop at the symphysis pubis. This can be assessed in several ways (Technique 10-16). One is manual muscle testing, which can detect bilateral weakness of adductor muscles that generally accompanies pubic symphysis restriction (Technique 10-17).

Correcting the sacral mechanics frequently also correct joint restriction in the lower lumbar spine and vice versa, but often these dysfunctions are treated sequentially. Normal spinal mechanics involves movement in three planes: flexion/extension, lateral flexion (side-bending), and rotation. The vertebrae must rotate away from the direction of side bending when lateral flexion is introduced into the spine. This is called neutral spinal mechanics (Fig 10-2). When lateral flexion is introduced into the spine already in flexion or extension, a central vertebral segment rotates toward the direction of side-bending to allow surrounding vertebrae to rotate away. This is called non-neutral spinal mechanics (Fig 10-3). Both of these patterns of function are part of the normal patterns of mobility of the lumbar spine.

The degree of mobility at each segment is controlled by the orientation of the facet joints. When the spine is in flexion, the facet joints are opened, and there is greater possible mobility. When the spine is in extension, the facet joints are approximated, and there is decreased possible mobility. When vertebral movement is restricted in the neutral posi-

TECHNIQUE 10-16

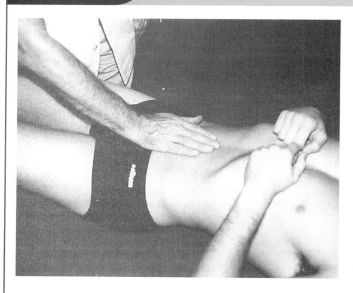

(A) Assessment of pubic symphysis alignment.

Reprinted with permission from Greenman PE. Principles of Manual Medicine, 3rd Ed. Baltimore: Lippincott Williams & Wilkins, 2003 (fig. 17.19), p. 350.

Pubic Symphysis Evaluation

The pubic tubercles are found by placing the hand gently on the patient's abdomen so that the middle finger is at the patient's navel and the heel of the hand is resting on the pubic bones or tubercles (**A**). In most cases, one pubic tubercle is superior or inferior to the other. This dysfunction is often caused by a habitual pattern of standing with one knee bent and the opposite leg straight. The examiner's index fingers may then be placed on the right and left pubic tubercles to establish their relationship to one another. For example, the left pubic tubercle may be superior to, or higher than, the right (**B**). Whichever the relationship, a simple maneuver can reposition the pubic tubercles and create symmetry in the pubic bones (**C**).

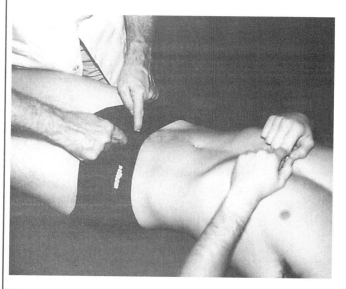

(B) Assessment of pubic symphysis alignment.

Reprinted with permission from Greenman PE. Principles of Manual Medicine, 3rd Ed. Baltimore: Lippincott Williams & Wilkins, 2003 (fig. 17.21), p. 350.

TECHNIQUE 10-16

Pubic Symphysis Evaluation *(Continued)*

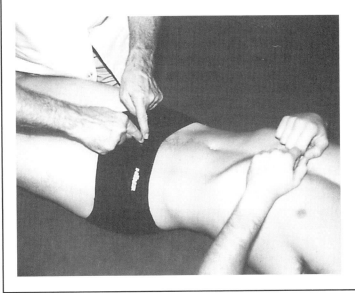

(C) Re-assessment of pubic symphysis alignment after treatment.

Reprinted with permission from Greenman PE. Principles of Manual Medicine, 3rd Ed. Baltimore: Lippincott Williams & Wilkins, 2003 (fig. 17.20), p. 350.

TECHNIQUE 10-17

Treating Pubic Symphysis Dysfunction

This is a muscle energy technique with the patient supine, with bent knees and feet placed together on the examination table. The clinician stands at the side of the patient, holding the patient's knees together (**A**). The patient is instructed to try to separate the knees against the clinician's resistance. This is repeated 2–3 times and held for 4–5 seconds each time. Then the clinician holds the patient's knees apart with a hand on each knee (**B**) or places the forearm between the patient's knees with the palm of the hand on one of the knees and the elbow on the medial aspect of the other knee. The patient is asked to try to bring the knees together against the clinician's resistance. This position is held for 3–5 seconds, and the exercise is repeated 2–3 times. Sometimes a small "click" can be heard and felt by the patient as the pubic symphysis repositions into balance.

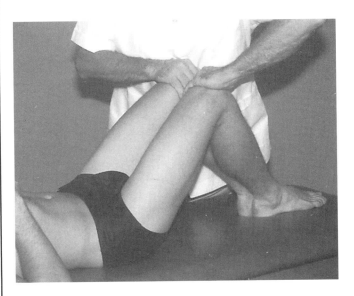

(A) Mobilization technique for the pubic symphysis.

Reprinted with permission from Greenman PE: Principles of Manual Medicine, 3rd Ed. Baltimore: Lippincott, Williams & Wilkins, 2003 (fig. 17.112), p. 392.

(continues)

TECHNIQUE 10-17

Treating Pubic Symphysis Dysfunction   (*Continued*)

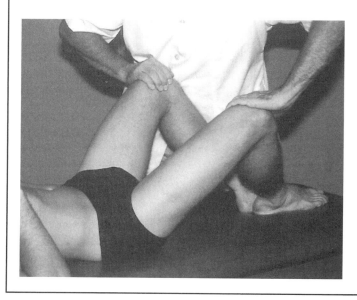

(B) Mobilization technique for the pubic symphysis.

Reprinted with permission from Greenman PE: Principles of Manual Medicine, 3rd Ed. Baltimore: Lippincott, Williams & Wilkins, 2003 (fig. 17.113), p. 392.

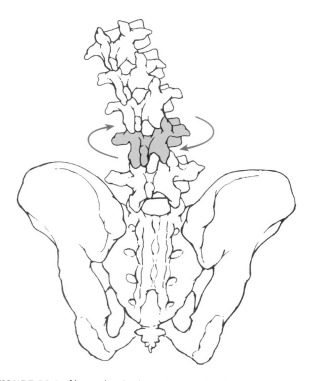

FIGURE 10-2. **Neutral spinal mechanics.** With the spine in left lateral flexion, the L4 body rotates to the right, toward the convexity.

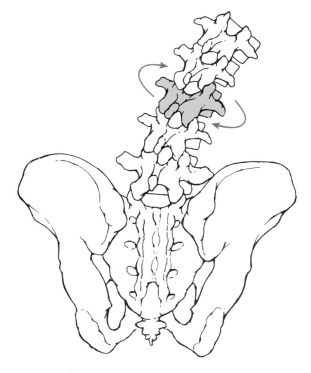

FIGURE 10-3. **Non-neutral spinal mechanics.** With the spine in right lateral flexion, the L3 body rotates right, toward the concavity.

tion (standing, or lying on the examining table), joint dysfunction or subluxation is present. For example, when one or several segments are fixed in lateral flexion and rotation when the patient is in a neutral position, the correction of this restricted mobility is often associated with decreased pain and an enhanced ability to release and elongate surrounding muscles. Some degree of disc bulging is a normal occurrence with lateral flexion of the spine. Therefore, it is logical to expect that, if myofascial shortening and hip hiking are reduced, and a segment or series of lumbar spinal segments are brought out of a position of fixed lateral flexion, the degree of disc bulging may be reduced. At the very least, compressive forces across the disc and the nerve root near the disc are decreased.

Hypermobility versus Hypomobility. When treating the patient with chronic low back pain, the issue of hypermobility versus hypomobility often arises. This section develops a framework for understanding these concepts, particularly with regard to the sacroiliac joint. In the spine, if there is restriction of normal mobility at one segment, there often will be a compensatory increase of movement at another level, for the body to carry out normal movements. Yet clinical findings in regard to the sacroiliac joint are often confusing. A patient who presents with a previous diagnosis of a hypermobile sacroiliac joint may, on examination, have significant hypomobility at that same sacroiliac joint. Response to tests for sacroiliac instability and difficulty with load transfer (35) indicate that often hypomobility of the sacroiliac joint prevents the mechanical locking that should occur during stance and that should confer stability to the sacroiliac joint. This inability to fully lock during stance phase is analogous to the mechanics of the knee. In the case of the knee, if the tibia cannot glide into sufficient extension, and is maintained in a partially flexed state, the normal locking during stance cannot take place, and there will be more demand on muscle and ligamentous structures to hold and guide the knee. Clinically, this knee joint dysfunction renders the knee less stable.

Similarly, the sacrum flares posteriorly when the leg on the same side is raised, but it should glide into extension and a normal locking position at the joint during stance phase. If this does not occur, there will be more stress on the ligaments and muscles to control movement during gait. Therefore, the clinician's first line of approach for such instability is to address all of the aspects of this inability to extend fully at the sacroiliac joint; the hypomobility should be addressed first. In the spine also, restoring mobility to hypomobile segments will decrease hypermobility of other segments and reduce the stresses on muscles and ligaments. In addition to the aspects of joint mobility in the pelvis described in this chapter, the femur dysfunction described in Chapter 11 is often a factor as well. Flexion stress to the sacroiliac joint produced by the shortened iliopsoas, either alone or in combination with the femur dysfunction, is important to treat but often is overlooked in patients with

sacroiliac instability. Other shortened muscles with myofascial trigger points also can produce the same effect, preventing restoration of normal mechanics. The standing motion palpation or the supine motion palpation procedure to assess sacral mobility described earlier in this chapter are helpful here, and the ability of the sacrum to go into extension (the locking position required for stability during normal gait) can be assessed at any one point in time, but successive treatments should result in increased ease of sacral mobility; therefore, repeated evaluations are necessary. In fact, test results for instability or difficulty with load transfer should progressively improve as the normal mechanics are restored.

In this discussion, the most common form of instability has been discussed, but in unusual instances normal mechanics cannot be restored, and the instability persists. In these cases, **prolotherapy** may be appropriate to increase ligamentous stability and support. Furthermore, significant trauma can result in actual tears to the joint capsule of the sacroiliac joint. Although this form of extreme instability is not responsive to manual treatment, the clinical picture that is emerging from current imaging and treatment programs is of such an identifiable syndrome that clinicians should recognize it and make appropriate surgical referrals.

The Disrupted Sacroiliac Joint Capsule. (Section by Shannon Goossen, AP, LMT, CMTPT and Arnold Graham Smith, MD, FRCS)

Whereas most sacroiliac joint (SIJ) dysfunction is treatable with conservative care, including manipulation and mobilization, manual myofascial therapy, trigger point injection, and other techniques, some patients have severe symptoms that are only temporarily resolved, are resistant to intervention, or are made worse by manual therapy techniques. Typically these patients have been to many physicians and therapists, but no one has successfully diagnosed and treated them. They have had numerous tests such as MRI, computed tomography (CT), x-ray, bone scan, and electrodiagnostic studies that have ruled out other disorders, or they have been treated for concurrent disorders, but severe and disabling posterior hip and buttock pain remains. Patients with such a history of failed interventions often seek some type of manual therapy to relieve their pain. For this reason, practitioners treating MPS and joint dysfunction must recognize the telltale signs.

Recent research and clinical investigation has clarified the clinical profile of patients with a disrupted SIJ capsule (36–40). Patients with a disrupted SIJ capsule can present with symptoms similar to myofascial pain arising from trigger points in the quadratus lumborum, gluteus medius, maximus, and minimus, piriformis, lumbar multifidi, and sometimes external oblique and hamstring muscles. They also may present with symptoms similar to the disordered hip complex (see Chapter 11), a herniated disc with S1 radicular pain, or other types of sacroiliac disorders. Symptoms include: buttock pain while turning over in bed, the need to sit on the opposite buttock to keep pressure off the affected side, and stabbing pain in the sulcus of the SIJ. Additionally, many patients state that the leg or knee on the affected side feels unstable. Many report it has already given way, causing them to fall and suffer other injuries that can complicate the diagnostic process. The buttock pain at night is often severe enough that sleep is disrupted. Pain levels increase with walking or sitting, and the patient typically cannot sleep on the affected side. They avoid common activities such as sitting at the table for meals, sitting at work or in the car, going to church, walking in the grocery store, standing to prepare meals, as well as sports activities, playing with children, and having sex with their partner. Almost all patients will point to the PSIS or the sacral sulcus as the location of their worst pain. Most state that pain medication does not help them much, or that the pain does not stop but that they mind it less.

Most patients report a traumatic event or a specific event that preceded the onset of symptoms. Traumatic events include motor vehicle accidents, often with the foot on the involved side bracing for the impact and thus transmitting shear forces to the SIJ. Patients also report slip and fall accidents, being dropped, a direct blow to the SIJ, or a pelvic fracture. The patient who has fallen often will report direct impact to the SIJ while in a twisted position. Nontraumatic or nonimpact events that preceded onset of pain include lifting while twisting, gynecologic surgery, pregnancy, labor, and delivery. Rheumatoid arthritis also may be a factor. Some patients report a vague and slow onset, in which case the practitioner needs to obtain a thorough history to detect previous traumatic injuries.

During history taking and examination, the clinician will notice that the patient unconsciously avoids sitting, standing, walking, or leaning on the affected side. The clinician often enters the examination room to find the patient sitting on the opposite buttock with the leg of the involved side extended. The clinician should proceed to perform a full evaluation for lower back conditions, joint dysfunction, and myofascial involvement, and the patient with a disrupted SIJ has some typical findings on standard tests. Tests such as side-bending with extension will stress all the posterior elements, so this test will be painful in patients with disrupted SIJ capsule as well as facet syndrome. Although all lumbar movements may be reduced, flexion will not cause sciatica as it does with a herniated disc. There will be no signs of motor, sensory, or reflex abnormalities in the lower extremities, and straight-leg raising will be normal (unless there are other concurrent disorders.) The patient often will be reluctant to stand independently or hop on the affected side. This is such a pathognomonic test that it is recommended to be performed during any examination of a patient with low back and buttock pain. Some patients attribute this difficulty to a knee problem, but results of examination of the knee will be normal (unless they have already fallen and injured the knee.) Patrick's (Fabere) test (see illustrations in Technique 10-16) generally will stress the SIJ and produce

increased pain. The pelvic thrust test is performed by flexing the knee of the supine patient to 90°, applying a force to the knee and quickly thrusting toward the pelvis. This test also will produce pain. With the patient prone over a pillow, palpating pressure over the SIJ will be painful. This can be compared with pain on palpation of the lumbosacral supraspinous ligament and, if both are painful, a concurrent pathologic condition may be present. (Probably because of the history of trauma, up to 35% of the patients eventually selected for arthrography have intercurrent spinal conditions.)

Even with a high degree of suspicion of disrupted SIJ capsule, a brief trial of comprehensive myofascial and articular care is recommended, much as described in this chapter. During the first two treatment sessions, the focus should be on dropping the elevated hip (usually on the involved side) and releasing trigger points. If the patient appears to benefit, on the next visit the disordered hip complex can be treated. Because joint mobilization of the pelvis often was a source of aggravation of pain, joint mobilization or gentle manipulation is only carried out if the patient is improving from the initial stages of this trial of conservative care. If the patient has the hallmark history, symptoms, and examination findings of disrupted SIJ capsule, generally there is no need to carry out a trial of comprehensive care for more than three visits. More of what is not working will not eventually work. Those patients with more conventional SIJ dysfunction will respond significantly and progressively to the program of comprehensive conservative care. The diagnosis of disrupted SIJ capsule is thus reached by exclusion and is verified by a positive SI arthrogram, and at least two therapeutic SI blocks.

The SI arthrogram is conducted under fluoroscopic control, using a 25-gauge needle to introduce contrast through the inferior pole of the joint. Noteworthy is that, sometimes during the contrast injection, the patient will report reproduction of the primary pain complaint. The spread of the dye throughout the joint space, producing an arthrogram, is verified by the use of the fluoroscopic imaging. Sometimes the contrast can be seen to leak through the fibrous portion of the SIJ into the S1 dorsal foramen. The contrast may track down the S1 nerve, or it may track anteriorly and contact the sciatic nerve where it lies over the front of the sacrum. Postarthrogram CT can be performed to review the tracking of the extravasated contrast. If the patient is a candidate for surgical intervention, the CT scan is used as an operative planning tool.

When arthrographic imaging confirms that the contrast is in the joint space, a therapeutic SI block is performed by injecting a small amount of steroid and bupivacaine hydrochloride and epinephrine, to produce an immediate analgesic effect. Patients may again report reproduction of the typical pain, followed by immediate relief. Amelioration of pain varies from instantaneous to an hour or two later. The length of time and degree of relief will depend on several factors, including the extent of leakage and disbursal of the medication, as well as the presence of intercurrent spinal conditions. The anesthetic effect wears off within 2 to 6 hours, but the steroid may provide longer relief, and the patient may be able to take walks and have an unbroken night of sleep for the first time in months or years.

After the arthrogram block, patients are asked to get off the x-ray table and walk, bend, stand, and hop on the leg on the affected side, or do an activity they generally cannot perform because of pain. The patient with a positive response to the block will demonstrate the ability to perform these activities, and this functional change is the most reliable indicator that the disrupted SIJ capsule has been a major source of pain and disability.

Once a successful SI arthrogram and block have been performed, confirmed by a second block, for the willing patient, surgical arthrodesis is indicated. These patients do not improve with conservative therapy. Patients unable or unwilling to live with their chronic SI pain should seek experienced surgeons who have good outcomes with SI fusions. When done correctly, the synovial portion of the joint is scraped clean, and the sacrum is fused to the pelvis on the affected side. Recovery from surgery and postoperative treatment and rehabilitation can take anywhere from 4 months to a year.

Myofascial therapists can play an important role by identifying patients who may have the disrupted SIJ capsule syndrome. They also can perform a trial of comprehensive conservative care and make appropriate referral of the patient whose condition does not respond to such care. They also can play an important part in postoperative rehabilitation, because these patients generally also had MPS that may need to be addressed for the best rehabilitative outcome.

Sensitized Spinal Segment. Another aspect of the relationship between the spine and the MPS has been postulated and explored clinically by Andrew Fischer, M.D., and his colleagues (41). They have observed and documented that a chronic pain condition with referred pain is accompanied by a sensitized spinal segment, which includes:

1. Paraspinal muscle hypertonicity at the level of that segment

2. Skin hypersensitivity in the dermatome emanating from that spinal level

3. A pattern of referred pain in the dermatome associated with that spinal segment

4. Muscles with active trigger points innervated from that spinal segment (**myotome**)

5. Inflammatory changes in connective tissues, such as tendons, emanating from that spinal segment (**sclerotome**).

Therefore, often it is necessary to treat and address spinal sensitization to achieve lasting improvement in chronic MPS. Fischer (42) recommends the use of paraspinous block injections and injection of anesthetic into the interspinous ligament, which he sees as the source of recurrent noxious input to the spinal segment. Fischer is using medical techniques to address the conditions traditionally treated manually by chiropractors and osteopaths: the spinal subluxation or the somatic dysfunction syndrome. Chiropractors and osteopaths are aware that they are treating not only a joint restriction, but the accompanying changes in muscle tone and function, nerve irritability, circulation, and inflammation and so on. It will be interesting to use Fischer's assessment criteria to compare manual (osteopathic and chiropractic) and medical approaches to the treatment of the spinal subluxation or dysfunction and the related sensitization.

Treating Lumbar Disc Disorders

Treating patients with lumbar disc disorders is similar to treating patients with low back pain, or back pain plus buttock pain with or without sciatica. The clinician identifies the patterns of myofascial and joint dysfunction, paying particular attention to attenuating the compressive forces across the lumbar spine. Although no rule exists regarding what myofascial and joint patterns will be found with a herniated disc, psoas muscle involvement is often overlooked, but it is of crucial importance. The disordered hip complex (see Chapter 11) and subluxations (articular dysfunctions) of the pelvis and lumbar spine are extremely frequent parts of the problem. To effectively attenuate the compressive forces of the myofascially shortened psoas muscle, the disordered hip complex must be treated. Other sources of sciatic nerve irritation need to be addressed as well, including that from piriformis muscle trigger points.

The usual effect of successful treatment of the patient with a herniated lumbar disc does not rely on putting the herniated nucleus pulposus back beneath the posterior ligament and within the annulus, or even that we physically displace the herniated disc material off the nerve root. These ideas have been taught in the past, and treatment methods based on these concepts appear to have been effective. Yet when MRI studies are repeated on recently asymptomatic patients, disc material may still be in the same location and not reduced or displaced. Months or years later, the herniated nucleus pulposus may no longer be in the same location; this may be caused by resorption or disintegration of the disc material. A difference exists as well between nucleus pulposus that herniates in continuity with the disc, and that which fragments. Material that fragments tends to disintegrate and move away more readily than herniation in continuity. Nevertheless, successful completion of treatment does not necessarily entail removing disc material from the nerve root. The successful treatment of lumbar disc disease, therefore, occurs because the compressive forces upon the disc and nerve root have been reduced, and the normal muscle and joint mechanics have been restored so as to reduce abnormal stresses on the herniated disc, allowing the edematous nerve root to shrink and heal. Patients are instructed to gradually increase their activities during the recovery phase. The clinician educates the patient in the *iceberg theory* of nerve healing, explaining that a substantial portion of the nerve fibers have to be inflamed for pain to rise above the pain threshold and be felt in the nerve. When the percentage of nerve irritation drops below the pain threshold, the patient may have a tendency to try to resume normal activity. Yet it will take very little in terms of increased activity to re-irritate the nerve fibers to the point that pain is again felt. If the patient can avoid re-aggravation until the degree of nerve irritation is progressively lessened, the scope of activity that will not reinitiate pain will probably broaden. Thus, the management of a lumbar disc herniation is different from the management of a lumbar strain or sprain, and the patient needs to be educated about the difference. Most patients with sprains or strains can use the pain level that they experience *during* activity as a guide to prevent re-injury. The patient treated for a herniated disc must be mindful of pain that may occur *after* activity. Specifically, the patient needs to avoid sitting for a prolonged length of time, needs to avoid heavy lifting, pulling, and pushing, and significant impact activities. If the patient is in significant pain and these functions do not increase the pain, then the diagnosis of lumbar disc herniation and radiculopathy needs to be reconsidered, even when MRI findings indicate a disc herniation.

It may be difficult to make progress when treating the patient with a major pain disorder in which the disc plays a part unless there is also some degree of pain control. For example, an epidural block or trigger point injections often help resolve the patient's problem when used in conjunction with conservative and manual techniques. Restoring regular sleep patterns also helps relax the muscles so healing can proceed. Under these circumstances, manual techniques remain a central feature of the patient's care, and they lessen the need for repeated epidural blocks or other invasive procedures. The clinician must monitor the function of the nerve and identify any progressive impairment of nerve function, to determine whether continued conservative care is appropriate. Although surgery may be required to preserve nerve function and relieve pain, laminectomies and spinal fusions are performed at a much higher rate in some parts of this country than in others, with no demonstrable improvement in outcomes, so a significant portion of these surgeries are likely unnecessary (43).

Surgical Complications and Postoperative Pain

There are patients who have serious and painful adverse effects from back surgery, sometimes permanent, such as proliferation of scar tissue. Nevertheless, most cases of "failed back surgery" are not actual failures. In fact, reflex changes and muscle weakness that may have prompted the surgery are often improved, even though pain persists. Although postsurgical pain can be so severe that it seems like the pain

before surgery, it often can be successfully treated with myofascial release techniques and the restoration of normal joint function. The most common postsurgical problems include a disordered hip complex that perpetuates hip and thigh pain, gluteus minimus trigger points that mimic L5 and S1 radiculopathy, and sacroiliac joint dysfunction and quadratus lumborum trigger points that both maintain buttock pain. When the remaining pain does not radiate down the leg or to the buttock, but is in the lumbar spine region, then trigger points in the abdominal, psoas, quadratus lumborum, and paraspinal muscles, or lumbar spinal joint dysfunction may be maintaining low back pain.

Patient Exercise and Home Care

A rehabilitation program includes exercises performed by the patient. Even the patient with a significant disc disorder can engage in exercise to assist in rehabilitation. A patient deconditioned by bed rest for 4 months with two herniated lumbar discs and significant pain can walk in water in a pool and perform gentle stretches at home. Patients with acute back pain usually still can perform some gentle stretches of the paraspinal muscles and quadratus lumborum muscles while seated, and supporting the torso while leaning forward and to each side (see Fig 11-10). The psoas muscle stretch, important to perform, can be done even while lying in bed, or kneeling with one knee up and shifting the pelvis forward into a gentle stretch (see Fig 11-9).

Buttock and torso muscles can be stretched with a simple leg-over stretch. A simple variation of this stretch can help correct a posterior flare of the sacrum. For example, in a patient whose left sacrum flares posteriorly, the stretch position is lying supine and moving the left leg across the right until the foot contacts the floor to the right of the torso. Then the patient places the heel of the left hand against the left side of the sacrum and presses the sacrum further into rotation, letting the left leg extend further along the floor to the right of the body (Fig 10-4).

Stretches should be performed slowly and held for at least 10 to 15 seconds and should be stopped short of increasing the patient's pain level. In acute conditions, it is best to perform stretches every 2 hours. It is helpful to have the patient perform stretches every 2 hours in chronic conditions, but 3 to 4 times per day, even twice per day, often will enhance rehabilitation.

Other recommended stretches will depend on evaluating which muscles are myofascially shortened, thereby contributing to the dysfunction and pain. If the patient has a disordered hip complex, or a tendency for this problem to recur, then stretches of the buttock muscles or groin muscles that take the flexed thigh into full external rotation should be avoided. Stretches for these same areas can be performed without the external rotation (see Figs 11-10 and 11-11).

Strengthening activities are used sparingly while the patient has significant myofascial trigger point pain. Abdominal strengthening is supposed to help patients with

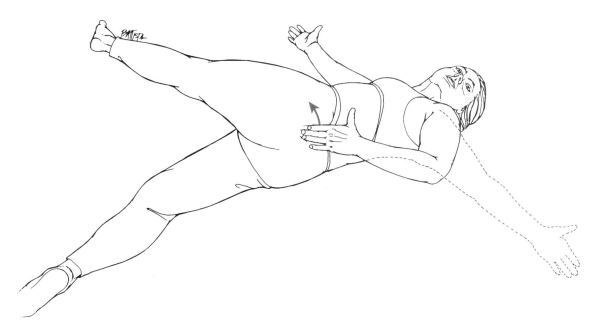

FIGURE 10-4. Leg-over stretch for torso and buttock muscles, with variation to help correct posterior sacral flare. If the sacrum flares posterior on the left (left sacral torsion), a leg-over exercise can be performed, and when the left leg is crossed over the torso, the left hand can press the sacrum forward, assisting toward normal mobility. The sacral assist is performed only to correct the dysfunctional side.

back pain, but many clinicians find that the abdominal and psoas trigger points are repeatedly aggravated unless the patient ceases the usual abdominal exercises that are designed to strengthen the oblique and rectus abdominis muscles. (For a further discussion of safe abdominal strengthening, see Chapter 12.) Likewise, it is possible to aggravate paraspinal muscles and quadratus lumborum muscle trigger points even if their trigger points are latent, if torso maneuvers against resistance are performed. Gentle progressive stabilization activities performed short of the patient's pain threshold are often safer and more easily tolerated by patients who have a significant myofascial component to their back pain. These activities are discussed well by Hyman and Liebenson (44) and involve using the muscles to provide stability while the spine is held in a position that minimizes the pain. Extension activities are very helpful exercises for some patients; others experience significant aggravation from extension, and thus should avoid these exercises.

Swimming with a straight flutter kick is an excellent exercise for most patients with back problems; it enhances the tone of abdominal, deep paraspinal, and gluteal muscles that can contribute to spinal stability. Most patients should build up to performing 15 to 30 minutes of swimming with a flutter kick 3 to 5 times per week..

Yoga can be very beneficial exercise for strength and flexibility. Patients with back problems have to be aware, however, that they need to stop stretching the muscles at the point that significant stress is placed on the joints, *even if they can go farther.* Thus, in the patient in whom there is a tendency for the sacrum to flare posteriorly (backward tor-

sion), seated forward bending activities cannot be performed with impunity. For example, in a patient seated on the floor leaning forward with the legs apart, a certain amount of forward bending will take place with stretch of the back and hamstring muscles and with the lumbar lordosis maintained. Once the limit of muscular stretch is reached, the sacrum will be induced to flare backward if the patient leans farther forward, and the lumbar lordosis will no longer be maintained. It will be difficult to treat the patient's sacroiliac joint dysfunction involving posterior sacral flare if this exercise is performed without sufficient care. The same cautions apply to lotus or other positions that place the femur in external rotation, if external rotation of the femur is a part of the patient's problem. In addition, Feldenkrais movements can gently encourage mobility of the pelvis and the lumbar spine that are very helpful for some patients. Tai chi also can be helpful with rehabilitation, when movements do not exacerbate pain; this exercise system promotes strength, coordination or controlled movement, and balance.

Patients with recurrent patterns of joint dysfunction may be able to learn to perform activities to address the usual patterns of their problem. For example, a patient with a recurrent anteriorly rotated right ilium can learn to perform the muscle energy release for that somatic dysfunction (see illustrations in Technique 10-14).

The Role of Perpetuating Factors

The evaluation of perpetuating factors is extremely important in designing a home care program for patients with back pain. It will be hard to stabilize the pelvis if the patient's habitual sleep position is lying partly on the side, but rolled almost prone, with one knee drawn up (a three-quarter position). It may even be necessary to have the patient place a brooch on their sleep wear, so the prone sleep position is uncomfortable.

The importance of good footwear and of orthotics in reducing the repetitive strain that contributes to recurrent back pain cannot be overestimated. Some patients have reasonably good orthotics, but the angle of the heel allows too much supination and does not properly direct the foot over the arch support during roll-through onto the forefoot. In these cases, piriformis, gluteal, and iliopsoas muscle trigger points may recur. By making a simple correction of the cant or angle of support of the heel, usually by only slightly elevating the outer edge of the heel of the orthotic, excessive supination at the heel is controlled, and the patient's weight is better directed over the arch of the orthotic. The patient's gait should be observed and footwear checked from time to time, because patients often adopt less supportive footwear in the summer, or when they have to wear boots in the winter.

A healthy diet, including minimizing high–glycemic index foods, reducing caffeine intake, introducing an optimal balance of omega-3 to omega-6 fatty acids, and drinking adequate amounts of water are all important for enhancing recovery. Addressing any medical conditions that may increase pain and inflammation is also important, such as those conditions that produce arthritis, such as Sjögren's syndrome, and allergies that involve high tissue histamine levels that contribute to inflammation.

Psychological Factors

It is often helpful for the patients with low back pain to assess sources of stress in their lives. If possible, they can make changes in such areas as lifestyle, work, and family relationships with counseling, if these are contributing to back pain. They also can learn coping and stress-management skills to deal with the stress factors that they cannot, or choose not to, avoid. A good emotional foundation is often important in finding stability and relief from low back pain. Interrupting the pattern of pain with myofascial and joint care techniques often enables patients to then recognize when the problem returns and what stress factors triggered the recurrence. Thus, manual care is not a crutch but rather a tool for investigating what needs to be addressed in a patient's emotional life.

CONCLUSION

Low back pain and its related conditions are challenging, because it can arise from a number of different tissues both at the site of pain and at a distance from the pain location; muscles with active trigger points and other tissues can refer pain into the back although they are located elsewhere.

Myofascial pain syndrome diagnosis and treatment, especially when coupled with diagnosis and treatment of joint restriction and dysfunction, are effective for most patients with back pain. Even when pain arises from nerve root injury or other structure dysfunction, there is generally some contribution of mechanical factors to the degree and severity of the patient's pain.

Clinicians should not consider any patient's low back pain to be nonspecific. Effective treatment requires a very specific diagnostic process to identify as many as possible of the factors in the patient's pain that can be controlled and treated. Effective unwinding of the pattern of myofascial and joint dysfunction usually results in changes in the patient's habitual pattern of joint problems or muscle problems that leads to recovery. In other words, in most patients, structural patterns are much more fluid than we have been taught. The clinician who is frequently repeating the same treatment procedures should look for the factors that have been missed either in evaluating mechanical dysfunction, assessing perpetuating lifestyle and activity factors, recognizing and addressing psychological stresses, or adequately treating other medical conditions. The diagnostic process is not performed at one time, but rather throughout the course of the patient's care, with changes of the treatment plan implemented according to the problems encountered in treatment and the progress of the patient.

TREATMENT PROTOCOL

1. **Evaluate and treat muscles that may be a source of low back pain, both local and referred, including the quadratus lumborum, the abdominals, the iliopsoas, the iliocostalis thoracis and lumborum, the longissimus thoracis, and the multifidi.**

2. **Evaluate and treat muscles that may be a source of buttock, pelvic, or leg pain, including the gluteus minimus, medius, maximus, the piriformis, obturator, iliopsoas, quadratus lumborum, iliocostalis lumborum, longissimus thoracis, multifidi, tensor fascia lata, and even portions of the quadriceps and hamstring muscles. Evaluate and treat the soleus muscle as well, as it can refer pain to the sacroiliac joint.**

3. **Palpate, evaluate, and treat dysfunctional joints that may be contributing to the pain, including the sacrum, the ilia, the pubic symphysis, the femur, and the lumbar spinal vertebrae. Assess the tenderness of the joints to palpation before and after treatment.**

4. *Muscles:* Evaluate and treat the muscles that are elevating one hip or anteriorly rotating it, including the quadratus lumborum, the abdominal obliques, and the iliopsoas. Evaluate and treat the muscles that may be lowering the opposite hip and posteriorly rotating it, including the hamstring and gluteal muscles. Addressing these muscles usually also will help to reduce lateral flexion, accompanying rotation, and scoliosis of the lumbar spine.

   Joints: Evaluate and treat dysfunction of the alignment and joint mobility of the ilia. Treat restrictions of normal lateral flexion and rotation of the lumbar spine.

5. *Muscles:* Evaluate and treat muscles that are increasing the sacral flare, including the piriformis and iliopsoas muscles.

   Joints: Evaluate and treat dysfunction of the alignment and joint mobility of the sacrum.

6. *Muscles:* Evaluate and treat muscles that decrease normal flexion of the lumbar spine including the paraspinal muscles, bilateral shortening of the quadratus lumborum, shortened hamstring muscles, and shortened psoas muscles.

   Joints: Evaluate and treat restriction of flexion of lumbar vertebrae.

7. *Muscles:* Evaluate and treat muscles that decrease normal extension of the lumbar spine, including shortened abdominals and shortened deep paraspinal muscles.

   Joints: Evaluate and treat restriction of extension of lumbar vertebrae.

8. Introduce appropriate specific stretching protocols, strengthening, stabilizing, and other exercises.

9. Evaluate and address other perpetuating factors, including work activities, sleep position, repetitive stress from gait problems, dietary factors, and emotional stress, as well as any contributing medical problems.

References

1. Magni G. The Epidemiology of Musculoskeletal Pain. In: Voeroy H, Merskey H, eds. Progress in Fibromyalgia and Myofascial Pain. Amsterdam: Elsevier, 1993:3–21.

2. Nachemson A, Waddell G, Norlund AI. Epidemiology of neck and low back pain. In: Nachemson A, Jonsson E, eds. Neck and Back Pain: The Scientific Evidence of Causes, Diagnosis, and Treatment. Philadelphia: Lippincott, Williams & Wilkins, 2000:165–187.

3. de Girolamo G. Epidemiology and social costs of low back pain and fibromyalgia. Clin J Pain 1991;7(suppl 1):S1.

4. Verhaak PF, Kerssens JJ, Dekker J, et al. Prevalence of chronic benign pain disorder among adults: a review of the literature. Pain 1998;77:231–339.

5. Fordyce W. Back Pain in the Workplace. Seattle: International Association for the Study of Pain, 1995:1–75.

6. Nachemson A, Vingard E. Assessment of patients with neck and back pain: a best evidence synthesis. In: Nachemson A, Jonsson E, eds. Neck and Back Pain: The Scientific Evidence of Causes, Diagnosis, and Treatment. Philadelphia: Lippincott, Williams & Wilkins, 2000:189–235.

7. Carlsson CA, Nachemson A. Neurophysiology of back pain: current knowledge. In: Nachemson A, Johnsson E, eds. Neck and Back Pain: The Scientific Evidence of Causes, Diagnosis, and Treatment. Philadelphia: Lippincott, Williams & Wilkins, 2000:149–187.

8. Olmarker K. The experimental basis of sciatica. J Orthop Sci 1996;1:230–242.

9. Olmarker K, Myers RR. Pathogenesis of sciatic pain: role of the herniated nucleus pulposus and deformation of the spinal nerve root and dorsal root ganglion. Pain1998;78:99–105.

10. Roberts S, Eisenstein SM, Menage J. Mechanoreceptors in intervertebral discs: morphology, distribution, and neuropeptides. Spine 1995;20:2645–2651.

11. Giles LGF, Harvey AR. Immunohistochemical demonstration of nociceptors in the capsule and synovial folds of the human zygapophyseal joints. Br J Rheumatol 1987;26:362–364.

12. Bogduk N. Clinical Anatomy of the Lumbar Spine and Sacrum, 3rd Ed. Edinburgh: Churchill Livingstone: 1997:133–136.

13. Fortin JD, Dwyer AP, West S, et al. Sacroiliac joint: pain referral maps upon applying a new injection/arthrography technique: part I: asymptomatic volunteers. Spine 1994;19:1475–1482.

14. Bogduk N. Clinical Anatomy of the Lumbar Spine and Sacrum, 3rd Ed. Edinburgh: Churchill Livingstone: 1997: 187–213.

15. Boden SD, Davis, DO, Dina TS, et al. Abnormal magnetic-resonance scans of the lumbar spine in asymptomatic subjects: a prospective investigation. J Bone Joint Surg Am 1990;72:403–408.

16. Simons DG, Travell JG, Simons LS. Myofascial Pain and Dysfunction, vol 1, 2nd Ed. Baltimore: Williams & Wilkins, 1999:913–970.

17. Travell JG, Simons DG. Myofascial Pain and Dysfunction, vol 2. Baltimore: Williams & Wilkins, 1992:28–459.

18. LeClaire R, Fortin L, Lambert R, et al. Radiofrequency facet joint denervation in treatment of low back pain. Spine 2001;26:1411–1417.

19. Waddell G. The Back Pain Revolution. Edinburgh: Churchill Livingstone: 1998.

20. Simons DG, Travell JG, Simons LS. Myofascial Pain and Dysfunction, vol.1, 2nd Ed. Baltimore: Williams &Wilkins, 1999:94–177.

21. Glossary Review Committee, Education Council on Osteopathic Principles, American Association of Osteopathic Medicine. Glossary of Osteopathic Terminology, 2002.

22. Deyo RA, Weinstein JN. Low back pain. N Engl J Med 2001;344:363–370.

23. Waddell G, Main CJ. A new clinical model of low back pain and disability. In: Waddell G, ed. The Back Pain Revolution. Edinburgh: Churchill Livingstone, 1998:223–240.

24. van Tulder MW, Ostelo R, Vlaeyen JWS, et al. Behavioral treatment for chronic low back pain. Spine 2000;25:2688–2699.

25. Gerwin RD. Myofascial and visceral pain syndromes: viscero-somatic pain representations. J Musculoskel Pain 2002;10(1/2):165–175.

26. Giamberadino MA, Affaititi G, Iezzi S, et al. Referred muscle pain and hyperalgesia from pain viscera. J Musculoskel Pain 1999;7(1/2):61–69.

27. Gerwin RD. A standing complaint: inability to sit: an unusual presentation of medial hamstring myofascial pain syndrome. J Musculoskel Pain 2001;9:81–93.

28. Bigos S, Bowyer O, Braen G, et al. Acute low back problems in adults. Clinical Practice Guideline No.14. Rockville (MD): Agency for Health Care Policy and Research, Public Health Services, US Department of Health and Human Services; 1994. AHCPR Publication No. (PHS) 95-0642.

29. Meade TW, Dye S, Browne W, et al. Low back pain of mechanical origin: randomized comparison of chiropractic and hospital outpatient treatment. Br Med J 1990;300:1431–1437.

30. Meade TW, Dyer S, Browne W, et al. Randomized comparison of chiropractic and hospital outpatient management for low back pain: results from extended follow-up. Br Med J 1995;311:349–351.

31. Giles LGF, Muller R. Chronic spinal pain: a randomized clinical trial comparing medication, acupuncture, and spinal manipulation. Spine 2003;28:1490–1503.

32. Vleeming A, Van Windergan JP, Dijkstra PF. Mobility of the sacroiliac joint in the elderly: a kinetic and radiology study. Clin Biomech 1991;6:161–169.

33. Strüresson B, Selvik G, Uden A. Movement of the sacroiliac joints: a roentgen stereophotogrammetric analysis. Spine 1989;14:162–165.

34. Jacob HAC, Kissling RO. The mobility of the sacroiliac joints in healthy volunteers between 20 and 50 years of age. Clin Biomech 1995;10:352–361.

35. Lee D. The Pelvic Girdle, 2nd Ed. Edinburgh: Churchill Livingstone, 1999:131–143.

36. Fortin JD, Aprill CN, Ponthieux B, et al. Sacroiliac joint: pain referral maps upon applying a new injection/arthrography technique. Part II: Clinical evaluation. Spine 1994;19:1483–1489.

37. Moore M. Diagnosis and surgical treatment of chronic sacroiliac arthropathy [abstract]. In Proceedings of the 7th annual North American Spine Society meeting: 1992 July 9–11: Boston: North American Spine Society: 1992:100.

38. Moore MR. Diagnosis and surgical treatment of chronic painful sacroiliac dysfunction. In: Proceedings of 2nd World Congress on Low Back Pain, San Diego, 1995.

39. Schwartzer AC, Aprill CN, Bogduk N. The sacroiliac joint in low back pain. Spine 1995;20:31–37.

40. Slipman CW, Sterenfeld EB, Chou LH, et al. The value of radionuclide imaging in the diagnosis of sacroiliac joint syndrome. Spine 1996;19:2251–2254.

41. Fischer A. Functional diagnosis of musculoskeletal pain and evaluation of treatment results by quantitative and objective techniques. In: Rachlin E, Rachlin I, eds. Myofascial Pain and Fibromyalgia, 2nd Ed. St. Louis: Mosby, 2002:145–173.

42. Fischer A. New injection techniques for treatment of musculoskeletal pain. In: Rachlin E, Rachlin I, eds. Myofascial Pain and Fibromyalgia, 2nd Ed. St. Louis: Mosby, 2002:403–419.

43. Davis H. Increasing rates of cervical and lumbar spine surgery in the United States, 1979–1990. Spine 1994;19:1117–1124.

44. Hyman J, Liebenson C. Spinal stabilization exercise program. In: Liebenson C. Rehabilitation of the Spine. Baltimore: Williams & Wilkins, 1996:293–317.

11 Hip and Groin Pain: The Disordered Hip Complex

Lucy Whyte Ferguson, DC
With contributions by David Simons, MD

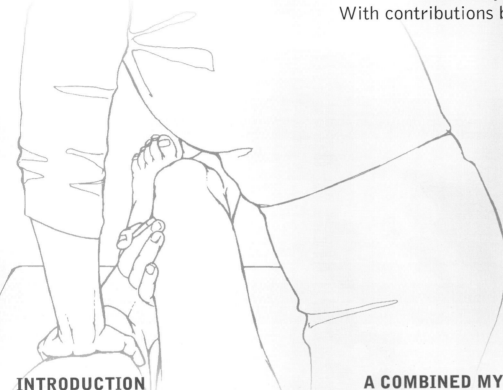

INTRODUCTION

Hip pain and groin pain are complex, challenging, and often baffling conditions for the clinician. Most conventional treatment approaches focus on identifying the painful or tender structure in the hip or groin and addressing the symptoms in isolation from surrounding structures. This chapter reviews existing research and treatment perspectives regarding both of these conditions. Two case histories are presented that demonstrate a myofascial model for evaluating and treating hip and groin pain. Finally, the chapter details a comprehensive myofascial approach that identifies and treats dysfunction in an interrelated set of muscles and joints as an interrelated system. The pathomechanics and pattern of clinical response show such consistency that this text groups musculoskeletal hip and groin pain into a single syndrome called **disordered hip complex**.

This new approach does not deny that identification of tender or painful tissue is important. Rather, it is based on the observation that *patients with both hip and groin pain present with remarkably similar patterns of muscle and joint dysfunction*. For the great majority of patients with *chronic groin pain*, treatment of the interrelated pattern of muscle and joint dysfunction using this new approach results in dramatic relief of pain within 3 weeks, and in completion of rehabilitation within another 3 weeks. For most patients with *chronic hip pain*, the course of treatment using this alternative model normally takes somewhat longer; pain can generally be relieved and function restored within 8 to 10 weeks. Patients with *both hip and groin pain* also generally respond within 8 to 10 weeks.

This chapter also addresses the limitations that osteoarthritis of the hip imposes on functional restoration. Although advanced osteoarthritis of the hip precludes functional restoration in many cases, the practitioner's challenge is to successfully intervene before arthritic changes progress to this stage. Restoring more normal joint and muscle function reduces the mechanical stresses on the hip and thus is likely to retard progression of osteoarthritis. A recommended protocol of treatment of muscle and joint dysfunctions that can bring about successful rehabilitation is provided at the end of the chapter.

GROIN PAIN: BACKGROUND

Groin injuries present a diagnostic and treatment challenge, because it is not unusual for symptoms to last for 6 months or more (1). Two percent to five percent of sports injuries are injuries to the groin (2). In a British study, 58% of professional soccer players gave a history of sports-related groin pain (2). In the National Hockey League, the rate of groin injuries in 1991/1992 was 12.99 per 100 players and rose to 19.87 per 100 players per year in the 1996/1997 season, re-

sulting in a conservative estimate of game loss of 25 player-games per year (3). In a study of Swedish soccer players, groin pain in 50% of the athletes persisted more than 20 weeks after the original injury (4).

Although the initial overload cause of groin pain is fairly clear, an accepted and effective course of treatment leading to rehabilitation is less clear. The cause of sports-related groin pain generally involves an overstretch of groin muscles, or a forced stretch into abduction while the athlete is adducting the leg. These injuries often do not respond to conventional care in the same way as stretch injuries do in other muscles in the body.

The Problem of Diagnosis

Differential diagnoses that may apply to patients who do not recover quickly after injury include inguinal hernia, neuralgia, disc disorder, facet disorder, spinal stenosis, osteitis pubis, tenoperiostitis, prostatitis, stress fracture of the femur or pubic bone, avulsion fracture (particularly in adolescents), iliopectineal or trochanteric bursitis, diverticulitis, abdominal aneurysm, and tumor (2,5–8) as well as the subject of this chapter, disordered hip complex. The difficulty and complexity of diagnosis become clear when it is noted that, in one study, 90% of 21 athletes with chronic groin pain were diagnosed with more than one "disease." Conflicting diagnoses were given to14% of these athletes by four of five specialists, with the diagnoses predominantly within each examiner's specialty (9,10).

For patients in whom established diagnoses have been ruled out and the pain continues, experts have searched for a new diagnostic entity. One such proposed diagnosis is "sportsman's hernia." A sportsman's hernia is a bulge in the posterior inguinal wall, regarded by one investigator as an incipient hernia. Eighty percent of chronic groin pain patients were found to have this bulge, and 93% of these were able to return to their sports activities after surgery (11).

Serious questions must be raised, however, about this approach to treating groin pain. Some investigators point out that herniography has identified actual (not sportsman's) hernias in 84% of symptomatic groins and 49% of *asymptomatic groins*. In addition, it has been suggested that the seemingly positive results of hernia surgery can be accounted for by rest and other conditions surrounding the surgery (9). Therefore, the clinical significance of hernia or incipient hernia in the patient with prolonged groin pain is not clear at this time. Other surgical procedures, such as Gilmore's groin surgery or the simpler surgery to repair a tear in the external oblique aponeurosis raise similar issues. Gilmore's groin describes groin disruption consisting of: 1) a torn external oblique aponeurosis causing dilation of the superficial inguinal ring; 2) a torn conjoined tendon; and 3) dehiscence between the inguinal ligament and the torn conjoined tendon, constituting the major injury (12). Although these conditions may exist, we might find that they would heal without surgery if the disordered hip complex is treated appropriately. Also, it appears that much of the confusion about diagnosis results from the failure of treatment approaches and the resultant search for a "magic diagnosis" that will explain previous treatment failure and afford a successful avenue of future treatment. Although it is important to be aware of possible complicating diagnoses, when groin pain results from musculoskeletal injuries, usually there is no need to search for other diagnoses, because most patients respond within 3 to 6 weeks to the comprehensive myofascial and articular treatment approach detailed in this chapter.

Conventional Treatment Approaches for Groin Pain

Conventional conservative care for groin pain initially involves the use of RICE: rest, ice, compression, and elevation; then later use of heat, passive stretch, range of motion, isometrics, support bandages, and nonsteroidal anti-inflammatory drugs (NSAIDs). When such conservative measures fail, steroid injection to the iliopsoas bursa (13) and to the adductor muscle or tendon may be performed. Adductor and iliopsoas tenotomy also have been proposed, and most athletes return to their sports after these procedures, but with some decrease in strength (14). Most clinicians do not perform surgery until a year has passed without sufficient rehabilitation. However, it is not unusual for rehabilitation to take 6 months or more, and patients who are still having problems after a year are not uncommon. Clearly, the conventional modes of treatment leave much to be desired. It is therefore worthwhile to ask whether other diagnostic and treatment avenues that could result in a shorter and less difficult period of rehabilitation are being overlooked.

In one interesting study, athletes who had been unable to participate in their sports for a mean time of 9 months because of groin injury and persistent groin pain were divided into two groups, one that received passive physical therapy modalities, and the other of which received those modalities but also engaged in an exercise program, starting with isometric exercises of the adductors and other gentle exercises and progressing to a more demanding set of exercises over a 10-week period. At follow-up, 4 months after the end of treatment, 79% of the athletes in the exercise group versus 14% of those in the physiotherapy-only group were without pain at clinical examination and could participate in sports at the same or a higher level of activity (as compared with before injury) without groin pain. The nature of the exercise program employed had certain interesting features: exercise was only performed within a pain-free range, adductor stretching was strictly avoided (presumably this meant not taking the thigh into external rotation as well as abduction, which is the most common position used for adductor stretch), but stretches of other lower extremity muscles, particularly the iliopsoas were recommended (15). The authors do not discuss why they have employed these features

in their rehabilitation program but state that they come from their clinical experience. The discussion of pathomechanics presented in the rest of this chapter will help clinicians to understand the underlying dynamics that affect choices regarding treatment and exercise.

In fact, very few researchers have investigated the functional changes in muscles and joints that take place with a groin injury so as to understand why the course of muscle recovery is prolonged. However, such studies could show an alternative and more successful course of rehabilitation. The following section reviews the sparse literature about pathomechanics, or pathofunction, in cases of chronic groin pain. Such a functional understanding of chronic groin pain forms the basis of the proposed alternative diagnostic and treatment model, presented later in this chapter, that relies on identifying and addressing myofascial dysfunction and accompanying joint dysfunction.

Pathomechanics of Groin Pain

Of over 100 articles on hip and groin pain, only a few include observations regarding muscle and joint dysfunction. Observations include:

- Groin pain can involve pain on passive hip movements, particularly flexion and internal rotation of the femur (13).

- Limitation of hip joint mobility and inhibition of muscle function are often part of the acute stage of groin injury (2).

- Lumbosacral or sacroiliac joint dysfunction, pelvic malalignment, and reduced internal rotation of the hip occur in significant portions of a population with osteitis pubis, a condition that is commonly seen as a repetitive trauma disorder associated with sports, such as distance running, rugby, or Australian-rules football (16).

- Spinal involvement at levels T9–L5 occurs in every case of nonacute groin pain; in most cases, manipulation of the spine reduced the groin pain or was necessary to render peripheral treatment effective (17).

These observations point to the importance of assessing and treating joint and muscle dysfunction in the rehabilitation of chronic groin pain.

HIP PAIN: BACKGROUND
Diagnosis and Clinical Features

Like groin pain, hip pain presents a complex clinical challenge. Differential diagnoses that may apply to the patient who does not recover quickly include degenerative joint disease of the hip, avascular necrosis (Legg-Calve Perthes disease), septic arthritis, trochanteric or ischial bursitis, spinal stenosis, degenerative disc disease, lumbar radiculopathy, lumbar facet imbrication, ankylosing spondylitis, rheumatoid arthritis, gout and pseudogout, slipped capital femoral epiphysis and avulsion fractures (seen in adolescents), coccyx fracture, and femur fracture, and of course disordered hip complex.

Nonmusculoskeletal conditions that can cause hip pain include hernia, aneurysm, atherosclerosis, meralgia paresthetica, thrombophlebitis, cellulitis, abdominal disease, and retroperitoneal pathologic conditions (18–20). Although x-rays are useful to confirm the diagnosis of degenerative joint disease, they do not identify or predict the severity of the patient's pain or dysfunction. For instance, x-rays of an asymptomatic patient may show major degeneration, whereas minimal changes may be seen on x-rays of a patient who is disabled (20). Thus, the relationship between degree of degenerative joint disease and pain is unpredictable.

The relationship between hip intra-articular fluid pressure and pain, however, is linear and predictable. Less pain is associated with pressures below 60 cm H_2O, and markedly increased pain is associated with pressures over 60 cm H_2O (21). Studies have shown that increased intra-articular fluid pressure, whether from synovitis or muscular and capsular constriction, can compromise both arterial circulation to and venous drainage from the head of the femur (21,22). In animals, such compromise for even a brief period (10 hours) causes changes in the femoral head and articular cartilage (23). Therefore, it appears likely that increased intra-articular pressure is a major predisposing factor to degenerative joint disease in the hip. Although the importance of muscular factors in increasing intra-articular fluid pressure is not addressed in any of these studies, the fact that iliopsoas tenotomy performed on cadavers resulted in a 50% decrease in intra-articular pressure may indicate the importance of the increased tension resulting from shortened muscles in contributing to increased intra-articular pressure and resultant degenerative changes (24). Furthermore, one study showed that, in patients with significant hip pathologic conditions, all of whom had advanced osteoarthritic hip degeneration and were scheduled for total hip replacement surgery, long-term pain relief (an average of 13 months' follow-up) was achieved with treatment of myofascial trigger points. Treatment included injection of active tender trigger points with 1% lidocaine, followed by physical therapy and a home stretching program. The following is the frequency of specific muscles found and treated: piriformis—20%, iliopsoas—18%, adductor longus—18%, gluteus medius—12%, gluteus minimus—12%, and other muscles—20%. Treatment was performed weekly for an average of 5.3 weeks, and only 5 of the original 21 patients proceeded to require hip replacement surgery (25). Because it has been established that hip pain increases with increased intra-articular pressure, and also that effective trigger point injection with a stretching program resulted in pain relief for a high percentage of the study participants, it appears likely that inactivation of the trigger

points and release of abnormal muscle tension contributed to that pain relief.

The positions that loosen the joint capsule and decrease intra-articular fluid pressure are 30° to 60° of flexion, 15° of abduction, and 15° of external rotation. It is probably for this reason that the patient with hip pain loses extension and internal rotation first, and often holds the leg in a partially flexed and abducted position (21,26). Shortening of the iliopsoas, the piriformis, and the obturators would also tend to increase flexion and external rotation. In dancers, approximately 40% of all injuries are to the hip and knee. In dancers, whose general flexibility was greater than nondancers, adduction and internal rotation were significantly restricted. A taut iliotibial band has been postulated as a factor in both knee and hip problems in dancers and as a factor in lateral snapping hip (27). Trigger points and muscle shortening in the tensor fascia lata are the most common causes of a shortened iliotibial band (ITB). Taut posterior gluteus maximus fibers with associated trigger points also can contribute to shortening of the ITB, and shortening of the adductor muscle group that affects the femur/hip angle can contribute indirectly as well. Understanding these dynamics and the relationship between increased intracapsular fluid pressure, myofascial involvement, pain, and degenerative arthritic changes in the hip joint will help the clinician understand the importance of providing treatment that will elongate myofascially shortened muscles and decrease pressures across the hip joint. Successful muscle elongation is thus a central aspect of restoring normal joint function and reducing pain, and any resulting decrease in intracapsular pressure may retard degenerative arthritic changes. To accurately assess the impact of myofascial intervention and treatment on arthritic degeneration obviously would require long-term research with appropriate control groups.

Muscle weakness of hip flexors also often accompanies hip pain. Most authors view muscle weakness as a direct response to pain. It also can be caused by reflex inhibition from a remote source such as myofascial trigger points or articular dysfunction, and it does so much more commonly than most clinicians realize. Histologic studies of the muscles of patients with hip pain and weakness have shown atrophy of both type I and type II muscle fibers (28). Others cite iliopsoas weakness and attribute that to an L1, L2 lesion and postulate that other muscles around the hip tighten in an attempt to compensate for the weakness and stabilize the hip (29). Nevertheless, we are in need of an alternative hypothesis because weakness is associated with hip problems, even when effort does not increase pain, and when there is no evidence of a nerve root lesion at the L1, L2 disc level. In fact, as will be shown, weakness is present when femur–hip **subluxation** is present, and there is generally a marked increase in strength when the femur–hip subluxation is corrected. (Subluxation is a chiropractic term that includes changes in normal joint mechanics and associated changes in features such as muscle tension, circulation, nervous system response, and lymphatic drainage. The term is thus akin to the osteopathic term "somatic dysfunction.") Likewise, resolution of associated trigger points also often results in immediate restoration of strength of an inhibited muscle. This alternative hypothesis, that weakness is directly associated with femur–hip joint dysfunction or subluxation or with myofascial trigger points, is discussed in more detail later in this chapter.

Three stages have been identified in the progression of hip degeneration and associated pain:

1. The *early stage* involves synovitis, hip pain and limp, and decreased range of motion, but with normal x-rays (20). This condition has been called "frozen hip." (At this stage, the pain and abnormal function may be primarily attributable to muscle shortening associated with myofascial trigger points, as is the case in most cases of "frozen shoulder." See Chapter 4.) Arthrograms show capsular retraction. Generally, the condition spontaneously resolves in 5 to 18 months (30). This type of hip problem may be similar to the irritable hip or acute transient synovitis seen in children.

   In children, septic arthritis and Legg-Calve-Perthes disease must be considered. Although most of these children have normal x-rays and blood tests, the medial joint space is slightly wider on the affected hip, and an accentuated capsular shadow is noticeable. The affected leg is flexed, slightly abducted, and externally rotated. Acute symptoms generally subside in 2 weeks with resolution in several more weeks. A small percentage of children have problems that persist for 6 months or more (31,32). Synovitis cannot account for all of the pain in children with irritable hip, because approximately 50% of these children do not have demonstrable effusion in the hip joint (33,34).

2. The *middle stage* of hip pain involves moderate hip stiffness, difficulty crossing the legs, and difficulty with abduction (as in sexual intercourse). At this stage, x-ray changes are usually minimal, although functional limitation is significant (20).

3. The *late stage* of hip pain is characterized by marked restriction of the hip, with less than 15° of internal rotation and 115° or less of flexion. Morning stiffness and nighttime pain are common. X-rays often show a significant decrease of joint space and osteophyte formation (35).

Conventional Treatment Approaches for Hip Pain

The challenge for the clinician is to successfully intervene during the early stages of hip pain and dysfunction and alter the progression of the disorder. Conventional therapy involves stretches, isometrics, active range of motion activities, long axis distraction, the use of NSAIDs, and various other treatment modalities. When these approaches are not successful, cortisone injection of muscles, tendons, or bursa is usually the next step. All too often, when conservative measures do not bring relief, the patient is advised to live with the current level of pain and dysfunction as well as possible, until pain and disability reach the point that warrants hip replacement.

A COMBINED MYOFASCIAL AND ARTICULAR APPROACH TO THE DIAGNOSIS AND TREATMENT OF HIP AND GROIN PAIN

When mechanics including *both* myofascial and articular dysfunction are thoroughly evaluated in patients with hip or groin pain, and treatment is provided to address these dysfunctions, rehabilitation is generally steady and progressive. (Note that we refer to the patient's complaint of pain in either the hip or the groin, although the site of pain is often not the source of pain. Much of the pain in the hip and groin is referred from adjacent or remote myofascial and articular structures.) The management and length of rehabilitation appears to be fairly consistent regardless of the patient's age or type of injury (e.g. sports injury, work injury).

The disordered hip complex involves a particular pattern of muscle "winding," including myofascially shortened iliopsoas, quadratus lumborum, gluteus minimus, tensor fascia lata, piriformis and other external rotators in the buttock, medial hamstring, oblique abdominals, adductor muscles, and the pectineus. The rectus femoris, vastus lateralis, and gluteus medius and maximus also may be shortened. The specific location of pain is often dependent on which one or several of these muscles have the most active trigger points; the pain often can be reproduced by palpation of these trigger points. Treatment or unwinding of the entire complex of shortened muscles is important to alter the disordered underlying mechanics. The disordered hip complex also involves subluxation or **joint dysfunction** in an interrelated set of joints. The femur is "jammed" or subluxated in external rotation and is often more prominent in the anterior and lateral portions of the hip joint than on the opposite side. Joint dysfunction also occurs in the sacroiliac joints, the lower thoracic and lumbar spinal segments, and sometimes in the pubic symphysis, tibia, talus, and lateral tarsals. The pathomechanics involving both muscle and joint dysfunction is remarkably similar, whether patients have hip pain, groin pain, or both hip and groin pain; hence the use of the general term *disordered hip complex*.

The treatment procedures described below are usually effective in alleviating pain, whether 1) by reducing mechanical irritation of the painful tissues or 2) by reducing pain referral into these tissues from the areas of muscle and joint dysfunction. The treatment protocol is designed to address *both* of these factors, and they are probably both important in the patient's rehabilitation from hip and groin pain.

The following case histories demonstrate the elements of disordered hip complex and the typical course of care and recovery.

CASE 11-1

Patient History

Mrs. B.L. was 67 years old at the time of her treatment for severe right hip and groin pain. She was 6 feet tall, of moderate weight. She had been treated 3 years previously for a shoulder joint disorder and suffered from rheumatoid arthritis, with at least 15 years of chronic pain in her knees, feet, shoulders, elbows, and wrists.

Three months before Mrs. B.L.'s initial visit for hip and groin pain, she had been laying kitchen linoleum floor tiles. Because of her long-standing problems with her knees, she laid the linoleum bent at the waist and swiveling from her hips, with her legs spread wide, to reach the floor. She subsequently experienced pain in her back that spread into her hip and groin and down her thigh. Electromyographic tests were normal. A magnetic resonance imaging (MRI) scan of the lumbar spine indicated degenerative disc disease at levels L3, L4 and L4, L5 with mild posterior spondylosis but no evidence of disc herniation. The patient also had multiple sacral meningoceles characteristic of Tarlov's syndrome, generally considered a benign and asymptomatic anomaly.

Symptoms

Mrs. B.L. presented for care of severe lateral hip pain radiating down her anterolateral thigh, and groin pain in the inguinal, adductor, and psoas areas. During the entire course of this painful disorder, she had been unable to bear full weight on the involved right leg and was forced to use a cane to walk. During the 3 weeks before treatment, pain in the region of the right sacroiliac joint and buttock recurred, and leg and groin pain worsened. Anti-inflammatory and muscle relaxant medications were of no benefit, and she reported that surgery directed to the sacral meningoceles was being recommended.

Examination Findings

Standing posture was distorted because of Mrs. B.L.'s inability to put weight on her right leg. Her right hip was elevated, and it continued to be elevated (cephalad) even when the patient was supine or prone. Internal rotation of the hip was 30°, and external rotation was 35°, with pain at the end of both movements. Extension was nil, with pain on attempting this movement. The leg was held in approximately 20° of flexion. Ninety degrees of flexion was possible and did not increase her pain. **Valsalva's Maneuver** and **Kemp's Test** of seated thoracolumbar compression were negative. Resistive manual muscle testing indicated mildly painful weakness of the right iliopsoas and right tensor fascia lata. There was tenderness in the lateral hip, but no focused tenderness at the trochanteric bursa. Active

tender trigger points were found in the right gluteus minimus and medius, piriformis, and tensor fascia lata muscles, as well as the right quadratus lumborum and lumbar erector spinae muscles. Diffuse groin tenderness was noted, with active tender trigger points in the oblique abdominal muscles, the iliopsoas, and the adductor group, including the pectineus, and the medial hamstring muscles.

Normal anterior-to-posterior and lateral-to-medial joint play in the right femur–hip joint was reduced. The head of the femur was situated in the anterolateral portion of the hip joint with anterolateral prominence of the femoral head compared with the opposite side. Normal sacroiliac joint play was restricted bilaterally, but was worse on the right and involved both the upper and lower portions of the joint. The right sacrum flared posteriorly. This means that the sacrum was palpably more posterior, with reduction of the depth of the sacral sulcus just medial to the posterior superior iliac spine when compared with the opposite side, and posterior-to-anterior joint play was reduced. When the patient was prone, not only were the right hip and buttock cephalad compared with the left, but the right buttock was raised further from the examining table (greater anterior-to-posterior distance) than the left. Extension and flexion joint play at L4, L5, S1 were reduced, with some tenderness in the posterolateral joint region. It was difficult to assess lateral flexion and rotational joint mobility because of the marked hip-hiking and concomitant rotation induced by the shortened right torso muscles.

Treatment

Treatment was directed toward reducing the pathomechanics of both the joints and muscles involved in the disordered hip complex, including restoring normal function to those structures involved in pain referral. Treatment involved spray-and-stretch myofascial release of the muscles of the torso, groin, buttock, and thigh. Technique for spray and stretch involved concurrent trigger point pressure release and other manual techniques for muscle elongation, with some focus on mobilization of the restricted joints at the same time. (This treatment technique is detailed more fully in the discussion section and Technique 11-4.) Postisometric relaxation or contract/relax was then performed on the right femur to increase external rotation (Technique 11-1), and the wishbone maneuver was performed to increase internal rotation (Technique 11-2). Internal rotation increased 15° after these releases, and external rotation increased 10°. Thus, normal mobility internal and external rotation were restored in the course of the first treatment session.

CASE 11-1   Continued

TECHNIQUE 11-1

Post-Isometric Relaxation (PIR) to Increase External Rotation of the Femur and Release Internal Rotator and Adductor Muscles

If the patient's right hip or groin is symptomatic, the beginning position for a PIR release is with the patient supine, the right hip flexed and thigh externally rotated, the knee flexed, and the right foot resting on the treatment table. The clinician's hand is placed over the thigh near the knee, and the other hand stabilizes the opposite anterior superior iliac spine (ASIS). The patient is asked to exert resistance, at 10% of normal available effort, as if to bring the thigh back toward the midline (out of external rotation). The clinician can control the degree of exertion by instructing the patient to give slight pressure against the clinician's pressure. The resistance is held for 4 seconds, and then the patient is asked to relax. The clinician also relaxes pressure and then takes up the slack in terms of increased external rotation. The procedure is often performed two or three times in succession, with improved external rotation on each repetition. A PIR release is generally performed before the wishbone maneuver, because extreme external rotation often stresses and resubluxates the femur or reestablishes the somatic dysfunction.

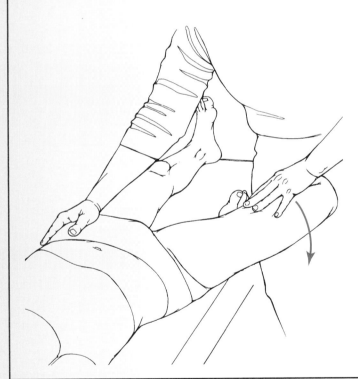

Post-Isometric Relaxation (PIR) release of the femur into external rotation. The patient lies supine with one leg extended and the leg on the side that is to be treated is flexed and the foot is placed flat on the table. That thigh is then gently glided into external rotation, and the clinician's hand contacts the inner side of that thigh, just above the knee. The clinician uses the other hand to stabilize at the opposite ilium. The patient is instructed to gently push medially with the flexed thigh, against the clinician's resistance. After a count of 4, the patient is instructed to relax, and the clinician glides the thigh into increased external rotation until tissue tension or resistance is felt. The maneuver is repeated 2 or 3 times to achieve increased external rotation without pain.

(continues)

CASE 11-1   Continued

TECHNIQUE 11-2

The Wishbone Maneuver

Traditional chiropractic and physical therapy methods of reducing subluxation or joint dysfunction of the femur include long axis distraction, long axis distraction with distraction thrust, and a drop thrust on the knee with the thigh flexed and internally rotated. Although these maneuvers are sometimes effective, they often are only partially so. In many cases, the patient's pain level or arthritis at the hip or knee renders these modes of adjustment inappropriate. The wishbone maneuver can be performed readily under these circumstances.

The wishbone maneuver involves lifting the thigh of the supine patient approximately 30°, abducting it approximately 15°, and internally rotating it as much as possible. In the starting position (**A**), the knees are approximately 12 to 18 inches apart. Then the patient exerts firm resistance with the lifted leg toward the stationary leg, while the clinician draws the thigh up and out in an arc, finishing abducted 30° to 50° and flexed 80° to 110° (**B and C**). The clinician moves the leg through the patient's resistance, but the patient should be instructed to allow movement while resisting, rather than fighting the clinician. *The low level of resistance typically applied in postisometric relaxation and contract-relax-release will not effectively alter the articular dysfunction of the femur in the acetabulum.* In fact, the resistance is submaximal only to the extent that the clinician can still move the leg without straining excessively. The proper level of pressure will become clear with practice: enough to achieve the desired effect and changes in joint and accompanying muscle function without injuring either the clinician or the patient. If the clinician only feels negligible resistance, a greater effort can be requested, or the procedure can be repeated. The effect of the strong eccentric contraction during the performance of this maneuver is to "screw" the hip more deeply and centrally into the "socket." If the patient has pain during this maneuver, the level of resistance can be kept within the patient's pain threshold. The effectiveness of the completion of the maneuver can be reassessed and, if necessary, the maneuver can be repeated. Generally, the pain will be less easily triggered and the patient will be more able to apply the necessary resistance with successive repetitions. Repeating the maneuver more than three times in a session would not, however, be advisable. Certainly treating the trigger points that are responsible for the pain is extremely helpful as well.

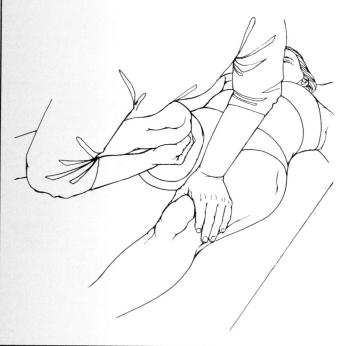

(A) Wishbone maneuver: Starting position. The clinician stabilizes the stationary leg, and grasps the patient's flexed thigh and knee against his or her torso, with the thigh internally rotated and approximately 30° of separation between the two knees. (The clinician's right hand is on the patient's right thigh, and the left hand is on the left thigh.) Care is taken to contact far enough from the knee with a broad contact using an open palm, that there is not direct pressure against tender medial knee tendons, and so that the flexed leg can be moved as a unit rather than producing torque at the knee. Stabilizing the leg against the clinician's torso often makes it easier to avoid torque at the knee.

CASE 11-1   Continued

TECHNIQUE 11-2

The Wishbone Maneuver (*Continued*)

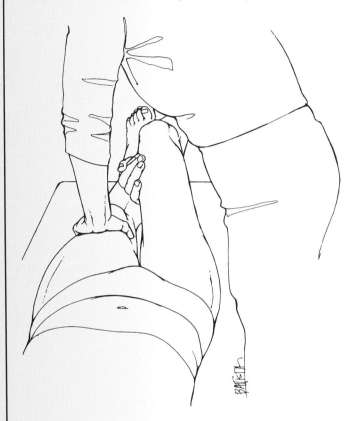

(B) Wishbone maneuver: Mid position. While the patient provides firm resistance, exerting pressure toward the opposite thigh, the clinician straightens up and steps back slightly to abduct the thigh.

Sometimes (approximately 20 % of the time), an audible release (popping or cavitation) occurs, but more often the clinician will evaluate the response by checking for improved range of internal rotation, improved joint play, and the most important indicator: improved strength in the muscle tests of the psoas and tensor fascia lata (and the rectus femoris if it was weak) immediately after the procedure. The changes in muscle strength observed after as compared with before this maneuver are dramatic. If only slight improvement occurs in muscle resistance, a repetition of the maneuver often will bring about a fuller muscle response, as well as further improvement in joint function. Although the procedure can be performed with a straight leg on the side being treated, it is often easiest for the clinician to achieve maximal internal rotation if the patient's knee is bent, and a bent knee is required if the patient has sciatica, a knee injury, or experiences pain on raising the straight leg.

The wishbone maneuver is an excellent method for stretching muscles, particularly the adductor group and the piriformis. However, the dramatic changes in muscle strength occur in muscles that include those that are not being directly stretched: the rectus femoris and the tensor fascia lata. Changes in strength thus may be attributable to changes in trigger point activity and reduced muscle dysfunction and pain, but they also are likely to be caused by a decrease of reflex spinal inhibition from the dysfunctional articulation as the joint function is improved.

It is much easier for the clinician to perform this maneuver on a treatment table that is bench height rather than usual massage table height. To treat the right hip, the clinician stands to the right of the supine patient, leans forward, and holds the right thigh against the chest with the right arm, while stabilizing the opposite hip with the left hand. Simply by straightening up from the leaning position and step-

(continues)

CASE 11-1   Continued

TECHNIQUE 11-2

The Wishbone Maneuver (*Continued*)

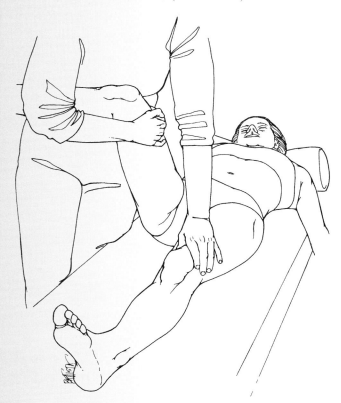

(C) Wishbone maneuver: Completion position. The clinician continues to straighten up and completes the procedure facing almost toward the patient's feet (rather than facing across the table as in the starting position). The thigh is slightly abducted from the vertical, and the clinician's contact on the flexed leg and thigh automatically brings the thigh into maximal internal rotation. The clinician straightens up until the thigh is flexed to at least 90°. Sometimes the thigh will need to be flexed to as much as 110° to feel the shift as the femur "screws into" the normal position in the acetabulum. The clinician who is experienced in this technique often can feel a subtle drop of the femur as it settles into the proper position.

ping backward and rotating to face the patient's feet, the thigh is automatically taken through the described arc. The clinician's position at the end of the maneuver is directly to the right of the patient's hip, facing the feet. This sequence is the best way for the clinician to avoid undue stress in the performance of this maneuver.

Unless there are perpetuating factors that continue to irritate the hip and associated muscles, home stretch exercises of the released muscles will be sufficient to assure maintenance of progress in terms of both the improved muscle strength and markedly improved hip mechanics. The patient may need to avoid repetitive clutch use in driving a car, and hiking uphill, because repetitive and sustained shortening of the psoas may reactivate trigger points. The patient is

instructed not to sit cross-legged, as in a partial Lotus, and not to use an external rotation position to achieve release of the adductors, because while the muscles are still shortened over the hip and groin, the stress of full external rotation positions (i.e., rotation to the end point) can easily resubluxate the femur and reestablish the disordered hip complex. For this reason, the patient is also advised to avoid the frog or whip kick while swimming. When the patient has progressed in treatment and the muscles around the hip and groin have elongated well, the patient can probably lift these restrictions.

(The wishbone maneuver was developed by the author through trial and error of various methods of using muscle effort while the limb is pivoted, to effect a change in articular function.)

CASE 11-1 Continued

Immediately after the wishbone maneuver was performed, the strength of the iliopsoas and tensor fascia lata muscles improved to normal response and the pain on muscle testing subsided completely. Five degrees of hip extension were also achieved with the combination of joint treatment and myofascial release. After 10 minutes of moist heat applied to the groin, thigh, buttock, and lower torso, mobilization of the lumbar spine and sacroiliac joints was performed. The patient experienced a marked reduction of pain after this treatment. The remaining pain tended to localize to the right adductor–pubic region.

After the initial treatment session, Mrs. B.L. began a prescribed regimen of gentle stretches, including stretches of the iliopsoas and quadratus lumborum, and other self-care techniques at home (detailed later in this chapter.) She started to bear more weight on the right leg. Within 12 days, she was able to walk about the house without a cane.

Mrs. B.L. was seen a total of nine times in 3 weeks. At this time, she still had some localized pain and tenderness in the upper adductor muscle but was walking

normally. Trigger point involvement was markedly reduced in the back, abdomen, buttock, groin, and thigh, but there was still localized trigger point involvement in the iliopsoas, pectineus, and the adductor magnus muscles. There was no restriction of hip or back range of motion, and there was no restriction in normal femur joint play, and only minimal sacroiliac and lumbar spine joint restriction. Mrs. B.L. then went out of town for 6 weeks and continued her stretching routine and swam regularly (performing flutter kick but avoiding the frog and whip kick, for reasons that are discussed below.) She had no recurrence of symptoms for 6 weeks, until, with the stress of a large family gathering, she lifted a turkey out of the oven and experienced an aggravation of her pain. She again had difficulty walking but was able to bear some weight on the right leg. After 2 weeks of resumed treatment, the condition resolved.

Follow-up

A year later, Mrs. B.L. reported no reoccurrence of hip and groin pain and no significant low-back problems.

CASE 11-2

Patient History

Mr. R.S. was a 45-year-old ski instructor who had pain in his right groin for 5 months, starting shortly after a ski fall in which he sprained the medial collateral ligaments of both knees. He was not sure exactly when the groin pain started, because his knees were so painful. He had injured his lower back in a motorcycle accident 25 years earlier but recovered with no major problems. He had a posterior dislocation of the right hip with three bone chips 20 years earlier. Surgery was not required, and again he recovered without major sequelae. He experienced chronic recurrent pain at the left thoracolumbar juncture since a fall 5 years earlier in which his back landed on a ski tip. In the most recent ski injury, his skis became entangled with someone else's, his legs were slightly spread apart, and he fell backwards. Before his boots released, he suffered a significant sprain to the inside of both knees, diagnosed as medial collateral ligament sprains. Within a month, using NSAIDs, support, and gentle stretches and exercises, the knees were much better. As his knee pain subsided, he noticed significant groin pain

that continued for 5 months before he came for treatment.

Symptoms

Mr. R.S. had right groin pain in the inguinal and adductor tendon region that, on bad days, extended into the lateral hip. He also had left low-back pain in the region of the thoracolumbar juncture. Although he continued to perform normal activities and exercises, he had been unable to find any stretches or activities that provided relief from the right groin pain.

Examination Findings

The right hip was elevated (raised cephalad) while standing. There was a C scoliosis of the spine, convex to the left, with the left 12th rib lower compared with the right than the disparity in hip height. The relative rib and hip height relationships were maintained with the patient supine and prone. Leg length discrepancy was identified as a major factor in the standing hip imbalance, but shortened muscles, particularly the shortened quadratus lumborum, were maintaining the imbalance

(continues)

CASE 11-2   Continued

in the supine and prone positions. Internal rotation of the right femur was reduced to 30°, and there was marked weakness of the right iliopsoas, tensor fascia lata, and quadriceps on resistive manual muscle testing. Much more resistance was noted in extension of the right hip than left, and the patient reported some pain at the end range of both internal and external rotation. Anterior to posterior and lateral to medial joint play of the right femur–hip joint was restricted.

Valsalva's maneuver, Kemp's seated thoracolumbar compression, and **Bechterew's** seated leg extension did not increase pain. There was bilateral sacroiliac restriction, with a posterior flare of the right sacrum and restriction of both upper and lower portions of the right sacroiliac joint. Extension joint play in the left lower thoracic region was significantly restricted and involved both the spine and the ribs. Anterior-to-posterior talus movement in the right ankle was also restricted, with dorsiflexion limited to 90°.

Bilateral quadratus lumborum muscles were shortened and had active trigger points, the left being much more tender than the right. Some trigger points also were found in the left lower erector spinae. Active trigger points were present in the iliopsoas, with exquisite tenderness over the common iliopsoas tendon. The external oblique muscles were shortened but minimally tender. Active trigger points were also present in the adductor muscles, the medial hamstring, the lateral portion of the piriformis, the gluteus minimus, and the tensor fascia lata.

Treatment

Treatment involved spray and stretch, performed with manual stretch and compression on all of the myofascially involved muscles. The wishbone maneuver was performed on the right hip to restore internal rotation and joint play, with immediate improvement in the strength of the psoas, tensor fascia lata, and quadriceps. Moist heat was then applied over the treated areas for 10 minutes. Afterwards, gentle manual stretching and trigger point pressure release was performed, as tolerated, over the iliopsoas, with the patient prone (Technique 11-3). Gentle side-posture right sacral osseous adjustment was performed, with ilium

TECHNIQUE 11-3

Prone Palpation of the Iliopsoas

The only easy place to palpate the iliopsoas is at the common iliopsoas tendon, where it attaches to the upper femur. The body of the iliopsoas can be palpated with the patient supine, by pressing into the abdomen and following the muscle as it angles medial, upward, and posterior, toward the lumbar spine. In patients who have other tender abdominal structures, palpating the muscle in this position and monitoring changes in muscle length and tension over time to chart therapeutic progress can be difficult. The patient's guarding and the tenderness of other abdominal structures can cause confusion. Therefore, prone palpation of the iliopsoas is recommended as an additional approach under these circumstances. Also, because trigger points are most readily palpated with the muscle on a partial stretch, it is often helpful to approach the muscle in various different positions, because different sets of trigger points may be palpated and treated in each position. The restoration of joint space or "drop-down" of the femoral head within the acetabulum is affected by the iliopsoas tension, and this also can be assessed easily in the prone position, and changes can be monitored from one visit to the next.

With the patient prone, the iliacus is palpated with the fingers around the anterior ilium and cupped into the recess just medial and deep to the bone. After palpating or treating the iliacus, the fingers are moved caudally, toward the common tendon of insertion at the top of the femur. Then the clinician, with the other hand, pulls the thigh into slight abduction and internal rotation, until the tension in the tendon is accentuated against the fingers of the palpating hand. In this position, it feels as though the tendon and muscle drop toward the anterior surface of the body, and the length of the psoas muscle can be palpated, following the line of tension, from the common tendon of insertion on the femur and following the line of tension to the lumbar spine, deep to the navel, and up toward the diaphragm. When there is marked resistance to soft tissue palpation in the lower groin, some of this resistance arises from the anteriorly subluxated femur and will decrease after the wishbone maneuver has been performed, and after moist heat application. This prone position is therefore useful not only for treatment, but also for monitoring progress. If the iliopsoas does not become progressively less

(continues)

CASE 11-2 Continued

TECHNIQUE 11.3

Prone Palpation of the Iliopsoas (*Continued*)

tender and more supple, aggravating factors need to be addressed, for example, excessive foot pronation, hip flexion activities such as mountain hiking that have been too intense for the patient's level of rehabilitation, and external hip rotation stresses that have resubluxated the femur.

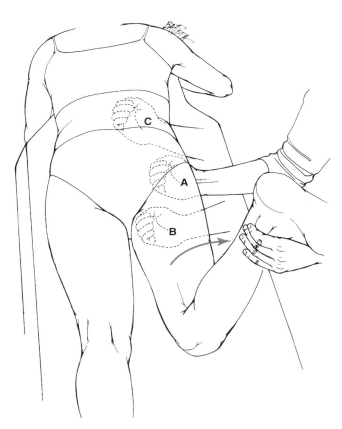

Prone palpation and trigger point pressure release treatment of the iliopsoas muscle. For the clinician learning this technique, it is easiest to start with the treating hand contacting the iliacus muscle just inside the anterior iliac border (A). The lower leg is guided laterally to produce internal rotation of the thigh, until the clinician can feel the increased tension in the bands of the iliacus muscle against the fingertips of the treating hand. The clinician treats tender knots in the taut bands of muscles simply by maintaining pressure with the finger tips while gently internally rotating the thigh and the treating hand gradually advances caudally, toward the insertion of the common iliopsoas tendon at the lesser trochanter (B). From this position, the clinician can follow the tension in the taut bands of the psoas muscle upward toward their origin at the lateral portion of each lumbar vertebra, near the navel and the diaphragm (C). Again, the treating pressure is created by maintaining the contact with fingertips of the treating hand and bringing the taut bands of the psoas muscle closer to the surface by internally rotating the thigh. The upward pressure does not require lifting the back of the treating hand off the table, but rather drawing the taut bands to the fingertips, until the clinician's upward pressure actually elongates the taut bands at each location of tender trigger points. The hand that stabilizes the flexed leg can gently provide a combination of traction, abduction, and internal rotation until the desired tension is achieved.

(continues)

CASE 11-2 Continued

adjustment on the opposite side to address the sacroiliac dysfunction identified in the examination. A "bear hug" type osseous maneuver was performed while rolling the patient back into a supine position, with a specific manual contact placed behind the patient at the left rib/thoracic juncture and with a gentle specific thrust, to restore normal spinal extension joint play and rib–thoracic joint play. An anterior-to-posterior osseous thrust was applied to the talus during ankle distraction and an anterior-to-posterior gentle thrust with an **activator** also was performed, as well as a rocking mobilization to improve foot dorsiflexion.

Mr. R.S. was re-assessed in the standing position at the end of the first treatment. Although lateral to medial joint play had improved, his right femur continued to appear more prominent laterally in relation to the torso and the center of gravity, and the right hip was still elevated. When a 7-mm. heel lift was placed under the left heel to level the pelvis, the patient noted an immediate decrease in right lateral hip discomfort. This factor of functional or actual leg length inequality was very significant in this patient's case, and it is likely that much of the correction of joint and muscle dysfunction would have been temporary, at best, if this perpetuating factor had not been recognized and dealt with initially. (A thorough discussion of the importance of dealing with this perpetuating factor appears in <u>Myofascial Pain and Dysfunction</u>, vol. 2, by Travell and Simon (36; pp. 45–63).)

The patient reported significant reduction of left thoracolumbar pain after the first treatment. When he was seen 2 days later, he still reported some groin pain. When he came for his third visit, 5 days after the initial treatment, his groin pain was reduced by 70%, and the tender distal iliopsoas tendon attachment could be more deeply palpated and gently stretched. Each visit included treatment of muscle and joint dysfunction as described. Because the strength of the tensor fascia lata and iliopsoas was well maintained after the first visit and joint play of the femur at the hip was much improved, the wishbone maneuver was performed only during the initial treatment session. By the fifth visit, 12 days after the initial visit, his groin pain was gone.

Follow-up

Mr. R.S. was seen 2 months later for a recurrence of thoracolumbar area back pain, but the hip and groin pain had not recurred.

An Overview of Disordered Hip Complex

Patients with new or persistent hip and groin pain of musculoskeletal origin generally present with a complex pattern of both muscle and joint dysfunction, which will be referred to as the disordered hip complex. Myofascial involvement generally includes the quadratus lumborum, gluteus minimus, tensor fascia lata, and piriformis muscles as well as other external rotators in the lower buttock, the abdominal obliques, iliopsoas, and adductor muscles including the pectineus, and the medial hamstring. Myofascial shortening also may occur in the rectus femoris and vastus lateralis as well as the gluteus medius and maximus muscles. Internal pelvic musculature also can be involved, including the obturator internus. (See Chapter 14: Pelvic Pain.) In some patients with myofascial shortening of the entire psoas including the T12 or L1 attachments, there is also a taut and tender diaphragm. Joint dysfunction involves the femoral head, the sacroiliac joints, the lower thoracic and lumbar spinal segments, and sometimes the pubic symphysis, and the tibia, talus, and lateral tarsals.

The clinician repeatedly finds a remarkably similar pattern of shortened muscles about the hip and groin in these patients, and significant effort is required to decrease the tension produced by these sets of taut muscles. Therefore, it is tempting to think of the muscle pattern as a guarding pattern. However, muscle guarding would require increased alpha motor neuron activity and active contraction or spasm. There is no evidence that alpha motor neuron activity is responsible for the muscle dysfunction being treated in most patients with chronic pain. In fact, the set of muscles involved are members of what has been termed a **functional unit.** Myofascial dysfunction in one muscle quickly affects the functions of the agonist and antagonist muscles, whether by creating an overload situation, causing reflex inhibition, or inducing development of trigger points in muscles that are a site of referred pain. This process of spread of myofascial dysfunction is so rapid that it is generally not necessary to ascertain which muscle became dysfunctional first, although early correction of "key" injured muscles can help to "unlock" the rest. The entire functional unit must be addressed. Unfortunately, unless the shortened muscles are lengthened as a group, myofascial therapy is unlikely to have lasting benefit. Furthermore, continued myofascial dysfunction maintains abnormal stresses on the joints that will preclude lasting restoration of normal joint function. By the same token, the abnormal joint mechanics are a major perpetuating factor in the myofascial dysfunction, and it is difficult to restore normal muscle length unless the joint function is also corrected. For example, achieving lasting lengthening of the iliopsoas muscle is difficult if significant femoral dysfunction is present (in the acetabulum.) Likewise, maintaining good mechanical function of the femur is difficult if the iliopsoas has not been lengthened.

Causes

Disordered hip complex can arise from any of the following:

- A fall on the hip or back

- A back injury from lifting

- A "groin pull" or strain of the adductor or iliopsoas muscles that occurs while kicking or falling

- Injury to or surgery to any part of the leg or foot that results in a need to hike the leg from the hip to clear the floor with the foot during ambulation

- Prolonged sitting with the thigh(s) flexed and externally rotated

- Intense practice to increase "turn-out" (dancers)

All of these events or situations are likely to activate myofascial trigger points and cause joint dysfunction. The myofascial trigger points are activated by either direct trauma, overload, or prolonged shortening.

Hip and groin pain also may occur in women after sexual intercourse, when the hips are flexed and externally rotated and the internal obturator is in a shortened position. In the latter stages of pregnancy, hip and groin pain may develop and, if severe, may make walking difficult. Severe foot pronation and accompanying eversion of the foot occasionally can cause the disordered hip complex, most commonly by activating trigger points in the iliopsoas and the adductor group. If excessive roll-out at the heel is present before the overpronation, trigger points in the lateral hip muscles can be activated including the tensor fascia lata, gluteus minimus, and piriformis. More commonly, however, hip and groin pain result from some other cause and are perpetuated by pronation and poor foot mechanics.

Cautions

Disordered hip complex also can arise in patients with a herniated disc, cauda equina syndrome, or spinal stenosis. In these situations, addressing the muscle and joint dysfunction in the hip can be a critical feature of effective conservative treatment. However, the patient also must be carefully monitored throughout treatment to ensure that neurologic compromise does not increase. (If neurologic compromise is progressive, the cause must be investigated, and invasive measures may be necessary.)

In children, septic hip must be considered. Children who have no other signs of illness (fever, malaise, elevated white blood count) can undergo a trial of the treatment approach described in this chapter. Under these conditions, children treated with this protocol generally respond more quickly than adults, with resolution within 2 weeks.

In traumatic injury, such as knee impact to the dashboard in a car accident, aseptic necrosis of the hip must be considered, even if no abnormality is visible in early x-rays.

In patients who have had hip replacement surgery, if the surgical hip is the site of joint dysfunction, a consultation with the surgeon is advisable to ascertain whether the hip can tolerate the various aspects of treatment, particularly resisted internal rotation, flexion, and abduction (the wishbone maneuver.)

The pathomechanics of the disordered hip complex also may be present in infants with hip dysplasia. In this case, we use very gentle techniques to elongate muscles and mobilize the hip joints, and we teach parents how to perform these gentle techniques at home. If the hip function cannot be normalized, the infant should be referred for other intervention, because the acetabulum will not form properly if the mechanical relationships cannot be normalized, and chronic problems producing much pain later in life can result from the failure to address this problem.

Symptoms/Pain Presentation

In disordered hip complex, the patient presents with pain in the groin or hip that may extend into the thigh. Pain radiation to the thigh and leg can be severe and can prevent weight-bearing on the leg while walking. Sometimes a clearly defined sciatica is present, including even sensory and motor deficits that follow clear nerve distributions, but more often the pain is diffuse and involves the anterior thigh as well as the lateral and posterior thigh, and is not dermatomal but generally can be accounted for by the sites of pain distribution from active trigger points. Regardless of whether there is nerve compromise, weight-bearing is usually restored after one or two treatments of the disordered hip complex, even when the patient has been unable to bear weight on the affected leg for weeks or months.

The patient also may present with weakness of hip flexors and with difficulty in climbing stairs or a buckling of the leg or knee. This weakness may be attributable to reflex inhibition arising from either joint dysfunction or myofascial dysfunction. The joint dysfunction that is most likely to cause this weakness is the femoral dysfunction at the acetabulum. The myofascial trigger points that are most commonly implicated are in the rectus femoris, vastus medialis, and vastus intermedius muscles, and these trigger points can be either active or latent (37). Pain in the back may accompany the hip and groin pain.

Asymptomatic disordered hip complex may accompany recurrent episodes of lower back pain, knee pain, ankle, or foot pain that are resistant to treatment efforts directed at the local problem. The joint dysfunctions that constitute the disordered hip complex and the muscle imbalances resulting from latent trigger points are likely to be involved. Restoration of normal joint and muscle function, as in the treatment of the disordered hip complex, may be critical to achieve long-term improvement in chronic recurrent back, knee, and ankle problems.

Myofascial Entrapments

The patient with disordered hip complex may have sciatica caused by myofascial involvement and shortening of the piriformis and other adjacent external rotators as the sciatic nerve passes through the sciatic notch. (Gluteus minimus trigger points also can mimic a sciatica, but this is not a case of true nerve entrapment.) Another entrapment associated with disordered hip complex is entrapment of the anterior lateral cutaneous branch of the femoral nerve (ALCB), causing **meralgia paresthetica**. Symptoms include pain or numbness of the lateral anterior thigh. In some individuals, the ALCB passes through the sartorius muscle just inferior to the anterior superior iliac spine and, thus, would be vulnerable to myofascial entrapment. Also, an aponeurotic expansion from the sartorius tendon at the anterior superior iliac spine attaches to the inferior border of the inguinal ligament, and myofascial shortening of the sartorius may depress the ligament and entrap the nerve. Myofascial shortening and thickening of the iliopsoas also may be a factor, because the muscle and the nerve both pass through the lacuna musculorum (38).

Relief of symptoms often can be provided by treatment of the sartorius. Iliopsoas release also may be helpful. However, to provide lasting relief from this disorder, treatment of the other elements of the disordered hip complex often is required, including addressing other myofascially shortened muscles and addressing the associated joint dysfunctions.

The evidence for another possible entrapment, traction neuropathy of the lumbar plexus because of its location within a shortened iliopsoas muscle, is discussed in Box 11-1.

Treatment

Understanding the three-dimensional mechanics of the disordered hip complex is essential to develop a successful program of treatment and rehabilitation. Two metaphors, the rubber band and the bowstring, can be used to conceptualize the disorder (and to describe the condition to patients.)

The Rubber Band Metaphor

The tightened anterior muscles, particularly the iliopsoas, can pull the femur into an abnormal anterolateral position within the joint. The metaphor for this dysfunction involves dolls that have legs attached to the torso by rubber bands. If the anterior rubber band is shortened, the top of the leg does not sit centered in the hip hole or socket (Fig. 11-1).

The Bowstring Metaphor

The bowstring metaphor helps explain the dynamics of the iliopsoas–adductor matrix. These muscles are taut and powerfully shortened in a disordered hip complex, and they act like the string of a bow. When the bowstring is drawn taut, powerful tension is set up in the bow (Fig. 11-2). If the medial pull of the adductors is significant, the tension forces will be reflected in the lateral hip, and the patient may have pain in the lateral hip involving the tendons, bursa, shortened iliotibial band, or lateral snapping hip. If the predominant pull is directed more anterior to posterior by tense hip flexors—the iliopsoas and rectus femoris—the tension effects are reflected into the sacroiliac joint, and the patient will have posterior flaring of the sacrum and a flexion pattern in the pelvis on the involved side (see Fig. 11-1) will be maintained.

This is a complex interrelationship between muscles and joints rather than a direct cause-and-effect relationship. The femur can be palpated as relatively more anterior and lateral in the acetabulum than the opposite hip. As long as the femur is not centered in the joint, the abnormal patterns of mobility or joint play will perpetuate both central and attachment trigger points in the iliopsoas muscle. It is often impossible to make progress in the release of the shortened and tender psoas muscle unless the femur dysfunction is also treated. Likewise, as long as the iliopsoas is so powerfully shortened, the normal joint mechanics cannot be fully restored. Regardless of whether the joint problem or the muscle dysfunction arose first in the sequence of injury (and both sequences are common), it usually is not productive to address the joint problem without addressing the muscle dysfunction, and vice versa. In fact, many patients seek treatment for chronic hip and groin pain who have had perfectly adequate treatment of the muscles or of the joint, but not of both. *The vicious cycle must be interrupted from both directions to achieve rapid and lasting improvements.*

Unfortunately, research and experimentation have not delineated the structures that hold the femur in an abnormal position with abnormal mechanics. However, the simple release of taut muscles frequently is not enough to restore normal hip function. Some researchers and clinicians have suggested contracture or winding of the joint capsule (21), but evidence is not sufficient at this point to draw such a conclusion. Patients who have had extensive treatment to address the muscle dysfunction and lengthen the involved muscles often experience easy retightening of the muscles until the subluxation of the femur in the acetabulum is addressed.

Evaluation of Muscles and Effects on Joint Function

In disordered hip complex, the matrix of myofascially shortened muscles appears to hold the femur too tightly in the joint and in external rotation, off-center in the socket. This disrelationship and dysfunction in joint play can be readily palpated by the skilled clinician, but it is not generally observable on plain x-ray films. Sometimes x-rays show a widening of the medial joint space in the affected hip, and capsular retraction is often visible on arthrography. The challenge is to decrease the compressive forces across the joint, which should reduce the patient's pain and also may improve circulation and possibly arrest the progression of degenerative osteoarthritic changes in the joint.

BOX 11-1

Is There a Psoas Syndrome?

Some patients with a severe and acute form of disordered hip complex appear to have direct nerve compromise arising from the shortened psoas. Usually they are unable to bear weight on the involved leg. Pain distribution is often into the anterior and lateral thigh and lower leg and sometimes the posterior thigh as well. Seated leg extension (Bechterew's test) is often painful. Although these findings of pain can be caused by myofascial and other problems, distal weakness of foot and ankle muscles and sensory changes may correlate with specific nerve involvement. The patients in whom the psoas syndrome is suspected appear not to have the degree of spinal restriction that typically accompanies lumbar nerve root compromise or disc disorder. They also may lack significant piriformis shortening or trigger point involvement, or only experience a slight improvement of symptoms when the piriformis is effectively treated or injected. But each of these patients has a very shortened psoas, and a markedly subluxated femur. The amount of palpable tension in the shortened psoas is quite remarkable. In these patients, the lumbar plexus, located in the body of the psoas muscle, and connected to the sacral plexus by the lumbosacral chord, may be under enough tension to produce a traction neuropathy.

Case Report

A 62-year-old diabetic woman was hospitalized for 2 weeks for severe left lateral hip and leg pain that disturbed sleep and precluded putting weight on the affected leg while walking. Left hip pain had been somewhat subacute, but a history of minor injury to the left knee seemed to provoke this episode of severe pain. Initial evaluation on admission suggested a piriformis syndrome, and injection of the piriformis did result in great improvement of hip function; however, the "radicular" pain persisted. The patient had an MRI that showed some mild degenerative joint disease, but no obvious nerve impingement or spinal stenosis. There was, however, a lighting up of the lumbar plexus in the left paraspinal space, indicating some edema of that structure. Patellar and Achilles reflexes were absent bilaterally, and the patient had decreased sensation in both lower extremities for many years secondary to the diabetes, so sensory examination was unreliable. Nerve conduction/EMG was performed to screen for diabetic neuropathy, and, surprisingly, fibrillation and positive wave activity was seen, suggesting a neuromyopathic process. This activity was seen in the tensor fascia lata, tibialis anterior, peroneus longus, extensor hallucis longus, and in the lateral gastrocnemius and biceps femoris, indicating active denervation in the left leg in the distribution of L5 and S1. The patient was treated with antibiotics for a presumed psoas abscess because she had an elevated sed rate in the 40s, although no elevation of white blood cell count nor any fever was seen. A computer tomography (CT) scan did not confirm the psoas abscess. The patient was put on a regimen of various pain medications, including multiple narcotics, and used a walker, gradually being able to put more weight on the left leg. Although she continued with some leg pain and limp, she was discharged from the hospital after 15 days. She was treated some months later for a chronic rather than an acute version of the disordered hip complex, with resolution of the hip, thigh, and leg pain after one treatment. After treatment, increased strength of both the iliopsoas and tensor fascia lata muscles, as well as ankle flexion and extension, was seen. Interestingly, another complicating factor was present in her disordered hip complex: she had markedly greater pronation of the left foot as compared with the right, and she had tender bumpy swelling of the tendons of origin of the anterior tibialis, along the left shin as well as a previous scar from injury to this same muscle, located just above the ankle, at the base of the belly of the muscle. She also had tender trigger points in this same muscle. Thus, the patient's nighttime lower leg pain appeared to be caused by shin splints and a related myofascial pain syndrome and was not demonstrably from any neuropathy, although the excessive pronation might have a relationship to the hip disorder.

Unfortunately, the complexity of this case and the time lapse between the acute condition and the identification and treatment of the disordered hip complex makes it impossible to draw any firm conclusions. The evidence is tantalizing and suggests the need for further research and documentation before any conclusions can be drawn regarding the psoas syndrome. However, perhaps raising the possibility of a psoas syndrome may increase the likelihood that such investigations will be performed.

Effective treatment involves correctly identifying the most severely shortened muscles and releasing these muscles first, then sequentially releasing the other muscles most responsible for joint compression and restriction at each stage of treatment. Attention also must be paid to the muscles with active trigger points that, on sustained palpation, are referring pain into the location of the patient's symptoms. Both these muscles and muscles with latent trigger points can cause *painful* restriction of range of motion. In the initial examination and throughout the course of treatment, the clinician should palpate to determine exactly those muscles that are restricting range of motion of the femur: specifically, those that restrict extension, those that restrict internal rotation, and those that encourage abduction or adduction. Rather than basing conclusions on the clinician's preconceived ideas, it is most helpful to identify the primary restrictive muscles by taking the femur to the end of joint motion and palpating the suspected muscles for relative tautness or tension. Obviously, if a muscle is at significant tension at the end of the range of motion, it may play a role in joint restriction. Conversely, if that muscle is not at significant tension at the end of the range of motion, then it does not play a role in the restriction of that range of motion. During the course of care, it is often necessary to

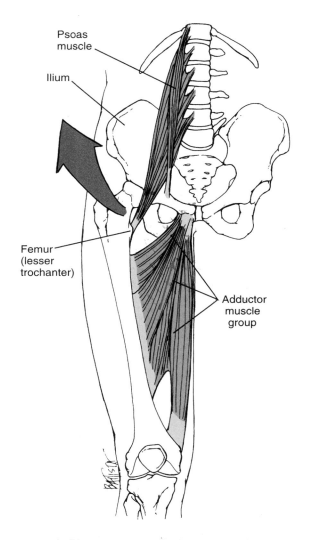

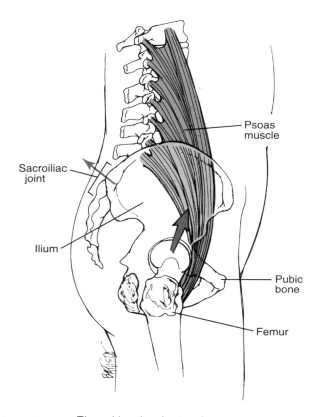

FIGURE 11-1. **The rubber band metaphor.** With the iliopsoas shortened, the femoral head does not center in the acetabulum, although it is still within the acetabulum. The shortened iliopsoas muscle angles forward over the pubic ramus and attaches to the lesser trochanter on the upper medial femur. Greater tension in the shortened muscle will thus pull the femur into the anterior portion of the joint. A reduction in anterior-to-posterior joint play often can be palpated by contacting the upper femur while the patient is supine. Often, the groin crease on the involved side will appear more shallow. The bowstring metaphor also applies here. The pull of the shortened iliopsoas reflects a stress posteriorly, to the sacroiliac joint. Often, the sacrum will flare posteriorly, and partial flexion rather than full extension and locking of the sacroiliac joint will result. For these reasons, when the patient is placed prone, the involved hip and buttock will be higher relative to the table than the uninvolved side.

FIGURE 11-2. **The bowstring metaphor.** The shortened iliopsoas and adductor muscles hold the femoral head compressed upward toward the lateral rim of the acetabulum. External rotation also is encouraged by the shortened iliopsoas and adductor muscles, because the iliopsoas attaches to the lesser trochanter at the medial femur, and portions of the adductor muscle attach from the pubic bone to the medial posterior femur. The combined shortening of the adductor and iliopsoas muscles reflects stress to the lateral hip, and can contribute to increased tension in the iliotibial band, tendonitis at the hip, and trochanteric bursitis. Thus, the medial tension and stresses need to be addressed to bring relief to the lateral structures.

reassess for muscles that may be restricting joint mobility. If the clinician has successfully released one set of taut muscles, then a different set of muscles may subsequently require treatment to restore full joint mobility.

The following sections describe suggested positions and modes of assessment of muscle and joint interaction and thus focus primarily on the *mechanical relationships*. Each section also discusses the most frequent patterns of muscle restriction.

Side-Lying Assessment. The principal player in restriction of hip extension appears to be a shortened iliopsoas. The rectus femoris can play a role as well. Extension of the straight leg shows the role of the iliopsoas, whereas extension of the bent leg demonstrates the rectus femoris contribution. Assessment of extension is easily accomplished with the patient side-lying with the symptomatic side up. The clinician blocks the backward movement of the patient's pelvis with the torso or knee and extends the patient's leg to tension (Fig. 11-3). Flexion of the underlying leg at the hip and knee is also helpful to stabilize the patient and reduce lumbar spine extension. The clinician compares the symptomatic side with the asymptomatic side. Often there is some restriction of extension at both hips, especially if the patient has had a forward bent **antalgic** posture.

This position also can be used to assess the muscular contributions to the hiking of the hip. A pillow can be placed under the pelvis to separate the rib cage from the pelvis, or the leg can be dropped backward, with the foot and lower leg off the edge of the table (with the under leg flexed and the ankle supporting the thigh or knee of the upper leg). When the ilium has dropped until the muscles are at tension, portions of the quadratus lumborum and the internal oblique abdominal muscles can be palpated, and their relative tautness and contribution to hip-hiking can be assessed (Fig. 11-4). When the leg is drawn forward, other portions of the quadratus lumborum and the external oblique abdominal tension can be assessed, again by feeling for restriction in the clinician's ability to press the hip away from the ribs. The rectus abdominis and erector spinae are part of the functional unit as well and can be palpated in this position, but they do not cause specific restriction of the range of motion (ROM) being assessed. The quadratus lumborum and internal and external abdominal oblique muscles are clearly the major muscles that restrict this movement.

It is important to perform a similar assessment of the muscles on the opposite side of the torso. Because of the hip-hiking, the lower thoracic and lumbar spine is often in a slight C-scoliosis, convex on the side opposite the hiked hip. The diagonal portions of the quadratus lumborum, particularly the iliolumbar fibers, are often shortened on the convex side as well, between the apex of the curve and the iliac crest (Fig. 11-5). Also, portions of the erector spinae on that side have usually shortened and will need to lengthen to allow the body to return to postural and functional balance.

In the side-lying position, the clinician can assess the tightening or cephalad compression arising from the gluteus minimus, medius, and tensor fascia lata. Long axis traction is placed on the femur to stretch directly across femoral joint, and the degree of tension in the posterior and lateral hip is assessed. Generally, the hip flexors (iliopsoas and rectus femoris) appear to be much more powerful in reducing joint space and joint play in the long axis direction than the gluteus minimus and medius and tensor fascia lata.

Supine and Prone Evaluation. Restriction of internal rotation can be assessed with the patient supine by rolling the entire leg internally (medially), or with the prone patient by bending the knee 90° and swinging the foot laterally, which also will internally rotate the thigh in this position.

Clearly, the taut iliopsoas is a major factor in decreasing internal rotation. Even after substantial elongation of the iliopsoas, however, the muscular restriction of internal rotation of the femur still can be significant. Generally, the remaining shortened muscle group that seems to play the most important role in further limiting internal rotation is the adductor group, including the pectineus. Although external rotation generally is not thought of as a function of this muscle group, the myofascially shortened muscle is a major factor in restricting internal rotation. The adductor longus arises just posterior to the pubic symphysis, and the pectineus, adductor brevis, and the uppermost part of the adductor magnus arise from the pubic ramus. All of these

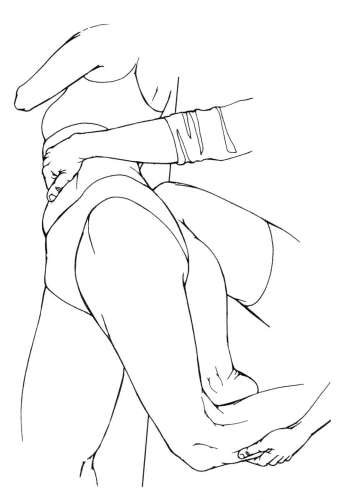

FIGURE 11-3. The side-lying position for evaluation and stretch release of the iliopsoas (and quadriceps) muscles. The clinician stabilizes the lumbosacral spine so that extension is focused at the hip. This is an ideal position in which to perform contract-relax-release and contract-relax-assist.

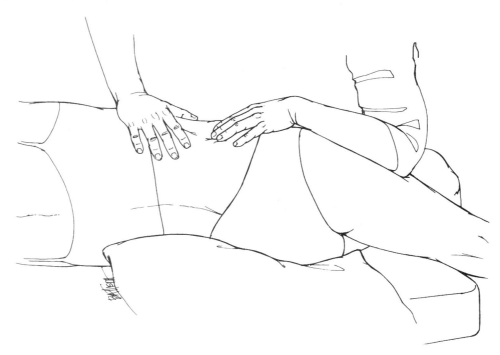

FIGURE 11-4. The side-lying position for evaluation and stretch release of the quadratus lumborum and internal oblique abdominal. A pillow is used under the waist, to enhance the separation of the rib cage from the pelvis. The leg should then be placed forward, and different taut bands will be palpated in the quadratus lumborum, and taut bands in the external oblique abdominal muscles will be easier to palpate. Contract-relax-release can be performed in this position, with the clinician stabilizing at the lower rib cage and the top of the ilium. The rib cage is passively stretched away from the ilium until tissue tension is reached, and then the patient is asked to contract (gently for a count of 4) and then release, and then the clinician stretches the ribs away from the iliac crest until a new barrier is reached, and the procedure is repeated.

adductor muscles attach to the posterior surface of the femur at different points along its posteromedial shaft (39). Accordingly, the shortened members of this muscle group can generate rotational forces by maintaining the posteromedial femur more anterior toward the pubic symphysis. Clinical experience indicates that the iliopsoas and adductors are primarily responsible for the restriction of internal rotation in 60% to 70% of hip and groin pain patients, with the piriformis and other external rotators in the buttock relatively slack at the end of internal rotation motion (assessed as described on pages 284–286). Only 30% to 40% have taut piriformis, gemelli, and obturators at the end of internal rotation motion, and in these patients, the role of the iliopsoas and adductor is still quite important, if not primary.

The semimembranosus and semitendinosus of the hamstring muscle group are also often taut and shortened along with the adductors. Medial hamstring involvement may become part of this functional unit, and thus the dysfunctional hip complex, because the hamstring is called on to balance the increased tension in the hip flexors. Whatever the reason, invariably the medial hamstring is shortened with trigger points in this hip complex.

With the patient prone, the relationship between tension in the iliopsoas, adductor, and medial hamstring (medial

muscles) and tension in the iliotibial band, tensor fascia lata, and other lateral buttock muscles can be assessed. Tautness in the gluteal muscles, piriformis, and iliotibial band can be palpated with one hand, while simultaneously slightly abducting and internally rotating the femur with the other hand (Fig 11-6). The degree of abduction and internal rotation that is necessary to create some slack in the iliotibial band can be assessed. Referring to the bowstring metaphor, this amount of slack in the medial muscles must be achieved in treatment to take strain off the lateral muscles.

Treatment Tips for Muscle Release. Once the clinician has identified the specific pattern of muscle involvement in each patient by the methods just described, the muscles can be treated. On subsequent visits, evaluation and treatment can be combined in each body position (side-lying, supine, prone) before moving on to the next body position.

When treating the abdominal-iliopsoas-adductor portion of the muscle matrix, the muscle stretching can be performed in the side-lying position. Care should be taken not to force the hip into excessive extension. The clinician should feel for the soft tissue barrier, and the patient should feel only muscle tension *but no pain*. Forced extension can recreate the joint dysfunction at the femoral head. The iliopsoas can then be treated in the prone position (see Technique 11-3). This is also an excellent position in which to monitor changes in tenderness and tautness of the iliopsoas throughout the course of treatment. In this position, as the iliopsoas releases over the course of successive treatments, the femur can be felt to "drop-down" in the socket. Precisely this increased space around the femoral head in the acetabulum makes it possible to establish and maintain normal hip mechanics.

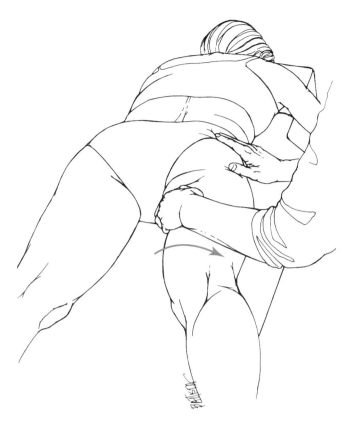

FIGURE 11-6. Hand positions to lengthen adductor and medial hamstring muscles at the medial thigh and reduce stress on the lateral hip structures. The clinician abducts and internally rotates the femur, and places a stretching or traction pressure on the taut bands of the adductor muscles. Because the different portions of the adductor attach at different portions of the posterolateral femur, this procedure is repeated with the hand at different positions along the inner femur. The clinician assesses the effects on the release of adductor tension on the tensor fascia lata, lateral portions of the gluteus medius and minimus, and the piriformis and associated external rotators in the lower buttock. Over successive treatment visits, the adductor muscle will need to be released sufficiently to reduce the stresses on the muscles attaching at the lateral hip, to effectively treat all of the members of this functional unit.

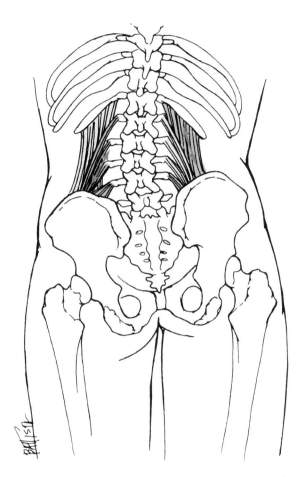

FIGURE 11-5. **Pattern of shortened muscles associated with hip-hiking.** On the side of the elevated hip, the iliocostal portions of the quadratus lumborum (highlighted in darker red on the side of the higher hip) are most severely shortened and will need to be lengthened to drop the hip down to a level position. However, if the pelvis levels, then the functional scoliosis will decrease; the spine will straighten. If the clinician does not sufficiently lengthen the iliolumbar portions of the quadratus lumborum (highlighted in darker red on the side of the lower hip), the tension in these muscles will *increase* with the leveling of the pelvis. To prevent the patient's pain from switching from one side to the other, the clinician will need to effectively treat the muscles on the involved (hip-hiked) side as well as the muscular compensations on the opposite side. To treat the side of compensation, the clinician places the pillow under the hip and then mobilizes (by pulling and pressing) the lumbar facet areas down and away from the iliac crest, while simultaneously pressing on the trigger points in taut bands of the iliolumbar portion of the quadratus lumborum.

If the iliopsoas is still fairly taut and shortened after prone treatment, the clinician can treat the patient supine with the thigh and knee flexed and the foot resting on the table. In this position, the clinician treats the iliopsoas by contacting taut portions of the muscle with moderate pressure and maintains this pressure while the patient gradually slides the leg into an extended position and then internally rotates the leg (Fig. 11-7). Another possible position for stretch is with the patient supine and dropping the involved leg off the table, but it may be best to avoid this position at first because it can be too stressful to the hip joint and can irritate the condition if the limb is not adequately supported by the clinician.

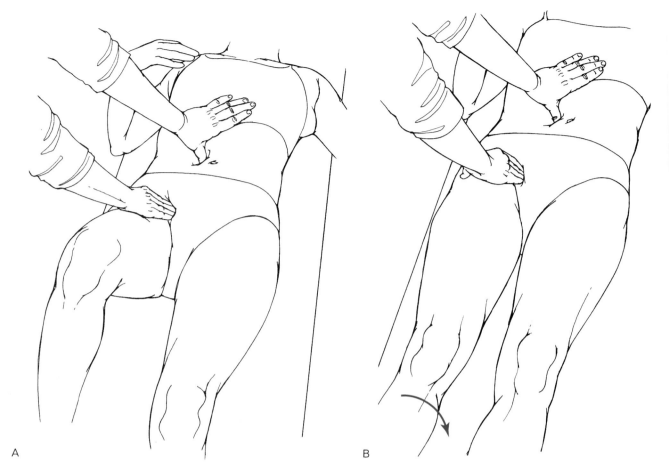

A   B

FIGURE 11-7. Level 4 or active myofascial release of the iliopsoas. **A.** Starting position. **B.** Ending position with leg extended and internally rotated. The contact is maintained on the taut bands in the upper and lower portions of the psoas muscle as pictured, or the lower hand may be placed on taut bands of the iliacus muscle as the foot slides slowly down the surface of the table until the leg is fully extended. The clinician then instructs the patient to turn the foot in toward the other foot as much as possible. (For an explanation of myofascial release, levels 1–4, see Chapter 6.)

When releasing the adductor muscle in the patient with the disordered hip complex, care must be taken not to put too much external rotation stress on the hip joint, or it may resubluxate. If subluxation recurs, the adductor will retighten with a vengeance within a few hours.

Recurrent subluxation of the femur and accompanying retightening of the adductor is, in fact, probably one of the features of disordered hip complex that results in very complicated and prolonged periods of recovery after hip and groin injury. The paradox occurs: *precisely the maneuvers that are being done to release tension in the adductor are often aggravating the femoral subluxation, thus perpetuating the entire condition.* These maneuvers generally involve taking the femur into external rotation. The initial femoral subluxation involved external rotation as well as loss of anterior to posterior and lateral to medial joint play. This was the nature of the lesion, and the clinician should avoid taking the femur back "into lesion." When the muscles around the hip are still fairly tight, the femur that is fully externally rotated can easily resubluxate. Within hours, the entire functional unit

of myofascial involvement often will recur as well, and the patient will feel no relief and often a worsening. Therefore, *the clinician should avoid taking the hip into full external rotation.* Other practitioners who are working with the patient concurrently should be advised about this as well, and the patient is advised to avoid these positions when sitting, sleeping, etc. The adductor can readily be stretched and treated with straight abduction or abduction with internal rotation. Most patients can return to full activity and external rotation positions as soon as sustained drop-down of the femur in the hip socket has occurred.

When treating the tensor fascia lata muscle to release tension of the iliotibial band, the clinician must be careful to avoid putting too much stress on the lateral hip. Some patients will tolerate significant adduction of the femur, and some will not. However, we can indirectly release much of the stress on the lateral hip by releasing the bowstring effect of the taut iliopsoas and adductor muscles. With this done, efforts to treat trigger points in the tensor fascia lata muscle will be much more successful.

Treatment Focused on the Muscles Involved in the Pain Pattern. This discussion has focused on addressing the muscles that make the most significant mechanical contribution to disordered hip complex. However, identifying and treating the specific myofascial trigger points that contribute pain to the hip or groin is also very important. In terms of evaluating the muscles involved in the patient's *pain*, the following sequence has been very helpful:

1. The patient identifies the exact locations of pain, and the clinician correlates these with the muscles likely to cause referral to these locations. (Volumes 1 and 2 of Myofascial Pain and Dysfunction: The Trigger Point Manual and the related wall charts are most helpful.)

2. Rather than examining the muscles right away, it is helpful for the clinician to check suspected muscles for *painfully* restricted range of motion (ROM.) Consistently, the muscle that has myofascial trigger points hurts before the muscle reaches full ROM. The trigger point may be active or latent, but the more active the trigger point, the less tolerant the muscle is to additional stretch tension at the end range of motion. This end range pain is likely caused by the attachment trigger points and the associated enthesopathy. According to current theory, the central trigger points in the muscle correspond with the contraction knots that create tension in the taut bands. When this tension is maintained over time, it causes an enthesopathy at the attachment of the taut fibers. This has been referred to as the attachment trigger point to distinguish it from the central trigger point (40).

3. When the muscle reaches the painful limit of stretch ROM, it is often enormously helpful to ask the patient: *Point to where it hurts.* The patient will usually point to the muscle with the most active myofascial trigger points in the muscle group that is being stretched. That muscle is then palpated for taut bands and trigger points. Often the patient points directly to the stretch-sensitive enthesopathy.

4. At this point, it is important to distinguish muscle spasm, which makes the whole muscle tense, from the trigger point tension caused by individually palpable taut bands. Generally this distinction can be made adequately by muscle palpation, but it also can be confirmed by electromyography (EMG), which can definitively identify whether the muscle is in spasm (41).

5. When the muscles that are painfully restricting ROM are palpated to identify trigger points and taut bands, it is an ideal situation to move right to treatment by lengthening the shortened muscle through **contract-relax-release**. The technique involves stretching the muscle to the point in the ROM where it is at its stretch barrier, tense but not painful. Then the patient is instructed to contract the muscle slightly against the clinician's counter pressure for a slow count of 4. The clinician thus can control the pressure exerted by the patient. Then the patient relaxes, and the relaxation may be augmented by respiratory expiration. The clinician waits a few seconds while the patient relaxes, and then draws the muscle through pain-free ROM until the new stretch barrier is encountered. This sequence can be performed three or four times, with progressive, but painless, lengthening of the muscle during each repetition.

A very useful variation of this technique is **contract-relax-assist.** The contraction and relaxation follow the description provided in the last paragraph. After the relaxation, however, the patient actively assists muscle elongation and stretch by contracting the antagonist muscle. This is a very useful technique to incorporate in the treatment, especially to work with those muscles that are not releasing readily with spray and stretch and manual trigger point pressure. Slight or 10% muscle contraction may recruit additional sarcomeres that are lengthened within the taut band to pull on the shortened sarcomeres that are within the contraction knot. The sarcomeres within the contraction knot are already at full tension in the starting position and cannot contribute significantly to the contraction. The contraction of the other sarcomeres within the taut band actually may help to undo some of the shortening of the sarcomeres within the contraction knot. In this way, the sarcomeres that were over-stretched in the taut band become less stretched, and the sarcomeres that were over-shortened in the contraction knot become less shortened. The resultant equalization is integral to the treatment of both the pain and dysfunction (40). The technique is also especially useful because the patient can incorporate the approach into an independent stretch program for home care. The patient should be instructed to use no more than slight or 10% effort and should have a sense of what constitutes slight effort from having performed contract-relax with the clinician's assistance. **Beware** *of a painful reaction that occurs if the trigger points in the antagonist are activated by this technique.* A progressive release of tightness back and forth between the agonist and antagonist generally results in effective release of both muscles and avoids this kickback reaction.

6. Education of the patient for home use of this technique involves showing the patient pictures of the muscle anatomy and of appropriate stretch positions, and explaining how the recommended stretch lengthens that muscle.

The following are the muscles most often referring pain to the hip or groin: Lateral hip pain can be caused by pain referred from the gluteus minimus, vastus lateralis, quadratus lumborum, gluteus maximus, piriformis, and tensor fascia lata muscles. It also can be caused by attachment trigger points and associated enthesopathy in the tendons that attach to the greater trochanter. The tensor fascia lata has been identified by Travell and Simons for its propensity to refer tenderness into the trochanteric bursa and to cause pseudotrochanteric bursitis as well as a deep ache in the hip (38). Piriformis trigger points can refer similar tenderness to the lateral hip and bursa. When trochanter bursa tenderness markedly improves in the course of one treatment session or by the next day (often 60% to 90% improvement), the condition is most likely pseudo-bursitis, because a true inflammatory tissue response does not ordinarily respond to care so quickly.

Likewise, trigger points in the external abdominal oblique, quadratus lumborum, adductor magnus, and iliopsoas muscles can refer and maintain pain in the groin area. The clinician should examine these muscles for trigger points that reproduce the patient's groin pain. Again, immediately after treatment or the next day, tenderness along the inguinal ligament and of the iliopsoas tendon or the adductor tendon often decreases significantly. When such rapid improvement occurs, it is likely that the pain represents pseudo-tendinitis. Some of the tenderness in the tendon can be referred tenderness, and some of the tenderness may be enthesopathy caused by attachment trigger points. Attachment trigger points in the external abdominal oblique muscles can account for the inguinal region tenderness, and attachment trigger points in the iliopsoas and adductor muscles can account for the tenderness in the respective tendons. Accordingly, treatment should be directed at releasing trigger points within the contraction knots in the taut bands located in these muscles and others that refer pain and tenderness into the groin as well as addressing the attachment trigger points. These manual therapy measures are often more effective than anti-inflammatory medication or cortisone injection in providing relief from chronic pain in the groin.

The specific myofascial release techniques used in treatment are presented in Technique 11-4.

Assessment and Treatment of Joint Dysfunction

The Femur. The treatment of muscle dysfunction and joint dysfunction go hand-in-hand when treating disordered hip complex. Central to the success of the treatment are both the ability to palpate joint dysfunction in the hip joint and the ability to restore normal joint function. With the patient supine or prone, the examiner can learn to feel decreased joint play, particularly in an anterior-to-posterior direction. The examiner also may be able to feel the prominence of the femur in the lateral hip. Internal and external ROM are easily assessed in the supine patient with the thigh and knee flexed to 90°. Changes in normal range of motion, when present, are clearly an important aspect of the joint dysfunction. (Normal internal rotation is 35° to 45°, and normal external rotation is 45°.)

However, the most reliable indicator of dysfunction of the femur in the acetabulum is weakness of the iliopsoas and tensor fascia lata muscles on manual resistive muscle testing. Severe joint dysfunction also often will cause generalized weakness of hip flexors, and the patient may describe the leg "giving way" on weight-bearing, such as going up stairs,

and arising from a chair. Although myofascial trigger points in the hip flexors also can be responsible for this weakness, the reflex inhibition from the articular dysfunction is a major factor in this weakness. Further discussion of "articular neurology" and the effects of joint dysfunction on muscle coordination is presented by Dvorak and Dvorak as well as Wyck and Polacec (42,43). Muscle testing before and after the wishbone maneuver, thus, is a reliable way to evaluate whether the desired change in articular function has been sufficiently realized. Improved joint play and an increase in ROM also result from effective treatment of the femoral dysfunction in the acetabulum.

Manual muscle testing of the psoas and tensor fascia lata muscles must be performed with considerable care; the clinician has a dramatic advantage over the patient because the clinician is standing over the supine patient, directing pressure against the patient's leg. The leg is a very long lever, and both the psoas and the tensor fascia lata are relatively small muscles. So as not to injure the patient, the clinician gradually exerts only enough pressure to see whether the patient can meet the testing pressure with a firm counter pressure. No matter how strong the patient's muscles, the clinician could easily overpower the patient, but no accurate results would come from such testing. The psoas muscle is tested with the femur flexed approximately 40° from the table, abducted approximately 45°, and externally rotated as far as can easily be accomplished. The patient is instructed to resist or maintain the leg in that position while the clinician contacts the medial lower shin and directs pressure laterally and inferiorly toward the table. The line of force should be imagined as that necessary to elongate the psoas muscle between its attachments at the lumbar spine and the inner upper femur. If the patient can meet the clinician's pressure with firm counter pressure, then the muscle is strong. To test the strength of the tensor fascia lata muscle, the leg is elevated approximately 45°, abducted 45°, and internally rotated as far as is easily accomplished. The clinician then contacts the outer shin and presses medially and inferiorly toward the table as though to elongate the tensor fascia lata between its attachments at the crest of the ilium and at the lateral upper femur. Again, if the patient can meet the clinician's pressure with a firm counter pressure, then the muscle is strong. If there is any question, the test can be repeated. If the muscle is weak, it will fatigue, but if it is strong, the second testing will be easier because the patient knows what to expect. If the clinician notices that the patient has a very strong quadriceps muscle and is clearly contracting that muscle during the performance of these tests, the clinician should lower the leg somewhat or increase abduction, until the quadriceps is placed at a greater relative mechanical disadvantage. If the patient has sciatica, and straight leg raising is painful, these muscle tests are performed with the knee bent. It is more difficult to achieve the direction of pressure required to test the psoas and tensor fascia lata muscles when the knee is bent than when the leg is straight, but the careful clinician generally can achieve accurate results. Accurate muscle testing

TECHNIQUE 11.4

Smorgasbord Approach to Myofascial Release

Many trigger point and muscle elongation techniques can be effectively employed together in a treatment sequence. The most important aspect of the approach is the use of whatever techniques are effective in elongating muscles, eliminating trigger points, and treating joint dysfunction. The following is an example of a treatment sequence most often used in the rehabilitation of patients with the disordered hip complex:

1. The patient is taken through a sequence of passive stretches in the treatment positions described in this chapter. This can be done with or without fluoromethane spray and stretch.

2. The clinician identifies and then holds taut muscle bands with one hand, focusing the stretch and manually pulling on the bands to increase the passive stretch.

3. The clinician identifies trigger points that are not readily releasing with the stretch and applies trigger point pressure release to these trigger points *during the passive stretch*.

4. The clinician also presses into the stiff joints to mobilize them, also *during the passive stretch*. For example, when the patient is in a side-lying position, with the upper arm raised and the upper hip lowered, the clinician can press with the hand or the elbow to increase extension or lateral flexion of the lumbar spinal segments, or to increase rib/spinal mobility.

   Because the most active trigger points are often in close proximity to the restricted joints, the same pressure used to release the trigger points also can be used to mobilize the joints *simultaneously*.

5. From passive stretch, the clinician can focus on muscles that need further elongation by proceeding directly to contract-relax-release and contract-relax-assist.

6. Moist heat then can be applied to all the muscles that have been treated, to assist in muscle relaxation. (There will be more effective psoas release during the moist heat if the wishbone maneuver is performed *before* the moist heat.)

7. After the moist heat, the clinician can "zero-in" on remaining taut bands and trigger points using whatever techniques are most effective with the particular patient:

   a. Further contract–relax techniques or trigger point pressure release

   b. Percussion technique (discussed in Chapter 4)

   c. Myofascial releases 3 & 4 (discussed in Chapter 6)

   d. Any of the techniques developed by Dejung for myofascial release (discussed in Chapter 14)

   e. Any other techniques that are effective in myofascial release

8. Remaining articular dysfunction then can be treated. Often the myofascial release techniques and joint mobilization that have already been performed will decrease the number of articulations that require further direct treatment. Also, the pressure or impulse required for release of joint restriction will be much less, so the joint treatment can be much gentler after myofascial release.

To perform these combined treatments, the clinician needs to keep in mind the patterns of trigger point involvement, taut muscle bands, and joint subluxation that have been identified in the examination or in the course of previous treatments. Although written examination notes are necessary for documentation, drawing the trigger points and taut bands, and marking the subluxated joints on a full-page body map, is an effective way to keep track of these patterns from one visit to the next.

---

is an art and can be used to assess the need for and the successful completion of the wishbone maneuver.

The wishbone maneuver has been found to be the most consistently useful and nontraumatic technique for restoring normal hip function (see Technique 11-2). Manual muscle testing of the iliopsoas and tensor fascia lata muscles (and the rectus femoris, if it is weak) is the best way to assess the successful completion of the wishbone maneuver. However, significant pain on gentle muscle testing indicates that myofascial pain and dysfunction also may be a factor in the muscle weakness. A clear correlation exists between femoral dysfunction and muscle weakness and the restoration of normal joint function and immediate increase

in strength. The wishbone maneuver clearly is likely to affect muscles as well as the hip joint, but this method of joint treatment is often critical to resolving the condition, even when every conceivable method of treating myofascial dysfunction has been tried by skilled practitioners without lasting result. *Thus, subluxation or joint dysfunction appears to be the most common cause of muscle weakness in patients with hip or groin pain.* When improved musculoskeletal function has been achieved, the muscles immediately will be markedly stronger than they were before the wishbone maneuver. Muscle testing can be performed on subsequent visits to assess the stability of the correction of the hip joint. In most patients, the wishbone maneuver does not need to be repeated on subsequent visits. If weakness does recur, the patient's activities and function need to be examined for perpetuating factors such as overuse of hip flexors, excessive lifting, excessive external rotation of the hip, and excessive pronation during ambulation. Other factors that can perpetuate the dysfunctional hip complex, particularly the myofascial dysfunction, include nutritional inadequacies, anemia, hormonal problems, and concomitant illnesses.

In patients with significant hip degeneration, hip dysfunction is very likely to recur. In these cases, it is generally safe to perform the wishbone maneuver repeatedly. For example, a patient in her mid-80s, with hip degeneration, fell, and pins were surgically installed to repair a fractured femur. During her long convalescence, medication reactions caused temporary dementia. She expressed a desire never to undergo such an experience again and refused to consider hip replacement. Over a period of several years, the wishbone maneuver and related procedures were performed once or twice per month. Each time she presented with approximately 15° of internal rotation. Each treatment resulted in an increase of 20°, for a total of 35° of internal rotation. Trigger points in the associated muscles were treated as well. She clearly felt that the treatment allowed her to continue to walk and perform her daily activities with much reduced pain.

A potential aggravating factor in some patients is the need to elevate the hip to clear the floor with the foot while walking. This need can result from knee or ankle injury and casting, but it is also a factor in patients with multiple sclerosis, postpolio syndrome, or other neurologic impairments. In these latter cases, the developing hip weakness is often seen by both the patient and the practitioner as a sign that the patient's nerve disorder is progressing. However, hip weakness may be associated with mechanical dysfunction of the hip joint, as described previously, rather than deteriorating nerve function. If the patient has neurologic impairment causing difficulty with dorsiflexion of the foot while walking, he or she may develop femoral dysfunction with the associated muscle weaknesses described previously. An easy way to differentiate neural weakness from weakness caused by mechanical hip dysfunction is to treat the mechanical disorder. If strength improves quickly in the muscles around the hip, the weakness probably was coming from the mechanical disorder. When the mechanical hip disorder is the source of the weakness, normal joint mechanics and normal muscle strength around the hip can be restored. If the hip disorder tends to return, prosthetic devices to assist dorsiflexion while walking can be introduced.

A curious paradox exists in patients with disordered hip complex. The femur can appear to palpation to be prominent anteriorly in the anterior portion of the joint, and can simultaneously appear to be prominent posteriorly, in the posterolateral buttock. To understand the basis of this apparent contradiction, the clinician must consider the fact that, when the head of the femur is rotated anterolaterally in the socket and the femur is maintained in external rota-

tion, the neck of the femur angles in a posterior direction rather than more directly lateral. Thus, the greater trochanter is often more prominent in the posterolateral buttock on the side of the disordered hip.

Accompanying the extreme rotation of the femur and prominence of the greater trochanter in the posterolateral buttock is shortening of the external rotators of the femur, including the piriformis, gemelli, and obturators. As these muscles are released and returned to normal length, with the patient prone, the greater trochanter can be felt to drop anteriorly and laterally. Frequently, release of the iliopsoas and adductor muscle tension results in a shift of the femur and, using the bow string metaphor, also release of the external rotators of the buttock also occurs, without much, if any, direct treatment of these muscles. For this reason, release of the iliopsoas and adductor muscles generally is performed first in the treatment sequence, and then any remaining tightness in the external rotators of the buttock is assessed and addressed.

The Pelvis. Numerous possible patterns of specific joint dysfunction of the pelvis, or pelvic listings, can be associated with a disordered hip complex. *However, the unifying features involve hypomobility in the upper and lower portions of the sacroiliac joint on the involved side, with significant posterior sacral flare.*

Joint dysfunction also may be evident in the sacroiliac joint contralateral to the disordered hip on initial examination, or it may become apparent after the treatment of muscle and joint on the side of the disordered hip. For further discussion of the pelvis, see Chapters 10 and 13. If major change occurs in the short term to correct pelvic asymmetry and restore normal hip and sacroiliac function on the involved side, the opposite sacroiliac joint may not tolerate and accommodate such major changes. A beginning practitioner may even see patients, having just received treatment on one side of the hip and pelvis, rise from the treatment table hobbled by pain in the opposite lower back or hip. Patients who have apparently tolerated a session of one-sided treatment often will arrive at the next session complaining of pain in the opposite side. Therefore, it is important to anticipate and address both joint restriction and shortened muscles that may not accommodate shifts in the symptomatic side. The contralateral structures that most often require attention include: the sacroiliac joint, the lower thoracic and rib joints, and the quadratus lumborum, iliocostalis lumborum, and longissimus thoracis muscles.

Frequently the lumbar spine restrictions will release in the course of treating the trigger points in the surrounding musculature and the sacroiliac joints. When this does not happen, the subluxations of the lumbar spine will need to be separately treated (See Chapter 10). Most frequently, the subluxation at the thoracolumbar juncture *will not be corrected* by treatment of the surrounding muscles and the sacroiliac joints, so this spinal area usually does need to be addressed separately.

Other Joints. Problems in the knee or ankle also can be associated with the treatment of disordered hip complex. When the foot is significantly externally rotated and pronated, this affects angulation of the knee and externally rotates the femur, thus affecting hip mechanics. Likewise, when the hip is externally rotated, and also may be raised to clear the foot in ambulation, the abnormal hip mechanics predispose to abnormal mechanics at the knee and ankle. These problems probably arise because the tibia, talus, and lateral tarsal mobility become well adapted to a gait with eversion of the foot and leg, but the joints are not taken through a normal full arc of movement during gait. For example, the everted leg does not normally place the tibia into a locked position of normal extension that would otherwise be part of bearing weight and then "pushing off." Furthermore, the everted leg does not place the foot into full dorsiflexion during the roll-through phase of gait. These joints thus maintain mobility to the extent that is required to walk with external rotation of the femur and foot eversion, but they often lack the full range of motion and joint play that are required to coordinate well in a gait with the leg and foot in a straighter position. Restriction in these joint areas may need to be addressed, to prevent the patient's pain from simply shifting from the hip and groin to the knee or ankle. Problems in foot mechanics are often a *major predisposing factor* in the development of the disordered hip complex, and this is a paramount reason to always assess the function of these joints in the course of treating the disordered hip complex. Evaluation and correction of foot mechanics, including the use of orthotics, is discussed in depth in Chapter 15, and correction of this perpetuating factor is often essential for full rehabilitation of the disordered hip complex.

Another joint area that must be addressed in a significant portion of patients is the pubic symphysis. Joint dysfunction or subluxation of the pubic symphysis usually is accompanied by bilateral adductor muscle weakness assessed by seeing whether the patient can maintain the legs together while the clinician manually attempts to sequentially abduct first one leg and then the other against the patient's resistance. The clinician must not exert excessive force during this test, but this muscle group is fairly strong, and any give rather than a full resistance is an indication of the need to address pubic symphysis subluxation. Pain is generally not experienced during this muscle test and, therefore, is not a factor in explaining the weakness that is observed. The restoration of proper joint mechanics usually results in immediate restoration of good adductor muscle resistance. (The use of these and other muscle tests to evaluate subluxation and joint dysfunction is a basic part of the chiropractic field of applied kinesiology.) Treatment of pubic symphysis dysfunction using Muscle Energy Technique is discussed in Chapter 10.

Lateral and anterior snapping hip have not been specifically addressed in this chapter, but clinical experience shows that effective treatment of the muscle and joint dysfunction involved in the disordered hip complex results in a cessation of the snapping in most patients and a reduction of the pain associated with snapping in all patients.

Patient Exercise and Home Care

At the outset of treatment, the clinician instructs the patient to perform gentle stretches of the iliopsoas and quadratus lumborum muscles (Figs. 11-8 and 11-9). Adductor stretches without external rotation are added on a subsequent visit (Fig. 11-10). Stretches of the lateral hip and buttock muscles (Fig. 11-11) may or may not be performed initially without pain, because of stress on the lateral hip in some of these stretch positions. The timing of adding these stretches depends on when they can be performed without pain. Stretches are performed at least three or four times per day, although some patients appear to derive benefit from even twice a day. Slow and careful use of the contract-relax-assist approach in stretching the muscles often brings about benefit with only two repetitions per day. Patients with acute but simple injuries are advised to stretch every 2 hours during their waking time. Patients with more severe injuries initially may be able to stretch very little without pain, and they are advised to apply cold to decrease edema from tissue trauma. After several days, they will be able to gently stretch the injured muscles more readily, but they should always avoid a painful range.

While side-lying, the patient can lie on a ball (tennis ball, racquetball, etc.) or on a roll of socks to put pressure on trigger points in the lateral buttock (Fig. 11-12). The patient should keep the ball in the upper buttock, pressing against any portion that is above the trochanter, but not significantly medial to it, to avoid compressing the sciatic nerve as it passes through the sciatic notch. The ball also can be used when the patient is supine to treat back muscles, particularly in the lower thoracic erector spinae. Lying on the ball is performed once a day. The patient does not roll around on the ball, but rather uses it to apply sustained trigger point pressure in one location (usually for 1/2–2 minutes) until an easing of pain and tension is experienced. The ball is then moved to the next spot where the technique is to be applied.

The patient's self-care includes the avoidance of activities that would aggravate the condition. The patient is advised to avoid long periods of sitting, particularly during the early stages of treatment. Sitting cross legged (as in a partial Lotus) is also to be avoided because the thighs should not be placed in full external rotation. The repeated stress on the hip flexors involved in driving with a clutch also is to be avoided. Some patients sleep on the side or nearly prone, with one hip hiked and the thigh and flexed knee drawn up and out to one side. This twisted sleep position makes effective treatment of the disordered hip complex much more difficult if not impossible. These patients often can maintain a more normal side-lying position and avoid undue tension on hip and buttock muscles during sleep, if a pillow is placed between the knees. In those patients who sleep supine, a few have become accustomed to allowing the affected thigh to flop out to one side. This aggravating position generally can be avoided by placing a thick pillow just lateral to the thigh of the straightened leg.

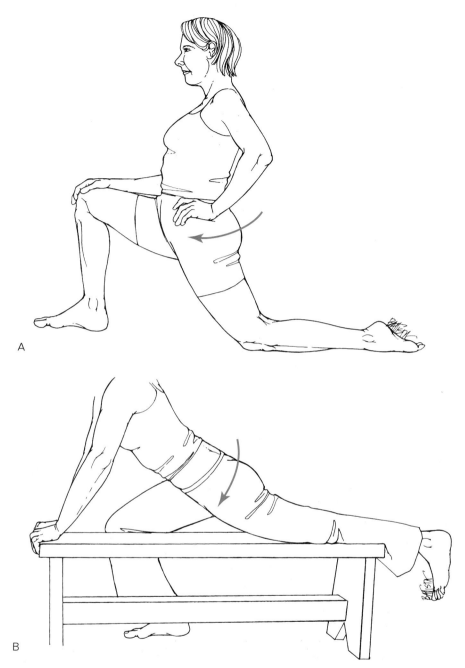

FIGURE 11-8. **Iliopsoas stretches. A.** Basic iliopsoas stretch. The patient kneels with one knee up and the other down. The upper torso can be steadied by placing one hand on the horizontal thigh, or on a piece of furniture nearby. Then the pelvis is taken forward into a lunge, until a comfortable stretch is felt in the psoas muscle on the side of the vertical thigh. Care is taken not to extend the lumbosacral spine to the degree of producing lower back pain. **B.** Advanced iliopsoas stretch (if the patient can tolerate more lumbosacral extension). With the upper torso staying fairly erect and the arms supporting, the standing leg is bent at the knee while a lunge is performed against a bench, coffee table, sofa, or bed. The pelvis is kept square to the bench, rather than rotating, and is lowered toward the bench until a gentle stretch is felt in the iliopsoas muscle but no pain is produced in the lower back. To perform contract-relax-release, the patient can press forward or against the bench with the horizontal thigh, and then can release and see whether the torso and groin can drop lower toward the bench.

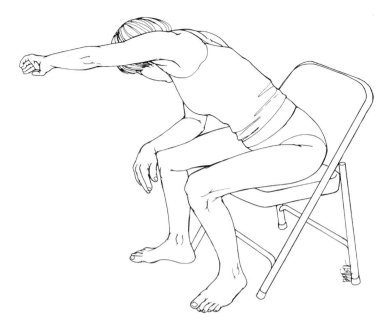

FIGURE 11-9. **Seated quadratus lumborum stretch.** The patient leans forward with the right elbow placed on the right thigh to support the weight of the torso and unload the lower back muscles. The left arm then reaches across in front as though reaching for a door handle located to the right of the patient, until a good stretch is felt between the rib cage and the hip. The hip is kept on the chair. The stretch is repeated toward the opposite side. To perform contract-relax-release, the patient can actually hold a door handle, and then can contract the quadratus muscle gently to resist the stretch. After relaxing, the patient can rotate the hips away from the door handle until the new barrier to stretch is felt, and the contraction and relaxation are repeated.

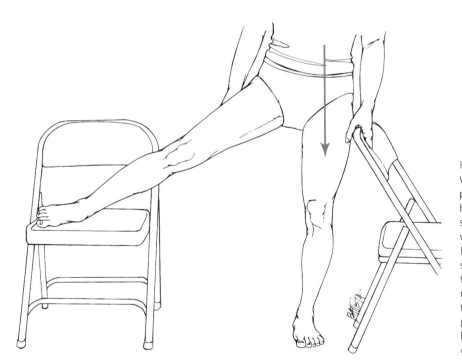

FIGURE 11-10. **Standing adductor stretch without external rotation of the femur.** The patient abducts one thigh to a comfortable height (chair height may be too high for some patients) with both feet facing forward. The hand on the side of the standing leg is placed on a chair or other furniture for stability. Then the standing knee is slowly flexed until a gentle stretch is felt in the inner side of the elevated thigh. The torso and the elevated leg are kept close to the same plane, rather than dropping the buttocks back, even if the torso cannot comfortably drop very far.

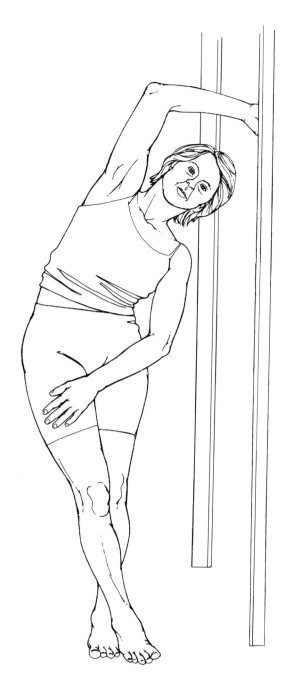

FIGURE 11-11. Standing tensor fascia lata and iliotibial band stretch. The patient stands next to a wall or doorway and crosses the foot that is away from the wall in front of and medial to the other foot. Then the patient leans toward the wall with the arm up and bows the body, until a gentle stretch is felt in the torso and hip. The torso is kept in the same plane with the legs, rather than dropping the buttock back or rounding the chest and head forward.

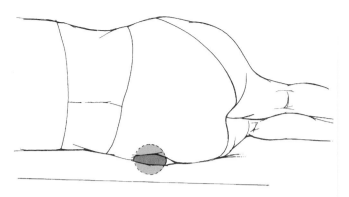

FIGURE 11-12. Using a ball while side-lying to treat trigger points in the lateral hip and buttock. It is often difficult for patients to stretch the tensor fascia lata and gluteal muscles effectively without pain, but self-treatment of trigger points can be performed by lying on a ball. The patient is instructed on the location of the sciatic nerve, to avoid placing the ball on the nerve and aggravating the pain. If the muscles are too tender to relax with the use of a ball, trigger point pressure release can be performed initially with a ball of socks or a hackey-sack.

If normal ambulation does not return within a few sessions, the patient is advised to walk in water at least chest high for 5 to 10 minutes, working up to 15 to 20 minutes three times per week. Flutter-kicking while swimming is also a good exercise for strengthening and stabilizing the hip and pelvis. Frog-kicking and whip-kicking generally should be avoided in the early stages of treatment.

When the patient has progressed well in treatment and wants to maintain improvements, an exercise can be prescribed that helps maintain internal rotation joint play and stretches external rotator muscles. To perform this maneuver for the right hip and associated muscles, the patient sits on the edge of a bench and lifts the right foot up beside the right buttock. With the thigh now in internal rotation, the patient rocks the right knee up and down toward the floor while attempting to keep both buttocks on the bench. If the knee is too uncomfortable, then the heel is placed further from the buttock (Fig. 11-13). This motion is performed with both hips, and the clinician notes any asymmetry. This exercise has been particularly useful to balance the exercise routines of dancers, who are constantly working with turn-out.

CONCLUSION

The complete pattern of muscle and joint dysfunction should be addressed to successfully treat patients with hip and groin pain. If done properly, treatment will result in a return of normal function and a healing of the tender and painful tissues in a fairly short period. Even if symptoms have been prolonged and unresponsive to traditional care, rehabilitation generally is complete in 3 to 10 weeks. As long as patients continue with home stretches and exercises, they usually are able to progress to and maintain nor-

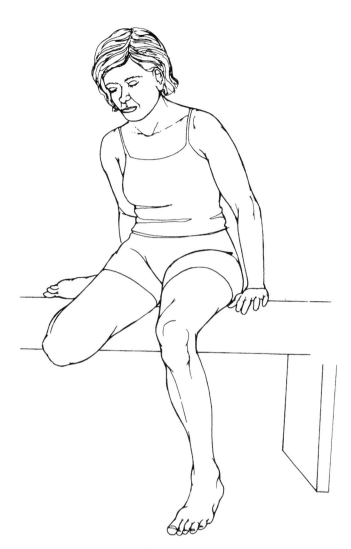

FIGURE 11-13. **Advanced internal rotation exercise.** The seated patient places the foot on the bench beside the buttocks, and drops the thigh forward, and rocks it gently up and down. The other foot is flat on the ground, and both buttocks are on or close to the bench.

mal pain-free activity. Treatments usually are performed twice per week or three times per week if ambulation is very difficult. However, sometimes good progress can be made with treatments once per week if the femoral release is maintained, and the patient performs home care and stretch retraining. Effective intervention early in the case of acute hip or groin injury prevents chronicity and usually requires a course of treatment lasting only 1 to 3 weeks.

Reoccurrence is not common and usually involves a clear re-injury. Patients with significant foot pronation, however, are likely to experience reactivation of the muscle and joint dysfunction if pronation is not sufficiently corrected. Some who were successfully treated experience recurrence of symptoms on seasonal change of footwear, such as the use of flip-flops or thong sandals.

Patients with significant osteoarthritis of the hip are likely to suffer repeated recurrences of the disordered hip complex. A 3- to 6-week trial of the therapies described is usually sufficient to ascertain whether conservative care can help the patient be reasonably comfortable and functional, or whether hip replacement would be advantageous.

TREATMENT PROTOCOL

In using this protocol, it should be remembered that no two patients are alike. The listed points are therefore guidelines to help ensure that the clinician takes a sufficiently comprehensive approach in the evaluation and treatment of the disordered hip complex to assure effective care.

1.   **Release the shortened torso muscles, usually the quadratus lumborum, internal and external obliques, and sometimes the latissimus dorsi, that are hiking the pelvis cephalad. Address the sacroiliac dysfunction that accompanies hip hiking and joint dysfunction in the lower thoracic and lumbar spine that accompanies this functional scoliosis.**

2.   **Treat the muscle dysfunction in the opposite side of the torso and the joint dysfunction in the opposite sacroiliac joint to ensure that these areas will be able to accommodate the leveling of the pelvis and the straightening of the scoliosis.**

3.   **Release the shortened iliopsoas and adductor group, including the pectineus muscle. Release the associated femoral restriction in the acetabulum, and restore normal anterior to posterior and internal rotation joint play. Assess the patient's response by muscle testing the psoas, tensor fascia lata, and rectus femoris before and after this procedure. Release the associated flaring of the sacrum and flexion pattern of the pelvis.**

4.   **Elongate the gluteus medius, gluteus minimus, tensor fascia lata, and quadriceps as necessary to assist in the drop-down of the femur within the hip socket. (The iliopsoas is also a major player in this aspect of joint function, and its tension should be released in several different positions to help in the drop-down.)**

5.   **Release the medial hamstring, as necessary, to restore normal function.**

6. Release the piriformis and other external rotators, as necessary, to restore the greater trochanter from its position of posterior prominence in the buttock into a more lateral position as internal rotation of the femur improves.

7. Restore normal joint function to the pubic symphysis, tibia, talus, and lateral tarsals, when dysfunction or subluxation in these joints is present.

8. Reassess and treat the trigger points in the tensor fascia lata, piriformis, gluteus minimus and maximus, quadratus lumborum, and vastus lateralis that are making muscles tense and may be referring pain and tenderness into the lateral hip.

9. Reassess and treat trigger points that are causing tension in the quadratus lumborum, abdominals, adductor magnus, and iliopsoas that may be referring and maintaining pain and tenderness in the groin. The diaphragm also may require treatment as part of the functional unit.

10. When necessary, evaluate and treat trigger points in the internal pelvic musculature. (See Chapter 13.)

11. Institute stretch retraining and a progressive return to normal activity and athletic pursuits.

12. Assess the patient's gait for excessive pronation. Some patients also have initial excessive supination at the heel strike and then roll into excessive pronation. Correction of this abnormal gait and also of Morton's toe syndrome often is important in stabilizing patients with hip and groin pain. Check for normal heel-to-toe roll-through, which may have been altered because of pain. Make sure that shoes are not too stiff, preventing normal roll-through.

13. Check sleep position as a perpetuating factor. The most problematic sleep position is lying partly on the side and partly on the stomach, with one knee drawn up.

14. Check relative hip height while the patient is seated and standing, not only on initial evaluation, but on subsequent visits as well. A difference in leg length may appear that was not discernible earlier in treatment, and correction may be required. Also, the treatment of the hip and pelvis may balance hip height in patients who previously had a functionally short leg or pseudo leg-length inequality. In such cases, correction needs to be removed. It is important in rehabilitation to balance weight distribution while seated and standing, so that the body does not have to continually compensate for an imbalance and muscles do not have to reshorten to perform this compensation.

References

1. Balduini F. Abdominal and groin injuries in tennis. Clin Sports Med 1988;7:349–357.
2. Karlssonn J, Sward L, Kalebo P, et al. Chronic groin pain in athletes. Sports Med 1994;17:141–148.
3. Emery CA, Meeuwisse WH, Powell JW. Groin and abdominal strain injuries in the National Hockey League. Clin J Sport Med 1999;9:151–156.
4. Tuite MJ, DeSmet AA. MRI of selected sports injuries: muscle tears, groin pain, osteochondritis desiccans. Semin Ultrasound CT MR 1994;15:318–340.
5. Ekberg O, Sjoberg S, Westlin N. Sports-related groin pain: evaluation with MR imaging. Eur Radiol 1966;6:52–55.
6. Thomee R, Karlsson J. Muscle and tendon injuries of the groin. Crit Rev Phys Rehabil Med 1995;7:299–313.
7. Makela JT, Kiviniemi H, Palm J, et al. The value of herniography in the diagnosis of unexplained groin pain. Ann Chir Gynecol 1996;85:300–304.
8. Uppington J, Warfield CA. Chronic pain in the perineum, groin, and genitalia. Hosp Pract 1988;23:37–52.
9. Fredberg U, Kissmeyer-Nielsen P. The sportsman's hernia-fact or fiction? Scand J Med Sci Sports 1996;6:201–201.
10. Ekberg O, Persson NH, Abrahamsson PA, et al. Longstanding groin pain in athletes. Sports Med 1988:6:56–61.
11. Malycha P, Lovell G. Inguinal surgery in athletes with chronic groin pain: the sportsman's hernia. Aust N Z J Surg 1992;62:123–125.
12. Williams P, Foster ME. Gilmore's groin—or is it? Br J Sports Med 1995;29:206–208.
13. Fortin L, Belanger R. Bursitis of the iliopsoas with pain as the only clinical indicator. J Rheumatol 1995;22:1971–1973.
14. Akermark C, Johansson C. Tenotomy of the adductor longus tendon in the treatment of chronic groin pain in athletes. Am J Sports Med 1992;20:640–643.
15. Holmich P. Rehabilitation for chronic groin pain in athletes. Int Sports Med J 2000;1:1–8 (internet).
16. Fricker PA, Taunton JE, Ammann W. Oseitis pubis in athletes. Sports Med 1991;12:266–279.
17. Chadwick P. The significance of spinal joint signs in the management of groin and patellofemoral pain by manual techniques. Physiotherapy 1987;73:507–513.
18. Schon L, Zuckerman JD. Hip pain in the elderly: evaluation and diagnosis. Geriatrics 1988;43:48–62.
19. Traycoff RB. "Pseudotrochanteric bursitis": the differential diagnosis of lateral hip pain. J Rheumatol 1991;18:1810–1812.
20. Brady LP. Hip pain: don't throw away the cane. Postgrad Med 1998;83:89–90, 95–97.
21. Goddard NJ, Gosling PT. Intra-articular fluid pressure and pain in osteoarthritis of the hip. J Bone Joint Surg Br 1988;70:52–55.

22. Arnoldi CC, Lemperg RK, Linderholm H. Immediate effect of osteotomy on the intramedullary pressure of the femoral head and neck in patients with degenerative osteoarthritis. Acta Orthop Scand 1971;42:357–365.

23. Tachdjian MO, Grana L. Response of the hip to increased intra-articular hydrostatic pressure. Clin Orthop 1968;61:199–212.

24. Soto-Hall R, Johnson LH, Johnson RA. Variations in the intra-articular pressure of the hip joint in injury and disease. J Bone Joint Surg Br 1964;46:509–516.

25. Imamura S, Riberto M, Fischer A, et al. Successful pain relief by treatment of myofascial components in patients with hip pathology scheduled for total hip replacement. J Musculoskel Pain 1998;6:73–89.

26. Eyring EJ, Murray WR. The effect of joint position on the pressure of intra-articular effusion. J Bone Joint Surg Am 1964;46:1235–1241.

27. Reid DC, Burnham RS, Saboe LA, et al. Lower extremity flexibility patterns in classical ballet dancers and their correlation to lateral hip and knee injuries. Am J Sports Med 1987;15:347–352.

28. Moritz U. Physical therapy and rehabilitation. Scand J Rheumatol 1982;43:49–55.

29. Mansour ES, Steingard MA. Anterior hip pain in the adult: an algorithmic approach to diagnosis. JAOA 1997;97:32–38.

30. Luukkainen R, Asikainen E. Frozen hip. Scand J Rheumatol 1992;21:97.

31. Koop S, Quanbeck D. Three common causes of childhood hip pain. Pediatr Clin North Am 1996;43:1053–1066.

32. Hughes RA, Tempos K, Ansell BM. A review of the diagnoses of hip pain presentation in the adolescent. Br J Rheumatol 1988;27:450–453.

33. Miralles M, Gonzales G, Pulpeiro JR, et al. Sonography of the painful hip in children: 500 consecutive cases. Am J Roentgenol 1989;152:579–582.

34. Royle SG. Investigation of the irritable hip. J Pediatr Orthop 1992;12:396–397.

35. Altman R, Alarcon G, Appelrouth D, et al. The American College of Rheumatology Criteria for the classification and reporting of osteoarthritis of the hip. Arthritis Rheum 1991;34:505–514.

36. Travell JG, Simons DG. Myofascial Pain and Dysfunction, vol 2. Baltimore: Williams & Wilkins, 1992:48–63.

37. Travell JG, Simons DG. Myofascial Pain and Dysfunction, vol 2. Baltimore: Williams & Wilkins, 1992:248–288.

38. Travell JG, Simons DG. Myofascial Pain and Dysfunction, vol 2. Baltimore: Williams & Wilkins, 1992:217–235.

39. Travell JG, Simons DG. Myofascial Pain and Dysfunction, vol 2. Baltimore: Williams & Wilkins, 1992:289–314.

40. Simons DG, Travell JG, Simons LS. Myofascial Pain and Dysfunction, vol 1, 2nd Ed. Baltimore: Williams & Wilkins, 1999:11–93.

41. Mense S, Simons DG. Understanding and measurement of muscle tone as related to clinical muscle pain. Pain 1998;75:1–17.

42. Dvorak J, Dvorak V. Manual Medicine, Diagnostics, 2nd Ed. New York: Stuttgart, New York: Thieme Medical Publishers, 1990:35–45.

43. Wyke BD, Polacek P. Articular neurology, the present position. J Bone Joint Surg Br 1975;57:401.

12 Abdominal Pain of Myofascial Origin

Mary L. Maloney, PT and Jill Maloney Newman, PT

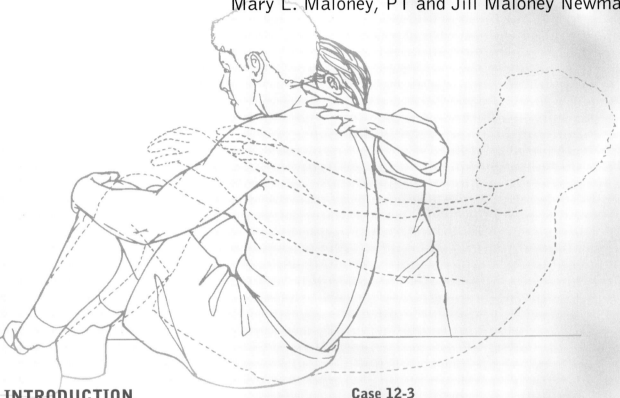

INTRODUCTION

"I have a stomach ache" is one of the most frequent complaints health care practitioners hear. Because the cause of abdominal pain is often difficult to determine, clinicians are challenged with a variety of possible diagnoses. A typical patient makes his or her way through the medical community, receives a diagnosis of visceral disease, and may be treated surgically. Often there may be persistent pain even after surgery, in which case abdominal pain becomes the primary symptom and the primary diagnosis.

Members of the medical community are just beginning to recognize the presence of a primary myofascial pain syndrome as the cause for persistent abdominal pain and in the absence of or after correction of visceral disease. The logical diagnostic step is a thorough evaluation of the abdominal musculature for the presence of trigger points that may explain the persistent pain and dysfunction. The medical literature regarding abdominal pain or visceral dysfunction and its treatment as a musculoskeletal disorder is very limited. The most notable exception is the information presented by Travell and Simons (1).

Although the focus of this chapter is the treatment of abdominal myofascial pain and dysfunction, joint **arthrokinematics** and biomechanical or visceral dysfunction are also important considerations. In no other area does this seem more relevant than the abdominal region, where it remains largely unknown among practitioners. The clinician faces a unique challenge: to identify dysfunction associated with the abdominal musculature and develop a comprehensive treatment plan that addresses the myofascial issues, paying appropriate attention to biomechanical and visceral components.

ABDOMINAL PAIN: BACKGROUND

Pain of muscular origin has been studied for many years. The large and somewhat confusing body of literature has slowly become more focused and specific with respect to both definitions and terminology. Travell and Simons define myofascial pain syndrome as "sensory, motor, and autonomic symptoms caused by myofascial trigger points"(2). Furthermore, some patients who have mechanical and systemic perpetuating factors seem to develop clusters of myofascial problems in several regions of the body, defined as chronic regional myofascial pain syndrome (3). Such conditions are characterized by the presence of myofascial trigger points. A myofascial trigger point is defined as a hyperirritable spot, usually within a taut band of skeletal muscle or in its fascia, that is painful on compression and that can give rise to characteristic referred pain, tenderness, and autonomic phenomena (2). The reference to autonomic phenomena becomes an especially important finding in the area of regional myofascial pain associated with the abdominal

muscles. However, the clinician must rule out visceral abnormalities before assuming that the cause of the dysfunction or pain is related to the abdominal muscle myofascial trigger points.

Few specific studies on the prevalence of myofascial pain as a specific diagnosis have been reported. Although not focusing on abdominal muscles, Skootsky, Jaeger, and Oye (4) reported that 30% of the visits to an internal medicine clinic by patients with a pain complaint satisfied the criterion for a clinical diagnosis of myofascial pain. Furthermore, 75% of these patients had pain for longer than 1 month (4). These statistics may be related to the poor rate of physician recognition of a myofascial pain syndrome diagnosis (4,5).

No specific literature is available on the size of the population with myofascial pain syndrome related to the abdominal regions, possibly because so much abdominal pain is related to visceral organ disorders. Such patients may have been examined by many tests and have had pain for many years. Their quality of life has deteriorated, and they have not found any solution to their problem. Patients often become conditioned to respond to questions about their abdominal pain by blaming it on a present or previous organ problem—for example, "Oh, that's my ulcer," or "Oh, that pain is from my [old] appendicitis scar." They may be reluctant to even touch the painful area, much less accept an alternative diagnosis.

Differential Diagnosis

Abdominal pain presents the clinician with a significant source of confusion. Myofascial trigger points in the abdominal muscles not only refer pain to the abdominal region but also can initiate visceral responses such as nausea, diarrhea, vomiting, and anorexia. Acting together, these causative factors can closely mimic serious disease. Also, visceral disease can activate abdominal trigger points, which may remain the source of discomfort long after the disease is resolved.

Abdominal pain is a broad complaint that may have various causes, falling into three major categories: non-abdominal disease, abdominal disease, and pain from myofascial trigger points. Health care providers must rule out other forms of disease-induced abdominal pain before progressing with treatment according to a myofascial approach.

NonAbdominal Disease

Nonabdominal diseases that may cause abdominal pain include coronary artery insufficiency, pneumonia, acute indigestion, herpes zoster, ruptured lumbar disc with nerve compression, diabetic acidosis, and abdominal migraine (1).

Abdominal Disease

Abdominal diseases also produce pain patterns that closely resemble those of myofascial pain. These include diaphragmatic hernia, peptic ulcer, gastric carcinoma, chronic cholecystitis, gallstone colic, ureteral colic, inguinal hernia, hepatitis, pancreatitis, appendicitis, diverticulitis, colitis, cystitis, and endometriosis. Other common medical problems are esophagitis, hiatal hernia with reflux, and spastic colon. Less frequent conditions that cause abdominal pain include aortic aneurysm, pancreatic carcinoma, bowel obstruction, ovarian cyst, and psychogenic pain. Also noted are abdominal epilepsy, amebiasis, hydronephrosis, and ascariasis infestation with bowel obstruction (1).

Myofascial Trigger Points

Myofascial trigger points can cause abnormal function in visceral organs. Likewise, the abdominal viscera can induce and perpetuate myofascial trigger points. Abdominal muscle trigger points have been reported to cause diarrhea, vomiting, colic, burping, **dysmenorrhea,** indigestion, and urinary bladder pain. This is known as a **somatovisceral** response. Conversely, the visceral organs have a profound effect on the muscular structure, which is referred to as a **viscerosomatic** response. As shown in Table 12-1, there is a link between certain visceral problems and myofascial trigger points (1). It would be reasonable to assume that the trigger points are activated by the visceral component but persist after the visceral component has resolved. Subsequent pain referral continues not from the visceral problem, but from the presence of the activated trigger points. After the patient has been cleared for the presence of disease, knowledge of myofascial trigger points can be applied to eliminate pain and restore function.

Conventional Treatment Approaches

Patients with complaints of abdominal pain initially present to their primary care physician, or to the hospital with acute pain problems. Usually a medical diagnostic work-up follows; leading to treatment that may include medication or surgical intervention. Unfortunately, elimination of the possible visceral causes of pain, either through invasive methods or with medication, does not necessarily mean that the pain will be eliminated. Rarely is the persistent pain associated with the presence of myofascial trigger points, either as the original cause or activated as a result of visceral disease.

If the abdominal pain is clearly related to trauma, the physician will also evaluate possible organ damage. Posttraumatic abdominal pain is usually treated with medication and rest but can include surgical repair of organ lacerations or punctures. The only standard follow-up treatment for the abdominal muscles involves a strengthening program often initiated in physical therapy. Abdominal strengthening continues to be done with patients who complain of chronic back pain, as well as with patients after direct trauma. Often patients are left with persistent pain.

TABLE 12-1
Referred Pain and Somatovisceral Symptoms from Abdominal Muscles

Trigger Point Location	Myofascial Referred Pain and Somatovisceral Symptoms
External oblique upper	Deep epigastric pain, abdominal pain across midline and quadrants. Heartburn and symptoms associated with hiatal hernia
External or internal oblique, lower lateral abdominal wall	Fingers of pain into abdomen, groin pain, testicular and ipsilateral lower quadrant pain
Internal oblique lower	Pain in groin and bladder region. Spasm of detrusor and urinary sphincter, urinary frequency and retention and chronic diarrhea
Transverse abdominal	Pain across upper abdomen and between anterior costal margins
Rectus abdominis upper	Horizontal pain across bilateral mid-back, pain across upper abdomen and ipsilateral quadrant. Precordial pain, nausea, epigastric distress; symptoms mimicking cholecystitis, peptic ulcer, and gynecologic conditions
Rectus abdominis, level of umbilicus	Diffuse abdominal pain aggravated with movement. Abdominal cramping; symptoms of intestinal colic
Rectus abdominis lower	Bilateral pain to sacroiliac region and horizontal pain to low back Dysmenorrhea
Right lower	Diarrhea; symptoms mimicking diverticulosis and gynecologic disease
Just above pubis	Spasm of detrusor and urinary sphincter causing urinary frequency and retention
Rectus abdominis, right lateral in region	Symptoms of acute appendicitis
McBurney's Point, other trigger points, region of McBurney's point	Pain in ipsilateral lower quadrant, right upper quadrant throughout abdomen, iliac fossa, iliacus muscle, and penis
Pyramidalis	Pain close to midline between symphysis pubis and umbilicus

Anatomy of the Abdominal Musculature

One of the characteristics of excellent clinicians is an understanding of anatomy. Knowledge of abdominal wall musculature enhances the clinician's ability to diagnose and treat abdominal pain. The muscles of the abdomen can be divided into two groups: the anterolateral muscles and the posterior muscles. The anterolateral muscles of the abdomen include: external obliques, internal obliques, transversus, pyramidalis, and rectus abdominis. The posterior muscles of the abdomen include the psoas major, psoas minor, iliacus, and quadratus lumborum. The first three posterior muscles fall within the pain referral zone of the abdominal muscles and usually are discussed with the lower extremity (6). The quadratus lumborum is usually discussed with the back muscles and, along with the other posterior muscles, refers to the abdomen. This shows the potential for the development and perpetuation of regional myofascial pain between the lower back and abdomen.

The individual muscles are discussed later in the chapter in the section on palpation, to provide the clinician with a clear picture of the anatomy while palpating each of the abdominal muscles. The trigger point location, the referred pain patterns, and the somatovisceral responses also are described in that context.

Dynamic Function

Although knowledge of muscle action from a static position is very important, clinicians must understand muscle function in a dynamic situation. Information regarding dynamic muscle function gives the clinician a more realistic view of muscle activity during the performance of normal daily activities. With this information, the clinician can develop more directed treatment goals and focus on function. Abdominal function during the dynamic process of posture; changes in trunk alignment; and gait are addressed in the evaluation section of the chapter.

Referred Pain Patterns

A discussion of myofascial pain of the abdomen necessitates a discussion of both somatovisceral and viscerosomatic reactions. A viscerosomatic response involves abdominal myofascial trigger points activated secondary to the presence of visceral disease. Somatovisceral responses include referred pain and visceral symptoms that occur secondary to the presence of trigger points in the abdominal musculature.

In general, referred pain from the abdominal musculature tends to be located in the same quadrants of the abdomen. Trigger points are capable of such somatovisceral responses as projectile vomiting, anorexia, nausea, intestinal colic, diarrhea, urinary bladder sphincter spasm, and dysmenorrhea. When the above symptoms occur with abdominal pain, the syndrome can strongly mimic visceral disease (see Table 12-1). Conversely, the activation of trigger points in the abdominal muscles may be secondary to the presence of disease. Diseases such as peptic ulcer, ulcerative colitis, **diverticulosis,** diverticulitis, and intestinal parasites are just a few of the conditions that may cause trigger point activation (1). Myofascial treatment of patients with trigger points activated by disease will not be effective until the underlying disease is treated by a physician.

A MYOFASCIAL AND ARTICULAR APPROACH TO THE DIAGNOSIS AND TREATMENT OF ABDOMINAL PAIN

Complete subjective and objective evaluations are necessary for establishing an effective treatment plan. A myofascial approach to the treatment of abdominal pain advocates complete rehabilitation with a multidisciplinary team to provide medical attention to the visceral problems. The treatment will specifically address specific problems unique to each patient, but the general approach is the same from patient to patient. Postural, mechanical, and soft tissue problems are corrected in all areas that may refer pain to the abdominal region. This is followed by a progressive strengthening and conditioning program and the correction of perpetuating factors. A more detailed discussion of evaluation and treatment follows the case histories.

In the case studies, range-of-motion (ROM) is measured as a percentage rather than in degrees. This is in response to recent requirements by insurance company treatment plans.

CASE 12-1

Patient History

Mr. M.P. is a 51-year-old, well-conditioned athlete who was ski racing at approximately 40 mph when he hooked his ski tip on a gate. He reported that his left leg was violently extended. The initial symptom of groin pain dis-

appeared without formal treatment in 3 to 4 weeks. He started on his own training program, including running, squats holding 90-lb weights, and skiing in heavy snow, all in the same day. By the end of the day, he could not lift his leg. He also reported that he tried to stay active but continued to lose strength in addition to having pain.

CASE 12-1 Continued

After resting for 3 months, he once again tried to start his training program. He stated that he was trying to do sit-ups with 4-lb weights and biking for more than 40 minutes. Pain increased and, again, functional range-of-motion and strength was lost. He continued in this pattern for over 3 years. His physician diagnosed a "strained sartorius, torn psoas with learned spasm response." Mr. M.P. had been to many other health care providers for treatment of the above diagnosis. The disciplines he explored included orthopedics, osteopathy, massage therapy, and physical therapy.

Symptoms

Approximately 31/2 years after the initial injury, Mr. M.P. presented with pain in the hip, groin, anteromedial thigh, testicle, and abdomen, all on the left side, and pain across the lower back. He reported that his pain increased with any lifting movements, rising from a deep chair, driving, doing supine pelvic tilts, and with work-related stress. He got temporary relief with the use of ibuprofen, ice, heat, and ischemic compression. He explained that he was no longer able to effectively manage his river outfitting business or perform his many rigorous physical activities.

Examination Findings

There were many deviations from normal. He had a forward and left side-bent posture with increased kyphosis, decreased lumbar lordosis with protruding abdomen, increased hip flexion, left iliac crest lower than right, left posterior superior iliac spine lower than right, and left anterior superior iliac spine higher than right. A left posterior rotated ilium was noted and confirmed by supine and standing tests.

Range-of-motion testing showed a 30% limitation of lumbar extension. Bilateral lumbar rotation and side-bending were each limited by 20%. There was pain only with lumbar extension. Mr. M.P. had full right hip motion, but left hip extension was limited to neutral position. Any active or passive movement into extension caused severe reproduction of all symptoms. Limited flexibility was noted, with tight left hamstrings, quadriceps, and iliotibial band. Strength testing indicated 2+/5 strength with pain in the abdominal muscles, 2+/5 strength with pain in the left iliopsoas, and 2+/5 strength with pain in the left hip adductors. Other hip motion tested within normal limits and without pain. No other arthrokinematic disorders were noted.

Palpation indicated active trigger points in the left rectus abdominis, left iliopsoas, left adductor magnus, left adductor longus, left external oblique, and left internal oblique. The primary trigger points were identified and located in the left external and internal obliques. Latent trigger points were identified in the rectus femoris and the quadratus lumborum.

Treatment

Treatment goals, discussed at length with the patient, focused on a return to functional activities of daily living and some athletic activities, but perhaps not to all of them as he had performed them previously.

Treatment was initiated at a frequency of twice each week. Spray-and-stretch techniques were applied to all the involved muscles. Muscle-energy techniques to correct **pelvic obliquity** were applied simultaneously with the stretching. Modalities such as pulsed short wave diathermy, electrical stimulation, and heat and ice were all used as adjuncts to manual therapy to induce relaxation and decrease pain. Mr. M.P. was immediately given a home stretching program and allowed to perform his general conditioning program only in the pool.

After treatment for 6 weeks, the symptoms were only partially resolved. He experienced relief from treatment and self-stretching but was unable to maintain pain-free status and gain strength. He moved away and was then seen only about once per month. The primary trigger points in the abdominal obliques could not be inactivated, and the other trigger points were perpetuated by the presence of the primary trigger points. Mr. M.P. had full hip and lumbar range of motion, normal postural alignment, and the pelvic obliquity had been resolved. Although pain persisted, he was able to return to his normal daily activities and running his business, but he could not tolerate any athletic activity.

Although Mr. M.P. resisted having trigger point injections, after 6 months of self- treatment without complete resolution, he agreed to injection therapy. Injections were performed on the external oblique, internal oblique, adductor, iliopsoas, quadratus lumborum, and rectus femoris over three different sessions. Each muscle was stretched and warmed immediately after the trigger point injection. Mr. M.P. continued his self-stretches and initiated a program using light weights, not in the pool.

Follow-up

Mr. M.P. was rechecked once per month for 3 months. At the end of his treatment, he reported that he had resumed all daily activities and job duties, and was now able to tolerate hiking, biking, and skiing.

CASE 12-2

Patient History

Ms. S.T., age 48 years, had a chief complaint of "pain at the bottom of my breastbone." She stated that she was not sure when it started, but that it had been there for at least 2 years. She described increased pain from sleeping for a long period in the fetal position, and with deep breathing. She had a long history of irritable bowel syndrome, for which she had been treated by her physician. The condition was now under control with the use of natural supplements and dietary restriction. She denied any history of abdominal trauma. She had previously been treated for a lumbar strain from a lifting injury, and a shoulder injury that was currently healing after a period of exacerbation. Ms. S.T. was cleared medically for other internal organ problems. Even when the irritable bowel syndrome was under control, she had persistent pain in the upper abdominal region.

Symptoms

Ms. S.T. complained of pain in the upper abdominal region, at the lower border of the sternum, extending along the border of the rib cage and sometimes all the way around to the upper back. She described increased pain when leaning back, taking a deep breath, changing position after prolonged flexion, and when lifting.

Examination Findings

Ms. S.T. had a forward-bent posture with increased kyphosis and depressed sternum. The lower abdominal region was slightly protruding. Range of motion was within normal limits in both hips and was limited in lumbar-thoracic extension by 50%, with complaint of increased abdominal pain. There was a significant depression along the rectus abdominis bilaterally during lumbar extension. Her abdominal strength was limited to 3/5, and she complained of pain with any attempt to perform a sit-up. Palpation indicated acutely active trigger points in the rectus abdominis muscles bilaterally, with referred pain into the xiphoid area and along the border of the rib cage. There was no evidence of active trigger points in the other abdominal muscles.

Treatment

The treatment goals were discussed with Ms. S.T., and treatment began at a frequency of 2 to 3 times per week. Spray-and-stretch techniques were immediately applied to the rectus abdominis muscles. Modalities included the use of ultrasound, electrical stimulation, and pulsed short wave diathermy. The most effective combination was found to be stretching techniques first, then ultrasound, followed by the Magnatherm. Self-stretching was initiated immediately, and the supine techniques were most effective. Posture education began, with emphasis on sternal elevation with proper head position and control of the lower abdomen. Cross-friction massage often was used as an adjunct to self-stretching at home, to deactivate the trigger points. After four treatments, she had total relief from all symptoms; however, any increase in activity would exacerbate the symptoms. At this time, prone self-stretching was initiated. She was able to tolerate 1 to 2 repetitions without any increase in shoulder pain. This provided a much more effective stretch and enabled Ms. S.T. to remain pain-free during normal daily activities. She continued to have discomfort when lifting or during aggressive activity in the gym. A strengthening program was initiated with sit-backs. Progression to abdominal curls started when the patient was able to complete 10 sit-backs. Ms. S.T. continued with her treatment until she could independently maintain her full activities without pain and perform all strengthening and stretching exercises without any problems. She was seen for a total of 5 weeks for 13 treatment sessions.

Follow-up

Ms. S.T. has had one recurrent episode, which she associated with an exacerbation of her irritable bowel syndrome during a very stressful period in her life. She continued under the care of her physician to control the symptoms of the irritable bowel syndrome. She was to treat any acute abdominal pain with self-treatment and exercise.

CASE 12-3

Patient History

Mrs. J.S. was a well-nourished 68-year-old, German woman with chief complaint of abdominal pain and denied the presence of any active disease or illness. She had an appendectomy at age 15, performed in Germany by an "old-fashioned, hometown doctor." She described the onset of a postsurgical infection, which required fur-

ther surgery and draining. She denied having had any history of trauma or intervertebral disc disorder.

Symptoms

Mrs. J.S. had had abdominal pain for over 1 year, located in the lower-right quadrant, extending into the groin, over the iliac crest, into the sacroiliac region. She had

CASE 12-3   Continued

difficulty standing and walking with erect posture. Furthermore, she had great difficulty transferring from lying down to sitting to standing.

Examination Findings

Mrs. J.S. had difficulty rising from her chair, removing her jacket, and walking in the treatment room. She stood in a forward-bent position, and both static and dynamic testing indicated a right anterior rotated ilium. Palpation showed the presence of active trigger points in the following muscles: right external oblique, right rectus abdominis, right iliopsoas, and right quadratus lumborum. The right iliocostalis thoracis, which can refer pain to the lower abdominal region, was examined at the T11 level and found to be negative for active trigger points. Her appendectomy scar was also palpated and found to be wide, dense, and tight. One area of the scar was indented to a depth of approximately a half inch and very adherent. Multiple acutely tender areas were palpated within the scar.

Treatment

Treatment was applied in the following sequence. Muscle-energy techniques were used to correct the ilial dysfunction. (Beginning therapists may find it useful to take a continuing education course to become more proficient in the treatment of articular dysfunctions.) Spray-and-stretch myofascial release was then performed on the quadratus lumborum, which was activated because of its shortened position from the ilial rotation and referred pain to the abdominal region. Spray-and-stretch techniques were applied to the psoas, which also perpetuated the anterior rotation. This muscle may have what is considered to be a satellite trigger point—that is,

a muscle that harbors an active trigger point because it lies within the referred pain pattern of the oblique muscles. Spray-and-stretch techniques were also used on the rectus abdominis and external oblique muscles.

Modalities for achieving increased pain relief and relaxation also were used. Pulsed short-wave diathermy was the modality of choice, because it penetrates deep enough to reach all of these tissues.

Although her pain decreased significantly, Mrs. J.S. continued to have persistent complaints. Scar releases were then performed. Longitudinal lengthening and broad stretching were followed by digital pressure exerted in the direction of the pain. The scar releases were only partially successful. As a result, a physiatrist with expertise in scar-tissue needling performed the final treatment—injection of the painful spots in and along the scar. Pain complaints decreased, mobility improved, and the results were lasting.

The last phase of rehabilitation was a strengthening program. Because Mrs. J.S. was markedly deconditioned, an aquatic therapy program was initiated to increase strength and endurance.

Follow-up

Mrs. J.S. did extremely well but had one last pain complaint. She described it as hip pain that occurred primarily when bearing weight. Manual hip joint compression increased the pain. An orthopaedic consultation and imaging studies indicated that joint space was narrowed and that a total hip arthroplasty was necessary. She received a total hip replacement and is currently pain-free and fully functional. Total treatment time, including the rehabilitation time from the total hip replacement, was 6 months.

An Overview of Abdominal Pain

Patients with the complaint of abdominal pain usually present with a combination of muscle and joint dysfunction, often with associated visceral symptoms that may require medical attention. Myofascial trigger points are usually located in abdominal muscles, the quadratus lumborum, iliocostalis thoracis, multifidus, the iliopsoas, and the adductor muscles of the hip. All muscles of the hip, thigh, and back must be palpated, together with the muscles of the abdomen, to detect the presence of secondary and satellite trigger points.

Joint dysfunction includes postural abnormalities, pelvic obliquity, rib mobility problems, and intervertebral disc disorders. All of these combine to change the static and dynamic function of the abdominal muscles and are

perpetuated by the patient in an effort to avoid pain. The myofascial, arthrokinematic, and perpetuating factors must be reversed and a self-management program of stretching and strengthening initiated to fully rehabilitate the patient.

Causes

Abdominal pain arises from a variety of causes, including:

- The presence of a visceral disease
- Acute direct trauma to the abdominal region
- Chronic trauma from occupation or postural deviations
- Sustained positioning in either a flexed or a twisted posture

- Breathing problems
- Trauma from a surgical procedure
- Scarring after a surgical procedure
- Structural problems, such as leg-length discrepancy
- The overuse or overactivity of the abdominal muscle

Cautions

Abdominal pain encompasses a great many possible diagnoses. Patients with abdominal pain, especially when it is associated with visceral complaints, must be fully evaluated from a medical perspective. Visceral causes of pain must be treated before the myofascial component is addressed.

Symptom/Pain Presentation

The patient with a regional myofascial pain syndrome involving the abdominal area usually presents with a variety of complaints. Typically, referred abdominal pain and some visceral symptoms are present. Pain may extend into the groin and genitals and even across the back (See Table 12-1).

Associated weakness of the abdominal muscles and poor posture may be present. Structural problems, such as leg-length discrepancy or a small hemipelvis, may be present. Arthrokinematic disorders of the spine, pelvis, hip, or ribs can occur.

Myofascial Entrapments

Nerve entrapment can also occur. The major nerve entrapment is of the anterior branch of a spinal nerve in the rectus abdominis muscle or sheath. It will refer pain to the lower abdominal and pelvic area and can mimic the pain from gynecological conditions in females (1).

Evaluation

An extensive and thorough evaluation will enable the clinician to establish a comprehensive problem list from which to set the treatment goals. It is important to have the patient participate in this process, so that the clinician's goals and the patient's goals are the same. It is also beneficial to recognize when the goals are unrealistic to either party in the treatment team. Current healthcare guidelines require that all goals be functional in nature and that all outcomes be measurable.

The scope of regional myofascial pain is wide and can affect any area of the body. Single areas should not be considered in isolation; rather, the whole body is viewed as a functional unit. The evaluation process is divided into subjective and objective portions. The clinician should be as specific as possible in the subjective part of the evaluation, because this will provide an initial clinical impression.

Subjective Evaluation:

The following outline of the subjective evaluation is intended to be a guide for the clinician and is in no way meant to limit the scope of this portion of the evaluation.

I. History
  A. Onset of pain
    1. Sudden
      a. Traumatic
      b. Nontraumatic
    2. Insidious
  B. Occurrence
    1. First time
    2. Previous episodes
      a. Number
      b. Intensity
      c. Frequency
    3. Previous treatment
  C. Pain complaints
    1. Location
    2. Nature
    3. Presence
      a. Constant
      b. Intermittent
    4. Intensity
    5. Aggravating factors
    6. Relieving factors
  D. Sleep quality
  E. Any other complaints
II. Lifestyle
  A. Effect of pain
  B. Activities of daily living
  C. Occupational activities
  D. Recreational activities
III. Personal Information
  A. Age
  B. Family and social factors
  C. General health
    1. Last physical
    2. Test results
    3. Medications
    4. Any other pertinent health information

Objective Evaluation

The clinician gains much of the information for the objective portion of the evaluation through both visual observation and tactile means. The clinician should establish a systematic approach for gathering facts and details in the most efficient manner. The following discussion focuses on the abdominal region, but the general process can be used for any problem.

Posture. In one of the most basic functions, standing, very little activity occurs in the muscles of the back, and only slight activity in the abdominals (7). Most of the activity is in the internal obliques, which are thought to primarily protect the inguinal canal. Furthermore, because the line of gravity passes very close to the axis of movement at L4, the force of gravity is counteracted by one set of muscles, either the back muscles or the abdominal muscles (7). Increasing the pull of gravity always increases the activity on one set of muscles, either the abdominals or the back muscles, depending on which side of L4 the line of gravity passes The abdominals stabilize the spine as a whole (7). Furthermore, the transverse abdominal muscle acts first, as all of the abdominal muscles are activated to stabilize the spine in advance of the use of the prime movers (1).

Posture and function are related and explain the presence of postural maladaptation with weakness and tightness. Chaitow and Liebenson describe a pattern of dysfunction studied by Janda (8). Janda named this dysfunction the lower crossed syndrome. In this condition, the abdominal and gluteal muscle groups are weak, whereas the back extensors (erector spinae) and the hip flexors are tight and shortened. This posture leads not only to weakening of the abdominal musculature but also to a tightening of the abdominals. The anterior thoracic region is depressed because the shortened abdominal muscles achieve a pull on the mobile structures of the rib cage toward the stable pelvis. Furthermore, the musculature is overused to support the sagging viscera, which should be supported by their own ligamentous structure. The imbalance creates tightness, weakness, overuse, and biomechanical abnormalities, all of which can influence the activation and perpetuation of trigger points and myofascial pain syndrome (8).

During the postural evaluation, the patient is observed from the right and left sagittal planes, as well as the anterior and posterior coronal planes. (Primary spinal curves and bony landmarks are examined as though the skin is not there.) Muscle mass is observed for size and appearance, and for indications of atrophy, weakness, or overactivity. Abdominal scars are noted. In the abdominal pain patient, the status of the thoracic and lumbar curves are noted, with special attention paid to sternal depression, protruding abdomen, and amount of hip flexion.

Motion Testing and Related Arthrokinematic Issues. Myofascial trigger points and articular dysfunction are both important and closely related components that need to be addressed to achieve full resolution of pain and return to function. Several authors have developed and promoted manual techniques that are extremely useful in understanding the physiology of articular dysfunction and performing mobilization techniques. Mitchell, Lewit, Grieves, and Greenman are from a variety of backgrounds and have all published material that recognizes the importance of muscles in treating articular dysfunction (9–12). Once recognized, the articular dysfunction can be treated with the mobilization technique that the clinician finds is most effective.

Both passive and active motion are examined. Individual joint motion, as well as segmental and regional spinal motion, are evaluated for both quantity and quality and palpated for the end feel. The effect of the motion on other areas is also noted. Evaluating the movement in both the weight-bearing and non–weight-bearing positions is helpful. Often the motion is controlled or affected by numerous other related structures or forces. This is most evident with abdominal wall pain and dysfunction. Discussing other structures possibly functionally related to the abdominal wall will enable the clinician to be thorough in evaluating motion. The abdominal musculature provides stability to the vertebral column. Thus, the abdominal muscles are affected by vertebral position, intervertebral disc disorders, pelvic obliquity, hip joint function, rib mobility, small hemipelvis, and leg-length discrepancies. General examples are provided below, to illustrate the effect on the abdominal musculature.

Vertebral Position. Generally speaking, the vertebral segments are evaluated for rotated, flexed, or extended positions. If any of these abnormalities are noted, the clinician may find that the patient's posture has been compromised such that the primary curves are changed and regional motion is affected. For instance, if upper lumbar segments are flexed, less available active flexion is present, and the patient will tend to lean forward to avoid pain. As a result, the abdominals are held in a shortened position, facilitating the activation or perpetuation of trigger points.

Intervertebral Disc Disorders. An intervertebral disc disorder is a significant problem for both the activation and perpetuation of abdominal trigger points. In the case of a lumbar intervertebral disc herniation, the postural compensations are usually severe, and the patient experiences responsive abdominal muscle tightening and weakness. The paraspinal muscles are antagonists to the trunk flexors and show increased activity when the flexors are painful and the load is anterior. The iliocostalis thoracis refers pain to the anterior rib cage and abdominal wall. The postural dysfunction, muscle overactivity, and tightening may induce and perpetuate abdominal pain. Furthermore, nerve root compression by the disc may cause radicular pain in muscles of the back and hip. Trigger points in these muscles are often activated or perpetuated by the presence of nerve root compression. Some of these muscles, such as the quadratus lumborum and iliopsoas, refer pain to the abdominal wall.

In addition, the abdominals may be overused to stabilize the lumbar spine.

Pelvic Obliquity. The pelvic girdle is evaluated for sacral and ilial position. Anterior and posterior iliosacral rotation with apparent leg-length discrepancies are identified. Pubic shears, ilial flares, as well as up-slips and down-slips, are noted. Sacral position is evaluated for nutation, counter-nutation, and torsion/rotations. Abnormal positions of the sacrum directly influence the motion of the lumbar spine and the position of the ilium. Primary attachments for the abdominals include the pubis and the ilium; therefore, pelvic obliquity and changes directly affect the function of the abdominal wall. For instance, in the presence of a right posterior iliosacral rotation, the patient will present in standing posture with the right ilium lower, the right posterior superior iliac spine lower, the right anterior superior iliac spine higher, and an apparent right shorter leg. In this case, the patient generally presents with increased weight-bearing on the right leg. The right hip will be in more flexion, shortening the iliopsoas. The quadratus lumborum and paraspinals are overused in spinal stabilization. The right-side abdominals are shortened from the posterior rotation of the ilium. Both the quadratus lumborum and the psoas minor refer pain to the lower abdominal area, and the function of the abdominals is compromised by their shortened position. The pelvic obliquity then becomes both a precipitating and a perpetuating factor of the abdominal discomfort.

Hip Joint Function. Muscle tightness, weakness, and bony abnormalities all affect the function of the hip joint. Referred pain from the hip musculature to the lower abdomen is common. Conversely, the external oblique refers pain to the groin and anteromedial thigh. In addition, abnormal hip function may influence posture, causing abdominal tightening and weakness. Both the hip and the abdominal musculatures are tight and overused secondary to weakness, activating and perpetuating trigger points. The abdominal muscles continue to refer pain to the hip, perpetuating the presence of secondary and satellite trigger points in the psoas major, psoas minor, iliacus, adductor magnus, and rectus femoris.

Rib Mobility. Occasionally, upper-quadrant abdominal pain results from abnormal mobility of the lower intercostal joints, a condition known as Tietze's syndrome (1). Also, severe hypomobility of the chest wall may exaggerate the normal abdominal breathing pattern. This may result in an overuse syndrome of the abdominal musculature.

Small Hemipelvis and Leg-Length Discrepancies. The small hemipelvis and leg-length discrepancies are structural in nature; their associated muscle imbalances are chronic and, at best, controlled. Symptoms most often occur on the long side. Postural deviations are significant and include anterior pelvic tilt and increased lumbar lordosis. The abdom-

inals become tight and weak, and the anterior hip musculature often becomes symptomatic.

Palpation. Thorough palpation of the abdominal musculature is necessary for determining the presence of active and latent trigger points. Palpation of the abdominal muscles presents a unique set of problems for both novice and experienced clinicians. Palpation in other areas allows the clinician to push against the bone or to feel the muscle between the thumb and fingers. In contrast, the clinician is forced to compress the abdominal muscle against the internal organs. The exception is the lateral portion of the oblique muscles, which can be palpated with a pincer technique, between the thumb and fingers along the flank. Patient positioning, technique, and knowledge of anatomy and fiber direction enable the clinician to fully evaluate the muscle for the presence of trigger points while avoiding the organ tissue. Clinicians may find it helpful to imagine the anatomy of the abdominal musculature while palpating each of the abdominal muscles. With either flat or pincer palpation, the clinician moves perpendicular to the fibers and explores the full length of the muscle in search of taut bands and trigger points.

Most clinicians agree that it is nearly impossible to identify trigger points in totally lax abdominal muscles. Some prefer to use flat palpation with the patient lying supine. The patient is then instructed to take a deep breath to passively stretch the abdominal muscle. Pincer palpation to grasp the muscle is also useful. The patient side-lies and places the top arm over the head with the top leg drawn back in extension at the hip. Both of these positions increase the abdominal muscle tension, thereby making it easier to differentiate the taut bands from other structures. If the patient cannot tolerate side-lying, supine with a lumbar support and the arms over the head might be a more comfortable position. In addition, asking the patient to take a deep breath may increase the tension and sensitivity of the abdominal muscles to palpation. The clinician may have to be creative to accommodate the individual patient's need. As long as abdominal muscle tension is maintained, an effective and efficient evaluation can be performed. Often a clinician finds that a combination of techniques and positions allows for the most complete inspection of this large group of muscles.

The anterior muscles of the abdomen comprise five separate muscles: the external oblique, internal oblique, transverse abdominis, rectus abdominis, and pyramidalis. In addition to these five muscles, an extensive fascial layer is continuous cranially with the subcutaneous fascia of the thorax, and caudally with that of the thighs and external genitals. As it changes into the fascia of the back, it gradually becomes tougher and less elastic (6).

Palpation of the external oblique, internal oblique, and transverse abdominis muscles is best achieved by using the pincer technique with the patient in the side-lying position. The patient is placed in a well-supported side-lying position with the arms over the head and the legs drawn back. The angle of the arm and leg can be changed to increase the tension on the different parts of the oblique muscles.

The external oblique is the largest of the three flat muscles. It arises from the external surfaces and interior borders of the lower eight ribs and inserts into the outer lip of the iliac crest to a broad aponeurosis at the final insertion into the linea alba (Fig. 12-1A). The muscle's action is compression of the abdominal contents to assist in urination, defecation, vomiting, childbirth, and forced exhalation. Acting together, both sides flex the vertebral column, whereas one side acting alone bends the vertebral column laterally and rotates it, bringing the ipsilateral shoulder forward. The external obliques are innervated by the branches of the 8–12 intercostal nerves and the iliohypogastric and ilioinguinal nerves (6).

The fiber direction of the external oblique is up and out. This is one side of a V. The internal oblique is located in the lateral and ventral parts of the abdominal wall under the external oblique. It arises from the fibers of the lateral half of the inguinal ligament, the nearby iliac fascia, the anterior two-thirds of the middle lip of the iliac crest, and the lumbar aponeurosis near the iliac crest. It inserts into the posterior portion of the cartilage of the last three or four ribs and, by means of the aponeurosis, makes its final insertion into the linea alba (Fig. 12-1B). The action of the internal oblique is consistent with the external oblique in compressing the abdominal contents. However, both sides acting together flex the vertebral column, whereas one side acting alone bends the vertebral column laterally and rotates it, bringing the contralateral shoulder forward (1,6). The internal obliques are innervated by branches of the 8–12 intercostal, iliohypogastric, and ilioinguinal nerves.

The fiber direction of the internal oblique is up and in. It is the opposite of the external oblique, and is one side of an upside-down V, or Λ (Fig. 12-1A,B).

Palpation of the trigger points may reproduce the patient's symptoms. The clinician must be sure to fully examine both the internal and the external obliques, because the referred pain pattern of the oblique muscles is not consistent from one patient to the next. The referred pain may project up to the chest, across the midline either straight or diagonally, or downward. Somatovisceral symptoms such as heartburn, epigastric pain, and signs associated with a hiatal hernia are usually related to trigger points in the upper

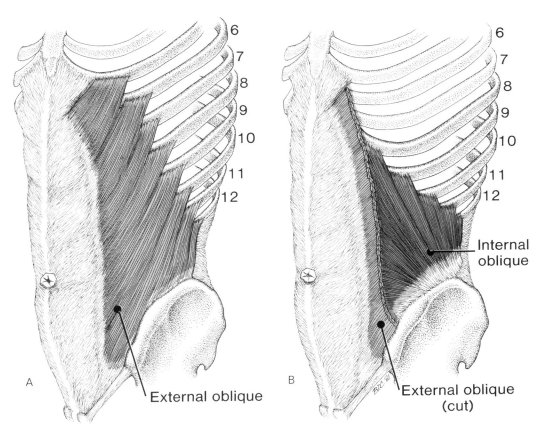

FIGURE 12-1. Attachments of two lateral abdominal wall muscles. A. The external oblique (light red). B. The internal oblique (dark red); the external oblique (light red) is cut.

Reprinted with permission from Simons DG, Travell JG, Simons LS. Travell & Simons' Myofascial Pain and Dysfunction: The Trigger Point Manual, vol 1: Upper Half of Body. 2nd Ed. Baltimore: Lippincott Williams & Wilkins, 1999 (fig 49.4), p. 947.

portion of the external oblique muscles (Fig. 12-2A). Pain into the groin and testicle may be induced from a trigger point in any one of the three layers of muscles in the lateral abdominal wall (Fig. 12-2B,C). Trigger points located along the pubis and inguinal ligament can cause increased irritability and spasm of the sphincter muscles. This may be related to urinary retention, urinary frequency, chronic diarrhea, and groin pain (Fig. 12-2D). The internal oblique or the rectus abdominis may harbor these trigger points as well (1).

The transverse abdominis, the most internal of the flat muscles of the abdomen, lies just under the internal oblique. It arises from the lateral third of the inguinal ligament, from the anterior three-fourths of the inner lip of the iliac crest, from the thoracolumbar fascia and the inner surface of the cartilage of the last six ribs. It passes horizontally and forward to end in an aponeurosis that fuses with that of the internal oblique to insert into the linea alba (Fig. 12-3) (6). The action of this muscle helps in compression of the

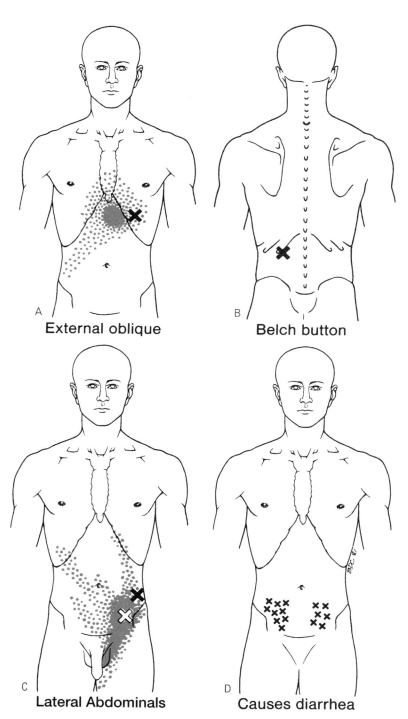

A **External oblique**

B **Belch button**

C **Lateral Abdominals**

D **Causes diarrhea**

FIGURE 12-2. Referred pain patterns (red) and somatovisceral symptoms (black X) of trigger points in the oblique (and possibly transverse) abdominal muscles. **A.** "Heartburn" from an attachment trigger point of the external oblique overlying the anterior chest wall. **B.** Projectile vomiting and belching from the "belch button," which is usually located in the most posterior abdominal wall musculature or in connective tissue and may be on either side. **C.** Groin and testicular pain, as well as chiefly lower quadrant abdominal pain, referred from trigger points in the lower lateral abdominal wall musculature of either side. **D.** Diarrhea from various trigger points in lower abdominal quadrant muscles (after Melnick).

Reprinted with permission from Simons DG, Travell JG, Simons LS. Travell & Simons' Myofascial Pain and Dysfunction: The Trigger Point Manual, vol 1: Upper Half of Body. 2nd Ed. Baltimore: Lippincott Williams & Wilkins, 1999 (fig. 49.1), p. 942.

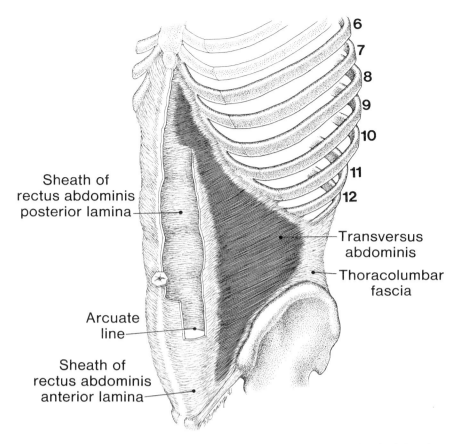

FIGURE 12-3. Attachments of the transverse abdominis muscle (red), which lies deep to the obliques.

Reprinted with permission from Simons DG, Travell JG, Simons LS. Travell & Simons' Myofascial Pain and Dysfunction: The Trigger Point Manual, vol 1: Upper Half of Body. 2nd Ed. Baltimore: Lippincott Williams & Wilkins, 1999 (fig 49.5), p. 948.

abdominal contents. It has a similar innervation to that of the internal oblique, except from branches of intercostal nerves 7–12 (6).

The fiber direction of the transverse abdominis is nearly horizontal toward the linea alba. This muscle refers pain between the costal margins. These trigger points are also located near the costal margins (1).

Thorough palpation of these muscles is done systematically by using the pincer technique. The direction is changed according to changes in the fiber direction of the muscles. The clinician must maintain a 90° angle to the fiber direction to identify all trigger points. Furthermore, palpation must be done carefully to keep the muscle away from the viscera and avoid exciting any deeper active trigger points. Care should be taken not to confuse skin tension with taut bands. Skin tension is felt as an overall surface tightness. A taut band is very specific and follows in the same direction as one of the muscles. The clinician should remember to probe deeply under the diaphragm and above the pubic bone. These areas are more difficult to examine, and extra care should be taken.

Once a taut band is identified, the clinician can track the band and locate the trigger point. By tracing the band with pincer palpation, internal organs can be avoided. The fiber direction will confirm the identity of the muscle.

Flat palpation is preferred for examining the rectus abdominis and pyramidalis. The patient may remain in the side-lying position to maintain adequate muscle tension. Flat palpation is a more difficult technique, because it is harder to avoid compressing organ tissue. Constant communication with the patient is necessary. If the taut band can be traced to locate a tender point that when palpated reproduces the patient's pain, an active trigger point has been located.

The rectus abdominis is a long muscle extending along the abdomen, separated from the opposite side by the linea alba. It arises by two tendons. The lateral tendon is larger and attached to the pubis. The medial tendon, which weaves with the opposite side, is connected with the ligaments covering the ventral surface of the symphysis pubis. The muscle is inserted by thin portions of unequal size into the cartilages of the fifth, sixth, and seventh ribs. Some fibers occasionally extend to the costoxiphoid ligament (Fig. 12-4). The action of this muscle is primarily to flex the lumbar portion of the vertebral column. It also helps compress the abdominal contents and tense the abdominal wall. The rectus abdominus is innervated by the same nerves as the transverse abdominis (6).

The rectus abdominis has fibers that are oriented vertically. Trigger points are most often, but not always, located in the upper portion, lower portion, or periumbilical area. Trigger points located above the umbilicus can refer pain to the middle back horizontally across. Somatovisceral symptoms include heartburn, nausea, vomiting, and indigestion. These trigger points are located around the xiphoid process. Travell reports that the left-sided trigger point is more often linked with epigastric pain and nausea (1). A left-side upper rectus abdominis trigger point also may induce precordial pain (Fig. 12-5A). When it is clearly established that the chest pain is not cardiac in nature, the myofascial symptoms are usually associated with the pectoralis muscles or the

sternalis muscles. However, examining the upper rectus abdominis to determine the source of the pain is important. In addition to same-quadrant pain, the rectus abdominis simulates the symptoms of cholecystitis, gynecologic disease, and peptic ulcer (1).

Trigger points in the rectus abdominis located around the umbilicus are likely to induce diffuse abdominal pain. The pain decreases with rest and increases with movement. Deep palpation often is required to locate these periumbilical trigger points. Somatovisceral responses include cramping or colic and the tendency to bend forward to minimize discomfort (1).

Trigger points in the lower rectus abdominis refer pain in a similar pattern to that of the upper rectus, that is, across the lower back and sacroiliac regions. The patient's description of horizontal pain is a helpful clue for distinguishing it from the vertical pain referred from the paraspinals or iliopsoas.

A trigger point in the right rectus near McBurney's point (located halfway between the anterior superior iliac spine and the umbilicus) is likely to induce symptoms simulating an acute appendicitis (Fig. 12-5B). Other trigger points in this area also may refer pain to the ipsilateral lower quadrant, the upper right quadrant, or throughout the abdomen. Sharp pain may be referred to the iliac fossa, the iliacus musculature, and the penis. The pain may mimic the symptoms of renal colic. A trigger point in the right lower rectus abdominis may cause diarrhea and symptoms of diverticulosis and dysmenorrhea. Somatovisceral symptoms associated with trigger points in the lower rectus abdominis include dysmenorrhea (Fig. 12-5C). This trigger point is located approximately halfway between the umbilicus and the pubis (1). A trigger point located just above the pubis may cause a spasm of the urinary sphincter (1).

The pyramidalis muscle is located in front of the rectus abdominis in the sheath of the rectus abdominis. It arises from the ventral surface of the pubis and from the pubic ligament, and terminates in the linea alba (Fig. 12-4). Innervated by branches of the twelfth thoracic nerve, this small muscle tenses the linea alba (6).

The fiber direction of the pyramidalis is down and out, like one side of an upside-down V, or Λ (Fig. 12-4). This is similar to the direction of the internal oblique. Palpation of this muscle is best achieved during palpation of the lower rectus and by changing the direction slightly to accommodate the direction of the pyramidalis. Trigger points in the pyramidalis refer pain close to the midline between the symphysis pubis and the umbilicus (Fig. 12-5D) (1).

Occasionally, the clinician will have difficulty distinguishing the pain elicited from palpation of an abdominal myofascial trigger point from that caused by an underlying visceral disease. Long describes a technique to assist in a differential diagnosis (13). The sensitive area is compressed with enough pressure to cause pain. The patient then raises the legs high enough to bring both heels off the table, and the tensed abdominal muscles should lift the palpating

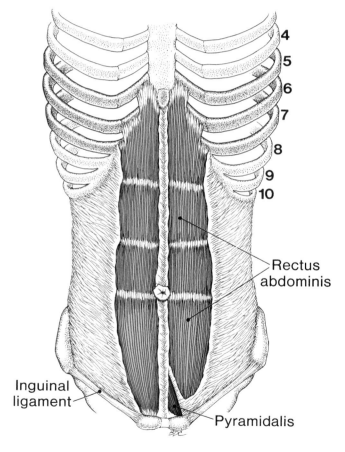

FIGURE 12-4. Attachments of the rectus abdominis muscle (light red), which connects the anterior rib cage to the pubic bone close to the symphysis, and attachments of the variable pyramidalis muscle (dark red), which lies just above the symphysis pubis within the anterior rectus sheath.

Reprinted with permission from Simons DG, Travell JG, Simons LS. Travell & Simons' Myofascial Pain and Dysfunction: The Trigger Point Manual, vol 1: Upper Half of Body. 2nd Ed. Baltimore: Lippincott Williams & Wilkins, 1999 (fig 49.6), p. 949.

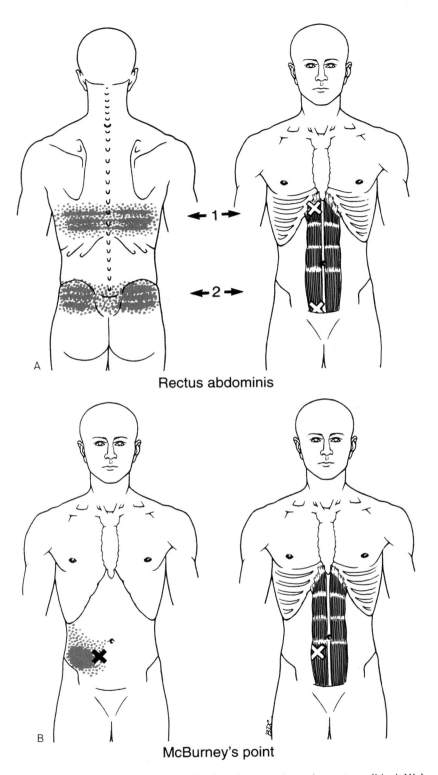

Rectus abdominis

McBurney's point

FIGURE 12-5. **Referred pain patterns (red) and somatovisceral symptoms (black X's) of trigger points in the rectus abdominis and pyramidalis. A.** Bilateral pain across the back, precordial pain, or a feeling of abdominal fullness, nausea, and vomiting can be caused by trigger points (1) in the right (pictured) or left upper rectus abdominis. A similar pattern of bilateral low back pain is referred from what is often an attachment trigger point (2) in the caudal end of the rectus muscle on either side. **B.** Lower right quadrant pain and tenderness may occur in the region of McBurney's point because of a nearby trigger point in the lateral border of the rectus abdominis.

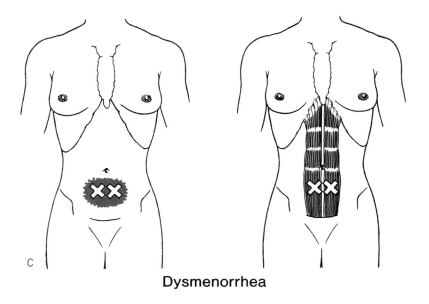

Dysmenorrhea

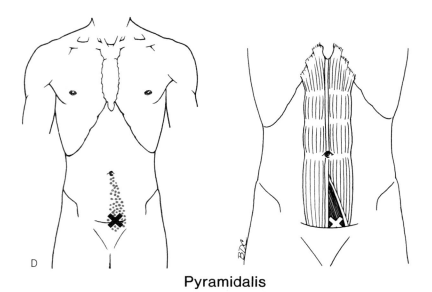

Pyramidalis

FIGURE 12-5. **Continued. C.** Dysmenorrhea may be greatly intensified by trigger points in the lower rectus abdominis. **D.** Referred pain pattern of trigger points in the pyramidalis muscle.

Reprinted with permission from Simons DG, Travell JG, Simons LS. Travell & Simons' Myofascial Pain and Dysfunction: The Trigger Point Manual, vol 1: Upper Half of Body. 2nd Ed. Baltimore: Lippincott Williams & Wilkins, 1999 (fig 49.2), pp. 944–945.

finger away from the viscera. The digital pressure on the muscle then increases. If pain increases, it originates in the abdominal wall; if it decreases, the pain source is within the abdomen. This is not considered a substitute for a physician's evaluation for the presence of visceral disease and should not be used as such.

During the palpation portion of the objective evaluation, the clinician may find it necessary to examine other muscle groups that refer pain to the abdomen. These associated trigger points include the quadratus lumborum, iliocostalis thoracis, multifidus L1–L5, adductor muscles of the thigh, and the iliopsoas. The clinician's ability to reproduce the patient's pain complaints will confirm the location of the primary trigger point.

Strength Evaluation. Most anatomy books describe the function of the rectus abdominalis to include flexion of the spine. However, a distinction must be made between standing and lying supine. The upper and lower parts of the muscle vary in activity (7). In standing with a back load, the rectus is active, but with the load anterior to the thighs, the rectus is silent. Most activity in the rectus is seen with flexion from the supine position and is in the first half of the movement. Trunk raising requires more effort than trunk lowering, and this is important in designing a strengthening program. Bilateral leg raising activates all of the abdominal muscles to stabilize the pelvis. Bearing down while holding the breath increases the activity of the obliques while the rectus is quiet (7). Standing flexion does not increase the activity of the rectus, and gravity is the major factor. Any increased muscle activity appears to be a response to attempts to further increase flexion (7).

Muscle strength is evaluated through manual muscle testing. Abdominal strength is tested, as well as the strength of the lower extremities and the other trunk muscles. Muscles with active trigger points are often weaker and painful on resistance. This also may give the clinician a clue regarding dynamic function as it relates to weakness. It is also an effective screening tool for the presence of a possible neurologic problem.

Gait Evaluation. Weakness and tightness in the trunk and the functionally related hip will be reflected in the patient's gait. These gait deviations and dysfunctions will perpetuate active trigger points and may induce other primary trigger points in remote areas. Gait deviations should be noted and correlated with tightness, weakness, and the presence of active trigger points to identify dysfunction in the abdominal region.

Graven-Neilsen, Svensson, and Arendt-Nielsen reported that the maximal voluntary contraction during muscle pain was significantly lower than the control (14). In addition, pain caused a decrease in the electromyographic output of the agonists and increased activity in the antagonists during dynamic contraction. They theorize that increased activity of the antagonists is a functional adaptation of muscles to limit movements. This may account for the role of abnormal biomechanics and weakness in the perpetuation of trigger points in chronic regional myofascial pain syndrome.

According to Perry, during walking, muscle activity becomes phasic (15). The abdominal muscles have two patterns. The activity of the external oblique muscle is intermittent, with low intensity through stance and peak actions during late mid-swing and early terminal swing. The rectus abdominis has a low level of continuous activity. Functionally, the back and abdomen control the alignment of the trunk over the pelvis. There is no significant deviation from normal walking movement until muscle weakness is severe.

Pain decreases the maximum voluntary contraction of the painful muscle and its agonists, whereas there is an increased activity of the antagonist. This accounts for the significant weakness and subsequent deviations in trunk alignment during dynamic function, seen in chronic pain patients. Static and dynamic posture and gait should always be important parts of the evaluation process to fully assess the level of dysfunction.

Treatment

Inexperienced clinicians may have to address one problem at a time. Experienced clinicians, however, will be able to combine treatments that address myofascial trigger points and arthrokinematic disorders simultaneously. The following discussion is presented as sequentially as possible, while not limiting the clinician who needs to adapt the examination to accommodate individual needs.

Active Trigger Points

The primary trigger points are treated first, using spray-and-stretch techniques (Technique 12-1). The primary trigger point is identified in the evaluation as the one that, when palpated, reproduces the patient's major pain complaint. There may be several primary trigger points in a chronic regional myofascial pain patient. These trigger points are not activated as a result of trigger point activity in another muscle (3). The original mechanism of injury may provide valuable information about the muscle first affected. These trigger points would most likely be located in the abdominal muscles. It is most effective to treat the primary trigger

---

TECHNIQUE 12-1

Abdominal Muscle Stretches

There are two major ways to stretch the abdominal muscles. The first positions, shown in the illustration below, are totally passive and stretch the rectus muscles. The patient lies supine on the table with the legs over the edge and supported about 2 feet below the hips. The spray is applied in parallel lines from the superior rectus downward over the involved muscles and pain referral zone. The rectus muscle stretch is enhanced by using a pillow to arch and support the back, by raising the arms, and by taking a deep breath to protrude the abdomen. The flexion position shown helps to relax the lumbosacral area, and the alternation between stretch and flexion helps achieve the desired full stretch while minimizing stress to the lower back.

Another position is used to stretch the oblique and transverse abdominal muscle fibers. The patient lies on the one side and lowers the opposite top shoulder back toward the table. Thoracolumbar and torso rotation is achieved. The spray pattern follows the direction of the muscle fibers and covers the pain referral zone. As the muscles release, the patient actively increases the stretch, without inducing pain. Again, the use of a pillow under the waist, elevation of the top arm (reaching up and back toward the table), and breathing deeply and protruding the abdomen all increase the stretch. This procedure is repeated for the other side, and often a series of alternating stretches achieves maximal stretch and minimizes discomfort.

(continues)

TECHNIQUE 12-1

Abdominal Muscle Stretches (*Continued*)

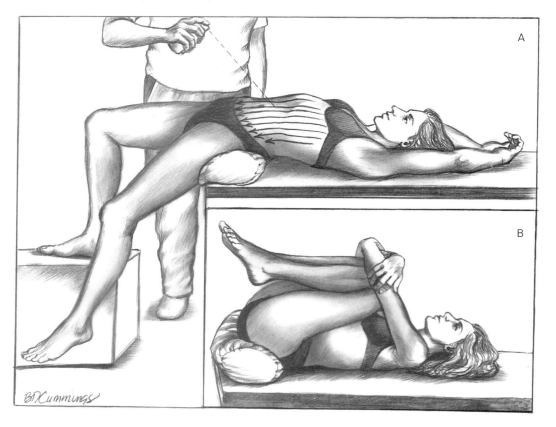

Stretch position and spray pattern (arrows) for trigger points in abdominal muscles on the left side of the body with follow-up full range of motion. **A.** The patient lies supine with the hip joint at the edge of the treatment table, and with the lower limbs extending over the end of the table. The hips are padded with a pillow. The arms are raised and one lower limb is supported on a stool or chair seat. The lower limb on the treatment side at first is supported by the stool or by the therapist to allow gradual stretch. After the operator initially applies vapo-coolant with sweeps in the caudal direction, the patient allows the lower limb on the treatment side (left) to hang free and then takes a very deep breath, allowing the downward-moving diaphragm to strongly protrude the relaxed abdominal musculature. This is a critical step to stretch the abdominal muscles effectively. As the patient completes the inhalation and begins to slowly exhale, sweeps of spray are applied in a caudal direction and extend to the attachment of the iliopsoas muscles, because that muscle (which often has trigger points) also is stretched by this procedure. *The procedure should be repeated for the contralateral abdominal muscles.* **B.** Bilateral knee-to-chest position that unloads stress that might have been placed on the lumbosacral spine. The patient assumes this position after release of the muscles on *both* sides of the abdomen. In this position, the abdominal muscles are fully shortened when the patient gently and fully exhales. To restore full functional range of motion, the patient should gently alternate between the fully stretched and the fully shortened position three times, one leg at a time.

Reprinted with permission from Simons DG, Travell JG, Simons LS. Travell & Simons' Myofascial Pain and Dysfunction: The Trigger Point Manual, vol 1: Upper Half of Body. 2nd Ed. Baltimore: Lippincott Williams & Wilkins, 1999 (fig. 49.7), p. 960.

point first, because it is the key point that influences the present satellite trigger points.

Environmental concerns have led to decreased use of fluoromethane spray and the substitution of other treatment techniques. An environmentally friendly vapocoolant spray has been developed for the application of intermittent cold and stretch. Another option has been to fill an examination glove with water and freeze it. The fingers can be detached and used as an applicator stick for the cold without any drips or deep pressure during the application over the referral pattern. Post-isometric relaxation (PIR), described by Lewit (10), also can be used, either with or without intermittent cold, to achieve trigger point release. This technique involves the use of isometric contraction of the muscle in tension followed by relaxation (10). This technique is somewhat difficult to apply to the abdominal muscles but possible by using a posterior pelvic tilt before the stretch.

Satellite trigger points are located in the muscles that lie within the pain referral zone of the muscle with the primary trigger point or located in the muscles that are functionally associated with the muscle that harbors the primary trigger point (2). These trigger points would most likely be located in the hip, thigh, and back. For purposes of clarification, trigger points that were classified as secondary are now identified as satellite. The clinician may need to address all of the associated trigger points that refer pain to the abdomen, including those in the quadratus lumborum, iliocostalis thoracis, multifidus, iliopsoas, and hip adductors (1).

Scar Releases

The clinician should be aware that scars also limit movement, and any scar should be examined with deep palpation for the presence of pain and adhesions or areas of resistance. The clinician may palpate with digital pressure along the scar, asking the patient to identify the most sensitive spots. Adhesions also may be detected by gently pinching and lifting up the scar. Areas of hyperalgesic skin may be located around the scar. To determine the extent of the hyperalgesic zone, the clinician should gently stretch the skin around the scar (16). The patient will complain of discomfort with the stretch. Any scar should be released to restore full mobility. More than one treatment may be required to restore full mobility. The age of the scar does not affect its ability to be released, but age is related to the amount of time or number of treatments needed to achieve full mobility.

There are several ways to release a scar, all of which are useful. The basic techniques are described in Technique 12-2. The effectiveness of these myofascial techniques is not limited to scars and can be used on any other areas identified as having tissue restrictions.

More broad stretches also may be performed. These are often effective when the surrounding tissue and underlying muscles are especially tight or sensitive. The palms are placed flat on the patient's skin across the scar. It may be more comfortable to cross the arms so that the pressure can be applied with the hypothenar eminences. The skin is stretched between the hands until no further mobility is achieved, and held until a release is achieved. The hands will feel as though they are sliding apart. The hands are then moved so that the next stretch is performed perpendicular to the first. If full mobility is not achieved, it may be necessary to finish with a stretch at a 45° angle.

If a scar has persistent minimal restrictions, skin rolling is a useful tool for achieving full mobility. The clinician simply pinches the scar between the thumb and fingers and rolls the tissue along the scar or into any area of restriction. If a scar remains adherent despite therapy, treatment by injection with a local anesthetic, or needling the most painful spots within the scar, may be necessary (10).

TECHNIQUE 12-2

Releasing a Scar

The first method is to palpate along the scar with one finger. The clinician asks the patient to identify the most painful areas. The finger is rotated on the sensitive spot, noting the most restricted direction. The digital tissue pressure is increased to move into the deeper tissue in the direction of greatest resistance. Pressure is held until the release is felt and the patient indicates reduced pain. The clinician continues in the same manner along the scar until all areas are released.

The second method is usually used as a more general scar release and is done with a pincer grasp. The hand is placed perpendicularly to the scar, the thumb on one side and the fingers on the other. The scar is gently pinched between the thumb and fingers, then lifted directly upward from the body. When the tissues release, the hand slowly moves back and forth perpendicular to the scar. It is important to keep the upward force on the scar while moving in either direction, and to be sure to wait for the tissue to release before moving in the other direction.

Arthrokinematic Dysfunction

The best result is achieved when the related arthrokinematic dysfunctions are treated at the same time as the active trigger points. These are treated very effectively with manual muscle-energy techniques and mobilization techniques. Clinical experience has shown that resolution occurs more quickly when any pelvic and sacral problems are addressed first in the sequence of treatment for arthrokinematic problems. The order of treatment for the pelvis and sacrum is as follows:

1. Pelvic shears
2. Up-slips or down-slips
3. Anterior or posterior rotations of the ilium
4. In-flares or out-flares of the ilium
5. Sacral nutation or counter nutation
6. Sacral torsion
7. Sacroiliac dysfunction

The next arthrokinematic disorder to address is vertebral position. In the lower lumbar segments, this is often closely related to sacral position. This combination is most often seen in the patient with back pain as well as abdominal pain. It may be necessary to address both the position of the sacrum and the altered vertebral segment in the same treatment to improve the result.

The presence of abdominal pain as a result of hip dysfunction is usually secondary to hip and groin pain. The abdominals usually have to be cleared to fully resolve groin pain. Hip tightness and weakness must be corrected to decrease the perpetuating factors secondary to abdominal pain.

Rib mobility usually causes more upper abdominal pain than lower abdominal pain. It is also easier to treat hypomobility than hypermobility. Hypomobility is treated easily with mobilization techniques. Breathing exercises are often effective in improving rib expansion.

Leg-length discrepancy and small hemipelvis are corrected with lifts appropriately placed to level the pelvis while sitting and standing.

The presence of a herniated intervertebral disc is a special case. In this situation, the centralization of symptoms becomes the primary goal. Extension exercises are very effective. Extension exercises also provide an excellent stretch for the abdominals. A herniated disc patient may require further neurosurgical consultation.

Physical Therapy Modalities. Several physical therapy modalities are used to help relieve myofascial abdominal pain. These can be used throughout the treatment process.

Ultrasound is an inaudible high-frequency acoustic vibration traditionally applied at a continuous or pulsed frequency to produce a thermal effect. Many clinicians find ultrasound an effective adjunct to intermittent cold and stretch to inactivate trigger points. No studies are known to demonstrate the specific effectiveness of ultrasound on the treatment of myofascial trigger points. Nielson describes the use of ultrasound on particularly resistant trigger points (17). The ultrasound is increased to the point of pain (not over 1.5 W/cm^2), then the intensity is decreased by half. The applicator is moved in a circular motion over the trigger point while the intensity is gradually increased over the next 2 to 3 minutes until the original pain intensity is reached. There is usually no further discomfort at this level, and the trigger point is less irritable.

High-volt galvanic stimulation (electrical stimulation) usually is used in combination with either heat or ice. This method is used to achieve increased relaxation and decreased inflammation, and to change pain perception. Clinicians commonly use this form after stretching or injections. Another clinically effective method involves the combination of electrical stimulation and pulsed ultrasound at a frequency of 0.8 to 1.5 W/cm^2. The electrical component is increased to an intensity that causes contraction and applied over the entire muscle. It is common for the patient to experience some increased discomfort over the trigger points; however, the sound head is constantly moving so as not to cause pain. The treatment is usually applied for approximately 5 minutes. This treatment reduces muscle tightness and trigger point irritability. Intermittent cold-and-stretch techniques are then applied and are often more effective than when applied without the combined ultrasound and electrical stimulation.

Moist heat is used after intermittent cold and stretch to warm the skin and to achieve greater patient relaxation. Short-wave pulsed diathermy is a deep-heat treatment that also may be applied after intermittent cold application. It involves the application of high-frequency electrical energy that is used to generate heat in body tissues as a result of the resistance of the tissues. The pulsed short wave diathermy is created by simply interrupting the output at consistent intervals. It is helpful for reaching tissues that are difficult to get at with other treatments. This method has proved very beneficial in the treatment of abdominal muscle pain.

Alternative Techniques for the Treatment of Trigger Points

Several alternative techniques are used to decrease active trigger points. These methods are primarily used with hypermobile patients. These are also used with patients who cannot tolerate stretching because of pain or complicating arthrokinematic dysfunctions. Included in this category are trigger point pressure release, myofascial release techniques (MRT), massage, and trigger point injection (18).

Patient Exercise and Home Care

The home exercise program is the most important part of the program, and it begins right away. The patient must be compliant to control symptoms and fully resolve the condition.

The passive stretch is initiated first. The patient is instructed not to lean into the stretch, causing contraction of the involved muscle. The stretch should be performed every waking hour; two to three repetitions are held for no longer than 10 seconds. Longer stretches may cause a rebound contraction or irritation. The home passive stretch for the abdominals is achieved in the prone position. The patient is first instructed to remain prone on the elbows, allowing the abdomen to sag, and use deep breathing (Fig. 12.6). The patient then advances to a press-up. The elbows are extended and the anterior superior iliac spine remains on the table. Initially, the patient is instructed to press up only to individual tolerance without causing pain. The cervical spine is held in a neutral position, but may be extended to increase the stretch. This stretch is often used in the clinic in place of the passive stretch described in Technique 12-1.

The patient is also encouraged to use other modalities and treatment techniques at home. These include heat, ice, self-massage, breathing exercises, and relaxation exercises.

Strengthening and Conditioning

A progressive strengthening program is necessary for the patient to resume normal daily activities without exacerbating the pain. Patients should start to strengthen their abdominal muscles when they are able to fully complete their stretching exercises without pain.

The gentlest strengthening exercise is the pelvic tilt. It increases the ability of the abdominals to stabilize the lumbar spine. The pelvic tilt is done in three steps. First, in the

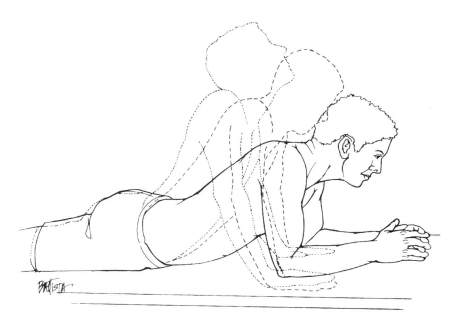

FIGURE 12-6. **A self-stretch for the patient's home exercise program.** The patient is prone on the elbows and allows the abdomen to sag. The patient advances to a press-up. The elbows are straightened, and the anterior superior iliac spine remains on the table. The patient is encouraged to let the abdomen sag and use deep breathing. The cervical spine can be extended to increase the stretch.

supine position the patient identifies the arch in the lower back (Fig, 12-7). Second, the lumbar spine is pressed into the floor, tilting the pelvis and flattening the arch. Third, a bridge is initiated, lifting the buttocks up while maintaining the pelvic tilt. When the patient can complete 10 of these exercises without pain, he or she advances to sit-backs and sit-ups.

In sit-backs, the eccentric contractions place relatively less of a load on the abdominal muscles. First, the patient is assisted to a sitting position (Fig. 12-8). Second, the patient lowers to the table in a slow and controlled curl-down, the hands first held at the hips, then at the abdomen, and then at the neck. The patient should pause and take a deep breath between repetitions. When the patient can perform 10 sit-backs without pain, progression to curls and sit-ups is appropriate.

In the abdominal curl, the patient lifts each vertebral level in order (Fig. 12-9). The arms are at the level of the hip, and the patient performs only a partial sit-up. When a

curl can be performed without pain, the patient can move to a full sit-up (Fig. 12-10). Occasionally, stabilization is required at the feet. Once they can be done independently, these exercises become part of the patient's home program.

A general conditioning program can be started when the patient is able to tolerate the abdominal strengthening exercises without pain. Overall conditioning may include both an aquatic program and a gym program.

Perpetuating Factors

Perpetuating factors must be addressed throughout the duration of care. A primary care physician may need to be included in the effective treatment of many of the perpetuating factors. Referrals to specialists may be necessary to detect and treat nutritional deficiencies, metabolic and endocrine inadequacies, psychological problems, and other health problems.

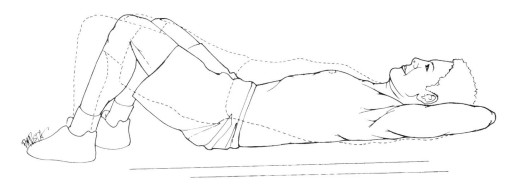

FIGURE 12-7. **Initial strengthening exercises for the abdominal muscles.** The patient lies supine with hips flexed, and identifies the arch in the lower back. The patient presses the lumbar spine into the table to flatten the arch. The patient then bridges up while maintaining the pelvic tilt and the flattened lumbar spine.

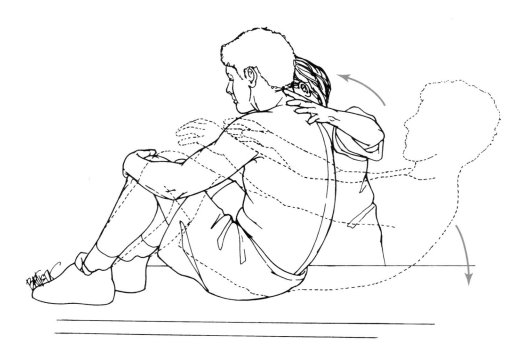

FIGURE 12-8. **A sit-back.** The patient is helped to sitting. The patient lowers to the table in a slow curl-down.

Continued mechanical dysfunction such as postural problems can perpetuate abdominal pain. The patient must be instructed in proper standing and sitting posture as it relates to job duties, daily activities, and other more strenuous physical activities. Ergonomic adjustments may be needed at the workstation.

Sleep deprivation or impairment often becomes a problem for chronic pain patients. Instruction in sleeping in a neutral position may be necessary but difficult. The hip-flexed position is usually the position of choice but needs to be avoided in patients with abdominal trigger points and tightness. The physician may be helpful in prescribing medication to aid sleep.

CONCLUSION

The treatment of the chronic regional myofascial pain patient is a long-term process that involves constant evaluation of the dysfunction. The goal is to achieve a balance between structure and function that can be independently maintained by the patient. The earlier the intervention, the more quickly the problem can be resolved, especially in the case of direct or acute trauma. Often, however, patients who experience abdominal pain describe a long history and may have associated medical problems, such as a history of surgery or trauma that has left them significantly deconditioned and with postural problems. A return to full function may

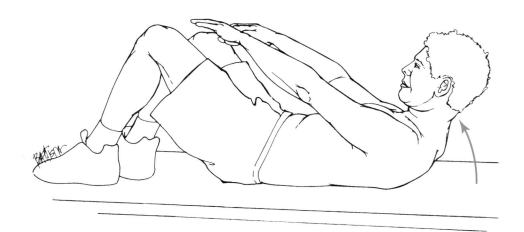

FIGURE 12-9. **An abdominal curl.** The patient curls up to a partial sit-up, with the knees bent.

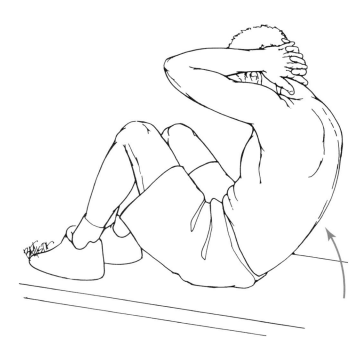

FIGURE 12-10. **A full sit-up.** The knees are bent and the neck is supported. This exercise may require stabilization at the feet.

take anywhere from a few weeks to several months, depending on the level of disability. The patient must be instructed and reminded to perform the home exercise program regularly to maintain functional status. The clinician must remember to act in a systematic fashion in applying treatment. But most of all, the clinician must be compassionate and patient, because progress may vary, and exacerbation of the patient's pain may occur with changes in activity.

TREATMENT PROTOCOL

1. **Allow for a medical evaluation, especially for those patients with concomitant visceral complaints.**

2. **Treat and release all muscles with active trigger points:**

   - Primary trigger points in the abdominal muscles

   - Secondary trigger points in the hip flexors (iliopsoas), lumbar paraspinals, iliocostalis thoracis, and multifidi

   - Satellite trigger points in the quadriceps, hip adductors, hip flexors, quadratus lumborum, and lumbar paraspinals

   - Remember that the primary complaint is abdominal pain, not hip and groin pain.

3. **Initiate a self-stretching program, starting with the muscles harboring the primary trigger points and slowly adding all of the muscles with associated** trigger points. Start with once every hour, but only one to two repetitions.

4. **Use physical therapy modalities as an adjunct for achieving greater relaxation, pain relief, and better releases.**

5. **Address and correct any arthrokinematic dysfunction, starting with those related to the ilium and then those related to the sacrum.**

6. **Correct positional problems of the vertebrae.**

7. **Assess for and address intervertebral disc disorders. Include neurosurgical consultation and use of extension exercises if appropriate.**

8. **Assess for the presence of leg-length discrepancy or small hemipelvis. Correct with lifts, if necessary.**

9. **Correct rib hypomobility, using gentle mobilization or breathing exercises.**

10. **Have the patient begin an additional strengthening program, starting with eccentric or lengthening contractions and progressing to concentric contractions. The use of a pool is highly recommended. Continue the stretching exercises, and be sure to evaluate the patient's performance of the exercises to see that they are done correctly.**

11. **Assess any perpetuating factors. Most important are posture, both static and dynamic. Discuss the patient's daily activities—at home, at work, and during recreation. Specifically look for signs of overuse and poor ergonomic position. Check the patient's sleep position for perpetuation of tightness. Discuss other metabolic or nutritional perpetuating factors with the patient and a physician, as needed.**

12. **Reassess for trigger points in primary and associated muscles.**

13. **Reassess for normal joint function.**

14. **Reassess the patient's medical status, with further medical consultation if necessary.**

15. **Ensure the patient's progressive return to normal activities at work, recreation, or athletics. Reinforce the importance of a continued stretching and strengthening program, and an overall conditioning program.**

References

1. Simons DG, Travell JG, Simons LS. Myofascial Pain and Dysfunction: The Trigger Point Manual, vol 1: Upper half of body. 2nd Ed. Baltimore: Williams and Wilkins, 1999:940–970.

2. Simons DG, Travell JG, Simons LS. Myofascial Pain and Dysfunc-

tion: The Trigger Point Manual, vol 1: Upper half of body. 2nd Ed. Baltimore: Williams and Wilkins, 1999:1–10.

3. Travell JG, Simons DG. Myofascial Pain and Dysfunction: The Trigger Point Manual, vol 2: The lower extremities. Baltimore: Williams and Wilkins, 1992:541–551.
4. Skootsky SA, Jaeger B, Oye RK. Prevalence of myofascial pain in general internal medicine practice. West J Med 1989;151:177–160.
5. Simons DG. Myofascial pain syndromes: where are we? where are we going?. Arch Phys Med Rehabil 1988;69:207–212.
6. Gray H, Gross CM, eds. Gray's Anatomy, 29th Ed. Philadelphia: Lea & Febiger, 1973:371–526. .
7. Basmajian JV, De Luca CJ. Muscles Alive: Their Functions Revealed by Electromyography, 5th Ed. Baltimore: Williams and Wilkins, 1985:252–264.
8. Chaitow L, Liebenson G. Muscle Energy Techniques. New York: Churchhill Livingstone, 1996:15–46.
9. Mitchell FL, Moran PS, Pruzzo NA. Evaluation and Treatment Manual Osteopathic Manipulative Procedures. Valley Park: Mitchell, Moran and Pruzzo Associates, 1979.
10. Lewit K. Manipulative Therapy in Rehabilitation of the Motor System London: Butterworth and Co. Ltd., 1985:177–191.
11. Grieve GP, ed. Modern Manual Therapy of the Vertebral Column. Edinburgh Churchill Livingstone, 1986:151–164.
12. Greenman PE. Principles of Manual Medicine. Baltimore: Williams and Wilkins, 1989:88–93.
13. Long C II: Myofascial pain syndromes, III: some syndromes of the trunk and thigh. Henry Ford Hosp Med Bull 1956;4:102–106.
14. Graven-Nielsen T, Svensson P, Arendt-Nielsen L. Effects of experimental muscle pain on muscle activity and coordination during static and dynamic motor function. Electroencephalogr Clin Neurophysiol 1997;105:156–64.
15. Perry J. Gait Analysis Normal and Pathological Function. New York: McGraw-Hill, 1992:131–140.
16. Manheim CJ, Lavett DK. The Myofascial Release Manual. Thorofare, NJ: Slack, Inc., 1989:95–162.
17. Nielsen AJ: Personal communication with Simons DG, 1981. In: Simons DJ, Travell JG, Simons, LS. Myofascial Pain and Dysfunction: The Trigger Point Manual, vol 1: Upper half of body. 2nd Ed. Baltimore: Williams and Wilkins; 1999;1:94–177.
18. Simons DG, Travell JG, Simons LS. Myofascial Pain and Dysfunction: The Trigger Point Manual, vol 1: Upper half of body. 2nd Ed. Baltimore: Williams and Wilkins; 1999;1:94–177.

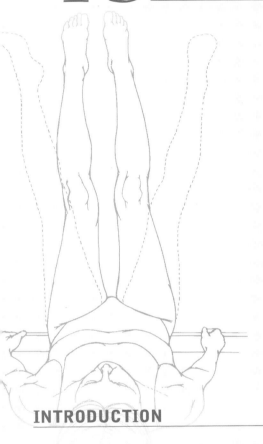

13

Chronic Pelvic Pain of Myofascial Origin

Rhonda Kotarinos, MS, PT

INTRODUCTION

PELVIC PAIN: BACKGROUND

Medical Diagnosis and Clinical Features
Conventional Medical Management

MYOFASCIAL APPROACH TO THE DIAGNOSIS AND TREATMENT OF CHRONIC PELVIC PAIN

Case 13-1
Case 13-2

Overview: Physical Therapy Management of Chronic Pelvic Pain

Causes

Cautions

Symptoms/Pain Presentation

Physical Therapy Evaluation

Myofascial Evaluation

Treatment of Pelvic Pain Syndromes

CONCLUSION

Treatment Protocol

APPENDIX 13.1

INTRODUCTION

Chronic pelvic pain is defined as the persistence of unexplained pain in the low abdominal and pelvic tissues without evidence of active disease (1). This actually is a very vague definition. As a result, many diagnoses have fallen under this definition. **Vulvodynia, vulvar vestibulitis,** dyspareunia, and pelvic floor tension myalgia are just a few of the more specific diagnoses that are considered chronic pelvic pain. Medical assessment of the patient complaining of chronic pelvic pain will be dictated by the specialty of the practitioner. The urologist will evaluate the lower urinary tract, and the gynecologist will evaluate the female reproductive organs; the gastroenterologist and colorectal surgeon will evaluate the lower digestive tract. Of course, the orthopaedic physician will look for a skeletal source of the pain. When these medical disciplines can find no pathologic conditions, as the definition dictates, they defer to psychiatry. Because there is no diagnostic evidence of an active disease process, the pain has to be "in your head." The common denominator, totally overlooked by most medical practitioners when evaluating a complaint of chronic pelvic pain, is the myofascial component.

PELVIC PAIN: BACKGROUND

Mathias et al. (2) did a telephone survey of 17,927 households to identify women between 18 and 50 years of age who had experienced pelvic pain. Of the eligible women, 14.7 % reported experiencing pelvic pain in the past 3 months. This indicates that 9.2 million women are suffering from pelvic pain. Sixty-one percent of that study group did not have a diagnosis to explain their pain. Fifty-five percent of the 14.7% that met the study criteria were sexually active. Of the sexually active group, 88% reported pain during or after intercourse most or all of the time (2).

In 1992, Baskin and Tanagho (3) reported on four patients with severe, persistent pelvic pain. All four patients had undergone multiple surgeries, including removal of the bladder, uterus, ovaries and fallopian tubes, with no resolution of their pain. The authors did note in their discussion that the pelvic musculature is a significant component in the functioning of the pelvic organs. The optimal functioning of the pelvic organs is dependent on the coordination between the pelvic musculature and the pelvic organs. The most important point of their discussion is "The pelvic muscular element, which could well be the source of pain, must be evaluated."(3)

Medical Diagnosis and Clinical Features

All patients, when they first see a physician, must undergo a history and physical examination. A patient with a pain complaint would not be handled any differently. Careful listening is extremely important because it will dictate the course of the physical examination and diagnostic workup.

History

Key points to be addressed in obtaining the history from a pain patient are the nature, intensity, and distribution of the pain. Specifically, the physician is looking for the descriptive characteristics and location of the pain.

A description of the onset of the pain is important, as is the behavior of the pain with regard to duration, changes, cyclicity, and any other factors that can modify the pain. This could include posturing, foods, bowel movements, micturition, menstruation, intercourse, and medications. The physician should listen carefully or directly ask about associated symptoms such as loss of appetite, defecation complaints (constipation or diarrhea), fatigue, or sleep disturbances. A detailed surgical, menstrual, and obstetric history should be obtained.

An assessment should be made regarding the impact of this pain on the patient's ability to function. The health care provider could objectively assess this by using the Functional Pelvic Pain Scale (FPPS) developed by Menard et al. (4) (Table 13-1). What have they had to stop doing in their life as a result of the pain? As difficult as it may be, the physician should also question the patient regarding possible physical or sexual abuse, currently or in the past.

Critical to the accuracy and thoroughness of the history is the quality of communication between the patient and the doctor. This will require scheduling time appropriately, so that the patient does not feel hurried. The physician should empathize with patients but not identify with them. Female patients may feel that a male physician may not be able to empathize as they describe their pelvic pain and how it impacts their life. The physician must be in tune to not only the verbal but the nonverbal communication of the patient. The most valuable skill of the health professional is the art of communication (5).

Physical Examination

The physical examination should include a general systems physical and neurologic assessment. A component of the physical assessment should be to ask the patient to point to where the pain is located. Usually, with chronic pelvic pain, the patient will use the whole hand to sweep the area of the lower abdominal wall. She may describe her pain as "in there," indicating deep within the vagina. A patient experiencing pelvic pain associated with urinary symptoms will place an open palm in the supra-pubic region and complain of pain in her urethra or bladder.

A standard abdominal assessment should be done to rule out obvious organomegaly or masses, as should a comprehensive gynecologic examination.

Laboratory studies required are dependent on the information gained from the history and physical examination. Possible laboratory studies may include cultures, serum chemistry, electrolyte, or specific enzyme studies, depending on the signs and symptoms of the individual patient. Likewise, diagnostic studies used by the physician will depend on the patient's symptomatology and the clinical

TABLE 13-1

Functional Pelvic Pain Scale

Name: _____   Date: _____

INSTRUCTIONS: Please fill out this form by placing an X in the box that best describes your pain when it is the WORST, even if it occurs at different times of your cycle.

If any of these functions *do not* apply to you, please write N/A (not applicable) in the box beside that function.

Function	0 No Pain, Normal Function	1 Some Pain with Function	2 Moderate Pain with Function	3 Severe Pain with Function	4 Incapable of Function Because of Pain
Bladder					
Bowel					
Intercourse					
Walking					
Running					
Lifting					
Working					
Sleeping					

Reprinted with permission from Menard C, Farrell JF, Seidel J, et al. Reliability and validity of the functional pelvic pain scale: a new measure of pelvic pain severity. Journal of SOGC. 1996;69–76.

findings of the physical examination. They may include x-ray, ultrasound, magnetic resonance imaging, or computerized axial tomography. Assuming the primary physician is an obstetrician/gynecologist, referrals may be made to other specialists in urogynecology, gastroenterology, neurology, orthopaedics, or anesthesiology.

Conventional Medical Management

Traditional medical management most commonly consists of pharmacotherapy and surgical therapy. The technical bulletin on chronic pelvic pain from the American College of Obstetricians and Gynecologists states that management of chronic pelvic pain should be focused on resolving the underlying cause of pain, and that it is not always necessary or even possible to determine a diagnosis before starting treatment (6). The general principles of pain management should be followed (Box 13-1).

Pharmacologic Management

Appropriate pharmacologic management may be difficult to establish. In chronic pain, multiple targets may be available to aim for with drug therapy. The World Health Organization promotes a three-step approach in determining the appropriate analgesics for the management of chronic pain (7). The first step in the management of the pain would be acetaminophen and nonsteroidal anti-inflammatory drugs. Low-dose opioid combinations such as acetaminophen and codeine or acetaminophen and hy-

drocodone or acetaminophen with oxycodone would constitute the second step. Stronger opioids would be used for the third step. These could include morphine, hydromorphone, or methadone.

If adequate pain control is not achieved with the three-step approach, adjuvant analgesic therapy may be considered. Adjuvant agents are not usually thought of as having analgesic properties. They do assist in maximizing pain control while lowering the required dosage of opioids.

The most common adjuvant agents used in chronic pain are tricyclic antidepressants. This classification of drugs has the largest body of literature in their use with **nociceptive** and **neuropathic pain** (8). The mechanisms underlying how tricyclic antidepressants work are unknown, but their effects are thought to be attributable to an increase in norepinephrine levels in the central nervous system (9). Selective serotonin reuptake inhibitors are a new class of antidepressants being studied for the management of chronic pain. The mechanism of action for the serotonin reuptake inhibitors is thought to be that the increased serotonin in the central nervous system has an effect on the pain-modulating system in the brain (10,11).

Anticonvulsants are the new group of drugs being studied as adjuvant agents for chronic pain. This group of adjuvant agents will treat the chronic pain that is characterized by bursts of spontaneous or shooting pain that may be the result of neural irritability or damage (12,13). The mechanism of action for drugs such as carbamazepine and phenytoin is that they are sodium channel blockers that inhibit the transmission of excitatory impulses (12).

BOX 13-1

Pain Management Principles

Use positive reinforcement and support.

- Placebos should not be used to assess pain.

- The placebo effect should be used to supplement other therapy through positive reinforcement.

Assess psychological factors early in the evaluation process.

- Coexisting depression or sleep disorders should be sought.

- The diagnosis of "psychogenic pain" should not be a diagnosis of exclusion. Rather, it should be made only when there are clear indications for it.

Treat the underlying disorder whenever possible.

- Pain receptors do not adapt, and under some circumstances, actually lower their thresholds, causing hyperalgesia.

Treat the pain promptly and continue on a regular basis.

- Treatment that effectively suppresses pain or that is not based on the need to re-experience pain gives the best results (e.g., patient-controlled analgesia for postoperative patients). Frequent, scheduled follow-ups are better than "as needed" visits.

Consider use of multiple treatment modalities in synergy.

- Different methods of treatment work by way of different routes (e.g., relaxation techniques, transcutaneous electrical nerve stimulation, physical therapy, vocational rehabilitation, biofeedback).

- The nuances of the treatments used should be understood (e.g., site of action, half-life, administration routes available, interactions).

- Combinations of medications that increase sedation without enhancing analgesia should be avoided.

Use narcotic drugs with caution.

- Tolerance and dependence may occur with long-term use.

- Narcotics should not be withheld if other therapies are ineffective.

Reprinted with permission from American College of Obstetricians and Gynecologists. Chronic Pelvic Pain: (Technical Bulletin No. 223). Washington, DC, May 1996. © ACOG.

Gabapentin, a newer antiepileptic drug, also is used to treat chronic pain. The proposed mechanism of action for gabapentin is related to the presynaptic or postsynaptic regulation of glutaminergic receptors or that it can potentiate the adrenergic function of gamma-aminobutyric acid (13).

Pharmacologic management of chronic pelvic pain also could have a hormonal component. Hormonal drug therapy may be used when there is a strong cyclic component to the pain. Association of cyclic pain with the menstrual cycle suggests a causal relationship with the female reproductive organs. Unfortunately, this is not always a correct assumption (14). Hormonal management may be as simple as oral contraceptives to regulate the menstrual cycle or can be as involved as full medical menopause.

Management of chronic pain, especially chronic pelvic pain, is difficult and very complicated. There is not a simple answer or a cookbook recipe to resolve the problems. In managing a patient with chronic pelvic pain, the health care practitioner must remember to treat the whole person and not only their complaint of pain. The treatment plan must be individualized to each patient's needs and reviewed frequently to enhance the outcome.

Surgical Management

Surgical management of chronic pelvic pain should be used only when there is a surgically correctable cause (14). Laparoscopy or laparotomy frequently is used in this patient population to diagnose and or treat **endometriosis.** Lysis of adhesions also may be performed when indicated. If no pain relief is achieved with these procedures, then one must carefully consider additional surgery.

Chronic pelvic pain is the operative diagnosis for 15% of all hysterectomies, and at least 50% of them are not successful. Studies show that hysterectomy or oophorectomy performed for chronic pelvic pain has a very poor long-term success rate. Hysterectomy is considered when a significant pathologic condition is not detected laparoscopically, or if the pain has persisted for more than 6 months, has not responded to pharmacologic management, and impairs the patient's normal function. All other means of conservative management should have been tried and all other possible causes ruled out before surgery. The physician must adequately communicate to the patient that hysterectomy may not cure her pain.

Pelvic vascular congestion as a result of pelvic varicosities can cause chronic pelvic pain in some women. This will be the only positive finding with diagnostic laparoscopy. Pelvic vein embolization is a surgical technique that can be done to treat the pelvic varicosities.

When pharmacologic management and pelvic surgery are unsuccessful in resolving the pain, surgery may be directed to the nervous system. Neurosurgery for chronic pelvic pain is attempting to interrupt the neural pathways that transmit pain in the pelvis. Neural procedures for chronic pelvic pain can include a laparoscopic uterosacral nerve ablation and a presacral neurectomy. Studies do indicate short-term favorable results with a presacral neurectomy for midline dysmenorrhea (15). For other chronic pelvic pain conditions, the long-term effects of the neural surgical procedures are extremely variable. The complication rate is also noted to be very high. The use of these procedures is therefore severely limited.

MYOFASCIAL APPROACH TO THE DIAGNOSIS AND TREATMENT OF CHRONIC PELVIC PAIN

There are many possible causes for chronic pelvic pain. Until recently, the musculoskeletal system was not considered as a causative factor in chronic pelvic pain. This may be related to the fact that there is not a dedicated medical discipline overseeing muscle in general, let alone the muscles of the pelvis. Very little time is spent in medical school addressing the muscles as a source of pain. Even less time is spent covering the relationship between skeletal muscle and the other systems of the body. The physician must evaluate all organ systems that could be contributing to pelvic pain and should at least screen the musculoskeletal system.

Little information is found in the literature on the musculoskeletal factors of enigmatic pelvic pain. What is available statistically supports the relationship between the musculoskeletal system and chronic pelvic pain in some patients. King et al. (16) found that 70% of their pelvic pain patients reported complete or significant relief of their symptoms when the musculoskeletal dysfunction found during the physical therapy evaluation was treated.

Very old literature also establishes a very close relationship between pelvic pain and dysfunction and the musculoskeletal system. In 1909, Joel Goldthwait (17) published an extensive article addressing the impact of the musculoskeletal system on conditions of the pelvis. He stated ". . . that the physician has a higher function than the mere treatment of local conditions . . ." and ". . . whatever solution of the problem we may have to offer must be offered only after due consideration, not of any one part or of any one use, but of the organism as a whole with regard to all its functions." (17) Herein lies the problem with chronic pelvic pain; the medical system at this time tries to treat the problem locally, for the most part ignoring the body as a functioning whole.

Travell and Simons (18) did address various myofascial pain syndromes that involve pelvic pain in Volume 1 of Myofascial Pain and Dysfunction. In this text, they discussed the abdominal trigger points that cause lower urinary tract complaints, groin pain, and dysmenorrhea and other diagnoses that could be associated with chronic pelvic pain (18). In Volume 2 of Myofascial Pain and Dysfunction, they discussed the association between pelvic pain and trigger points located within the adductor muscle group as well as the internal and external pelvic floor muscles (19). These remain the most comprehensive sources of information regarding trigger points, which can be components of chronic pelvic pain.

CASE 13-1

Patient History

Mrs. S. was a 41-year-old female accounting professor who complained of right pelvic and groin pain for the past 9 months. The activities that were out of the ordinary for her routine at the time of the onset of her pain were a trip to Disney World and painting her house. Her first medical visit was to her gynecologist, who stated that it was a muscle pull and to go home and rest. The pain was constant, with no change occurring with rest. She spent her holidays in misery. She returned to her gynecologist, who then ordered a computed tomography (CT) scan. With regard to the reproductive system, the workup was negative. A hemangioma was found on the liver. Her gynecologist referred her to a surgeon. He chose to do an exploratory laparoscopy. He found and repaired a left inguinal hernia. No significant findings were present on the right. Two weeks after the surgery, the pain returned. She returned to the surgeon, who sent her back to her gynecologist, stating that he believed the source of her pain was ovarian. Treatment choices offered by her gynecologist at this time, 9 months after the onset of her pain, were surgery to remove the ovary (even though there was no documented pathologic condition), medical menopause, and to see a psychiatrist. A friend told her about physical therapy for pelvic pain. When she requested a referral to physical therapy, he refused. Physical therapy support came from her family practice physician.

Symptoms

Mrs. S. complained of pain in the right anterior lower abdominal wall, in the area of the inguinal ligament. For the most part, it was very circumscribed, but with increased irritability would radiate in the groin and down the medial aspect of the right thigh. There was also a burning sensation from the inside. The pain worsened with driving and crossing her legs. She was able to golf and ride her bike, but was unable to keep up her normal lower extremity strength training secondary to increased pain. There was no problem with prolonged standing; she therefore had no problems with work.

CASE 13-1   Continued

Examination Findings

Postural screening findings were noncontributory to the evaluation. Gross strength assessment of the lower extremities indicated a slightly decreased level of strength with the hip girdle muscles. They were still within a good to normal grade. The patient stated that she felt she could have done better on the right, but she was afraid of pain. Gross hip range of motion was overall within normal limits bilaterally. Stiffness or resistance to passive motion was noted in all planes of motion of the right joint. Overpressure into right hip internal and external rotation was uncomfortable but did not reproduce her pain. The abdominal wall assessment did indicate a **diastasis recti** of three to four fingers at the umbilicus and two to three fingers below the umbilicus. Above the umbilicus, the separation was at least three fingers. The lower and upper abdominal strength ranged from a fair to good grade, respectively, in spite of the altered insertion of the abdominal muscles.

Myofascial assessment of the entire anterior and posterior lower quadrant indicated extensive myofascial and connective tissue restrictions on the right. Taut bands were noted in the right iliopsoas and the adductors. An internal examination also showed taut bands and tenderness in the obturator internus and piriformis. The primary trigger point was found in the obturator externus. On palpation, the patient shouted, "That's it, that's my pain." With provocation of her pain, she remembered that while painting her hallway she used her right leg to support herself while hanging over the railing of the stairway.

Treatment

Treatment involved some form of deep heat, ultrasound to the right femoral triangle or short-wave diathermy to the entire right lower trunk and hip, followed by myofascial and connective tissue manipulation to the right anterior lower quadrant. Trigger point release techniques with contract/relax and reciprocal inhibition of the right hip internal and external rotators also were used. At the first visit, the patient was taught an exercise to correct her diastasis recti and hip girdle stretching. This included a hamstring and adductor stretch. Ice massage was done to the anterior hip and groin area after treatment. The patient noted significant improvement in her pain after the first visit, but it was reactivated after prolonged driving. Treatment focused on trigger point release of the primary trigger point in the obturator externus after deep heat.

A gentle stretching exercise program was gradually transitioned to a progressive strengthening program as the irritability of the trigger point decreased. After each visit, the patient was asked to slowly resume her normal activities and to stop any activity that caused her pain. Each activity that caused her pain was then analyzed at the next visit and broken down into components. Exercises were then developed to address each component. The patient was discharged from physical therapy to an independent home program. She had resumed her normal routines with no limitations.

Follow-up

During a telephone interview with the patient approximately 2 years after her last visit, the patient stated that she had not had a recurrence of her pain and that she had resumed all of her activities.

CASE 13-2

History

Mrs. G. was a 36-year-old woman with the complaint of right-sided deep pain with deep penetration and thrusting with intercourse. She was 8 weeks status post vaginal hysterectomy with bilateral salpingo-oophorectomy for menorrhagia. Before surgery, she had no history of dyspareunia. Mrs. G. was medically released at 6 weeks after surgery to resume intercourse. Her first attempt was very painful, to the point of not being able to complete. Repeated attempts did not improve the situation. Changing sexual position did not improve her dyspareunia.

Symptoms

The pain with attempted intercourse was sharp but also achy. The ache would persist after intercourse for several hours. Because intercourse was usually attempted at bedtime, there was minimal limitation of her other functional activities.

Examination Findings

Postural screening, movement evaluation, and the muscle strength assessment were all essentially noncontributory to the significant clinical findings. An active trigger point was found in the right obturator internus

CASE 13-2   Continued

during the internal myofascial evaluation. This correlated well with her complaint of her pain with intercourse when her legs were positioned in external rotation and abduction at the hip. Speculation as to the mechanism of injury would probably be the positioning of the lower extremities in the stirrups during the hysterectomy.

Treatment

Initially, myofascial manipulation and trigger point release were the primary components of treatment. Once the tenderness of the obturator internus was decreased with the above techniques and the trigger point could be easily localized, an injection was done. Immediately after the injection, internal myofascial manipulation was done, combined with therapeutic exercise of localized manual stretching and active concentric and eccentric contractions of the right obturator internus. As the irritability of the trigger point decreased, progressive strengthening was initiated. The patient was discharged from physical therapy after eight visits. She was completely pain-free with intercourse in all positions and had resumed her presurgery workout routine.

Follow-up

A retrospective chart review indicated that, at her regular 1-year gynecology visit, the patient had no complaints of pain.

Overview: Physical Therapy Management of Chronic Pelvic Pain

Causes

One of the most frustrating aspects of chronic pelvic pain is that usually the cause is unknown. Endometriosis is a possible cause. But all too often the endometriosis is diagnosed while looking for the source of pain; it is then treated medically and surgically, with no significant decrease in pain; therefore, the endometriosis was not the source of pain. A lower urinary tract infection could be the inciting event in the development of chronic pelvic pain. The pain that is normally felt with an acute, culture-proven urinary tract infection may persist, even after a cure culture has been done.

Frequently pelvic pain also may start after an unrelated surgical procedure such as a hysterectomy, an anti-incontinence procedure, or surgery to correct a pelvic organ prolapse. Retractors used in the abdominal cavity during surgery may irritate the iliopsoas and cause trigger points to develop. Trigger points in the iliopsoas may develop functionally and go undiagnosed as sources of pelvic pain. Many times these trigger points may be mistaken for ovarian dysfunction. While discussing surgery, one must not overlook episiotomies as a possible source of chronic pelvic pain and more specific dyspareunia.

Cautions

Most patients have had an extensive medical workup before being evaluated for physical therapy. On occasion, if the pain appears to have a strong neuropathic component, the clinician may refer the patient to a urogynecologist for neurophysiologic testing of the pudendal nerve.

The evaluation performed by the clinician must increase or decrease the patient's pain. If this is not accomplished, then the likelihood of myofascial therapy being beneficial is minimal. The clinician may be the one health care provider who will assess all of the systems and their integration to diagnose at least the musculoskeletal sources of pelvic pain. When medical disciplines and physical therapy approaches are to no avail, the patient may be considered for neural modulation.

Symptoms/Pain Presentation

Chronic pelvic pain is a general diagnostic label that covers many pelvic pain disorders. Vulvodynia will present as an intense burning pain in the superficial tissues that are innervated by the pudendal nerve. This will include burning on the external skin as well as a burning and itching sensation within the vagina. Vulvar vestibulitis, a subset of vulvodynia, is described as an intense burning pain when the vulvar tissues are touched. Penile penetration or the insertion of a tampon will cause the patient to complain of a ripping or tearing pain associated with an intense burning sensation. Usually, with vulvar vestibulitis, if the tissues are not being touched, the patient will not experience any pain.

Dyspareunia, pain associated with intercourse, can be experienced during penetration, or with thrusting, or both. It is also used to describe the pain felt after intercourse, which may or may not be accompanied by pain during intercourse. Pain with penetration is usually described as very sharp with burning, ripping, or tearing sensations. The pain of thrusting can be sharp, aching, or described as a deep pressure into a bad bruise. Postcoital pain will be described as an intense aching or soreness, sometimes with severe burning and occasional sharp stabs.

Chronic pain associated with urinary complaints has many different presentations. Some patients will only experience an intense sharp pain in the urethra with the onset or termination of urination. This can be associated with trigger points in the urethral sphincter muscles. Other patients may complain of intense suprapubic aching on bladder filling with a constant sense of urge. Their only pain-free moments may be during urination. Frequency may then become a very debilitating component of the pelvic pain syndrome.

Incontinence is not usually associated with pelvic pain but can present as stress or urge or mixed incontinence as a result of the dysfunction that can develop in the pelvic floor muscles in response to pain. If the levator ani or the urethral sphincter muscles have trigger points, they may not function normally within their reflex capacities. With stress incontinence, this would mean that the reflex contraction of the pelvic floor during times of increased intra-abdominal pressure is not sufficient to maintain the increased urethral pressure required for continence. Urge incontinence would occur if the trigger points altered the pelvic floor's reflex response required to inhibit the bladder contraction that is signaling urge. In mixed incontinence, both situations occur.

Patients who present with left or right anterior lower abdominal/pelvic pain will complain of a constant dull aching. Sharp and stabbing pain may develop with certain functional activities.

Cyclic characteristics of the pain will establish a link to the female reproductive system and hormonal cycle. Unfortunately, this may establish a false relationship. A physical therapy evaluation should be considered on all patients about to undergo a surgical procedure for lower abdominal/pelvic pain when there is not an obvious diagnostic cause that warrants surgery. Many young girls will present with this pain to a pediatric gynecologist. A thorough physical therapy evaluation would be prudent to rule out a myofascial origin of the pain. One visit with a knowledgeable physical therapist may prevent the young patient from starting down a long path of unwarranted invasive procedures.

Physical Therapy Evaluation

A comprehensive physical therapy evaluation has been discussed elsewhere in this book and within other reference resources (20). This comprehensive evaluation would include a thorough evaluation of the lumbosacral spine, pelvic ring, and its articulations. Articular dysfunction of the lumbosacral spine and pelvic ring could be perpetuating factors of myofascial trigger points in the pelvic musculature. This section focuses on the myofascial assessment for chronic pelvic pain.

The key elements of the subjective examination are the location and description of the symptoms, the behavior of the symptoms, special questions, and the history. Specific information to be gained regarding the location and description would be the area and depth of pain and the area of greatest intensity. The patient should be asked whether there is pain, stiffness or tightness, or both. The patient should describe the sensations that are felt—pain, tingling, numbness, or all three. The type of pain and all of its variations also should be described. The descriptions of pain might include burning, cramping, stabbing, aching, throbbing, bruised, raw, open wound, ground glass, and razor blades, to name a few.

The behavior of the symptoms is another element of the subjective examination. The patient should be questioned about pain over a 24-hour period. The clinician should ascertain how the symptoms vary from awakening in the morning through a normal day to bedtime. A determination also must be made as to what aggravates the pain and what eases the pain. Documenting specific functional limitations can serve as objective measures of progress. This could include sitting tolerance (decreased with vulvodynia), standing tolerance, and duration of walking. With some of the pain syndromes, activity could be very limited. In vulvar vestibulitis, the functional limitation may only be the inability to use tampons or to engage in intercourse.

Also to be covered in the history is the patient's reasoning for seeking treatment at this time. The clinician should ask patient how long the pain has been experienced. An attempt should be made to determine what was the inciting event and how it has changed over time. All previous treatments should be disclosed, as well as whether they were beneficial. When multiple symptoms are present, it may be helpful for the patient to prioritize their symptoms. Which complaint would they want resolved first?

After the history has been obtained, the patient is asked to fill out pain diagrams and a visual analog pain scale (Figs. 13-1 and 13-2). The International Pelvic Pain Society has developed a comprehensive pelvic pain intake form. This form can be used by physical therapy practitioners, with minor changes for each individual practice (Appendix 13-1)

A screening postural evaluation is performed and is progressed to a more detailed evaluation based on the findings of the screening. A postural evaluation usually is considered as only a structural assessment. Attention is given to postural conditions, such as a leg length discrepancy, that could be a perpetrator of myofascial trigger points within the pelvic musculature. However, a more comprehensive approach will incorporate the myofascial system into the postural evaluation by looking at the muscle asymmetry, connective tissue asymmetry, and muscular activity as it relates to the abnormal structural findings. During the postural evaluation, special attention should be given to the soft tissue to help direct the more detailed soft tissue evaluation.

An active movement evaluation of the spine and the extremities provides dynamic information that can be correlated with the postural findings and the soft tissue evaluation. When focusing on a myofascial assessment, the active range of motion evaluation initially should direct the examiner to look regionally and then segmentally (21). The regional assessment typically will show myofascial abnormalities, whereas the segmental evaluation will identify joint dysfunction. Specific joint or muscle length evaluation will be done based on the information gained from the active movement evaluation, to direct the evaluation to a more specific joint or muscle length. The range of motion of the components of the lower quadrant is assessed. The focus is primarily on the range of joint motion and the range of muscle length of the hip girdle. The range of joint motion and

Pelvic Pain Chart

Name (last, first, m.i.) : _____

Date pain charted: _____

Perceived pain index (PPI):   0   1   2   3   4   5   6   7   8   9   4   10
                           (none)   (worst)

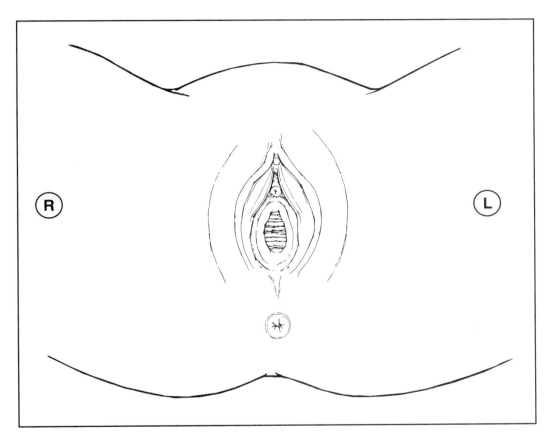

B = burning pain
S = stabbing pain
N = numbness
I = itching

FIGURE 13-1. **Pelvic pain chart.** The patient is asked to indicate the location of pain or other symptoms on this diagram.

Body Pain Chart

Name (last, first, m.i.) : _____

Date pain charted: _____

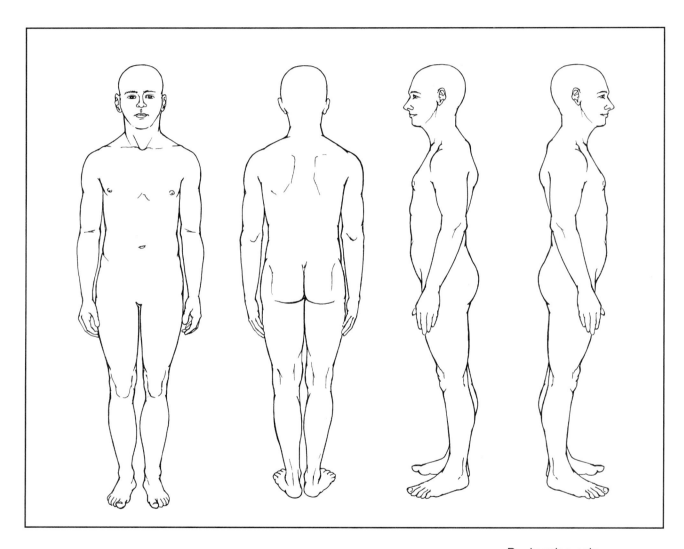

B = burning pain
S = stabbing pain
A = aching pain
N = numbness
I = itching
P = pins & needles

FIGURE 13-2. **Body pain chart.** The patient is also asked to indicate locations of pain, numbness, or other symptoms on a full body chart.

muscle length assessment is only a screening examination to determine factors associated with the pelvic myofascial dysfunction. Special attention may be given to the hip flexors, hamstrings, hip rotators, and the abdominal wall.

Gross muscle strength will be tested in all of the lower quadrant muscle groups. When doing the strength assessment, the examiner must determine whether the weakness present is a true weakness or a function of inhibition of the muscle as a result of a trigger point. True weakness within a muscle may be the source of the overload that caused the trigger point in that muscle or an associated muscle.

Special attention needs to be given to the assessment of the abdominal wall. Diastasis recti is a common problem that can compromise the strength and function of the abdominal wall musculature. Diastasis recti is a separation of the rectus abdominis muscles at the linea alba. The most common precipitating cause is pregnancy. In adults, diastasis recti is also seen in obese, hypersthenic males and in patients with chronic obstructive lung disease. Diastasis recti is normally seen in children up to the age of 2 years.

The insertion of the external oblique, internal oblique, and transversus muscles is altered when there is a diastasis recti. This therefore compromises the function of the abdominal wall and can be the precipitating factor in the development of trigger points in the abdominal musculature. An extensive advertising campaign usually starts in January for weight loss and getting into shape for summer. Many people start an inappropriately aggressive abdominal strengthening exercise program. Trigger points then develop in the abdominal wall musculature, causing somatovisceral responses, including frequency, urgency, and possibly pain. Thus, a higher volume of patients complaining of urinary frequency and urgency will be experienced in the spring. Their primary complaint is of feeling as though they have a constant sense of pressure or urge. At times, the symptoms can be so severe that they feel as though they have a urinary tract infection, even though the cultures are negative. Information gained while taking their history indicates that just before their symptoms started they had initiated an aggressive abdominal strengthening program. Almost

universally, this group of patients has a diastasis recti that should have been corrected before starting an abdominal strengthening program.

The commonly accepted procedure to examine a patient for diastasis recti is as follows: "The patient assumes a supine position. The examiner places the fingertips of one hand on the linea alba of the abdomen near or at the umbilicus and palpates the area. The patient is then requested to raise her head and shoulders from the table. With contraction, as the muscles shorten, they approach the midline. At this point, the examiner gauges the extent of the separation with the number of fingertips that fit between the recti bellies" (22).

This author does vary from this procedure slightly. The generally acceptable range for the width of the linea alba between the rectus bellies is from 0.5 cm to 2.5 cm (23). The widest natural separation is above the umbilicus, and the narrowest is below the umbilicus. Below the umbilicus, the rectus bellies may fuse, obliterating any evidence of the linea alba. One must keep in mind that these anatomic measurements were made on cadavers. The cadavers were not asked to raise their head and shoulders. Therefore, if the examiner is palpating at the umbilicus and the recti bellies are felt approaching the midline from a wider resting position yet close to within two fingers' separation, this clinician believes that a diastasis is present. From a functional anatomic standpoint, the rectus bellies should be at no more than a two-finger separation whether they are at rest or contracted. A diastasis recti should be corrected with exercise before a progressive abdominal strengthening program is initiated (Fig. 13-3).

The foundation of the assessment for chronic pelvic pain of a myofascial origin is the soft tissue evaluation. The soft tissue to be evaluated includes skeletal muscle, connective tissue, and the neural tissue. The focus on this section of the chapter covers primarily the assessment of the skeletal muscle associated with chronic pelvic pain syndromes. Trigger point examination of skeletal muscle is emphasized. The examination of the connective tissue and

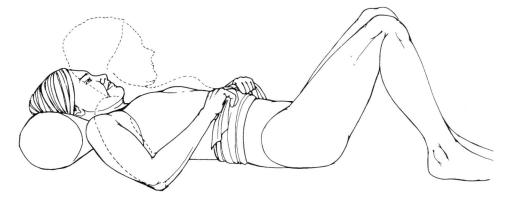

FIGURE 13-3. Diastasis recti correction exercise. The patient lies on the back with the knees bent and the feet flat. A sheet or cloth is placed around the waist, crossed as if tying a knot. The head is raised with the chin towards the chest. This position is held for a count of 5, exhaling during the count. This is repeated 10 to 30 times per session, two sessions per day.

neural tissue are very important and should not be neglected. Information regarding connective tissue evaluation and treatment can be found in publications by Elizabeth Dicke and Maria Ebner (24,25). In his text on the mobilization of the nervous system, David Butler covers adverse neural tension theory, evaluation, and treatment (26).

Myofascial Evaluation

The muscle groups to be examined for trigger points in a chronic pelvic pain patient are determined by the patient's symptoms and the evaluation results up to this point. From an external approach, the muscles most often involved will include the abdominal muscles, iliopsoas, obturator externus (see case study 13-1), gluteal muscles, adductors, and the piriformis. The internal examination will be of the muscles of the superficial and deep urogenital diaphragm, levator ani, obturator internus (see case study 2), coccygeus, and the piriformis.

Simons et al. (27) state that "the presence of exquisite tenderness at a nodule in a palpable taut band" is the most reliable diagnostic criterion for detecting a trigger point in a muscle. When palpation or needle penetration of the trigger point reproduces the patient's clinical pain complaint, it is considered an active trigger point. A characteristic pattern of referred pain and a local twitch response are features typically found with a trigger point (27). With internal palpation of the pelvic musculature, the local twitch response would be felt and not visually observed.

Autonomic phenomena associated with trigger points are localized vasoconstriction, **sudomotor activity, lacrimation, coryza,** salivation, **pilomotor activity,** and proprioceptive disturbances (27). Sudomotor activity, lacrimation, salivation, and coryza are phenomena that involve glandular activity. Trigger points in the lower trunk may have their autonomic impact on the glands of that region, Skene's glands, Bartholin's gland, and so forth. Many pelvic pain patients complain of excessive vaginal discharge, frequently sending them to the doctor thinking that they have a yeast infection or some form of vaginitis. Most of the time their cultures are negative. Unfortunately, they are treated empirically and often develop contact dermatitis from the unnecessary medication.

Abdominal wall myofascial trigger points are strongly associated with somatovisceral and viscerosomatic effects. This is especially evident in the pelvic pain population that also has urinary complaints. Active trigger points along the suprapubic rim involving the insertions of the rectus abdominis, internal oblique, and transversus can cause increased sensitivity and spasms of the urinary bladder and urinary sphincter. This results in the patient potentially experiencing urinary urgency and frequency, urinary retention, or pain (18). Trigger points in the lateral aspect of the inguinal ligament area also can create urinary complaints. Trigger points in the inferior lateral internal oblique attachments may be associated with the urethral pain of urethral syndrome.

Gynecologic pain complaints also can be associated with trigger points in the lower abdominal muscles. Many patients with lower abdominal or pelvic pain are diagnosed with endometriosis. All too often medical management of the endometriosis does not resolve the patient's pain complaints. Myofascial trigger points, unfortunately, are not even considered as possible causes of the various pelvic pain syndromes. This could be a possible explanation for the confusion that develops when a patient diagnosed with endometriosis has minimal disease but is totally disabled by pain, and the patient with extensive disease has no pain. In many cases, the endometriosis is probably not the source of their pain.

Pelvic pain is considered to be extremely perplexing, especially when traditional medical management has not been able to locate and resolve the source of pain. The solution to enigmatic pelvic pain may be found in part by considering the reciprocal somatovisceral and viscerosomatic effects of myofascial trigger points. An acute visceral disorder, such as a culture-positive urinary tract infection, can produce a trigger point in a somatic tissue (usually the abdominal wall musculature or connective tissue). This would represent a viscerosomatic effect. This trigger point can persist long after the acute urinary tract infection has been cured with oral antibiotics, causing the patient to continue to experience the symptoms of an acute urinary tract infection: a somatovisceral effect.

A flat palpation or pincer palpation technique can be used to examine the abdominal wall musculature. Flat palpation is usually more effective along the bony attachments of the abdominal wall to locate attachment trigger points. A pincer technique can be used to locate central trigger points within the bellies of the muscles. Either technique can be used at the linea alba. Increasing the abdominal muscle tension during the examination may assist the examiner in distinguishing a tender trigger point from possible organ pathologic conditions. Several methods of increasing the abdominal muscle tension have been described (18). They include raising both legs several inches above the table surface, elevating the head and shoulders as if doing a partial sit-up, or doing both at the same time. While the examiner palpates the most tender area of a taut band, producing pain, the patient is asked in one of several ways to increase the tension in the abdominal wall. As the tension in the abdominal wall increases, if the pain increases, this indicates the presence of a trigger point. If the pain decreases, the source of the pain may be visceral.

Attachment trigger points of the external oblique muscle may be found along the inferior aspect of the rib cage, along the iliac crest or at its attachment at the midline into the linea alba. If the patient is placed in a supine position with her legs flexed, the abdominal muscles will be on slack, making it easier to perform a pincer evaluation.

Internal oblique trigger points associated with chronic pelvic pain are most frequently found along the muscle's attachments at the lateral aspect of the inguinal ligament, on the iliac crest at the anterior and inferior to the anterior superior iliac spine and the pubic crest. Palpation can start at the anterior superior iliac spine moving inferiorly along the iliac to the pubic arch. At times, the nodule of the trigger point will roll under the finger as if it were a pea. Care must be taken to not use a flat palpation on the pubic bone itself. This could definitely be painful but not from a trigger point. The periosteum is a very highly innervated structure, and prolonged point pressure can be painful. Other diagnoses that could cause pain with palpation include osteitis, osteomyelitis, and rheumatoid arthritis.

Flat palpation at the midline of the pubic crest can be used to locate attachment trigger points of the rectus abdominis. Flat or pincer palpation can be used to locate trigger points in the lower portion of the muscle from the umbilicus to the symphysis or at its medial borders along the linea alba. Trigger points in these areas are most commonly associated with various pelvic pain syndromes.

Respiration While examining the abdominal wall for trigger points, the examiner should take the time to evaluate the patient's respiratory pattern. Paradoxical breathing is frequently found in chronic pelvic pain patients.

With inhalation, the diaphragm contracts, pushing the abdominal contents down into the pelvis. As the lung volume increases in the lower chest, the abdominal wall should protrude. This is a very simple description of diaphragmatic breathing. During paradoxical breathing, the chest and abdominal functions counter each other. In paradoxical breathing, during inhalation, the chest moves up and out while the abdomen moves up and in. This elevates the diaphragm, causing a decrease in lung volume.

Fear of pain during breathing as a result of stretching the rectus abdominis with trigger points inhibits normal diaphragmatic breathing, causing the patient to establish a paradoxical breathing pattern. Because the abdominal wall muscles and the pelvic floor muscles work synergistically and reciprocally during breathing, paradoxical breathing can occur as a result of trigger points in the pelvic floor muscles.

Determining what has occurred to establish this pattern is not always easy. Some patients actively contract their abdominal walls for the purpose of looking slimmer. If the abdominal wall is actively contracting, there will be a reflex contraction of the pelvic floor. If the pelvic floor is actively contracted, there is a reflex contraction of the abdominal wall muscles (28). This prolonged excessive muscle activity could cause or perpetuate a trigger point. Resolving the trigger points is easy compared with trying to break the patient's habit of the active contraction of either muscle group.

Examination of the Intrapelvic Muscles Examination of the intrapelvic muscles may be done vaginally or rectally. The pelvic muscles can be divided into three layers: perineal muscles, pelvic diaphragm, and pelvic wall muscles. The superficial perineal muscles to be examined would include the ischiocavernosus, bulbocavernosus, and the superficial

transverse perinei. The deep perineal muscles would not be distinguishable on palpation but would include the transversus vaginae, compressor urethra, and urethrovaginal muscle. Muscles of the pelvic diaphragm would include the levator ani and the coccygeus. The pelvic wall muscles would be the obturator internus, piriformis, and possibly the iliopsoas. On a vaginal examination, the clinical correlation of bony landmarks would be the posterior pubic bones, anterior linea terminalis, symphysis pubis, obturator foramen, and ischial spine. During the rectal examination, the bony landmarks would be the ischial spines, anterior surface of the coccyx and sacrum, sacrococcygeal joint, margins of the sciatic foramen, and the sacrospinous ligament.

The **lithotomy position** or semiprone in the Sim's position can be used for a rectal examination. It is difficult to examine both sides of the pelvis with one hand. Therefore, it is advisable to examine the patient with the hand that will supinate toward the side to be examined and use the other hand to examine the other side. The external anal sphincter, the levator ani, coccygeus, and the piriformis can be evaluated during a rectal examination.

A rectal examination can be distressing regardless of whether there are trigger points. Care must be taken to minimize the patient's distress. A water-based lubricant should be applied to the gloved finger and to the anal orifice if needed. To minimize distress and protective guarding by the patient, the examiner may ask the patient to bear down (as if initiating a bowel movement) as the examining finger is slowly inserted into the anal orifice. At this time, the examiner should check the anal orifice for internal hemorrhoids. If present, these may be a perpetuating factor of anal sphincter trigger points.

Palpation of the external and internal sphincters can be accomplished by gently flexing the fingertip. Withdrawing the finger halfway allows for gentle palpation of the external anal sphincter at every one-eighth of a circle for trigger point tenderness. As with trigger point examination in other skeletal muscles, the examiner is looking for the most tender area within a taut band. Contraction of that muscle while palpating the trigger point will increase the pain. The examiner may find that patient's ability to bear down or eccentrically contact the muscle is limited as a result of the limitation of stretch range of motion caused by the trigger point. If external anal sphincter trigger points are present and too acute, they may need to be inactivated before a more thorough rectal evaluation of the pelvic muscles can be completed.

The pelvic wall and pelvic diaphragm muscles are the next layer to be evaluated during a rectal examination. The posterior aspect of the levator ani, puborectalis, and iliococcygeus is easier to assess rectally. The examining finger should palpate the posterior medial borders of the levator ani for trigger points and then move from the perineal body superiorly across the posterior aspect of the mid-belly of the levator ani up to the sacrospinous ligament. Methodically sweeping the finger in a 180° arc from posterior to anterior at successively higher levels will allow the examiner to fully assess the levator fibers for trigger points (29). When palpating the lateral and anterolateral aspects of the levator, the examiner must be careful to distinguish which muscle the positive findings are in—the levator ani or the underlying obturator internus. This can be determined by asking the patient to actively contract the pelvic floor. The command could be to squeeze the examining finger or do what you would do to stop the flow of urine. This should isolate the levator ani. While palpating the obturator internus, the examiner would ask the patient to abduct the hip on the side being examined if in a hook-lying position or to externally rotate the hip if the lower extremity on the side being examined were in full extension. Mild resistance would be applied during each of these actions to enhance the response.

The coccygeus lies lateral to the sacrococcygeal joint overlying the sacrospinous ligament. The firm fibers of the sacrospinous ligament under the coccygeus make it easier to palpate for taut bands and trigger points. Isolated contraction of the individual muscles of the pelvic floor is next to impossible (30). The coccygeus flexes and abducts the coccyx. To elicit an active contraction, the examiner would ask the patient to squeeze around the examiner's finger while the examiner is palpating the coccygeus for provocation of trigger points. Trigger points in this muscle frequently refer pain to the coccyx. Trigger points in the levator ani and gluteus maximus also can be responsible for pain in the coccyx. Coccygodynia, therefore, can have a myofascial origin (19).

The pelvic wall muscles that can be examined rectally for trigger points are the obturator internus and the piriformis. The obturator internus originates from the obturator foramen and can be palpated from an anterior lateral approach. Using the arcus tendineus fascia as a landmark, the examiner will be able to palpate the muscle with only the rectal wall between the examining finger and the muscle. Below the arcus tendineus, the examiner has to use active contraction, as previously described, of either the levator ani or the obturator internus to determine the source of the taut bands and trigger points.

The examination just described was from a rectal approach, which of course is the only route for an examination of the intrapelvic muscles of a man. A rectal examination would be required to evaluate the external anal sphincter and the more posterior pelvic diaphragm and pelvic wall muscles in a woman. A vaginal examination is definitely more comfortable and preferred to examine the levator ani, deep and superficial urogenital diaphragm, and the anterior pelvic wall muscles.

In the man, the urogenital muscles would be examined from an external approach. Palpation of these muscles could be performed with the patient in a hook-lying position, supporting his testicles. The bulbocavernosus can be examined by a gentle pincer technique along the length of the muscle during a vaginal examination. Bulbocavernosus

trigger points may cause penetration dyspareunia as well as vaginal aching. Ischiocavernosus examination also is accomplished vaginally. Palpation is performed with the fingertip just inside the pubic rami, with pressure applied along the length of the muscle from the pubic arch to the medial aspect of the ischial tuberosity. Trigger points in the ischiocavernosus refer pain to the perineum and to the clitoris. The transverse perinei originates at the ischial tuberosity and inserts into the central tendon of the perineum. These muscles can be examined externally in both sexes. With counter pressure applied, by a finger in the rectum or vagina, the examination of the transverse perinei is easier to execute.

The perineal body is a wedge-shaped mass that separates the vagina from the anal canal. Muscles of the superficial and deep urogenital diaphragm insert into the perineal body. This includes the bulbocavernosus, ischiocavernosus, superficial transverse perinei, transversus vaginae, compressor urethrae, and the urethrovaginal muscle. Acute trigger points within the perineal body can cause the urethral pain and sensory complaints associated with the diagnosis of urethral syndrome. A combined vaginal and rectal examination in the woman may allow for easier location of trigger points within the perineal body.

If a female patient has been severely traumatized, the musculature may be very taut and abnormally easily palpable at the **introitus.** Tenderness at the introitus may create a **vaginismus**-like condition in which severe pain precludes further examination. In this case, a topical anesthetic may be added to the lubricant, and initial treatment of this musculature with gentle digital pressure will progressively reduce tenderness until the patient is able to tolerate fuller treatment of the intrapelvic muscles.

Biofeedback Evaluation A more objective evaluation of the function of the levator ani and or the external anal sphincter can be accomplished by surface electromyography or pressure biofeedback. This examiner prefers to use pressure biofeedback. Conditions involving increased tone or spasms certainly do exist, but this does not constitute the majority of this clinician's patient population. By the time the patient is seen, the muscle tension coming from electrogenic muscle contraction has generally abated, and the patient is left with a shortened muscle, commonly referred to as a **contracture** (31,32). Active protective guarding or passive shortening as a result of muscle inhibition or the development of taut bands with trigger points can result in muscle shortening. The resultant contracture can be a possible source of pain but is a definite source of decreased function of the muscle.

The ability of a muscle to contract and relax simply defines the function of a skeletal muscle. During an active contraction of a muscle, two factors are related to the force generation by the muscle. Passive tension is attributable to the stretching of the connective tissue elements, and active tension is from the actual stimulation of the contractile units of the muscle (33). The key element of the length–tension relationship of a muscle is that the force of the muscle contraction declines on either side of the optimal length of the muscle. Over-stretching or excessive shortening will compromise the function of a muscle. In the pelvis, this becomes critical because of the interaction of the pelvic floor musculature and the functioning of the lower urinary tract and gastrointestinal system.

An initial transvaginal or transrectal pressure assessment is done to determine the force of the pelvic floor contraction in centimeters of water pressure. Treatment is then provided to release the trigger point and the associated myofascial and connective tissue restrictions. The transvaginal pressure evaluation is repeated after treatment. An objective parameter is then available to document change in the function of the muscle as related to treatment. Typically, the force generated from a pelvic floor contraction will increase significantly after trigger point release and myofascial and connective tissue manipulation (Fig. 13-4).

Treatment of Pelvic Pain Syndromes

Manual Therapeutic Approaches for the Treatment of Myofascial Trigger Points

Manual therapeutic approaches can go by many different names. Manual approaches could include myofascial manipulation, myofascial release, myotherapy, shiatsu, acupressure, and strain/counterstrain, to name a few. All of these techniques may be extremely beneficial in the management of trigger points associated with pelvic pain. Myofascial manipulation, as defined by Cantu and Grodin (21), has been found to be very effective as a manual approach to the treatment of muscular trigger points. Their definition of myofascial manipulation is "the forceful passive movement of musculo-fascial elements through its restrictive direction(s), beginning with its most superficial layers and progressing into depth" (21). Trigger point pressure release as described by Simons, Travell, and Simons (34) is a more tissue-specific form of myofascial manipulation.

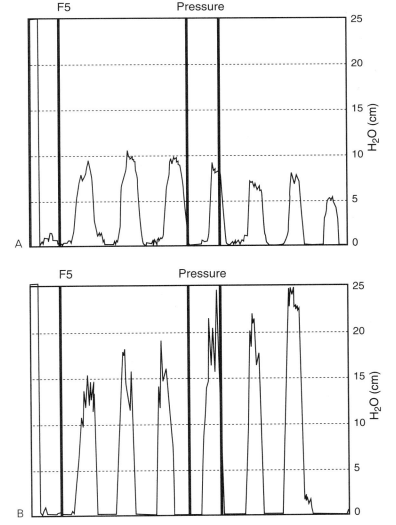

FIGURE 13-4. A diagrammatic representation of peak transvaginal pressures in cm H_2O before and after treatment of myofascial trigger points. **A.** Pretreatment pressures. **B.** Post-treatment pressures.

Trigger point pressure release attempts to release the over-shortened sarcomeres of the contraction knot of a trigger point. This is accomplished by applying a steady, increasing; nonpainful pressure to a trigger point until a resistance is felt within the tissue. This pressure is maintained until the resistance releases. The pressure applied by the clinician will increase again until the next layer of resistance is met. This process continues until there is no resistance palpated within the tissue; the trigger point is released.

One can enhance the trigger point release by incorporating various active exercise techniques to facilitate a lengthening, relaxation, or inhibition reaction of the muscle in which the trigger point is found. Contract/relax is an exercise technique frequently combined with trigger point release. Knott and Voss (35) described contract /relax in their text on proprioceptive neuromuscular facilitation. They described its use for patients with marked decreased range of motion with no active motion available in the agonistic pattern. The technique involves an isotonic contraction of the antagonist against maximal resistance (35). Contract/relax is the basis of Lewit's and Simons' (36) post-isometric relaxation technique. In post-isometric relaxation, the shortened muscle is contracted isometrically against resistance and then encouraged to lengthen passively during the voluntary relaxation phase (36). In the pelvis, the finger would passively lengthen the levator ani in the area of the trigger point. The patient then would be asked to contract their pelvic floor against the resistance of the clinician's finger. Commands could include "squeeze around my finger," "tighten up," "pull up," or "do a Kegel." The finger would be maintaining resistance in the area of the trigger point for 3 to 10 seconds. The patient is then asked to relax or stop contracting. During the relaxation, the clinician gently takes up the slack that develops within the muscle as a result of the increased range of motion. Reciprocal inhibition is another active exercise technique that can enhance the lengthening of muscle fibers shortened by a trigger point. An active contraction of one muscle causes a reflex inhibition of the antagonist. Reciprocal inhibition works very nicely for trigger points in the obturator internus. While doing trigger point pressure release in trigger point of the obturator internus, the clinician would ask the patient to adduct the hip on the involved side. Because the obturator internus abducts the hip when it is flexed at 90°, adduction would be its antagonistic motion, thereby inhibiting the obturator internus and facilitating the lengthening of the muscle fibers and releasing the trigger point. Reciprocal inhibition of the levator ani would be accomplished by asking the patient to attempt to initiate urination or defecation. While the pelvic floor is lengthening, the clinician would be performing trigger point release. Repeated active contraction is performed to incorporate the changes into function.

The Use of Injections in Pelvic Pain Syndromes

According to Simons, Travell, and Simons (34), three different injection approaches may be used for the inactivation of trigger points: injection with a local anesthetic, dry needling, and injection with botulinum toxin A (34). Trigger point injections using a local anesthetic are most commonly used in the treatment of chronic pelvic pain.

Injection techniques for the external muscles that can refer symptoms into the pelvis are covered in extensive detail in Travell & Simons' Myofascial Pain and Dysfunction, volume I (Upper Half of the Body), second edition, and volume II (Lower Half of the Body) (18,19). Injection of the most common internal pelvic muscles associated with pelvic pain syndromes is described in further detail below.

Simons et al. (34) raise the question: what determines whether a trigger point is injected? Should manual techniques or injection treat the trigger point? It is most useful to combine both manual techniques and injections. Some of the pelvic pain syndromes have allodynia and hyperesthesia of the external and internal tissues as components of the syndrome. Usually patients will be treated by manual techniques first, then injected once the trigger points are easily isolated. Reflex and direct desensitization with manual techniques may take several visits before injections are performed. Manual treatment is performed immediately after all injections. Using trigger point injections sooner rather than later seems to decrease the number of physical therapy visits required to release the trigger point and to resolve the patient's pain. Thus, a combination of manual and injection techniques is often the best approach.

Precise localization of the trigger point is always imperative to successful injections. Locating internal trigger points within the levator ani or obturator internus requires extremely skillful palpation. Eliciting a local twitch response is difficult enough when you have the benefit of visualization, but definitely more difficult when only relying on the sense of touch. In this clinic, the physical therapist locates the trigger point first, and the injection is then done by a physician. Unfortunately, many trigger points of the levator ani and obturator internus muscle bellies are not easy to reach with a needle, because a significant portion of their muscle bellies are extremely anterior and medial. The trumpet used to do a pudendal nerve block is used to inject trigger points in the more posterior and deeper aspects of the levator ani and obturator internus. To reach the more anterior and medial trigger points, the pudendal trumpet is modified. A flexible plumber's pipe bender is used to angle the trumpet for a more precise localization of the needle into the muscle. Trigger point injection may be performed rectally on male patients. A needle guide used for prostate biopsies can be used as a guide for a transrectal injection of a pelvic trigger point. *Editor's note: The trigger point can be located rectally, by digital exam and injection can be performed from the outside, perianally.*

The patient is seen by the physical therapist immediately after the injection for myofascial manipulation and neuromuscular reeducation of the involved muscles. The local anesthetic used is 0.25% bupivacaine (Marcaine). Usually up to 5 mL will be injected into each trigger point.

The needle is inserted and moved within the trigger point region to locate the sensitive loci, as described by Hong (37). Each sensitive locus is injected. The patient's positioning depends on the location of the trigger point. Deeper trigger points will require the lithotomy position with stirrups. As described previously, a pudendal trumpet may be used to reach the deeper trigger points. More superficial trigger points can be reached in a hook-lying position on a regular examination table.

Modalities Used in Treating Pelvic Pain

Many therapeutic modality options are available to the clinician who treats pelvic pain. This clinician seldom uses anything other than manual techniques and therapeutic exercise. When modalities are used, it is to enhance the effect of the manual techniques and therapeutic exercise.

Thermal Modalities Therapists frequently use ultrasound to inactivate trigger points. Unfortunately, no controlled studies support this effect on trigger points. Hong (38) did find that ultrasound did have the ability to increase the pain threshold of an active myofascial trigger point. With this in mind, ultrasound may be beneficial in preparing the tissues for myofascial manipulation and enhance the effectiveness of the myofascial manipulation. This is an assumption, supported by anecdotal evidence, and needs to be proved by controlled studies.

Deep heat also could be provided by short-wave diathermy. The local effects of the diathermy would be increased tissue temperature and vasodilation resulting in an increase in the caliber of the blood vessel but also an increase in patent vessels. Increased arterial flow would promote improvement in the nutrition of the area, whereas the increased venous flow would facilitate the elimination of the local metabolic by-products. Like ultrasound, short-wave diathermy may serve to decrease the pain threshold of active myofascial trigger points and to facilitate the tissue changes associated with myofascial manipulation. Superficial heat also can be used before myofascial manipulation to prepare the tissues for the manual work as well as to calm and comfort the patient.

Ice can be used for pain relief because of its numbing effect. It also may help with any posttreatment soreness or discomfort. Sweeping strokes of ice can have the same effect as a vapo-coolant spray in the release of a trigger point.

Electrical Stimulation Many electrical modalities are available to choose from when treating pelvic pain. They include transcutaneous electrical nerve stimulation (TENS), interferential, microcurrent, and high-volt pulsed galvanic stimulation. This clinician uses high-volt pulsed galvanic most often. Trigger point regions are known to have impaired circulation (38). The autonomic phenomena of trigger points can be associated with trophic changes in the region of the trigger point and its referral zone. With this circulatory compromise associated with trigger points, high-volt pulsed galvanic stimulation can be used for promoting increased blood flow. Direct sympathetic activation is one theory to explain the modulation of the microcirculation by high-volt pulsed galvanic stimulation.

Treatment of Accompanying Articular Dysfunction

The clinician should address the articular dysfunctions identified in the examination. These would include dysfunctions involving the lumbar spine, sacrum, coccyx, and pubic symphysis, as well as the femur. In-depth discussion of treatment approaches for these dysfunctions is presented in Chapters 10 and 11.

Patient Exercise and Home Care

The exercise approach for the pelvic pain patient is broken down into two segments: localized, which is exercise specific to the pelvic floor, and global, which is exercise addressing the musculoskeletal dysfunction in the lower back and hips, including external pelvic muscles, and imbalances of the body as a whole. The focus with the global exercise program may be to the lower trunk and hip girdle, but before discharge should address a full general conditioning program.

Most pelvic pain patients are found to have shortened pelvic floor muscles commonly referred to as contractures. Exercise of the pelvic floor is initially focused on restoring it to its normal resting length. Eccentric exercise is the major component of the exercise program utilized to achieve this goal. Passive stretching of the pelvic floor through myofascial manual techniques or active-assisted stretching may be used as needed. Active-assisted stretching can be accomplished by the utilization of the Valsalva maneuver. This needs to be very closely monitored secondary to the negative impact that excessive use of the Valsalva maneuver can have on the support structures of the pelvic organs.

Also, the patient is asked to focus on what action they take to initiate urination. Initially, this is a relaxation response, but an eccentric contraction or lengthening of the pelvic floor is also executed. The patient may be asked to attempt to initiate urination again after urination is completed. Care is taken to reinforce to the patient that they should not bear down to initiate urination. What the patient is being asked to do is to relearn the active component of urinary control without the reflex factor of a full bladder.

Proprioceptive neuromuscular facilitation may be used to enhance the ability to lengthen the pelvic floor. This is accomplished by having the patient in a supine position with knees pulled to the chest with slight abduction at the hips. By resisting the flexion and abduction component of this position, the pelvic floor can be inhibited (Fig. 13-5). Inhibition will decrease the reflex activity that may be partially responsible for holding the pelvic floor in a shortened position. Once the patient has a good sense of the eccentric contraction, the exercise command used is "drop your

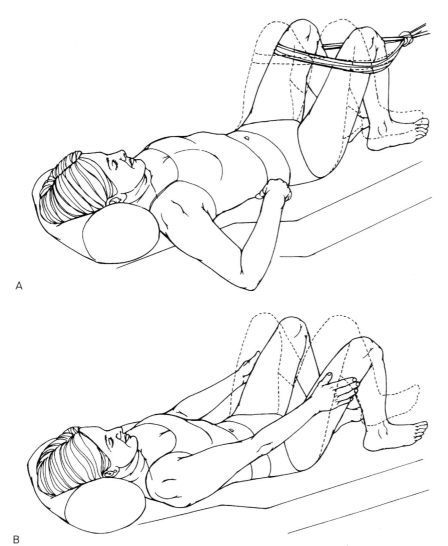

FIGURE 13-5. **Proprioceptive neuromuscular facilitation technique to inhibit the pelvic floor musculature. A.** The patient is supine with the knees bent and the feet flat, and a stretch band is placed around the knees and the other end is fixed at a point caudal to the patient, keeping the band horizontal. The patient inhibits the pelvic floor musculature by flexing and abducting against the resistance of the stretch band. **B.** The resistance to abduction and flexion can be provided by the patient, contacting the anterior-lateral aspect of the thighs with the hands.

pelvic floor". This is held for a count of 5 and then the patient is asked to stop dropping their pelvic floor. Early in the reeducation process, the patient may use proprioceptive inhibition first, followed by active eccentric contractions. Each of these is held for a count of 5 and repeated five times at least twice per day. Patients who have had shortened pelvic floor muscles should always precede their concentric contraction with an eccentric contraction. As a result of tissue memory, repeated concentric contractions may result in an inappropriately maintained shortened state. The command for this would be to "drop your pelvic floor, hold for a count of 5, squeeze your pelvic floor, hold for a count of 5, and then relax." They would build this series up to 30 repetitions. The goal is to achieve and maintain the ideal resting length of the levator ani so that it will function optimally in terms of length–tension relationship.

Exercise to the lower trunk and hip girdle would be focused on correcting the dysfunctions that were identified during the examination and followed with a general conditioning program. Correcting the length/strength muscle imbalances is paramount. Short muscles need to be lengthened. and long muscles need to be shortened. Strengthening exercises are introduced progressively and upgraded to a full conditioning program once the imbalance has been corrected.

When dealing with the lower trunk, specifically the abdominals, diastases recti should be fully corrected before a progressive abdominal strengthening program is started. The adductors and the gluteus maximus muscles need to be lengthened and inhibited before their strengthening (Fig. 13-6). This is secondary to the fact that they are part of the functional unit of myofascial involvement that accompanies chronic pelvic pain and urinary complaints. Shortened hip

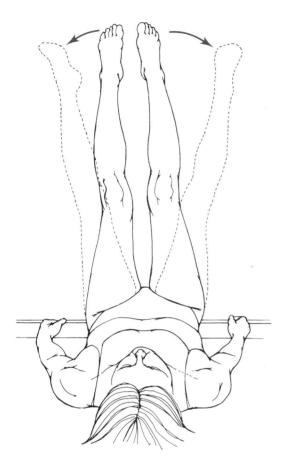

FIGURE 13-6. **Adductor lengthening activity.** The patient lies with the buttocks against a wall and the lower extremities flexed at 90° and resting on the wall. The legs are gradually separated, still resting against the wall.

flexors are also typical in pelvic pain patients and need to be lengthened (Figs. 13-7 and 13-8). Most often the hip external rotators are short and need to be lengthened. But it is not that uncommon to see excessively long external rotators that need to be shortened. All trigger points need to be resolved as the clinician progresses the patient through the exercise program.

Stress is a very important component of flare-ups. Instead of clenching the teeth, the pelvic pain patient clenches the pelvic floor. Once they can feel that this is occurring, they can learn to actively reverse the process. As patients improve, they are encouraged to do things that have, in the past, increased their pain. As they have gone through treatment, they have learned which self-management techniques and exercises have been able to decrease their pain. As they improve, they can practice and develop the ability to desensitize the tissue response so that they can engage in an increasing range of activities in the future without pain.

Relaxation therapy can be extremely beneficial. The clinician should not hesitate to refer the patient out for relaxation or stress management classes. The holistic benefit for this has a definite overflow to the pelvic floor. Working on eccentric pelvic floor exercises is usually sufficient to reverse muscle shortening that may be present in a pelvic pain patient. Biofeedback also may be helpful.

Self-management techniques that the patient may use include stretching, ice, aerobic activity, self myofascial and connective tissue manipulation, as well as desensitization and stress loading. Trial and error determines which technique is the most successful in reducing pain. As the pain is resolving, the patient is progressed into trying to find activities that provoke pain and then using the self-determined pain relief techniques to stop the pain. As this is repeated, the stimulus that is required to provoke the pain becomes greater, and less effort on the patient's part is required to turn the pain off. In summary, patients are actively participating in decreasing the severity and frequency of pelvic pain.

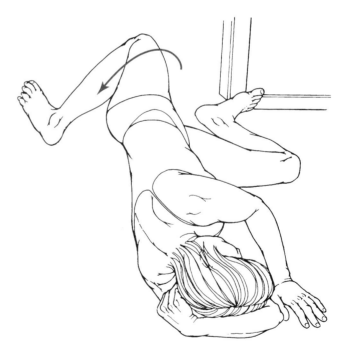

FIGURE 13-7. **Quadriceps stretch.** This exercise is performed with the patient resting on the floor in a doorway. The inferior knee is drawn up toward the chest, with the foot stabilizing against the door frame. The patient pulls the other heel toward the buttocks until a comfortable stretch is felt in the front of the thigh, then the thigh is moved into extension. This position is held for 15 to 30 seconds. The exercise is repeated 6 to 8 times on each side. This exercise is performed once or twice per day.

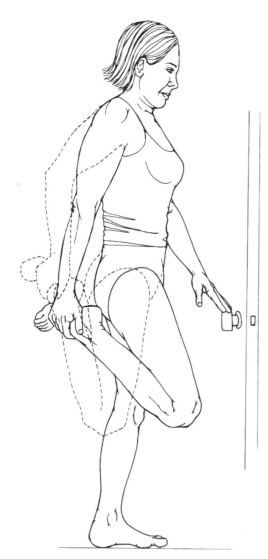

FIGURE 13-8. **Standing hip flexor stretch.** The patient stands on the left leg and holds onto something for balance. The right knee is bent, and the patient grasps the ankle. The abdominal muscles are tensed to stabilize the pelvis and to prevent increased lordosis. This position is held throughout the exercise. The right knee is extended backwards without moving the pelvis. This position is held for 15 to 30 seconds. Then the patient relaxes and repeats the exercise 6 to 8 times with each leg.

CONCLUSION

The June 2000 issue of *Good Housekeeping* contained an article entitled "A Private Agony," in which the author stated, "Women with chronic pelvic pain know how hard it is to treat. Finally [there are] breakthrough therapies for one of medicine's most baffling conditions." The author also describes the ongoing problems with management of chronic pelvic pain. Fortunately, the article does at least allude to the possibility that chronic pelvic pain may have musculoskeletal origins, and thus other possible treatment options (39).

Physicians are slowly becoming aware of the services that can be provided by health care providers who specialize in the management of musculoskeletal dysfunction. When treating chronic pelvic pain, one must remember to treat the patient as a whole. Global management will address the major musculoskeletal problems that could have an impact on pelvic pain. Myofascial trigger points that have pain referral patterns to the pelvis would have to be resolved. The localized management of the local tissues in the pelvis, just described, would be addressed, including myofascial trigger points, connective tissue restrictions, and adverse neural tension, all of which can be directly related to the patient's complaints. Correction for a small hemipelvis and leg length discrepancy and other perpetuating factors would need to be addressed as well. With this comprehensive approach, patients who have had chronic pelvic pain for years can experience relief and resolution of chronic pain.

TREATMENT PROTOCOL

1. **Desensitize all allodynic tissues. Initially, this can be accomplished indirectly, by using reflexive approaches when treating skin and superficial tissues, and connective tissue release and trigger point release in tissues that are not the primary location of the patient's pain. Our understanding is that these approaches operate via the autonomic nervous system to decrease the sensitivity of the allodynic tissues. Direct stress loading of the allodynic tissues would start when the sensitization has decreased. This may include behavioral modification techniques, such as timed voiding, to address the sensitization of the bladder when frequency and urgency is associated with pelvic pain.**

2. **Release connective tissue restrictions throughout the entire lower quadrant with special focus to those areas (Head's zones) related by referral to the pain problem. In other words, address the viscerosomatic and somatovisceral reflexes associated with the noted connective tissue restrictions.**

3. **Release all trigger points, using trigger point release techniques and trigger point injections. The external muscles most often involved in pelvic pain are the abdominal muscles, the iliopsoas, adductors, obturator externus, gluteal muscles, and piriformis. The intrapelvic muscles requiring evaluation and treatment include the superficial and deep urogenital diaphragm, levator ani, obturator internus, coccygeus, and the piriformis. Utilizing injections, sooner rather than later, to treat trigger points in the internal pelvic muscles can facilitate the recovery process. Post-isometric relaxation and reciprocal inhibition are very appro-**

priate when the pain is acute. As the pain becomes more localized, injections should be considered.

4. **Correct all muscle imbalances in the lower quadrant.**

5. **Normalize the pelvic floor function. Lengthen before strengthening if the pelvic floor is found to be short, and strengthen if there is only weakness of the pelvic floor.**

6. **Address joint problems at the sacroiliac joints, the pubic symphysis, the sacrococcygeal joint, and the femur function at the acetabulum, if any of these are found to be a problem.**

7. **Establish a comprehensive general conditioning program. This should address aerobic fitness, strength, and flexibility from a holistic approach.**

References

1. Enigmatic pelvic pain (Editorial). Br Med J 1978;6144:1041.
2. Mathias S, Kupperman M, Leberman R, et al. Chronic pelvic pain: prevalence, health-related quality of life and economic correlates. Obstet Gynecol 1996;87:321–327.
3. Baskin L, Tanagho E. Pelvic pain without pelvic organs J Urol 1992;147:683–686.
4. Menard C, Farrell JF, Seidel J, et al. Reliability and validity of the functional pelvic pain scale: a new measure of pelvic pain severity. Journal of SOGC 1996;18:69–76.
5. Travell J. Chronic myofascial pain syndromes: mysteries of the history. Adv Pain Res Ther 1990;17:129–136.
6. American College of Obstetricians and Gynecologists. Chronic Pelvic Pain: (Technical Bulletin No.223). Washington, D.C., copyright ACOG, May 1996.
7. Montauk S, Martin J. Treating chronic pain. Am Fam Physician 1997;55:451–460.
8. Oneghena P, Van Houdenhove B. Antidepressant induced analgesia in chronic nonmalignant pain: a met-analysis of 39 placebo controlled studies. Pain 1992;49:205–219.
9. Bushnell T, Justin D. Choosing the right analgesic: a guide to selection. Drug 1993;46:394–408.
10. Rani R, Naaidu M, Prasad M, et al. An evaluation of antidepressants in rheumatic pain conditions. Anesth Analg 1996;83:371–375.
11. McQuay H, Carroll D, Glynn C. Low dose amitriptyline in the treatment of chronic pain. Anesthesia 1992;47:646–652.
12. Macdonald R, Kelly K. Mechanisms of action of currently prescribed and newly developed antiepileptic drugs, Epilepsia 1994;35:s4l.
13. Singh L, Field M, Ferris P, et al. The antiepileptic drug gabapentin (Neurontin) possesses anxiolytic-like and antinociceptive actions that are reversed by D-serine Psychopharmacology 1996;127:1–9.
14. Baskin L, Tanagho E. Pelvic pain without pelvic organs J Urol 1992;147:683–686.
15. Black W. Use of presacral sympathectomy in the treatment of dysmenorrhea: a second look after twenty-five years. Am J Obstet Gynecol 1964;89:16–22.
16. King P, Myers C, Ling F, et al. Musculoskeletal factors in chronic pelvic pain. J Psychosom Obstet Gynecol 1991;12:87–98.
17. Goldthwait J. The relation of posture to human efficiency and the influence of poise upon the support and function of the viscera. Boston Med Surg J 1909:CLXI (24): 839–348.
18. Simons D, Travell J, Simons L. Myofascial Pain and Dysfunction: The Trigger Point Manual, vol 1, 2nd Ed. Baltimore: Williams and Wilkins, 1999:940–970.
19. Travell J, Simons D. Myofascial Pain and Dysfunction: The Trigger Point Manual, vol 2. Baltimore: Williams and Wilkins, 1992:289–314, 110–131.
20. Baker P. Musculoskeletal Problems in Chronic Pelvic Pain: An Integrated Approach. Philadelphia: W. B. Saunders, 1998;215–240.
21. Cantu R, Grodin A. Myofascial Manipulation: Theory and Clinical Application. Gaithersburg, Maryland; Aspen Publishing, 1992.
22. Webster J. Textbook of Diseases of Women Philadelphia W. B. Saunders Company, 1907:682–697.
23. Williams P, Warwick R, eds. Gray's Anatomy, 36th Ed. Philadelphia: W. B. Saunders, 1980:556–558.
24. Dicke E, Schliack H, Wolf A. A Manual of Reflexive Therapy of the Connective Tissue. Scarsdale: Sidney S. Simon Publishers, 1978.
25. Ebner M. Connective Tissue Manipulations. Melbourne, FL: Robert and Kreiger Publishing Company, 1987.
26. Butler D. Mobilization of the Nervous System. Melbourne: Churchill Livingston, 1991.
27. Simons D, Travell J, Simons L. Travell and Simons' Myofascial Pain and Dysfunction: The Trigger Point Manual, vol. I Upper Half of Body, 2nd Ed. Baltimore: Williams and Wilkins, 1999;11–93.
28. Floyd WF, Silver P. Electromyographic study of patterns of activity of the anterior abdominal wall muscles in man. J Anat. 1950;84:132–145.
29. Thiele G. Coccygodynia and pain in the superior gluteal region. JAMA. 1937;109:1271–1275.
30. Basmajian J. Muscles Alive: Their Functions Revealed by Electromyography, 2nd Ed. Baltimore: Williams and Wilkins, 1967:265–286.
31. Fischer E. Discussion on terminology, in an exploratory and analytical survey of therapeutic exercise project. Am J Physiol Med 1967;46: 1054.
32. Simons D, Mense S. Understanding and measurement of muscle tone as related to clinical muscle pain. Pain 1998;75:1–17.
33. Jones D, Round J. Skeletal Muscle in health and Disease: A Textbook of Muscle, vol 3: Physiology. Manchester: Manchester University Press, 1990:19–40.
34. Simons D, Travell J, Simons L. Travell and Simons' Myofascial Pain and Dysfunction: The Trigger Point Manual, vol. I: Upper Half of Body, 2nd Ed. Baltimore: Williams and Wilkins, 1999;94–177.
35. Knott M, Voss D. Proprioceptive Neuromuscular Facilitation: Patterns and Techniques, 2nd Ed. New York: Harper and Row, 1968:188.
36. Lewit K, Simons D. Myofascial pain: relief by post isometric relaxation. Arch Phys Med Rehabil 1984;65:452–456.
37. Hong C. Considerations and recommendations regarding myofascial trigger point injection. J Musculoskel Pain 1994;2:29–57.
38. Hong C. Immediate effects of various physical medicine modalities on pain threshold of an active myofascial trigger point. J Musculoskel Pain 1993;1:37–53.
39. Umansky D. A private agony. Good Housekeeping. June 2000, vol 230:74.

APPENDIX 13-1

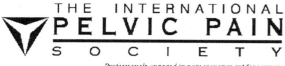

THE INTERNATIONAL
PELVIC PAIN
S O C I E T Y
Professionals engaged in pain management for women.

Pelvic Pain Assessment Form

Physician: _____

Initial History and Physical Exam

Date: _____

Contact Information

Name: _____   Birth Date: _____   Chart Number: _____

Phone: Work: _____   Home: _____

Is there an alternate contact if we cannot reach you? _____

Alternate contact phone number: _____

Information About Your Pain

Please describe your pain problem: _____

What do you think is causing your pain? _____

What does your family think is causing your pain? _____

Do you think anyone is to blame for your pain? ❑ Yes   ❑ No   If so, who? _____

Do you think surgery will be necessary? ❑ Yes   ❑ No

Is there an event that you associate with the onset of pain? ❑ Yes   ❑ No   If so, what? _____

How long have you had this pain? ❑ < 6 months   ❑ 6 months – 1 year   ❑ 1 – 2 years   ❑ > 2 years

For each of the symptoms listed below, please "bubble in" your level of pain over the last month using a 10-point scale:

0 – no pain   10 – the worst pain imaginable

	0	1	2	3	4	5	6	7	8	9	10
How would you rate your present pain?											
Pain at ovulation (mid-cycle)	O	O	O	O	O	O	O	O	O	O	O
Pain level just before period	O	O	O	O	O	O	O	O	O	O	O
Pain (not cramps) with period	O	O	O	O	O	O	O	O	O	O	O
Deep pain with intercourse	O	O	O	O	O	O	O	O	O	O	O
Pain in groin when lifting	O	O	O	O	O	O	O	O	O	O	O
Pelvic pain lasting hours or days after intercourse	O	O	O	O	O	O	O	O	O	O	O
Pain when bladder is full	O	O	O	O	O	O	O	O	O	O	O
Muscle/joint pain	O	O	O	O	O	O	O	O	O	O	O
Ovarian pain	O	O	O	O	O	O	O	O	O	O	O
Level of cramps with period	O	O	O	O	O	O	O	O	O	O	O
Pain after period is over	O	O	O	O	O	O	O	O	O	O	O
Burning vaginal pain with sex	O	O	O	O	O	O	O	O	O	O	O
Pain with urination	O	O	O	O	O	O	O	O	O	O	O
Backache	O	O	O	O	O	O	O	O	O	O	O
Migraine headache	O	O	O	O	O	O	O	O	O	O	O
What would be an acceptable level of pain?	O	O	O	O	O	O	O	O	O	O	O

What is the worst type of pain
that you have ever experienced?

❑ Kidney stone   ❑ Bowel obstruction   ❑ Migraine headache
❑ Labor & delivery   ❑ Current pelvic pain   ❑ Backache
❑ Broken bone   ❑ Surgery
❑ Other _____

Demographic Information
Are you (check all that apply):
    ❑ Married   ❑ Widowed   ❑ Separated   ❑ Committed Relationship
    ❑ Single   ❑ Remarried   ❑ Divorced
Who do you live with? _____

Education: ❑ Less than 12 years   ❑ High School graduate
             ❑ Bachelor's degree   ❑ Postgraduate degree

What kind of work are you trained for? _____
What type of work are you doing? _____

Health Habits
Do you get regular exercise? ❑ Yes   ❑ No   Type: _____
What is your diet like? _____
What is your caffeine intake (number per day, include coffee, tea, soft drinks, etc.)? ❑ 0   ❑ 1–3 ❑ 4–6 ❑ >6

How many cigarettes do you smoke per day? _____   How many years? _____
Have you ever felt the need to cut down on your drinking? ❑ Yes   ❑ No
Have you ever felt annoyed by criticism of your drinking? ❑ Yes   ❑ No
Have you ever felt guilty about your drinking, or about something you said or did while you were drinking? ❑ Yes   ❑ No
Have you ever taken a morning "eye-opener" drink? ❑ Yes   ❑ No

What is your use of recreational drugs? ❑ Never used ❑ Used in past, but not now ❑ Presently using ❑ Choose not to answer
      ❑ Heroin   ❑ Amphetamines   ❑ Marijuana
      ❑ Barbiturates   ❑ Cocaine   ❑ Other _____
Have you ever received treatment for substance abuse? ❑ Yes   ❑ No

Coping Mechanisms
Who are the people you talk to concerning your pain, or during stressful times?
      ❑ Spouse/Partner   ❑ Relative   ❑ Support Group   ❑ Clergy
      ❑ Friend   ❑ Doctor/Nurse   ❑ Mental Health Professional   ❑ I take care of myself

How does your partner deal with your pain?
      ❑ Doesn't notice when I'm in pain   ❑ Takes care of me   ❑ Not applicable
      ❑ Withdraws   ❑ Feels helpless
      ❑ Distracts me with activities   ❑ Gets angry

What helps your pain?   ❑ Meditation   ❑ Relaxation   ❑ Lying down   ❑ Music
                       ❑ Massage   ❑ Ice   ❑ Heating pad   ❑ Hot bath
                       ❑ Pain medication ❑ Laxatives/enema ❑ Injection   ❑ TENS unit
                       ❑ Bowel movement ❑ Emptying bladder ❑ Nothing
                       ❑ Other _____

What makes your pain worse? ❑ Intercourse   ❑ Orgasm   ❑ Stress   ❑ Full meal
                       ❑ Bowel movement ❑ Full bladder   ❑ Urination ❑ Standing
                       ❑ Walking   ❑ Exercise   ❑ Time of day ❑ Weather
                       ❑ Contact with clothing ❑ Coughing/sneezing ❑ Not related to anything
                       ❑ Other _____

Of all of the problems or stresses in your life, how does your pain compare in importance?
          ❑ The most important problem   ❑ Just one of several/many problems

Menses

How old were you when your menses started? _____

Are you still having menstrual periods? ❏ Yes   ❏ No

Answer the following only if you <u>are</u> still having menstrual periods:

Periods are: ❏ Light   ❏ Moderate   ❏ Heavy   ❏ Bleed through protection

How many days between your periods? _____

How many days of menstrual flow? _____

Date of last menses? _____

Do you have any pain with your periods? ❏ Yes   ❏ No

Does pain start the day flow starts? ❏ Yes   ❏ No

Starts _____ days before flow starts: ❏ Yes   ❏ No

Are periods regular? ❏ Yes   ❏ No

Do you pass any clots in menstrual flow? ❏ Yes   ❏ No

Bladder

Do you experience any of the following:

Loss of urine when coughing, sneezing, or laughing? ❏ Yes   ❏ No

Frequent urination? ❏ Yes   ❏ No

Need to urinate with little warning? ❏ Yes   ❏ No

Difficulty passing urine? ❏ Yes   ❏ No

Frequent bladder infections? ❏ Yes   ❏ No

Frequency of nighttime urination: ❏ 0–1   ❏ 2 or more   Volume: ❏ Small   ❏ Medium   ❏ Large

Frequency of daytime urination: ❏ 8 or less   ❏ 9–15   ❏ >16   Volume: ❏ Small   ❏ Medium   ❏ Large

Do you still feel full after urination? ❏ Yes   ❏ No

Bowel

Is there discomfort or pain associated with a change in the consistency of the stool (i.e., softer or harder) ? ❏ Yes   ❏ No

Would you say that at least one-fourth (_) of the occasions or days in the last 3 months you have had any of the following (Check *all* that apply)

❏ Fewer than three bowel movements *a week* (0–2 bowel movements)

❏ More than three bowel movements *a day* (4 or more bowel movements)

❏ Hard or lumpy stools

❏ Loose or watery stools

❏ Straining during a bowel movement

❏ Urgency – having to rush to the bathroom for a bowel movement

❏ Feeling of incomplete emptying after a bowel movement

❏ Passing mucus (white material) during a bowel movement

❏ Abdominal fullness, bloating, or swelling

[1] The Functional Gastrointestinal Disorders, Drossman, et al. Chapter 4, "Functional Bowel Disorders and Functional Abdominal Pain". 1994.

Gastrointestinal/Eating

Do you have nausea?   ❏ No   ❏ With pain   ❏ Taking medications

❏ With eating   ❏ Other _____

Do you have vomiting?   ❏ No   ❏ With pain   ❏ Taking medications

❏ With eating   ❏ Other _____

Have you ever had an eating disorder such as anorexia or bulimia? ❏ Yes   ❏ No

Short-Form McGill

The words below describe average pain. Place a check mark (✓) in the column which represents the degree to which you feel that type of pain. Please limit yourself to a description of the pain in your pelvic area <u>only</u>.

What does your pain feel like?

Type	*None (0)*	*Mild (1)*	*Moderate (2)*	*Severe (3)*
Throbbing	_____	_____	_____	_____
Shooting	_____	_____	_____	_____
Stabbing	_____	_____	_____	_____
Sharp	_____	_____	_____	_____
Cramping	_____	_____	_____	_____
Gnawing	_____	_____	_____	_____
Hot-Burning	_____	_____	_____	_____
Aching	_____	_____	_____	_____
Heavy	_____	_____	_____	_____
Tender	_____	_____	_____	_____
Splitting	_____	_____	_____	_____
Tiring-Exhausting	_____	_____	_____	_____
Sickening	_____	_____	_____	_____
Fearful	_____	_____	_____	_____
Punishing-Cruel	_____	_____	_____	_____

Melzack, R: The Short-Form McGill Pain Questionnaire, Pain 30:191–197, 1987

Which statement(s) below best describes how you cope with the pain? Check all that apply
- ❏ I count numbers in my head or run a song through my mind
- ❏ I just think of it as some other sensation, such as numbness
- ❏ I pray to God it won't last long
- ❏ I do something active, like household chores or projects
- ❏ I ignore it as best I can
- ❏ I tell myself to be brave and carry on despite the pain
- ❏ I tell myself that it really doesn't hurt
- ❏ I worry all the time about whether it will end
- ❏ I take pain medication
- ❏ Other

SF-36

In general, would you say your health is: ○ Excellent   ○ Very Good   ○ Good   ○ Fair   ○ Poor

Compared to one year ago, how would you rate your health in general now?
- ○ Much better now than one year ago
- ○ Somewhat better now than one year ago
- ○ About the same as one year ago
- ○ Somewhat worse now than one year ago
- ○ Much worse than one year ago

The following items are about activities you might do during a typical day. *Does your health now limit you in these activities? If so, how much?*	Yes, limited a lot	Yes, limited a little	No	Not limited at all
Vigorous activities, such as running, lifting heavy object, participating in strenuous sports				
Moderate activities, such as moving a table, pushing a vacuum cleaner, bowling, or playing golf				
Lifting or carrying groceries				
Climbing several flights of stairs				
Climbing one flight of stairs				
Bending, kneeling, or stooping				
Walking more than a mile				
Walking several blocks				
Walking one block				
Bathing or dressing yourself				

During the *past 4 weeks*, have you had any of the following problems with your work or other regular daily activities *because of your physical health*?

Cut down the amount of time you spent on your work or other activities O Yes O No
Accomplish less than you would like O Yes O No
Were limited in the kind of work or other activities O Yes O No
Had difficulty performing the work or other activities (for example, it took extra effort) O Yes O No

During the *past 4 weeks*, have you had any of the following problems with your work or other regular daily activities *because of any emotional problems* (such as feeling depressed or anxious)?

Cut down the amount of time you spent on work or other activities O Yes O No
Accomplished less than you would like O Yes O No
Didn't do work or other activities as carefully as usual O Yes O No

During the *past 4 weeks*, to what extent has your physical health or emotional problems interfered with your normal social activities with family, friend, neighbors, or groups?

O Not at all   O Slightly   O Moderately   O Quite a bit   O Extremely

How much bodily pain have you had during the past 4 weeks?

O None   O Very mild   O Mild   O Moderate   O Severe   O Very severe

During the past 4 weeks, how much did pain interfere with your normal work (including both work outside the home and housework)?

O Not at all   O A little bit   O Moderately   O Quite a bit   O Extremely

These questions are about how you feel and how things have been with you *during the past 4 weeks*. For each question, please give the one answer that comes closest to the way you have been feeling. How much of the time during *the past 4 weeks*:

	All of the time	Most of the time	A good bit of the time	Some of the time	A little of the time	None of the time
Did you feel full of pep?						
Have you been a very nervous person?						
Have you felt so down in the dumps that nothing could cheer you up?						
Have you felt calm and peaceful?						
Did you have a lot of energy?						
Have you felt downhearted and blue?						
Did you feel worn out?						
Have you been a happy person?						
Did you feel tired?						

During the *past 4 weeks*, how much of the time has your *physical health or emotional problems* interfered with your social activities (like visiting with friends, relatives, etc.?

O All of the time   O Most of the time   O Some of the time   O A little of the time O None of the time

How TRUE or FALSE is each of the following statements for you?

	Definitely True	Mostly True	Don't Know	Mostly False	Definitely False
I seem to get sick a little easier than other people					
I am as healthy as anybody I know			.		
I expect my health to get worse					
My health is excellent					

Personal History

What would you like to tell us about your pain that we have not asked? Comments: _____

_____

_____

What types of treatments have you tried in the past for this pain?   ❏ Acupuncture   ❏ Homeopathic medicine ❏ Physical
therapy

❏ Anesthesiologist	❏ Lupron, Zoladex, Synarel	❏ Psychotherapy
❏ Anti-seizure medications	❏ Massage	❏ Rheumatologist
❏ Antidepressants	❏ Meditation	❏ Skin magnets
❏ Biofeedback	❏ Narcotics	❏ Surgery
❏ Birth control pills	❏ Naturopathic medications	❏ TENS unit
❏ Danazol (Danocrine)	❏ Nerve blocks	❏ Trigger point injections
❏ Depo-Provera	❏ Neurosurgeon	❏ Other _____
❏ Family Practitioner	❏ Nonprescription medicine	
❏ Herbal medication	❏ Nutrition/diet	

What physicians or health care providers have evaluated or treated you for chronic pelvic pain? Include all healthcare professionals, whether they were physicians or not. Do you have any objections to me contacting these healthcare providers? ❏ Yes   ❏ No

Physician/Provider	City, State

Who is your primary care physician? _____

Please list all surgical procedures you've had (*related to this pain*):

Year	Procedure	Surgeon

Please list all other surgical procedures:

Year	Procedure		Year	Procedure

Please list pain medications you've taken for your pain condition in the past 6 months, and the physicians who prescribed them (use separate page if necessary):

Medication	Physician	Did it help?
		❏ Yes ❏ No
		❏ Yes ❏ No
		❏ Yes ❏ No
		❏ Yes ❏ No
		❏ Yes ❏ No
		❏ Yes ❏ No
		❏ Yes ❏ No
❏ I have written more medications on a separate page		

Have you ever been hospitalized for anything besides surgery or childbirth? ❑ Yes   ❑ No   If yes, explain: _____

Have you had major accidents such as falls or back injury? ❑ Yes   ❑ No
Have you ever been treated for depression? ❑ Yes   ❑ No   Treatments: ❑ Medication   ❑ Hospitalization   ❑ Psychotherapy

Birth control method: ❑ Nothing   ❑ Pill   ❑ Vasectomy   ❑ Hysterectomy
                             ❑ IUD   ❑ Rhythm   ❑ Diaphragm   ❑ Tubal Ligation
                             ❑ Condom   ❑ Other: _____
Is future fertility desired? ❑ Yes   ❑ No

How many pregnancies have you had?_____
Resulting in (#): _____ Full 9 month _____ Premature _____ Abortions (miscarriage) _____ # living children
Any complications during pregnancy, labor, delivery, or post partum period?
        ❑ 4° Episiotomy   ❑ C-section   ❑ Post-partum hemorrhaging
        ❑ Vaginal lacerations ❑ Forceps   ❑ Medication for bleeding
        ❑ Other: _____

Has anyone in your family ever had: ❑ Fibromyalgia   ❑ Chronic pelvic pain   ❑ Scleroderma
                                           ❑ Endometriosis   ❑ Lupus   ❑ Interstitial cystitis
                                           ❑ Cancer   ❑ Depression   ❑ Irritable Bowel Syndrome
                                           ❑ Recurrent Urinary Tract Infections

Place an "X" at the point of your most intense pain.
Shade in all other painful areas.

Sexual and Physical Abuse History
Have you ever been the victim of emotional abuse? This can include being humiliated or insulted. ❑ Yes   ❑ No   ❑ No answer

		As a child (13 and younger)		As an adult (14 and over)	
	Circle an answer for <u>both</u> as a child and as an adult.				
1a.	Has anyone ever exposed the sex organs of their body to you when you did not want it?	Yes	No	Yes	No
1b.	Has anyone ever threatened to have sex with you when you did not want it?	Yes	No	Yes	No
1c.	Has anyone ever touched the sex organs of your body when you did not want this?	Yes	No	Yes	No
1d.	Has anyone ever made you touch the sex organs of their body when you did not want this?	Yes	No	Yes	No
1e.	Has anyone ever forced you to have sex when you did not want this?	Yes	No	Yes	No
1f.	Have you had any other unwanted sexual experiences not mentioned above? If yes, please specify: _____	Yes	No	Yes	No

2	When you were a child (13 or younger), did an older person do the following?				
a.	Hit, kick, or beat you?	Never	Seldom	Occasionally	Often
b.	Seriously threaten your life?	Never	Seldom	Occasionally	Often
3	Now that you are an adult (14 or older), has any other adult done the following:				
a.	Hit, kick, or beat you?	Never	Seldom	Occasionally	Often
b.	Seriously threaten your life?	Never	Seldom	Occasionally	Often

Leserman, J., Drossman, D., Li, Z: The Reliability and Validity of a Sexual and Physical Abuse History Questionnaire in Female Patients with Gastrointestinal Disorders. Behavioral Medicine 21:141–148, 1995

Physical Examination – For Physician Use Only

Name: _____   Chart Number: _____

Height: _____   Weight: _____   BP: _____   LMP: _____   Temp: _____   Resp: _____

ROS, PFSH Reviewed: ☐ Yes   ☐ No   Physician Signature _____

General: ☐ WNL   ☐ Walk   ☐ Facial expression
              ☐ Color   ☐ Alterations in posture   ☐ Other _____

┌───┐
│ *NOTE: Mark "Not Examined" as N/E* │
└───┘

HEENT ☐ WNL _____   ***Chest*** ☐ WNL _____   ***Heart*** ☐ WNL _____   ***Breasts*** ☐ WNL _____

Abdomen
☐ Non-tender   ☐ Incisions   ☐ Trigger Points   ☐ Ovarian point tenderness
☐ Inguinal tenderness ☐ Inguinal bulge   ☐ Suprapubic tenderness ☐ Other _____

Back
☐ Non-tender   ☐ Tenderness   ☐ Altered ROM   ☐ Alterations in posture

Extremities
☐ WNL   ☐ Edema   ☐ Varicosities   ☐ Neuropathy   ☐ Range of motion

Neuropathy
☐ Iliohypogastric   ☐ Ilioinguinal   ☐ Genitofemoral   ☐ Pudendal   ☐ Altered sensation

EGBUS/Vagina
☐ WNL   ☐ Lesions
☐ Wet prep:
☐ Local tenderness:
☐ Vaginal mucosa:
☐ Posterior fourchette:
☐ Discharge:
Cultures:
        ☐ GC   ☐ Chlamydia   ☐ Fungal   ☐ Herpes

Unimanual pelvic exam
☐ WNL   ☐ Cervix
☐ Introitus   ☐ Cervical motion
☐ Uterine-cervical junction ☐ Parametrium
☐ Urethra   ☐ Vaginal cuff
☐ Bladder   ☐ Cul de sac
☐ R ureter   ☐ L ureter
☐ R inguinal   ☐ L inguinal
☐ Muscle awareness   ☐ Clitoral tenderness

Patient rates allodynia produced by Q-tip for each circle (0-4). Total Score: _____

Rank muscle tenderness on 0-4 scale
☐ R obturator _____
☐ L obturator _____
☐ R piriformis _____
☐ L piriformis _____
☐ R pubococcygeus _____
☐ L pubococcygeus _____
☐ Total pelvic floor score _____

Bimanual pelvic exam
  Uterus:
   ☐ Absent
  ☐ Tender   ☐ Non-tender
  Position   ☐ Anterior   ☐ Posterior   ☐ Midplane
  Size   ☐ Normal   ☐ Other _____
  Contour   ☐ Regular   ☐ Irregular   ☐ Other _____
  Consistency   ☐ Firm   ☐ Soft   ☐ Hard
  Mobility   ☐ Mobile   ☐ Hypermobile   ☐ Fixed
  Support   ☐ Well supported   ☐ Prolapse

Adnexae
  Right   Left
   ☐ Absent   ☐ Absent
   ☐ WNL   ☐ WNL
   ☐ Tender   ☐ Tender
   ☐ Fixed   ☐ Fixed
   ☐ Enlarged _____ cm   ☐ Enlarged _____ cm

Rectovaginal
  ☐ WNL   ☐ Nodules   ☐ Guaiac positive
  ☐ Tenderness   ☐ Mucosal pathology   (negative with
  ☐ Not examined   quality control)

Trigger Points

Fibromyalgia

Assessment: _____

_____

Diagnostic Plan: _____

_____

Therapeutic Plan: _____

_____

14 _Knee Pain_

Jan Dommerholt, PT, MPS, and Christian Gröbli, PT

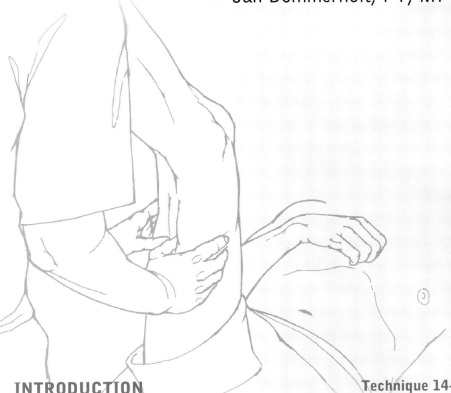

INTRODUCTION

In recent years, much attention has been paid to the knee and its specific disorders. Textbooks and articles describe the medical management and rehabilitation of common knee injuries, including osteoarthritis, patellofemoral dysfunction, bursitis, and ligamentous and meniscal injuries. In spite of the overwhelming number of publications on knee pain, most of the literature is fairly subjective in nature and demonstrates little consensus among experts (1).

Knee pathologic conditions often are associated with muscle weakness, restricted range of motion, and referred pain (2). Although these clinical features are the primary characteristics of myofascial trigger points, few texts include myofascial pain syndrome (MPS) as a source of knee pain. The potential contributions of trigger points to muscle and knee dysfunction are generally not appreciated; however, according to Travell and Simons, trigger points frequently are involved in knee pain (3). In their study of overlooked physical diagnoses in chronic pain patients, Hendler and Kozikowski concluded that MPS is the most commonly missed diagnosis (4). Muscles with trigger points may alter normal biomechanics of the knee because of functional shortening of the muscle. The mechanical dysfunction and the referred pain patterns from trigger points into the knees may be the actual cause of persistent knee pain and should be considered in the differential diagnosis. Instead, tendinitis and bursitis are viewed as the most frequent repetitive stress injuries at the knee. In this chapter, "myofascial pain" refers to pain caused by trigger points in skeletal muscles.

KNEE PAIN: BACKGROUND

Hahn and Foldspang (5) concluded that the prevalence of knee pain is associated with the type, amount, and duration of sports participation. However, knee pain and injuries occur not only in athletes, but also in the general population (5). Knee pain was positively associated with a history of jogging and competitive gymnastics. In active athletes, 54% had chronic knee pain and 34% had recurrent knee pain. In a study of former elite athletes, 52% of soccer players, 31% of weight lifters, 21% of runners, and 17% of shooters described having knee pain at least once per month (6). Dannenberg et al. reported that in their prospective study of 1,638 recreational bicyclists, the most common overuse injury was knee pain, whereas in another study of elite British bicyclists, knee pain was the second most common problem after low back pain (7,8). Female athletes involved in jumping and cutting sports, such as volleyball, basketball, and soccer, suffer serious knee injuries five times more often than male athletes. This pattern has been associated with a decreased use of the hamstring muscles during landings, exposing the anterior cruciate ligaments to excessive stress patterns (9–11).

Past knee injuries and occupational physical activities are associated with knee pain and dysfunction in later life (6,12). Of 390 elite Israeli infantry recruits, 15% were found to have anterior knee pain. Six years later, half of the knees were still symptomatic, whereas in 8% of the originally symptomatic knees, the pain was severe (13). Sobti et al. (14) found that 50% of elderly women reported complaints of knee pain and stiffness that were thought to be the result of previous work activities. In addition, obesity was positively associated with the risk of pain or stiffness at the knee and hip. Almost half of carpet and floor layers were found to have thickening of the prepatellar and superficial infrapatellar bursa associated with knee pain in kneeling postures, compared with only 7% of house painters (15). Osteophytes of the patella were significantly more common in this population (16). In general, occupations that involve knee bending and heavy lifting, such as mining, construction work, and carpentry, are at increased risk of knee pain (17).

In a British community setting, the overall prevalence of knee pain was 28% based on a mail survey (17). In northern Finland, the prevalence of chronic knee pain was 18.5% among adolescents and 3.9% among children (18). Bergenudd and colleagues reported that in a middle-aged Swedish population the prevalence of knee pain was 10% (19). In another British study, 27.6% of women older than age 55 reported knee pain, whereas Lamb et al. reported that in a cross-sectional analysis of 769 older women (mean age 77.8 years; range, 65–101 years), 53% had recent knee pain with approximately one-third rating the pain as "severe" (20,21). An American study indicated that 18.1% of U.S. men and 23.5% of U.S. women aged 60 years and older reported knee pain, with the highest prevalence found among 85- to 90-year-old men (23.7%) and women (30.0%) (22).

Diagnosis and Clinical Features

History

Rehabilitation of the knee joint and its related structures must be based on a thorough understanding of the functional anatomy and biomechanics of the knee under normal and pathologic circumstances.

To establish an accurate diagnosis, a structured approach that includes a comprehensive history, static and dynamic examination, and functional tests must be followed. The history will establish whether an injury was caused by a traumatic event or followed a more insidious onset. In case of trauma, it is important to assess the direction and magnitude of forces delivered to the knee, because this may point the clinician to the most likely injured structure(s).

A significant blow to the lateral aspect of the knee, a **valgus force** pattern, may damage the medial collateral ligament, the medial meniscus, or the medial joint capsule. A medial blow, a **varus force** pattern, may injure the lateral collateral ligament, the lateral meniscus, the lateral joint capsule, or perhaps the popliteus tendon (Fig. 14-1). The anterior cruciate ligament is frequently injured after either

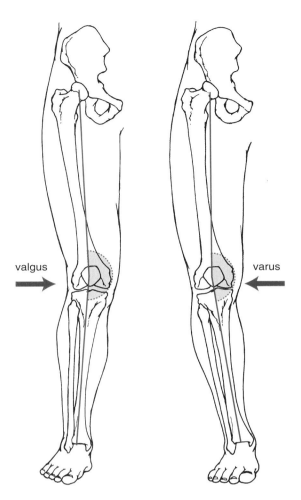

FIGURE 14-1. Valgus and varus force patterns. Valgus forces (lateral toward medial) produce a medial displacement of the knee. Varus forces (medial toward lateral) produce a lateral displacement of the knee.

a significant valgus force to the knee combined with external rotation of the tibia or a varus force combined with internal rotation of the tibia. The patient often recalls an audible "pop" followed by immediate swelling and loss of function.

The posterior cruciate ligament may be injured by falling on a flexed knee or when the knee hits the dashboard of a car in a frontal collision, both resulting in a forceful posterior displacement of the tibia. Twisting of the knee may result in tears of the menisci.

The clinician must determine the location of the pain complaint, realizing that a subjective complaint of pain does not always indicate the source of dysfunction. Localized pain may be referred from other regions or structures; for example, anterior knee pain may be associated with dysfunction of the vastus medialis muscle (23). In general, the intensity and nature of musculoskeletal pain varies with certain movements or activities, and most patients are able to indicate what activities, positions, or remedies make their pain worse or better. Constant pain that does not alter with

movement or changes in position may indicate a serious pathologic condition such as metastases to the bone. Are recurrent problems with buckling of the knee, effusion, pain at rest, or locking of the knee present? Has the patient been treated for similar complaints previously? If so, what was the course of treatment? Did the patient take medications, or follow a course of physical therapy or chiropractic? What previous treatments were successful?

Examination

The examination should include an assessment of the degree of effusion and muscle atrophy. Effusion is commonly seen with many structural lesions of the knee, including meniscal tearing, cruciate ligament tears, and synovitis. Hemarthrosis may imply an acute cruciate ligament tear or patellar dislocation. Localized swelling may be attributable to a variety of causes, including bursitis, Osgood-Schlatter disease, meniscal cysts, Baker's cysts, lipomas, degenerative joint disease, or tumors. Severe and persistent swelling may require further diagnostic studies to rule out serious pathologic conditions. Atrophy is common with all internal knee injuries and can be appreciated by visual inspection. The vastus medialis is particularly prone to atrophy after a lesion of the anterior cruciate ligament. Atrophy is also common after immobilization or with decreased activity levels. Atrophy of the vastus medialis facilitates abnormal lateralization of the patella and problems with patellar tracking.

Clinical Evaluation

In this era of evidenced-based medicine, establishing an accurate baseline and measuring the patient's status before and after intervention is important. For the knee, osteokinematic movements can be determined easily by measuring active and passive range of motion. Arthrokinetic movement is more difficult to quantify and is plagued by poor interrater reliability. Active range of motion tests should be performed under non–weight-bearing and weight-bearing conditions and must include the low back, hip, knee, and ankle joints. Osteo-kinetic movements may be restricted by pain, effusion, adhesions, scar tissue, meniscal tears, or arthritic changes. More specifically, clinicians should determine the end feel, which is defined as "the quality of resistance that the clinician feels when passively taking a joint to the clinical limits of range" (24). An abnormal end feel in the knee also may indicate adhesions, scar tissue, or meniscal tears. Pain-restricted range of motion of the knee is usually indicative of myofascial trigger points either in the quadriceps muscles with painful knee flexion or in the hamstring muscles with painful knee extension.

Evaluating the stability of the ligamentous system through a series of tests, such as the **Lachman test** (anterior cruciate ligament), **valgus tests** (medial capsule, medial collateral ligament, anterior and posterior cruciate ligaments), **varus tests** (lateral capsule, lateral collateral ligament, anterior and posterior cruciate ligaments), the **anterior and posterior drawer tests** (anterior and posterior cruciate ligaments), the **sag test** (posterior cruciate ligament), and the **lateral pivot shift test** (anterior cruciate ligament, arcuate complex, and lateral capsule), is critical. Meniscal dysfunction can be evaluated with the **McMurray test** and **Apley's compression test.** The integrity of the joint surfaces can be assessed with the **patellofemoral grinding test,** even though this test frequently elicits false-positives. Functional tests may include squatting, jumping, and running, specific work tasks, sport-specific activities, and an analysis of the patient's gait and ability to negotiate stairs.

Another measurement is the so-called quadriceps angle (Q angle), the angle formed between the vectors for the combined pull of the quadriceps femoris muscle and the patellar tendon. The Q angle can be visualized by drawing a line from the anterior superior iliac spine to the center of the patella and from the center of the patella to the anterior tibial tuberosity (Fig. 14-2). The Q angle can be measured in both the standing position and supine; it is usually slightly greater in standing (25). A Q angle in excess of 15° to 20° frequently

is cited as a reliable risk indicator for patellofemoral pain, chondromalacia patellae, knee extensor dysfunction, and patellar subluxation, although little scientific evidence exists to support this notion (26–30). Q angles are not necessarily bilaterally symmetric, but they nevertheless may provide some initial clues in determining the nature of patients' problems (31,32). When reporting the Q angle, defining the protocol used for the measurement is important, because procedures have not been standardized (30).

Next, the clinician performs strength tests. Most clinicians perform manual muscle tests in which the patient is asked to contract a specific muscle or group of muscles against gravity or against resistance applied by the examiner. If more objectivity is desired, the clinician may use a hand-held dynamometer. Muscle strength can be compromised by effusion, joint dysfunction, pain, and shortened antagonistic muscles (33). After the strength assessment, the clinician proceeds with palpation of the femorotibial condyles, the collateral ligaments, and the muscles. When indicated, the process may include a neurologic assessment, proprioceptive testing, and other specific tests, including x-rays and magnetic resonance imaging (MRI).

Lower Extremity Alignment

Assessment of lower extremity alignment is relevant, because malalignments can cause or contribute to the patient's problem. Prolonged subtalar joint pronation may result in prolonged tibial internal rotation during weight-bearing, which can affect the mechanics of both the knee and the hip, including the screw home mechanism (Fig. 14-3). During the gait cycle, the tibia needs to externally rotate in midstance. Excessive subtalar joint pronation may limit the tibia in its capacity to externally rotate, causing a compensatory internal rotation of the femur, an increased Q angle, and compression of the patella on the lateral femoral condyle (34–37). The compensation at the hip joint may in some instances reduce the risk of knee injury (38).

The most common cause of injuries to the anterior cruciate ligament is abnormal pronation, which in the sports medicine realm has been referred to as a "deceleration injury" (11). Extreme subtalar joint pronation also can stress the popliteal and pes anserine tendons, especially in runners. The popliteal muscle is an internal rotator of the tibia on the femur; however, during the stance phase, the muscle becomes an external rotator of the femur on the tibia. Correction of excessive subtalar joint pronation with a foot orthotic, therefore, may decrease patellofemoral pain and reduce tendon stresses (39). The effect of foot position on quadriceps muscle activation continues to be controversial (40–42).

Simons, Travell, and Simons emphasized that one of the more common structural inadequacies is leg-length discrepancy (43). Although leg-length discrepancies are commonly reviewed in relation to low back pain, the knee also may be exposed to increased stresses. Individuals with a leg-length discrepancy may compensate by excessive supination of the subtalar joint on the shorter side, resulting in an

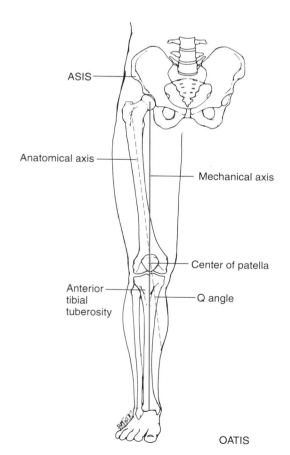

ASIS

Anatomical axis

Mechanical axis

Center of patella

Anterior tibial tuberosity

Q angle

OATIS

FIGURE 14-2. Q angle. The Q angle is the angle of displacement between a line drawn from the anterior superior iliac spine (ASIS) to the center of the patella, and a line drawn from the center of the patella to the anterior tibial tuberosity.

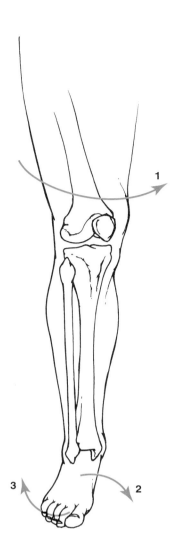

FIGURE 14-3. **Subtalar pronation.** Excessive subtalar pronation results in tibial, femoral, and hip internal rotation, external rotation of the foot, a valgus position of the knee, and an increased Q angle.

increase of forces to the lateral knee joint, or by excessive pronation on the longer side (44). Others may circumduct the longer limb during the gait cycle, or externally rotate the shorter limb, causing increased valgus forces to the knee. Efforts to maintain the pelvis level will result in exaggerated plantar flexion and chronic overuse of the quadratus lumborum, gluteal, and lower extremity muscles on the short-limb side. If the pelvis is not maintained level, a compensatory lumbar scoliosis will follow.

Careful analysis will identify the cause of the leg-length discrepancy and direct the corrective measures. Leg-length discrepancies can be either structural or functional. A structural leg-length discrepancy is the result of true differences in length of the tibia or femur, whereas a functional leg-length discrepancy may be caused by tightness of the hip capsule, unilateral innominate rotation, or muscle imbal-

ances, including shortening of a quadratus lumborum muscle, iliopsoas muscle, or hip adductors (45–47).

Differential Diagnosis

In the differential diagnosis, all potential causes of knee pain should be considered. Knee pain may be associated with hip fractures or total hip replacements, or as complications of surgical procedures such as intramedullary tibial nailing (48–53). It may be the result of neuromas, nerve damage, cysts, or ganglions, or it may accompany medical illnesses, such as juvenile ankylosing spondylitis (54–58). D'Haens et al. described a case of severe knee pain as the main symptom of systemic cytomegalovirus infection in an ulcerative colitis patient (59). Braverman et al. reported a case of avascular necrosis of both knees secondary to hydrocortisone enemas used in the treatment of inflammatory bowel disease, whereas Cohen et al. found a correlation between non–insulin-dependent diabetes and anserine bursitis (60,61). According to Strobel and Stedtfeld, diseases of the S1 and S2 spinal roots and of the sacroiliac joints also should be considered, especially with a posterolateral disc herniation (62).

Traditional Treatment Approaches

With most serious ligamentous knee injuries and instabilities, whether surgical repair is indicated is subject to debate. Although the treatment approaches vary for the various knee pathologic conditions, most rehabilitation programs follow certain principles. During the early phase after acute injury or postsurgically, the emphasis is usually on protecting the knee from further damage, control of edema, and active or passive range of motion as tolerated. Electrotherapy, ultrasound, heat or cold, and gentle mobilizations are included to reduce pain and swelling and to restore early function. Already during the initial phase of the rehabilitation program, the healing tissues need to be exposed to controlled stresses to promote the remodeling process. In subsequent stages, the patient will increasingly participate in strengthening exercises, flexibility and endurance training, movement re-education, proprioception training, and eventually functional training. Patients are introduced to both open and closed kinetic chain activities, plyometrics, and concentric and eccentric muscle training. In flexion and extension open kinetic chain activities, the foot is allowed to move freely through space with the quadriceps muscles generating knee extension and the hamstring muscles generating flexion. Arthrokinematically, the concave tibial plateau moves along the convex femoral condyles, with roll and slide occurring in the same direction. An example of an open kinetic chain activity is isotonic knee extension (Fig. 14-4).

During closed kinetic chain flexion and extension, the quadriceps and hamstring muscles cocontract, because the foot is maintained on the floor or on another surface, creating a multi-articular kinetic chain. Arthrokinematically, the convex femoral condyles move along the concave

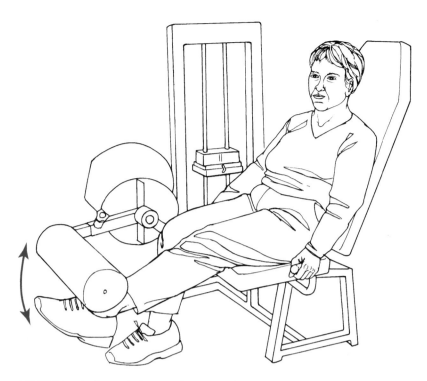

FIGURE 14-4. **Open-chain exercise.** The left quadriceps is undergoing strengthening by using an open-chain exercise in which the foot is not fixed, but moves, in contrast to the closed chain exercise with the foot fixed in Figure 14-5.

tibial plateau, with roll and slide occurring in the opposite direction. Examples of closed kinetic chain activities are wall slides and the leg press (Fig. 14-5).

Hypomobile patellofemoral, tibia-femoral, and tibia-fibular joints are mobilized. At various stages, the patient may be advised to wear a knee brace or foot orthotics or use patellar taping. Perpetuating factors are addressed through-out the rehabilitation program. Medical management may include analgesics, a course of nonsteroidal anti-inflammatories if there is bursitis, tendonitis, or synovitis, or local infiltration with lidocaine or corticosteroids. Infectious bursitis may require antibiotic treatment. Persistent effusion may be managed with iontophoresis, intra-articular injections of steroids, or with joint aspirations.

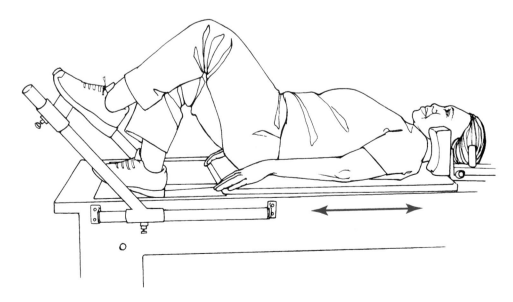

FIGURE 14-5. **Closed-chain exercise.** Closed kinetic chain strengthening of the lower extremity, showing the foot stationary and the body moving on the sliding board.

A MYOFASCIAL APPROACH TO THE DIAGNOSIS AND TREATMENT OF KNEE PAIN

At some point, most knee injuries have a myofascial component. Myofascial dysfunction can be the cause of knee pain, or it may accompany other sources of knee pain. MPS is characterized by the presence of trigger points within a taut band of muscle that can be assessed only by careful palpation. Throughout the interview, the clinician should consider whether the described pain complaints match any of the common myofascial referred pain patterns. Many of the commonly described symptoms of knee dysfunction may in fact be attributable to trigger points. For example, spontaneous buckling of the knee is often thought to be attributable to a variety of causes, including ligamentous or meniscal lesions, retropatellar or femorotibial osteoarthritis, loose bodies, or atrophy of the quadriceps after prolonged immobilization; however, it also may be attributable to trigger points in the vastus medialis or vastus lateralis.

It is not unusual to see patients with persistent knee pain after completion of typical rehabilitation programs. A common problem is that patients are instructed to participate in progressive strengthening programs before relevant trigger points are inactivated. When trigger points are not addressed, failure to progress with strengthening exercises, or continued complaints of pain, may be interpreted as "malingering" or as psychogenic. These patients may be discharged from therapy as maximally medically improved in spite of having significant pain problems. Simultaneously, the patient may develop pain-related fear and avoidance behavior, which is an important feature of the development of chronic musculoskeletal pain (63). In a study of discharged patients with persistent knee pain after a total knee arthroplasty, an 87.5% reduction in pain was achieved after an average 12 sessions of manual trigger point therapy combined with myofascial trigger point injections (64).

CASE 14-1

Patient History

At the time of her initial evaluation, Ms. S.T. was a 33-year-old married homemaker and professional designer. She was referred by her family practitioner for evaluation and treatment of complaints of anterior knee pain bilaterally with unknown origin. The pain started 10 months ago, shortly after the birth of her son. Her medical history was noncontributory. The patient was a recreational skier who also liked to work out in a fitness center. Before this referral, she had already completed 24 physical therapy sessions elsewhere, however, with no noticeable decrease in pain. Physical therapy included electrotherapy, massage therapy, and muscle strengthening.

Initially, the patient did not recall any precipitating events before the onset of pain. Later, she speculated that childbirth may have been contributory, because the pain started shortly after she delivered her baby. Ms. S.T. had not participated in any stressful activities, including sports activities, at that time. On further questioning, she described the birth process. Her labor lasted approximately 3 hours, during which she was positioned on her back with her feet in stirrups. Based on the patient's report, her knees were in approximately 90° flexion. In this position, she was able to exert enough force to push. She recalled that during her labor, she experienced a sudden sensation of severe fatigue in her thigh muscles.

Symptoms

The patient described her pain as being behind the patellae, right side more than left. The pain increased with most activities, especially descending and ascending stairs and with squatting. The pain decreased almost immediately during rest. She experienced pain on rising in the morning, which would dissipate after a few minutes. She did not have pain at night.

Examination Findings

Ms. S.T. rated her pain as a 4 out of 10 on a visual analog scale. Visual inspection showed a moderate valgus position of both knees during weight-bearing in standing, as well as during gait. In supine, the knee joint had normal passive range of motion without any pain in the end ranges. The end feels were normal. Actively, she could squat only to approximately 110° of knee flexion. There were no signs of local inflammation, bursitis, or infection. Laboratory studies were negative for any infectious disease process, or systemic inflammatory or metabolic disease. Valgus and varus stress tests were negative, as were the Lachman test, the anterior and posterior drawer tests, and the lateral pivot test, indicating that there was no instability of the knee. The McMurray tests and Apley's compression tests were negative, ruling out meniscal pathologic conditions. Patellar mobility was normal. The peri-patellar tissues were slightly loose. The patient had a normal Q angle of 12° measured in supine with the feet in a neutral position. She complained of pain with the patellofemoral grinding test and with gentle pressure over the upper and lower poles of the patellae; however, this was not consistent with her usual pain.

(continues)

CASE 14-1   Continued

Myofascial trigger points in the bilateral vastus lateralis and vastus medialis muscles were identified, which reproduced her usual knee pain with manual palpation. Muscle strength was normal and graded as 5/5. The quadriceps muscles appeared to be dystrophic bilaterally. Both rectus femoris muscles had slightly restricted flexibility. Ms. S.T. had normal range of motion in other joints, including the spine, in spite of a slight S-scoliosis.

Treatment

Because manual stimulation of the myofascial trigger points in the vastus lateralis and medialis reproduced the patient's pain, the treatment focused initially on inactivating these trigger points. The patient was seen by a physician and a physical therapist familiar with trigger point therapy. The trigger points were treated with manual trigger point therapy and dry needling. Because of pain during functional activities, the patellae were taped using McConnell's taping technique for patellofemoral dysfunction (65). With the taped knees, Ms. S.T. was able to actively bend the knee with only minimal discomfort. After four treatments, the patient reported that

the pain was approximately 40% less. She started a progressive closed kinetic chain conditioning program using a leg press and a stair climber. The patient was taught how to apply the tape before exercising. She performed active stretches for the rectus femoris muscles.

Although the patient had previously completed 24 physical therapy sessions without any relief of pain or increase in functional activities, she was pain-free and able to return to full activity after only 12 sessions that included the treatment of trigger points. Prior clinicians had not considered trigger points in the etiology of the patient's pain complaints, yet it is reasonable to conclude that MPS was the most likely cause of her pain. The patient's pain was reproduced only by manually stimulating the trigger points. Pressure over the patellae was also painful but did not reproduce the patient's pain.

Follow-up

Six months after the conclusion of therapy, the patient reported that she was still pain-free and able to participate in all functional and recreational activities.

CASE 14-2

Patient History

Mr. F.B. was a single 40-year-old developmental psychologist of average weight and height. Three weeks before his initial visit, the patient was involved in a skiing accident, during which he injured his left knee. In the emergency room, radiologic examination did not indicate any structural problems. Although he was able to walk, he complained of medial knee pain. He was provided with a lateral-medial stabilizing knee brace. Further treatment was not considered at that time. Although the patient modified his activity level considerably, the pain worsened during the next 2 weeks and spread into the posterior knee and the proximal aspect of the patella. The patient noticed that the mobility of the knee decreased as well. Both flexion and extension were restricted. He consulted with an orthopaedic surgeon, who diagnosed a partial rupture of the medial collateral ligament by using diagnostic ultrasound. The patient was referred to physical therapy. He had treated his knee with over-the-counter anti-inflammatory creams. Mr. F.B.'s medical history was noncontributory.

Symptoms

According to the patient, initially the pain was localized only in the medial aspect of the knee, especially during flexion and in the end range of extension. After a few weeks, the pain spread into the back of the knee and the patella. The pain occurred during both weight-bearing and non–weight-bearing activities. The patient described that he could not squat or bend his knee because of severe pain. The pain increased with ascending and descending stairs and at nighttime whenever he rolled over on his side. The patient described the pain as a sudden sharp, shooting pain. Occasionally the patient experienced a sensation of overall pressure on the knee and pain in the proximal aspect of the patella.

Examination Findings

The patient rated his pain as a 5 out of 10 on a visual analog scale. He was diagnosed with a medial collateral ligament lesion. The ultrasound examination did not show any meniscal tears. There were no fractures or

(continues)

other bony injuries. During the first visit, the patient's passive knee flexion was 100°, and knee extension was −10°. Both flexion and extension had a definite endpoint that was characterized by severe pain. He was unable to squat. Passive axial rotations of the knee joint were unremarkable; however, the patient described medial knee pain with compression of the joint in 90° flexion in the prone position.

Valgus tests were not performed, to avoid additional stress to the medial collateral ligament and the medial capsule. The **ballottement test,** during which the patella is manually pushed into the femoral trochlear groove, was negative; however, the **fluctuation test** was positive, indicating minor knee joint effusion (66). During the fluctuation test, the knee is placed in a position of 15° of flexion. The examiner assesses the shifting of synovial fluid by "milking" the suprapatellar bursa (66). Myofascial trigger points were identified in the popliteus muscle and in the rectus femoris. The popliteus trigger points reproduced the posterior knee pain; the rectus femoris trigger points reproduced the patellar pain. The medial knee pain could not be reproduced with palpation of myofascial trigger points. The patient's gait pattern was characterized by a noticeable limp, decreased stride length on the left, and a significantly shorter left stance phase.

Treatment

The patient was treated in physical therapy, with the initial objectives of improving the mobility of the knee and reducing pain. Therapy consisted primarily of manual soft tissue mobilization. Passive and active stretching of the quadriceps muscles was performed within the patient's pain tolerance. After three sessions, exercises to improve muscle endurance were included for the quadriceps and hamstring muscles, using closed chain activities. The trigger points in the popliteus and rectus femoris muscles were treated with trigger point therapy. Seven weeks postinjury, normal mobility was restored after eight sessions of physical therapy with an average frequency of twice weekly. The pain in the medial aspect of the knee and the sensation of pressure had resolved. There were no further signs of intra-articular swelling. However, the pain in the posterior aspect of the knee and the patella were reduced by only 50%. The patient was treated for three more visits, emphasizing trigger point therapy and overall conditioning, including strength training for the quadriceps, hamstrings, and calf and foot muscles. After a total of 11 visits, the patient complained only of minimal pain at the tip of the patella, at which point he was discharged from therapy with a home conditioning program in place.

Follow-up

Three months after his discharge, the patient reported that he was pain-free and that he had resumed his previous activity level.

An Overview of Knee Pain

When patients present with knee pain, the contributions of myofascial trigger points should be considered. The case histories illustrate that myofascial trigger points can cause knee pain even in the absence of a traumatic event. Case 14-1 describes how primary MPS with anterior knee pain developed after prolonged isometric contractions of the quadriceps muscles. Case 14-2 shows that MPS should be included in the differential diagnosis, even when there is a distinct injury, such as a partial rupture of the medial collateral ligament or a tear in the anterior cruciate ligament.

Usually within 2 weeks of an acute knee injury, active trigger points can be observed. Familiarity with referred pain patterns around the knee helps clinicians identify the structures involved and develop an effective treatment plan. Knee pain may be referred pain from more proximal or distal structures. Trigger points that may refer pain to the knee are often located in the quadriceps, the hamstrings, the sartorius, the popliteus, the adductors longus, brevis, and magnus, the gluteus minimus, the plantaris, and the gastrocnemius muscles (Figs. 14.6–14.13). With persistent knee pain, the mechanical effects of taut bands on the knee structures should be considered as well.

Biomechanical Considerations of Myofascial Trigger Points

The knee is an unstable joint, with both ginglymoid (hinged) and trochoid (pivot) articulations, that requires a significant degree of stability to accommodate loads equivalent to many times the individual's body weight (67). The knee joint obtains this stability primarily through a coordinated pattern of muscular, ligamentous, cartilaginous, and osseus structures. At the same time, the knee joint must have enough mobility to allow such movements as walking, running, dancing, squatting, and kneeling (68). Myofascial dysfunction is one of the contributing factors to altered knee biomechanics and instability, in addition to dysfunction of the cruciate–meniscus complex and the patellofemoral joint.

TECHNIQUE 14-1

Trigger Point Compression

Dejung's compression technique is basically the same as trigger point compression, as described by Simons, Travell, and Simons, although the amount of pressure may be slightly greater. Dejung's trigger point compression may be painful. After identifying the trigger point, the clinician applies localized compression over the trigger point either manually or with the TriggerPointer™, a wooden tool specially developed for this purpose. The pressure is maintained until the trigger point releases.

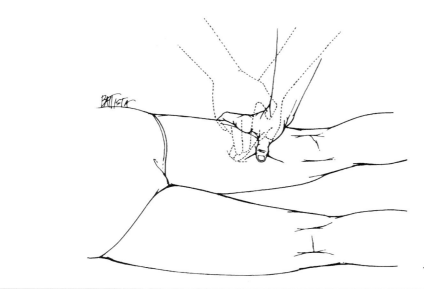

Trigger point compression.

Other texts and articles review the anatomy and biomechanics of the cruciate–meniscus complex and the patellofemoral joint in detail, so this material is not included in this chapter (45,62,69–74).

Taut bands in the hamstring or quadriceps muscles likely alter the mobility and biomechanics of the menisci and the patella, respectively. Considering that knee joint motion is accompanied by simultaneous co-activation of the quadriceps and hamstring muscles, any mechanical discrepancy in either muscle group will affect the resultant joint motion and possibly influence joint stability. For example, a taut band in the biceps femoris muscle may not only limit terminal extension of the knee, but also may decrease the ability of the biceps to cocontract during knee extension. To appreciate the possible mechanical effect of taut bands, the clinician must gain a thorough knowledge of the muscle, including its origins, insertions, and functions. The semimembranosus muscle will serve as an example.

The Semimembranosus Muscle

The semimembranosus muscle is the main posteromedial muscle. It is a bi-articular muscle, innervated by the tibial component of the sciatic nerve. The muscle originates from the ischial tuberosity and has multiple attachments at the posterior aspect of the knee. Fowler and Lubliner described five insertions of the semimembranosus muscle (67):

- A posteromedial tendinous insertion to the tibia and the posterior horn of the medial meniscus

- A medial tendinous insertion to the tibia deep to the superficial medial ligament

- A posterior fibrous attachment that blends with the posterior capsule and forms the oblique popliteal ligament

- A posteromedial fibrous attachment that forms the posterior oblique ligament

- A medial fibrous attachment that forms the superficial medial ligament.

Kim et al. identified a tendinous branch of the semimembranosus muscle inserting into the posterior horn of the lateral meniscus in more than 43% of the knees dissected (75).

The semimembranosus muscle reinforces the posteromedial aspect of the knee capsule. It can flex and internally rotate the tibia on the femur and pull the posterior horn of the medial meniscus posteriorly during flexion of the knee (67). According to Kim et al., the semimembranosus can pull the posterior horn of the lateral meniscus posteriorly as

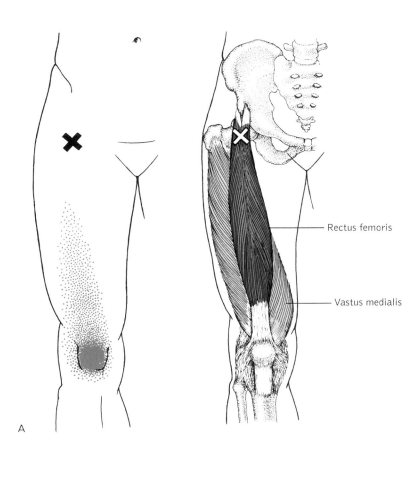

Rectus femoris

Vastus medialis

A

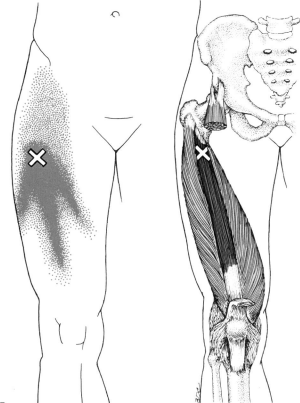

B

FIGURE 14-6. Trigger point pain referral patterns from trigger points in the quadriceps muscle. A. Referral patterns of trigger points in the rectus femoris muscle. B. Referral patterns of trigger points in the intermedius muscle.

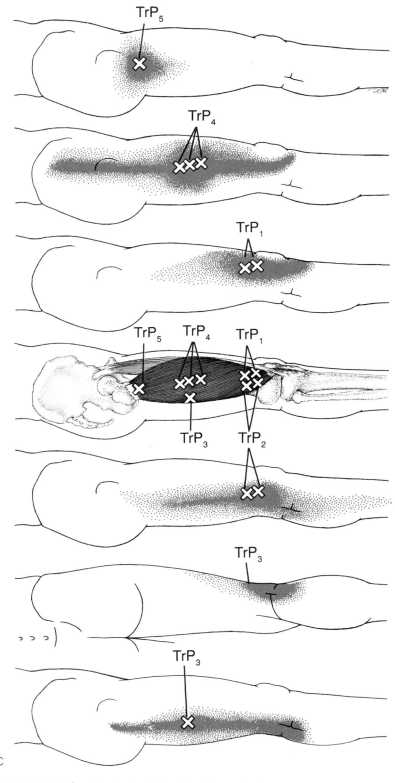

FIGURE 14-6. **Continued. C.** Referral patterns of trigger points in the vastus lateralis muscle.

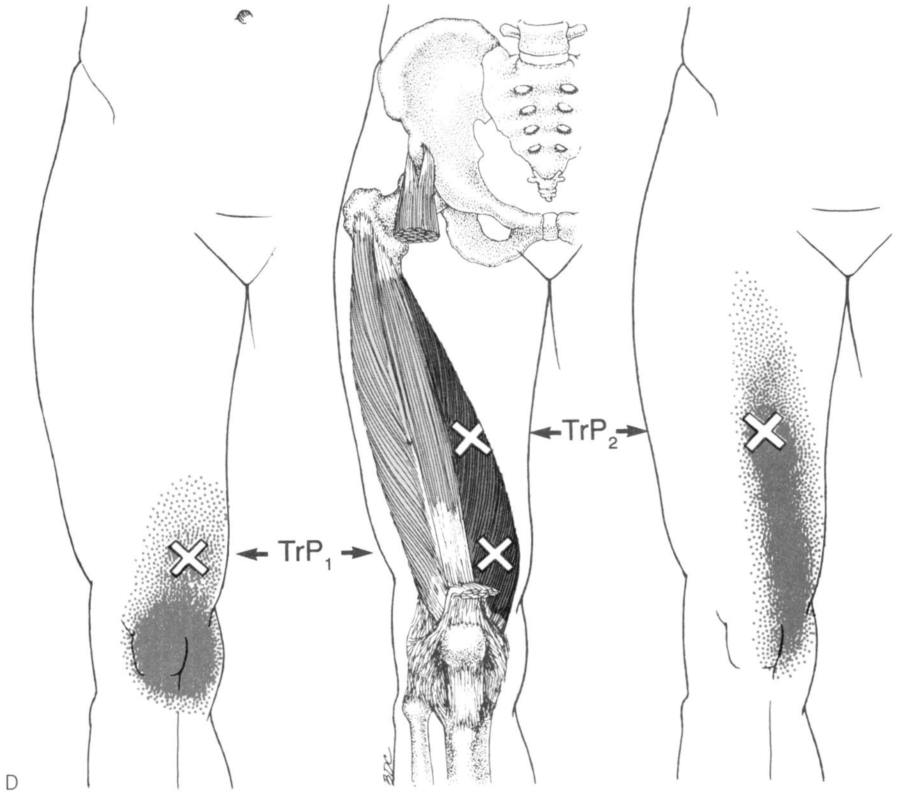

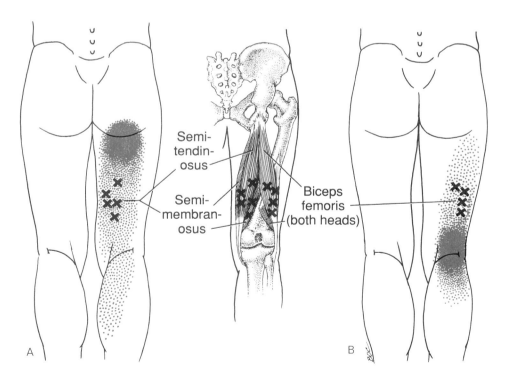

FIGURE 14-6. **Continued. D.** Referral patterns of trigger points in the vastus medialis muscle. The X's represent regions where trigger points are commonly found. The solid area represents the more common pain referral zones, and the stippled areas represent less common pain referral zones. Reprinted with permission from Travell JG, Simons DG. Myofascial Pain and Dysfunction: The Trigger Point Manual, vol 2: The Lower Extremities. Baltimore: Lippincott Williams & Wilkins, 1993 (figs. 14.1–14.4), p. 250–253.

FIGURE 14-7. Trigger point pain referral patterns from trigger points in the hamstring muscles. The X's represent regions where trigger points are commonly found. The solid area represents the more common pain referral zones, and the stippled areas represent less common pain referral zones. Reprinted with permission from Travell JG, Simons DG. Myofascial Pain and Dysfunction: The Trigger Point Manual, vol 2: The Lower Extremities. Baltimore: Lippincott Williams & Wilkins, 1993 (fig. 16.1), p. 317.

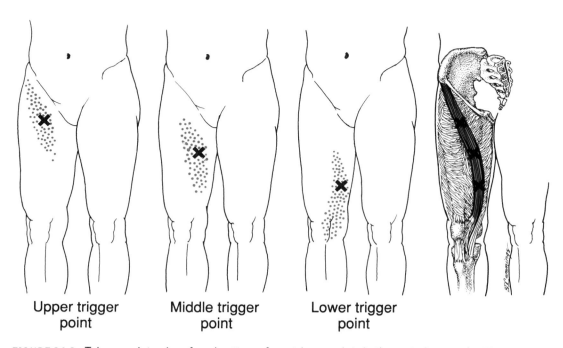

Upper trigger
point

Middle trigger
point

Lower trigger
point

FIGURE 14-8. Trigger point pain referral patterns from trigger points in the sartorius muscle. The X's represent regions where trigger points are commonly found. The solid area represents the more common pain referral zones, and the stippled areas represent less common pain referral zones. Reprinted with permission from Travell JG, Simons DG. Myofascial Pain and Dysfunction: The Trigger Point Manual, vol 2: The Lower Extremities. Baltimore: Lippincott Williams & Wilkins, 1993 (fig. 12.6), p. 227.

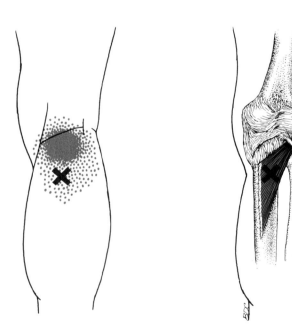

FIGURE 14-9. Trigger point pain referral patterns from trigger points in the popliteal muscles. The X's represent regions where trigger points are commonly found. The solid area represents the more common pain referral zones, and the stippled areas represent less common pain referral zones. Reprinted with permission from Travell JG, Simons DG. Myofascial Pain and Dysfunction: The Trigger Point Manual, vol 2: The Lower Extremities. Baltimore: Lippincott Williams & Wilkins, 1993 (fig. 17.1), p. 340.

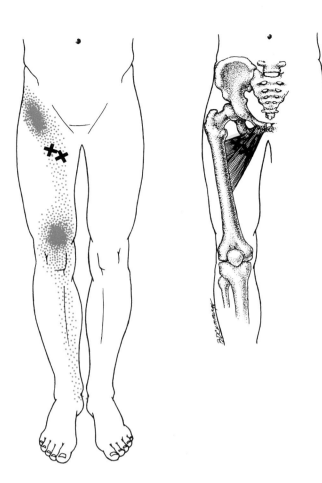

FIGURE 14-10. **Trigger point pain referral patterns from trigger points in the adductor longus and brevis muscles.** The X's represent regions where trigger points are commonly found. The solid area represents the more common pain referral zones, and the stippled areas represent less common pain referral zones. Reprinted with permission from Travell JG, Simons DG. Myofascial Pain and Dysfunction: The Trigger Point Manual, vol 2: The Lower Extremities. Baltimore: Lippincott Williams & Wilkins, 1993 (fig. 15.1), p. 291.

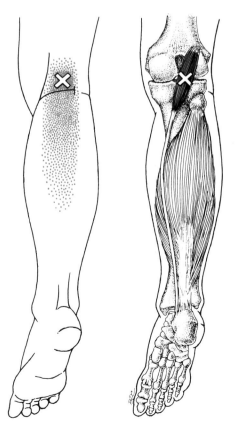

FIGURE 14-11. **Trigger point pain referral patterns from trigger points in the plantaris muscles.** The X's represent regions where trigger points are commonly found. The solid area represents the more common pain referral zones, and the stippled areas represent less common pain referral zones. Reprinted with permission from Travell JG, Simons DG. Myofascial Pain and Dysfunction: The Trigger Point Manual, vol 2: The Lower Extremities. Baltimore: Lippincott Williams & Wilkins, 1993 (fig. 22.3), p. 430.

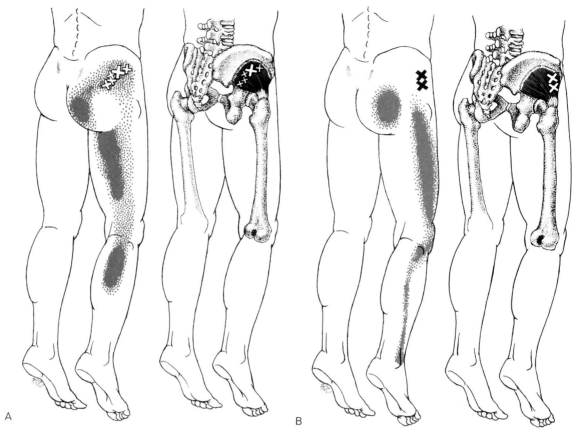

FIGURE 14-12. **Trigger point pain referral patterns from trigger points in the gluteus minimus muscle. A.** The referral pattern from posterior gluteus minimus trigger points. **B.** The referral pattern from anterior gluteus minimus trigger points. The X's represent regions where trigger points are commonly found. The solid area represents the more common pain referral zones, and the stippled areas represent less common pain referral zones. Reprinted with permission from Travell JG, Simons DG. Myofascial Pain and Dysfunction: The Trigger Point Manual, vol 2: The Lower Extremities. Baltimore: Lippincott Williams & Wilkins, 1993 (figs. 9.1, 9.2), p. 169.

well, a function that usually is attributed exclusively to the popliteus muscle (75). Under normal circumstances, the menisci move anteriorly during extension, because of contraction of the quadriceps muscle and the passive force exerted by the femoral condyles and the menisco-patellar ligaments. A taut band with myofascial trigger points in the semimembranosus muscle alters the normal functions of the muscle and exerts abnormal forces on the various knee structures. A shortened semimembranosus muscle may maintain the menisci in a relative posterior position, even during extension of the knee. Trigger points in the semimembranosus muscle, therefore, may increase the likelihood of meniscal injury. The menisci can be injured when they are not able to follow the movement of the femoral condyles.

A taut band in the semimembranosus muscle may limit the muscle's flexibility and contractile ability, causing muscle imbalances around the knee, which in itself may contribute to injury or dysfunction. Because of the shortening, the quadriceps muscles may become weaker as well

(33). Concentric contraction of the hamstrings to bring the knee into flexion may be weaker from trigger points. The gait cycle may be altered because of pain associated with trigger points and taut bands, as well as the limited ability of the muscle to contract eccentrically. Antalgic gait patterns with a noticeable limp from pain secondary to trigger points in the hamstrings are commonly observed. In their combined functions, the hamstrings assist in extending the hip. Taut bands in the hamstrings may limit the patient's ability to stand erect because of decreased hip stability and a flexed knee position and may contribute to posterior rotation of the involved innominate. Shortened hamstrings also may provide increased posterior pull to the proximal tibia. It is not clear whether this has any impact on the efficiency of the ligamentomuscular protective reflex initiated by mechanoreceptors in the anterior cruciate ligament. Under normal circumstances, the receptors in the ligament trigger contraction in the hamstrings, when the ligament is subjected to forces beyond its physiologic strain limits. Even with normal flexibility, active and pas-

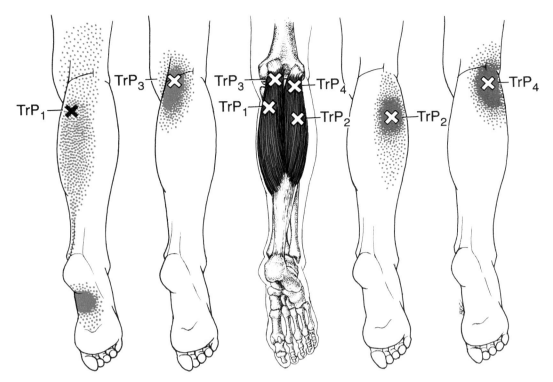

FIGURE 14-13. **Trigger point pain referral patterns from trigger points in the gastrocnemius muscles.** The X's represent regions where trigger points are commonly found. The solid area represents the more common pain referral zones, and the stippled areas represent less common pain referral zones. Reprinted with permission from Travell JG, Simons DG. Myofascial Pain and Dysfunction: The Trigger Point Manual, vol 2: The Lower Extremities. Baltimore: Lippincott Williams & Wilkins, 1993 (fig. 21.1), p. 399.

TECHNIQUE 14-2

Compression of the Trigger Point Zone with Local Stretch

This technique involves a combination of trigger point compression and a slow manual stretch of the trigger point area in the direction of the muscle fibers. The objective is to stretch the contracted muscle fibers at the level of the trigger point. This kind of localized stretching cannot be accomplished with more generic muscle stretches. The technique is used interchangeably with other techniques to inactivate a trigger point and to increase the local circulation. This technique is usually painful.

The clinician places the muscle in a slightly stretched position, then locates a clinically relevant trigger point. Realizing the direction of the muscle fibers, the clinician applies deep compression over the trigger point. While maintaining the compression, the fingers slowly move in the direction of the muscle fiber to stretch the fibers at the trigger point. As the stretch is directed at the trigger point zone only, the total distance over which the muscle is being stretched is usually only approximately 2 cm. For most patients, the use of a small amount of massage oil is recommended.

sive insufficiency is present at the hip and knee, which is increased when taut bands are present in the hamstring muscles. Because the hamstrings are bi-articular muscles, they cannot fully contract or be fully stretched across the knee and hip simultaneously (76).

During the stance phase of walking and running, the hamstrings provide stability to the knee and the hip. During push-off, the hamstrings cocontract with the quadriceps muscles. During the swing phase, the hamstrings act eccentrically and decelerate the swinging leg. Hamstring injuries are often related to ballistic actions during the late swing phase and the take-off phase (45). Taut bands and trigger points restrict the hamstrings in any of these functions.

Other Muscles

Similar biomechanical considerations can be developed for any of the other muscles around the knee; for example, taut bands with trigger points in the popliteus muscle may keep the lateral meniscus in a relative posterior position, even during knee extension. Taut bands with trigger points in the iliopsoas and rectus femoris muscles may maintain the hip in a flexed position. The adductor muscles may keep the femur in an adducted position, thereby changing the joint reaction forces at the knee. Trigger points in the

TECHNIQUE 14-3

Myofascial Release

This technique is similar to what is often described as myofascial release. The main objective is to improve the mobility of the connective tissue structures and fascia. The myofascial release stretch is not painful. Most patients experience myofascial release techniques as reasonably pleasant. From that perspective, alternating the more painful techniques with myofascial release is recommended.

The clinician places the muscle in a neutral or slightly stretched position. The clinician must use a flat surface of the hand, either the base or palm of the hand, the dorsal aspect of the proximal phalangeal bones, or the thumb, depending on the size of the muscle. The clinician uses one hand to pre-tense the muscle and skin. With the other hand, he exerts light pressure into the superficial fascia. While the light pressure is maintained, the tissues are stretched manually, usually in the direction of the muscle fiber; however, the stretch can be applied irrespective of the direction of the fibers.

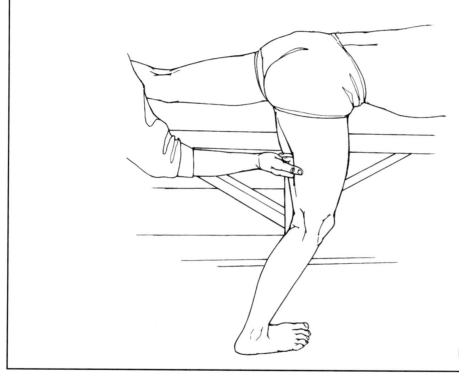

Myofascial release.

gluteus maximus and tensor fascia latae may cause shortening of the iliotibial band (IT band). This shortening may contribute to the high incidence of patellofemoral pain among dancers, in whom posteriorly displaced IT bands, especially during deep knee bends, result in excessive lateral deviation of the patella (77). Trigger points in the vastus lateralis also can cause lateral deviation, whereas trigger points in the iliopsoas and hip adductor muscles can result in abnormal stresses on the tensor fascia latae muscle and the IT band.

Other factors need to be considered as well, such as training errors or altered training habits, sudden increases in running speed or distance, and changes in dance repertoire, dance style, or floor surface (78). A change in footwear may cause an increase of force attenuation from decreased shock absorption in the new shoes. Different shoes also may alter the mechanics of the subtalar joint and result in excessive pronation, increased stress to the patellofemoral articulation, and trigger points in the vastus medialis.

Runners are exposed to greater risk of injury if they habitually run on transverse grades or crowned roads, which can result in either increased subtalar pronation for the uphill foot or supination for the downhill foot (28). Running on transverse grades, or downhill running, has also been associated with IT band friction syndrome, patellofemoral dysfunction, and muscle imbalances. The IT band acts as a femorotibial ligament; the band is a strong lateral stabilizer of the knee. When the knee is in 0° to 30° of flexion, the IT band is an extensor of the knee. At 40° to 145° of flexion, the IT band functions as a flexor (67). During downhill run-

TECHNIQUE 14-4

Muscle Play

This technique is similar to the osteopathic concept of muscle play. The objective is to improve the intermuscular mobility of two neighboring muscles. This technique may release possible connective tissue adhesions between muscles. The technique is especially important when the neighboring muscles are each other's antagonists. Technique 4 is usually painful.

The clinician places the muscles in a neutral or more relaxed position. He places his finger tips in between two muscles. He asks the patient to contract the muscles alternately by slowly moving the respective limb or body part. This facilitates further penetration of the clinician's fingers in between the muscles. The clinician may attempt to gently slide the fingers along the muscles to further improve muscle play. Excessive stress on the clinician's finger joints and collateral ligaments must be avoided.

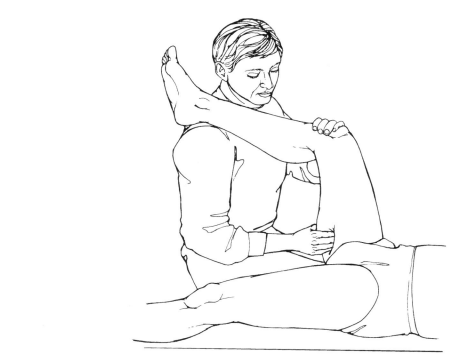

Muscle play.

ning, the contact forces between the IT band and the lateral femoral condyle may be increased, because usually the knee is kept in a few degrees of flexion (37,68).

Causes

Myofascial trigger points can develop after direct trauma to the lower extremity, such as in motor vehicle accidents or athletic events, when muscles can be suddenly overstretched. Other common causes of trigger points include prolonged repetitive activities, such as running, cycling, or dancing; prolonged mechanical stresses or awkward postures; joint pathologic conditions; and psychological stress (79). The diagnostic process must include the usual differential diagnostic considerations and rule out other pathologic processes. In the examination of a patient with knee pain, considering only MPS and the biomechanical contributions and referred pain patterns of trigger points is inadequate. The clinician always should consider ligamentous, meniscal, and capsular injuries, patellofemoral joint dysfunction, bursitis, tendinitis, neurodynamic dysfunction, and other disease processes, including Osgood Schlatter, degenerative joint disease, tumors, and complications from the ankle, hip, and low back regions.

Many chronic conditions, such as osteoarthritis and rheumatoid arthritis, are accompanied by trigger points, and the pain may be the result of both the arthritic condition and the trigger points. In osteoarthritis, weakness of the quadriceps muscles often results from decreased alpha-motoneuron excitability. Rheumatoid arthritis may feature swelling, morning stiffness, a hard end feel, pain on motion, and atrophy of the quadriceps muscle. Both muscle weakness and atrophy can result in myofascial trigger points, which can give rise to another source of pain in the involved knee.

Symptom/Pain Presentation

Most patients are not aware that their knee pain may be attributable to distant myofascial trigger points, and they act surprised when manual stimulation of a proximal trigger point in the rectus femoris muscle, for example, mimics their anterior knee pain. Especially in chronic pain patients, the reproduction of pain can be therapeutic by itself, because previous practitioners may not have been able to reproduce the pain. During a clinical examination, it is common to elicit referred pain patterns that are irrelevant for the patient's complaint. The patient's recognition of the elicited pain helps determine which muscles need to be treated. Referred pain from trigger points is often described as "deep tissue pain" of a dull and aching nature, which makes it often indistinguishable from pain originating in other structures around the knee.

Myofascial trigger points in the quadriceps muscles can contribute to other, more commonly diagnosed pain problems, such as patellofemoral pain and patellar tendinitis. Trigger points in the gluteus maximus and tensor fascia latae can contribute to IT band friction syndrome.

A detailed history and accurate physical examination are the key components to diagnosis in determining the source of the pain complaint and the functional deficits. Myofascial pain is often misdiagnosed as patellofemoral pain, medial plica syndrome, or pain secondary to bursitis. Patellofemoral pain is felt in the anterior knee and is exacerbated by prolonged knee flexion and activities, including sitting, squatting, and stair climbing. It is diagnosed by careful palpation and mobilization of the patella, such as passive lateral glides and compression of the patella.

Plicae are embryonic synovial folds that are frequently present, although they are rarely symptomatic. There are three plicae: the infrapatellar, suprapatellar, and medial patellar plica. The medial plica is the least often present; however, it most frequently causes knee problems. Patients with medial plica syndrome complain of anterior knee pain.

Bursitis does not appear to be as common as often suggested other than in serious athletes and ballet dancers or after direct trauma. Superficial bursitis, deep infrapatellar bursitis, and prepatellar bursitis may feature swollen painful bursae, especially with compression, and are seen after direct trauma to the anterior knee or after prolonged kneeling. Pes anserine bursitis is seen in serious runners and cyclists, who typically complain of medial tibial pain.

Patellar tendinitis is common in volleyball players and other jumping athletes, who may complain of pain at the insertion of the patellar tendon into the inferior pole of the patella. IT band friction syndrome is often seen in cyclists and runners and is especially associated with downhill run-

---

TECHNIQUE 14-5

Therapeutic Stretching

Following the previous techniques or dry needling/injection therapy, the treated muscles should be stretched. Stretching will facilitate maintenance of the newly gained muscle length and possibly improvement as well. The clinician may combine stretching with hold–relax or post-isometric relaxation techniques. By letting the patient gently contract the muscle before stretching, a greater gain will be accomplished. Once the muscle is stretched, the local circulation can be restored (see Fig. 14-20).

---

ning. The pain is usually located at the lateral aspect of the knee. Osteochondritis dissecans involves a lesion of the subchondral bone and the medial joint surface cartilage. The pain presentation varies greatly. Patients may describe pain throughout the entire knee or only at the medial aspect. It may be aggravated by activities or be present at rest. The diagnosis is confirmed by plain film x-rays and bone scans. Arthritic pain is often described as posterior knee pain. There may be moderate to severe effusion and restricted range of motion, usually in a capsular pattern. Sharp pain may be caused by an entrapment of a loose body, or it may indicate a synovial impingement. Many patients describe crepitus over the anterior knee, which usually is asymptomatic and nonspecific with regard to knee pain. A recent study suggested that anterior knee pain may originate primarily in the fat pad and medial retinaculum, based on the significantly higher distribution of substance P nerve endings in these structures (80).

Treatment

Myofascial trigger points are identified by systematic palpation of the muscles. As Simons, Travell, and Simons have outlined, myofascial trigger points are always located within a taut band of muscle (43). Taut bands should be differentiated from general muscle spasms, which can be defined as electromyographic (EMG) activity and the result of increased neuromuscular tone of the entire muscle (81,82). A taut band is a localized contracture within the muscle, without activation of the motor endplate (83). Taut bands and the trigger points can be identified by manual palpation perpendicular to the direction of the muscle fibers. Identifying trigger points requires both training and experience. Although it is not difficult for skilled and experienced clinicians to distinguish myofascial trigger points, it may still be difficult to determine which structure is primarily responsible for the pain. Unfortunately, few medical schools, or schools for chiropractic, physical therapy, or other disciplines, include adequate training in the identification of myofascial trigger points.

Evaluation and Treatment of Muscles

When examining a patient with knee pain, the clinician should systematically palpate those muscles that may harbor taut bands and trigger points, because they may cause increased mechanical tension on the various knee structures, as well as referred pain. Commonly, all muscles of a particular functional unit develop trigger points. The functional muscle unit includes a muscle's agonists and antagonists. Depending on the function, muscles may be part of various functional units. All skeletal muscles can develop taut bands and myofascial trigger points, and patients may present with trigger points that are not directly related to the actual pain complaint. Referred pain, by itself, is not specific to myofascial trigger points. Other tissues may also refer pain to the knee, including the skin, periosteum, the IT band, the sacroiliac region, or even healthy muscles in the hip and thigh (84). To improve the specificity of the diagnosis, the patient must recognize the pain elicited by pressure on the trigger point. Pain elicited with range-of-motion testing is another possible indication of MPS, although, again, it is not specific to MPS. Evidence indicates that neurodynamic tests, such as the slump test, also may be positively correlated with injury of the hamstring muscles and restricted range of motion (85).

After establishing which muscles are involved, the clinician must determine any mechanical perpetuating factors that may contribute to the formation or persistence of the trigger points (43). Any muscle that can alter the position of the femur should be considered in the analysis. Normal function of the hip is a critical component of knee rehabilitation. Other structural and mechanical factors need to be corrected, including altered gait patterns, leg-length discrepancies, poor shoe wear, and excessive subtalar joint pronation or supination. Particular attention should be paid to stressful training habits, athletic performance, posture, and repetitive motions.

Inactivation of trigger points involved in knee dysfunction can be performed with the patient positioned in supine, side-lying, or prone. Over the last 60 years, several assessment and treatment approaches have emerged independently of each other, both in Europe and in the United States, including myofascial trigger point therapy (United States), neuromuscular technique or NMT (United Kingdom), neuromuscular therapy, also abbreviated as NMT (United States), and manual trigger point therapy (Switzerland). These approaches share many similarities and have common goals and objectives. The general guidelines for treatment of myofascial trigger points have been described in detail by Travell and Simons and may include trigger point compression, spray and stretch, contract–relax or post-isometric relaxation, muscle energy techniques, massage therapy, strain and counterstrain, myofascial release, and electrotherapeutic modalities (3,43). Invasive techniques include superficial and deep dry needling and direct injection of a local anesthetic, saline, or botulinum A toxin into the trigger points.

The Swiss rheumatologist and psychologist, Beat Dejung, has developed a systematic seven-step treatment approach commonly referred to as manual trigger point therapy (86–88). These techniques appear in Technique boxes 14-1 to 14-7, throughout the chapter. Dejung's protocol combines sustained trigger point compression, manual stretching of the trigger point zone, myofascial release of the muscle and its connective tissues, muscle play techniques, a therapeutic stretching program, a self-stretching home program, and superficial and deep dry needling (89–91). These techniques are used interchangeably based on the specific findings, the patient's response, and the patient's tolerance. In a typical 30-minute treatment session, multiple muscles and trigger points can be treated. The patient's tolerance to treatment is probably the most important parameter in determining how many muscles can be treated. Compression, localized stretching, and the muscle play technique can be painful and should be combined with myofascial release, massage therapy, and gentle stretching. As Simons, Travell, and Simons have outlined, the clinician should use the least amount of pressure required to inactivate the trigger point. They now advocate using the osteopathic barrier concept in which painful stimuli are avoided. No one approach appears to be more effective than the next. After the manual treatments and dry needling, the clinician stretches the treated muscles. The patient is instructed in a home program, initially consisting of muscle stretches and correction of posture. Patients may apply trigger point gentle compression as well. Dejung's approach aims to decrease nociceptive activity, muscle contractures, and local edema, and to improve local circulation and the intramuscular and intermuscular mobility.

As with any treatment plan addressing pain problems, treatment can be divided into a pain-control phase and a training or conditioning phase. During the pain-control phase, inactivation of the trigger points and restoration of normal muscle length are the main short-term goals. Once these goals have been accomplished, the patients start a conditioning program to restore muscle strength and endurance, proprioception, and functional activities, including a return to sports participation. Throughout the treatment process, the clinician should educate the patient about causes, perpetuating factors, and self-management. Patients must learn to modify their behaviors and avoid overloading the muscles without resorting to total inactivity.

Persons with chronic myofascial knee pain often require extensive treatment not only of the muscles around the knee, but also of the hip and back muscles. Perpetuating factors are even more relevant and need to be addressed. Chronic pain patients may have developed pain-related fear and avoidance behaviors. They often are deconditioned, move with guarded movements, and may have developed a sense of hopelessness (63). Chronic pain patients tend to be fearful of the conditioning phase and tend to "hold on to their pain." However, motivating these patients to actively participate in the rehabilitation process by performing mus-

TECHNIQUE 14-6

Home Stretching Program

This technique constitutes a home stretching program. The patient learns no more than three to five stretches in one session. The clinician must review the stretches with the patient during follow-up visits. Although different thoughts exist regarding the ideal duration of muscle stretching, in clinical practice holding a stretch for up to 20 seconds appears to be effective (see Figs. 14-14–14-16).

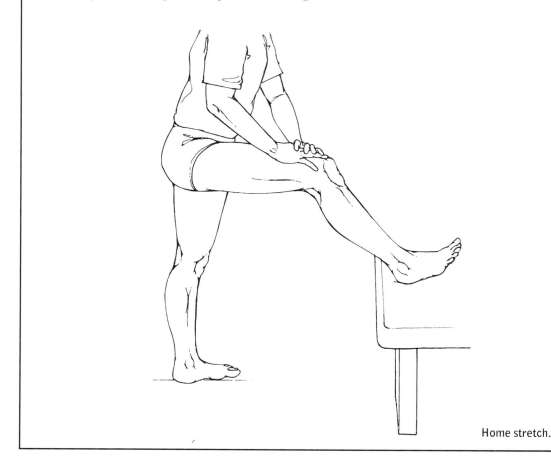

Home stretch.

cle stretches, followed by restoration of normal muscle functioning and optimal movement patterns, is important.

Assessment and Treatment of Joint Dysfunction

A common feature of knee joint injuries is weakness of the quadriceps muscle, which Stokes and Young have termed *arthrogenous muscle weakness* (92). Quadriceps weakness can occur after immobilization or with joint effusion (93,94). Articular structures, including the anterior cruciate ligament, feature multiple mechanoreceptors that provide information about joint position and joint movement (95–98). Any damage to these articular knee structures likely decreases the excitability of quadriceps alpha-motoneurons and gamma-motoneurons, resulting not only in a decrease of quadriceps activation, but also in decreased sensitivity of the muscle spindles and impaired proprioception (99–102).

Treating MPS around the knee, therefore, must include treatment of the joint by either manual mobilization, taping, or, in some cases, surgical correction (100,103,104). Surgery may be indicated when other articular structures are damaged, such as the menisci, in addition to the anterior cruciate ligament. The rehabilitation program also should include proprioceptive training. Loss of proprioceptive acuity actually may lead to premature arthritic changes.

Important in Case 14-1 is that the treatment was not limited to simply inactivating myofascial trigger points. Because the patient presented with abnormal patellar tracking during weight-bearing, the patellofemoral joint dysfunction had to be addressed. Under normal circumstances, the patella is in a slightly lateral position when the knee is fully extended. With flexion, the patella moves medially as it engages the trochlear groove (105). In this case, the patient presented with an increased genu valgum and Q angle in

TECHNIQUE 14-7

Dry Needling

Dry needling consists of superficial dry needling and deep dry needling. Superficial dry needling is usually painless and involves inserting an acupuncture needle in the subcutaneous tissue overlying the trigger point. Deep dry needling involves placing an acupuncture needle directly into the trigger point and may be painful. With deep dry needling, a local twitch response must be elicited.

Superficial dry needling: The clinician identifies the trigger point. The clinician then inserts an acupuncture needle into the subcutaneous tissue over the trigger point. The needle is angled at approximately 45°. The needle is left in place for at least 30 seconds, up to as long as 10 minutes, depending on the patient's response.

Deep dry needling: The clinician identifies the trigger point and then inserts an acupuncture needle into the trigger zone. Eliciting a local twitch response is the verification of the correct placement of the needle. Because multiple trigger points may be present within one particular trigger zone, it is important to inactivate as many trigger points as possible without withdrawing the needle from the skin.

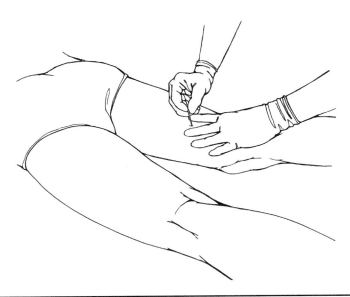

Dry needling.

standing, which may have predisposed the patella to deviate laterally. Treatment with either taping or inactivation of the myofascial trigger points alone probably would not have been successful. By combining trigger point therapy and patellar taping, the patient's pain was reduced in a few visits, allowing her to start a conditioning program and return to full function in a few weeks.

Patient Exercise and Home Care

Patients must be instructed in appropriate stretches of the involved muscles, immediately after the inactivation of trigger points. The therapist may provide the patient with written instructions for stretches for the quadriceps muscles, the hamstring muscles, the hip adductors and abductors, and the calf muscles (Figs. 14.14–14.16). Where appropriate, the home program also may include stretches for the gluteal muscles and the low back muscles, including the quadratus lumborum and paraspinal muscles. Initially, patients are advised to discontinue any sports participation, deep knee bends, full squats, or strengthening exercises, because these tend to exacerbate myofascial trigger points. Once the myofascial trigger points have been inactivated, the home program may include progressive strengthening exercises, proprioceptive training, plyometrics, and cardiovascular conditioning similar to any other knee rehabilitation program.

CONCLUSION

Patients with acute knee pain who present only with myofascial trigger points are relatively easy to treat. By using a combination of methods to inactivate the trigger points, followed by a progressive exercise program with initial stretching and subsequent strengthening and proprioceptive training as needed, most patients are able to return to their previous level of functioning in 2 to 6 weeks. Patients with chronic knee pain usually require more time. Patients with chronic ailments, such as advanced osteoarthritis, are likely to experience recurring myofascial dysfunction.

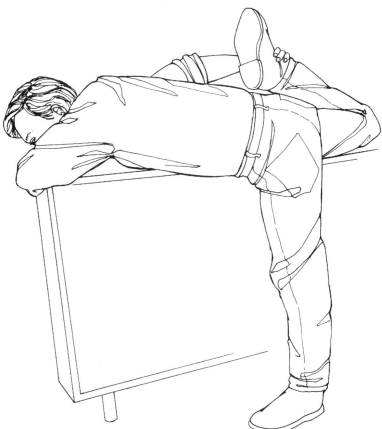

FIGURE 14-14. **A self-stretch of the right quadriceps muscle.** The left leg with the foot on the floor maintains the pelvis in a posterior rotation, as the stretch will otherwise move the pelvis into an anterior rotation.

Including the assessment of myofascial trigger points in the overall examination and evaluation is important. Most of the commonly recognized knee problems feature myofascial dysfunction in addition to the more obvious problems. In some cases, myofascial trigger points may have contributed to the onset of the orthopaedic problem, whereas in other cases, the trigger points may have developed after the onset of the orthopaedic problem. In the latter scenario, the duration of the rehabilitation program depends predominantly on the primary diagnosis. The treatment of trigger points as part of the rehabilitation program may reduce the associated pain complaint and facilitate a speedier return to function.

TREATMENT PROTOCOL

1. **Inactivate the clinically relevant trigger points.** As stated, several different treatment approaches have emerged that all seem to be able to accomplish the task. In this chapter, Dejung's approach was described. Trigger points that may refer pain to the knee are often located in the quadriceps, the sartorius, the hamstrings, the popliteus, the adductors longus, brevis, and magnus, the gluteus minimus, the plantaris, and the gastrocnemius.

2. **After trigger point inactivation, elongate the involved muscles.**

3. **Correct any biomechanical perpetuating factors, such as excessive pronation, leg-length discrepancies, innominate rotations, altered gait patterns, and poor shoe wear.**

4. **Correct any incorrect training habits, athletic performance, posture, and so on.**

5. **Once trigger points are inactivated and muscle length is restored, evaluate joint function of the ankle, knee, hip, and low back. Correct joint dysfunction as indicated.**

6. **Focus on developing normal muscle strength and endurance.**

7. **Develop a progressive home program.**

8. **Throughout the rehabilitation program, pay attention to medical issues, such as possible other contributing diagnoses, metabolic perpetuating factors, adequate medication prescriptions, and so on.**

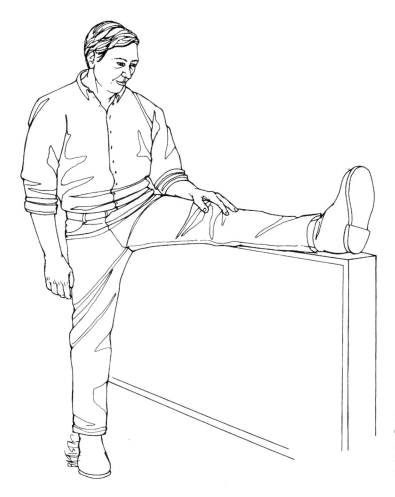

FIGURE 14-15. **A self-stretch of the left hamstring muscles.** The back is straight rather than bent forward. The right foot on the floor keeps the pelvis in anterior rotation, as the stretch will otherwise move the pelvis into posterior rotation.

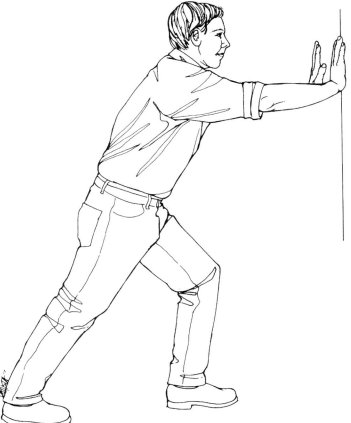

FIGURE 14-16. **A self-stretch of the right gastrocnemius muscle.** The right knee is straight, and the heel is on the floor. The back is kept straight.

Manual Myofascial Release Techniques for Specific Muscles Involved in Knee Pain

Editorial Note by Lucy Whyte Ferguson, DC

The quadriceps femoris muscle group (rectus femoris, vastus medialis, vastus intermedius, and vastus lateralis) is readily stretched with the patient side-lying. The thigh is drawn into extension, and the heel is drawn toward the buttock to progressively flex the knee as much as the patient's comfort allows. Vapocoolant spray can be used, and the contract–relax technique is also effective. With the patient supine, specific trigger points can be contacted and released with trigger point pressure release. For release of trigger points that have not readily released with the patient supine, it is often helpful to combine trigger point pressure with active elongation of the quadriceps with the patient prone. For example, using a small amount of cream lubricant, the clinician reaches one hand under the thigh just above the knee, and contacts with firm pressure the trigger points in the vastus medialis, intermedius, or lateralis (Fig. 14-17).

The clinician directs the patient to flex the knee by taking the heel toward the buttock. The clinician maintains the contact during the active stretch of the muscle; the clinician's contact contributes localized resistance to the stretch, and the trigger point appears to be drawn out and the tissue elongated in this manner. The procedure is repeated three or four times. The same technique can be applied to the rectus femoris by contacting higher in the thigh on the appropriate trigger points. Sartorius trigger points can be released in this way also, by contacting the trigger points in the anteromedial thigh during the active stretch.

The adductor longus, brevis, and magnus can be stretched with the patient supine and the thigh abducted. Trigger point pressure release can be used in this position as well. Combining these methods with contract–relax technique is particularly effective. The

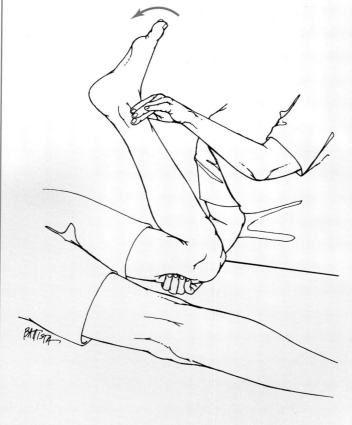

FIGURE 14-17. Myofascial release of trigger points in the vastus medialis muscle. The patient is prone; the clinician firmly contacts trigger points and applies local resistance as patient stretches the muscle by slowly approximating the heel to the buttock.

patient lies supine, and the clinician draws the extended leg into abduction and stands between the leg and the treatment table, supporting the leg with one hand, and contacting the trigger point with the other hand (Fig. 14-18). The clinician uses pincher palpation to locate and compress the trigger point and instructs the patient to contract the leg against the clinician's resistance gently for approximately 4 seconds. Then the patient is instructed to release and take the leg further out into abduction. The trigger point pincher contact is maintained during the stretch phase, and the tissue between the clinician's fingers can be felt to elongate and become less knotted. This procedure is repeated three or four times, with the leg further abducted at each repetition, and the clinician shifting body position away from the treatment table as necessary to provide resistance to the patient's contractions.

Trigger points that do not release easily can be addressed with percussion technique, discussed more fully in Chapter 4. For the adductor muscles, this can be performed with the patient either supine or prone. For example, in a prone position, the patient's thigh can be abducted until tension is palpable in the bands of the adductor muscle group. Internally rotating the thigh also can be helpful to bring the taut bands to tension. The patient's thigh will probably rest on the edge of the table, but it can be supported on the seated clinician's thigh if necessary. The clinician uses one hand to palpate the taut bands, traction them further, and contact the remaining trigger points. The clinician's contact provides increased tissue traction at the location of the trigger point (Fig. 14-19). Then the clinician moves the contact hand just distal to the trigger point, while maintaining tissue traction, and uses the other hand to perform percussion on the trigger point with a reflex hammer. As the muscle tissue elongates during the percussion, the tractioning hand takes the muscle tissue into further stretch, thus taking up the slack, until the trigger point location is reassessed and can no longer be palpated.

The hamstring muscle group can be effectively stretched with vapo-coolant spray and contract–relax with the patient supine and the thigh flexed at the hip. Prone trigger point pressure release is also effective. The trigger point compression can be combined with the muscle stretch and contract–relax technique with the patient supine. The clinician stands at the side of the table facing the head of the table, with the patient's straight leg resting on the clinician's shoulder. The clinician advances toward the head of the table until the limit of the patient's thigh flexion has been reached (Fig. 14-20). Then the clinician instructs the patient to let the knee bend slightly. The slight slacking of the hamstring muscle group allows the clinician to locate particular taut bands and trigger points selected for treatment. The clinician uses a small amount of cream lubricant and

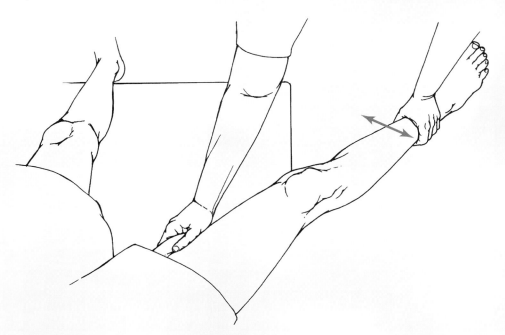

FIGURE 14-18. **Myofascial release of trigger points in the adductor longus, brevis, and magnus muscles.** The patient is supine and the clinician supports the abducted leg with one hand and presses on trigger points and pulls on taut bands a pincher contact. The contact is maintained while the patient contracts for 4 seconds and then relaxes.

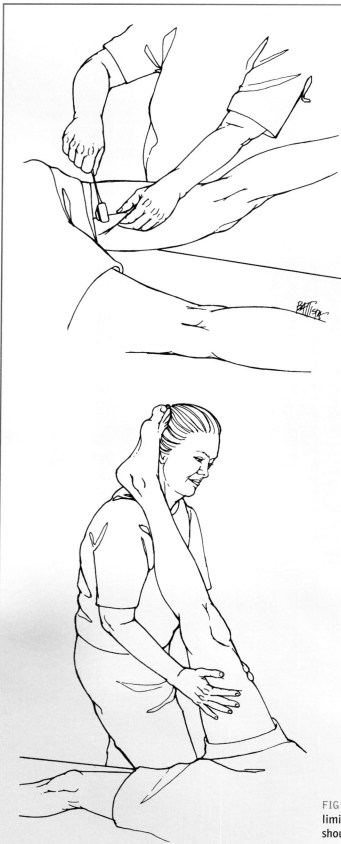

FIGURE 14.19. **Myofascial release of trigger points in the adductor with the patient prone, and the thigh abducted and internally rotated.** The clinican uses pincher contact to press on and pull trigger points, then moves contact hand just distal to the trigger point while maintaining tissue traction. The clinician performs percussion on the trigger point with the other hand. As the trigger point releases, the contact hand draws out and lengthens the taut band.

FIGURE 14-20. **Passive hamstring muscle stretch to the initial limit with the patient supine and the leg resting on the clinician's shoulder.**

places a firm contact against the trigger points with fingers of one or both hands (Fig. 14-21). The patient is then instructed to straighten the knee and press the extended leg against the clinician's shoulder for approximately 4 seconds. Then the clinician instructs the patient to relax the extended leg. The clinician waits a few seconds for the relaxation and then advances toward the head of the table, thus further flexing the thigh with the leg extended (Fig. 14-22). The procedure is repeated three or four times, with contact on the trigger points maintained throughout, to provide local tissue elongation. Each time that the patient is asked to allow the knee to slightly flex, the clinician re-checks to see that the finger compression contact is on the most knotted remaining portion of the group of trigger points being treated, and then proceeds with the contract–relax.

Myofascial release of the gastrocnemius muscle is discussed in the Heel and Arch Pain Chapter, pages (405–407). The key to effective release of the popliteus and plantaris muscles is the ability to correctly locate the muscle and its trigger points. With the patient prone, the popliteus is more easily palpated under the gastrocnemius if the patient gently rolls the calf slightly medially and laterally. The popliteus can be felt to slightly tense and relax during the patient's movement. By the same token, the plantaris can be localized by having the patient gently evert and invert the ankle. These small movements will not significantly activate the relaxed gastrocnemius, and the trigger points in the deeper muscles can be located and released, with trigger point pressure release, percussion, or any other technique.

The key to effective trigger point treatment is often the combination of a series of techniques, as in the techniques developed by Dr. Beat Dejung.

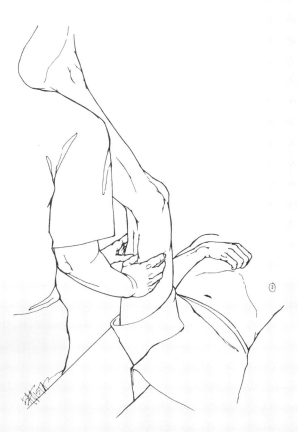

FIGURE 14-21. Patient slightly bends knee while clinician firmly contacts trigger points selected for specific treatment.

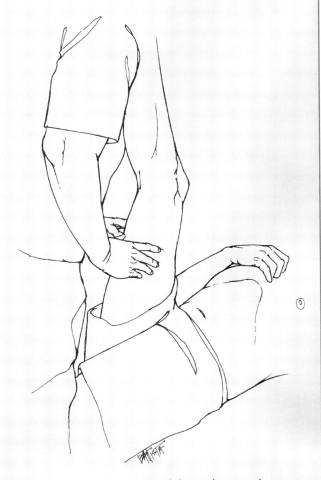

FIGURE 14-22. Patient straightens knee and presses against clinician for 4 seconds, then releases. Clinician then advances toward the head of the table until a new limit is reached. Sequence is repeated 3 or 4 times.

References

1. Cutbill JW, Ladly KO, Bray RC, et al. Anterior knee pain: a review. Clin J Sport Med 1997;7:40–45.

2. Lohman EB III. Diagnosis and management of patellofemoral pain. Orthop Phys Ther Clin North Am 1998;7:367–396.

3. Travell JG, Simons DG. Myofascial Pain and Dysfunction: The Trigger Point Manual, vol 2. Baltimore: Williams & Wilkins, 1992.

4. Hendler NH, Kozikowski JG. Overlooked physical diagnoses in chronic pain patients involved in litigation. Psychosomatics 1993;34:494–501.

5. Hahn T, Foldspang A. Prevalent knee pain and sport. Scand J Soc Med, 1998;26:44–52.

6. Raty HP, Kujala UM, Videman T, et al. Lifetime musculoskeletal symptoms and injuries among former elite male athletes. Int J Sports Med 1997;18:625–632.

7. Callaghan MJ, Jarvis C. Evaluation of elite British cyclists: the role of the squad medical. Br J Sports Med 1996;30:349–353.

8. Dannenberg AL, Needle S, Mullady D, et al. Predictors of injury among 1638 riders in a recreational long-distance bicycle tour: Cycle across Maryland. Am J Sports Med 1996;24:747–753.

9. Hewett TE, Lindenfeld TN, Riccobene JV, et al. The effect of neuromuscular training on the incidence of knee injury in female athletes. a prospective study. Am J Sports Med 1999;27: 699–706.

10. Hewett TE, Stroupe AL, Nance TA, et al. Plyometric training in female athletes. decreased impact forces and increased hamstring torques. Am J Sports Med 1996;24:765–773.

11. Ramus L. A training program for the prevention of ACL injuries in female athletes. in sports medicine in the 21st century: issues of impairment. 8th Annual Mid-American Sports Medicine Symposium, 2000, Ypsilanti, MI.

12. Cooper C, McAlindon T, Coggon D, et al. Occupational activity and osteoarthritis of the knee. Ann Rheum Dis 1994;53:90–93.

13. Milgrom C, Finestone A, Shlamkovitch N, et al. Anterior knee pain caused by overactivity: a long term prospective followup. Clin Orthop 1996;331:256–260.

14. Sobti A, Cooper C, Inskip H, et al. Occupational physical activity and long-term risk of musculoskeletal symptoms: a national survey of post office pensioners. Am J Ind Med, 1997;32:76–83.

15. Kivimaki J. Occupationally related ultrasonic findings in carpet and floor layers' knees. Scand J Work Environ Health 1992;18: 400–402.

16. Kivimaki J, Riihimaki H, Hanninen K. Knee disorders in carpet and floor layers and painters. Scand J Work Environ Health 1992;18:310–316.

17. O'Reilly SC, Muir KR, Doherty M. Occupation and knee pain: a community study. Osteoarthritis Cartilage, 2000;8:78–81.

18. Vahasarja V. Prevalence of chronic knee pain in children and adolescents in northern Finland. Acta Pediatr 1995;84:803–805.

19. Bergenudd H, Nilsson B, Lindgarde F. Knee pain in middle age and its relationship to occupational work load and psychosocial factors. Clin Orthop 1989;245:210–215.

20. McAlindon TE, Cooper C, Kirwan JR, et al. Knee pain and disability in the community. Br J Rheumatol 1992;31: 189–192.

21. Lamb SE, Guralnik JM, Buchner DM, et al. Factors that modify the association between knee pain and mobility limitation in older women: The Women's Health and Aging Study. Ann Rheum Dis 2000;59:331–337.

22. Andersen RE, Crespo CJ, Ling SM, et al. Prevalence of significant knee pain among older Americans: results from the Third National Health and Nutrition Examination Survey. J Am Geriatr Soc 1999;47:1435–1438.

23. Cesarelli M, Bifulco P, Bracale M. Quadriceps muscles activation in anterior knee pain during isokinetic exercise. Med Engl Phys 1999;21:469–478.

24. Patla CE, Paris SV. E1 Course Notes; Extremity Evaluation & Manipulation. 1996, St. Augustine: Institute of Physical Therapy.

25. Woodland LH, Francis RS. Parameters and comparisons of the quadriceps angle of college-aged men and women in the supine and standing positions. Am J Sports Med 1992;20:208–211.

26. Brody DM. Running injuries. Clin Symp, 1980;32:2–36.

27. Huberti HH, Hayes WC. Patellofemoral contact pressures: the influence of q angle and tendo-femoral contact. J Bone Joint Surg Am 1984;66: p.715–724.

28. Messier SP, Pittala KA. Etiologic factors associated with selected running injuries. Med Sci Sports Exerc 1988;20:501–505.

29. Goldberg B. Patellofemoral malalignment. Pediatr Ann 1997;26: 32–35.

30. Livingston LA. The quadriceps angle: a review of the literature. J Orthop Sports Phys Ther 1998;28:105–109.

31. Livingston LA, Mandigo JL. Bilateral within-subject Q angle asymmetry in young adult females and males. Biomed Sci Instrum 1997;33:112–117.

32. Livingston LA, Mandigo JL. Bilateral Q angle asymmetry and anterior knee pain syndrome. Clin Biomech (Bristol, Avon) 1999;14:7–13.

33. Janda V. Muscle strength in relation to muscle length, pain, and muscle imbalance, in Harms-Ringdahl K, ed. Muscle Strength Edinburgh: Churchill Livingstone, 1993:83–91.

34. Lutter LL. Injuries in the runner and jogger. Minn Med 1980;63: 45–51.

35. D'Amico JC, Rubin M. The influence of foot orthoses on the quadriceps angle. J Am Podiatr Med Assoc 1986;76:337–340.

36. Powers CM, Maffucio R, Hampton S. Rearfoot posture in subjects with patellofemoral pain. J Orthop Sports Phys Ther 1995;22:155–159.

37. Tiberio D. The effect of excessive subtalar joint pronation on patellofemoral mechanics: a theoretical model. J Orthop Sports Phys Ther 1987;9:160–165.

38. Lafortune MA, Cavanagh PR, Sommer HJ, et al. foot inversion-eversion and knee kinematics during walking. J Orthop Res 1994;12: 412–420.

39. Eng JJ, Pierrynowski MR. Evaluation of soft foot orthotics in the treatment of patellofemoral pain syndrome. Phys Ther 1993;73: 62–70.

40. Gough JV, Ladley G. An investigation into the effectiveness of various forms of quadriceps exercises. Physiotherapy 1971;57:356–361.

41. Signorile JF, Karcsik D, Perry A, et al. The effect of knee and foot position on the electromyographical activity of the superficial quadriceps. J Orthop Sports Phys Ther 1995;22:2–9.

42. Hung Y, Gross MT. Effect of foot position on electromyographic activity of the vastus medialis oblique and vastus lateralis during lower-extremity weight-bearing activities. J Orthop Sports Phys Ther 1999; 29:93–104.

43. Simons DG, Travell JG, Simons LS. Myofascial Pain and Dysfunction: The Trigger Point Manual, vol 1, 2nd Ed. Baltimore: Williams & Wilkins, 1999.

44. Donnatelli R. Abnormal biomechanics, in Donnatelli R, ed. The Biomechanics of the Foot and Ankle. Philadelphia: FA Davis, 1990:32– 65.

45. Reid DC. Sports Injury Assessment and Rehabilitation. New York: Churchill Livingstone, 1992.

46. Mitchell FL. Elements of muscle energy technique, in Basmajian JV, Nyberg R, eds. Rational Manual Therapies. Baltimore: Williams & Wilkins, 1993:285–321.

47. LeVeau B. Hip, in Richardson JK, Iglarsh ZA, eds. Clinical Orthopaedic Physical Therapy Philadelphia: Saunders: 1994: 333–398.

48. Hammer SG. Hip fracture presenting as knee pain in an elderly patient. Am Fam Physician 1996;54:872.

49. McCormack D, Mulcahy D, McElwain J. Knee pain after tibial nailing. J Bone Joint Surg Br 1996;78:511.

50. Guss DA. Hip fracture presenting as isolated knee pain. Ann Emerg Med 1997;29:418–420.

51. Court-Brown CM, Gustilo T, Shaw AD. Knee pain after intramedullary tibial nailing: its incidence, etiology, and outcome. J Orthop Trauma 1997;11:103–105.

52. Khan NQ, Woolson ST. Referral patterns of hip pain in patients undergoing total hip replacement. Orthopedics 1998;21: 123–126.

53. Yu SW, Tu YK, Fan KF, et al. Anterior knee pain after intramedullary tibial nailing. Chang Keng I Hsueh Tsa Chih 1999;22:604–608.

54. Pinar H, Ozkan M, Akseki D, et al. Traumatic prepatellar neuroma: an unusual cause of anterior knee pain. Knee Surg Sports Traumatol Arthrosc 1996;4:154–156.

55. Frey Law LA, Haftel HM. Shoulder, knee and hip pain as initial symptoms of juvenile ankylosing spondylitis. J Orthop Sport Phys Ther 1998;27:167–172.

56. Tennent TD, Birch NC, Holmes MJ, et al. Knee pain and the infrapatellar branch of the saphenous nerve. J R Soc Med 1998;91:573–575.

57. Noda M, Kurosaka M, Maeno K, et al. Case report ganglion cysts of the bilateral cruciate ligaments. Arthroscopy 1999;15:867–870.

58. Siebert CH, Kaufmann A, Niedhart C, et al. The quadriceps tendon cyst: an uncommon cause of chronic anterior knee pain. Knee Surg Sports Traumatol Arthrosc 1999;7:349–351.

59. D'Haens G, Suenaert P, Westhovens R, et al. Severe knee pain as the single symptom of CMV infection in acute ulcerative colitis treated with cyclosporine. Inflamm Bowel Dis 1998;4:27–28.

60. Cohen SE, Mahul O, Meir R, et al. Anserine bursitis and non-insulin dependent diabetes mellitus. J Rheumatol 1997;24:2162–2165.

61. Braverman DL, Lachmann EA, Nagler W. avascular necrosis of bilateral knees secondary to corticosteroid enemas. Arch Phys Med Rehabil 1998;79:449–452.

62. Strobel M, Stedtfeld H-W. Diagnostic evaluation of the knee. New York: Springer Verlag, 1990.

63. Vlaeyen JW, Linton SJ. Fear-avoidance and its consequences in chronic musculoskeletal pain: a state of the art. Pain 2000;85: 317–332.

64. Feinberg BI, Feinberg RA. Persistent pain after total knee arthroplasty: treatment with manual therapy and trigger point injections. J Musculoskel Pain 1998;6:85–95.

65. McConnell JS. The management of chondromalacia patellae: a long term solution. Aust J Physiotherapy 1986;32:215–223.

66. Greenfield BH. Sequential evaluation of the knee, in Greenfield BH, ed. Rehabilitation of the Knee: A Problem-Solving Approach. Philadelphia: FA Davis, 1993:43–65.

67. Fowler PJ, Lubliner J. Functional anatomy and biomechanics of the knee joint, in Grifin LY, ed. Rehabilitation of the Injured Knee. St Louis: Mosby, 1995:7–19.

68. Winkel D, Matthijs O, Phelps V. Diagnosis and Treatment of the Lower Extremities. 1997, Gaithersburg: Aspen Publishers, 1997.

69. Engle RP. Knee Ligament Rehabilitation. New York: Churchill Livingstone, 1991.

70. Greenfield BH. Rehabilitation of the knee: a problem-solving approach, in Wolf SL, ed. Contemporary Perspectives in Rehabilitation. Philadelphia: F.A. Davis, 1993.

71. Scott WN. The Knee. St. Louis: Mosby, 1994.

72. Griffin LY. Rehabilitation of the Injured Knee. St. Louis: Mosby, 1995.

73. Mangine RE. Physical Therapy of the Knee, 2nd Ed. New York: Churchill Livingstone, 1995.

74. Fulkerson JP. Disorders of the Patellofemoral Joint. Baltimore: Williams & Wilkins, 1997.

75. Kim YC, Yoo WK, Chung IH, et al. tendinous insertion of semimembranosus muscle into the lateral meniscus. Surg Radiol Anat 1997; 19:365–369.

76. Kreighbaum E, Barthels KM. Biomechanics: A Qualitative Approach for Studying Human Movement. New York: MacMillan, 1985.

77. Winslow J, Yoder E. Patellofemoral pain in female ballet dancers: correlation with iliotibial band tightness and tibial external rotation. J Orthop Sports Phys Ther 1995;22:18–21.

78. James SL, Bates BT, Osternig LR. Injuries to Runners. Am J Sports Med 1978;6:40–50.

79. Witonski D. Anterior Knee Pain Syndrome. Int Orthop 1999; 23: 341–344.

80. Witonski D, Wagrowska-Danielewicz M. Distribution of substance-P nerve fibers in the knee joint in patients with anterior knee pain syndrome. a preliminary report. Knee Surg Sports Traumatol Arthrosc 1999;7:177–183.

81. Janda V. Muscle spasm: a proposed procedure for differential diagnosis. J Manual Med 1991;6:136–139.

82. Mense S. Pathophysiologic basis of muscle pain syndromes, in Fischer AA, ed. Myofascial Pain: Update in Diagnosis and Treatment. Philadelphia: Saunders, 1997:23–53.

83. Hong C-Z. Pathophysiology of myofascial trigger point. J Formos Med Assoc, 1996;95:93–104.

84. Scudds RA, Landry M, Birmingham T, et al. The frequency of referred signs from muscle pressure in normal healthy subjects (abstract). J Musculoskel Pain 1995;3(Suppl 1): 99.

85. Butler DS. Mobilization of the Nervous System. Melbourne: Churchill Livingstone, 1991.

86. Dejung B. Die Behandlung "Chronischer Zerrungen". Schweiz Ztschr Sportmed, 1988;36:161–168.

87. Gröbli C. Klinik Und Pathophysiologie Von Myofaszialen Triggerpunkten. Physiotherapie 1997;32:17–26.

88. Gröbli C, Dommerholt J. Myofasziale Triggerpunkte; Pathologie Und Behandlungsmöglichkeiten. Manuelle Medizin 1997;35: 295–303.

89. Dejung B. Die Verspannung Des M. Iliacus Als Ursache Lumbosacraler Schmerzen. Manuelle Medizin 1987;25:73–81.

90. Dejung B. Triggerpunkt- Und Bindegewebebehandlung—Neue Wege in Physiotherapie Und Rehabilitationsmedizin. Physiotherapeut, 1988;24:3–12.

91. Grosjean B, DeJung B. Achillodynie—Ein Unlosbäres Problem? Schweiz Zeitschr Sportmed, 1990;38:17–24.

92. Stokes M, Young A. The contribution of reflex inhibition to arthrogenous muscle weakness. Clin Sci 1984;67:7–14.

93. Fahrer H, Rentsch HU, Gerber NJ, et al. Knee effusion and reflex inhibition of the quadriceps. a bar to effective retraining. J Bone Joint Surg Br 1988;70:635–638.

94. Shakespeare DT, Stokes M, Sherman KP, et al. Reflex inhibition of the quadriceps after meniscectomy: lack of association with pain. Clin Physiol 1985;5:137–144.

95. Freeman MAR, Wyke B. Articular reflexes at the ankle joint: an electromyographic study of normal and abnormal influences of ankle joint mechanoreceptors upon reflex activity in the leg muscles. Br J Surg 1967;54:990–1001.

96. Johansson H, Sjolander P, Sojka P. A sensory role for the cruciate ligaments. Clin Orthop 1991;268:161–178.

97. Schutte MJ, Dabezies EJ, Zimny ML, et al. Neural anatomy of the human anterior cruciate ligament. J Bone Joint Surg Am 1987;69: 243– 247.

98. Zimny ML, Schutte M, Dabezies E. Mechanoreceptors in the human anterior cruciate ligament. Anat Rec 1986;214:204–209.

99. Barrett DS. Proprioception and function after anterior cruciate reconstruction. J Bone Joint Surg Br 1991;73:833–837.

100. Beard DJ, Kyberd PJ, Fergusson CM, et al. Proprioception after rupture of the anterior cruciate ligament. an objective indication of the need for surgery? J Bone Joint Surg Br 1993;75:311–315.

101. Hurley MV. The effects of joint damage on muscle function, proprioception and rehabilitation. Manual Therapy 1997;2:11–17.

102. Hurley MV, Rees J, Newham DJ. quadriceps function, proprioceptive acuity and functional performance in healthy young, middle-aged and elderly subjects. Age Ageing 1998;27:55–62.

103. Warmerdam A. Arthrokinetic therapy: improving muscle performance through joint manipulation, in Proceedings of the 5th International Conference of the International Federation of Orthopaedic Manipulative Therapists, Vail, 1992.

104. Warmerdam A. Manual Therapy: Improve Muscle and Joint Functioning. Wantagh: Pine Publications, 1999.

105. Nissen CW, Cullen MC, Hewett TE, et al. Physical and arthroscopic examination techniques of the patellofemoral joint. J Orthop Sports Phys Ther 1998;28:277–285.

15 Heel and Arch Pain

Richard M. Kushner, DPM, and Lucy Whyte Ferguson, DC

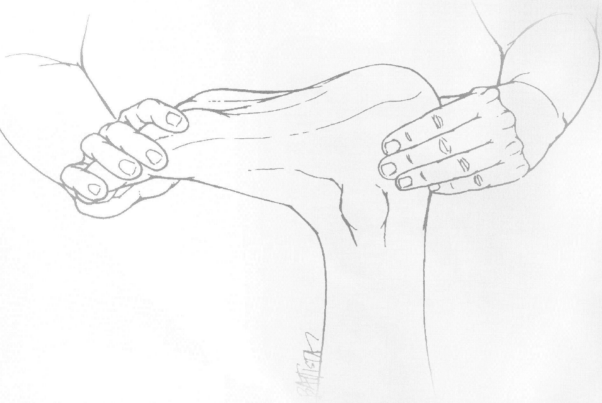

INTRODUCTION

Clinicians of different specialties are frequently called on to diagnose and treat aspects of heel and foot pain. These problems range from Achilles tendinitis to plantar fasciitis to neuromas, and include primary nerve entrapments such as tarsal tunnel syndrome. Heel spur syndrome and plantar fasciitis are among the most common of these problems and give rise to heel pain and pain in the arch of the foot. Although these conditions often have been treated as local syndromes, pain in the heel and arch often are caused by referred pain from trigger points in the intrinsic muscles of the foot and from the calf muscles. Myofascial trigger points in the intrinsic muscles of the foot and the calf muscles result from biomechanical dysfunctions in gait. Therefore, these myofascial trigger points generally cannot be successfully treated unless the biomechanical dysfunction is also addressed. Entrapment or compression of the calcaneal branch of the posterior tibial nerve, known as **Baxter's neuritis,** also can cause heel pain that behaves somewhat like heel spur syndrome, but is treated differently, with specific myofascial release techniques or a nerve block, if necessary.

Heel and arch pain often become chronic problems because they are difficult to treat, and because patients often delay seeking professional help for long periods, because pain waxes and wanes. Patients often try home remedies recommended by friends or relatives. The situation is often further complicated by ineffective treatment efforts that may include faulty foot orthotics, improper or faulty shoe gear, improper stretching exercises, and nonprescription medications. Regardless of the initiating circumstances, these conditions constitute a biomechanically perpetuated pathologic condition.

One study showed that 15% of all adult patients seen by podiatrists for foot pain had painful heels, and 73% of heel pain was a result of **heel spur syndrome** (1). Heel and arch pain can cause difficulty walking, necessitating alteration in gait, and affecting normal body mechanics.

Heel and arch pain typically present as a cramping, tight, or sharp pain that develops suddenly or insidiously. The most significant finding in **plantar fasciitis** and heel spur syndrome is point tenderness along the medial longitudinal arch and at the insertion of the fascia and intrinsic muscles to the anterior edge of the medial calcaneal tuberosity. The pain is often worse on putting weight on the feet after sitting for a period, or on arising in the morning. This condition is termed **post-static dyskinesia.**

Trigger points of the foot and calf often develop as a result of microtrauma arising from multiple causes. Chronic injury to the foot can arise from faulty biomechanics, improper shoe gear, or obesity, and it can be affected by the walking surface and the type of daily activity or job. The diagnostic and treatment challenge is not only to properly ad-dress the myofascial trigger point involvement, but also to comprehensively address the causes that gave rise to the trigger points in the first place. With such comprehensive care, this condition can be treated quickly and effectively, rather than lingering as a chronic condition.

HEEL AND ARCH PAIN: BACKGROUND

Little exists in the literature regarding heel pain before 1900. However, Zacharie in 1860 described patients with heel pain who had "greater pain in the morning than after standing or walking one or two hours" (2). Plettner, in 1900, recorded the incidental finding of an inferior calcaneal spur on a patient's radiograph (3). Baer, in 1906, had six patients who had both painful heel spurs and a history of gonorrheal infections (4). He theorized that all heel spurs were caused by gonorrheal infection (4). These plantar spurs were attributed to a venereal cause during most of the early part of the 20th century, and many symptomatic "gonorrheal spurs" were surgically treated, with poor postoperative results (5). This thinking changed by the early 1940s, and consideration was given to biomechanical factors and the repetitive pull of the plantar fascia and musculature on the calcaneus as the cause of heel pain (5,6).

Diagnosis and Clinical Features
Heel Pain

Although heel pain is often referred to as heel spur syndrome, the *presence of a heel spur is not essential to the diagnosis or treatment.* In fact, heel spur formation can occur with or without noticeable discomfort. The patient often endures some discomfort, or adjusts to it, choosing to "wait it out." The very existence of a heel spur indicates that an inflammatory process has occurred or, with pain, is occurring (Fig. 15-1). Conversely, inflammation and pain can occur with or without the radiologic presence of heel spur formation (7). Diagnosis and treatment therefore depend on the location and nature of the pain, rather than on the presence or absence of a heel spur.

Plantar Fasciitis

The pain that occurs at the anterior edge of the medial calcaneal tuberosity is often referred to as plantar fasciitis and can reflect chronic inflammation, but it can occur in the absence of what are usually considered to be hallmarks of chronic inflammation. LeMelle, Kisilewicz, and Janis compared the tissues of two patients with chronic heel pain who had surgery for resection of a heel spur and plantar fascia release (8). The fascia of the first felt thick and dense and had histologic changes typical of chronic inflammation: fibrovascular hyperplasia, fibrocartilaginous degeneration, accentuated perivascular spaces,

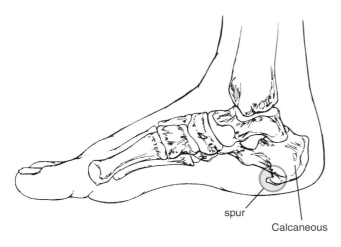

FIGURE 15-1. **Calcaneal heel spur.** The presence or size of a heel spur does not necessarily correlate with the presence of pain. Whereas the normal calcaneus has a fairly smooth and rounded anterior border, a heel spur extends *horizontally* into the location of tendon or fascial insertion onto the calcaneus. (The patient usually expects that a heel spur would be a *vertical* structure because the pain feels like stepping on the end of a nail.)

and fibroblastic proliferation. The fascia of the second patient did not feel thick or dense and had normal histologic architecture without significant pathologic changes. The problems of the patient with or without significant inflammation can be addressed with a myofascial and biomechanical approach.

Other Causes of Heel Pain

Other conditions than plantar fasciitis and heel spur can cause heel and arch pain. Posterior tibial nerve entrapment causes both heel and arch pain. Heel pain can occur rarely in autoimmune disease such as ankylosing spondylitis or atrophy of the plantar calcaneal fat pad. Athletes who have trained rigorously can suffer recurrent trauma from kicking and repeated heel trauma, which can cause sclerosis of the calcaneus, making it very dense, similar to that which occurs in the pubic symphysis of gymnasts who constantly roll on this structure. In calcaneus sclerosis, standing for more than 10 minutes at a time can be extremely uncomfortable.

Conventional Treatment Approaches for Treatment of Heel Pain

Conventional treatment of heel pain has generally focused on treating the local area of pain, with the use of heel cups and arch supports, steroid injections, nonsteroidal anti-inflammatory drugs (NSAID), physical therapy, and night splints. Cortisone injections into the region of the medial tubercle of the calcaneus (Fig. 15-2), especially when repeated, can result in the irreversible loss of adipose tissue. Heel pain can be treated conservatively for as long as 2 years. If no improvement occurs, surgical treatment is considered, but only after the patient is fully advised about the potential risks (9). When partial fasciotomy is performed, the medial column stability is compromised, and the arch structures from the first metatarsal through the first cuneiform to the talus tend to collapse. Other potential complications of surgery include infection and nerve and blood vessel damage (9).

A MYOFASCIAL APPROACH TO THE DIAGNOSIS AND TREATMENT OF HEEL AND ARCH PAIN

Foot biomechanics. The biomechanical function of the foot must be understood to appreciate the effectiveness of the myofascial and mechanical approach to heel and arch pain. Knowledge of the anatomy of the foot, and an understanding of the effect of repetitive forces on the foot, are also important. Twenty-six bones are found in the foot, with multiple joints that are involved in normal foot function. The functions of four of these joints are critical to normal mechanics of gait: the ankle, subtalar, midtarsal, and the first metatarsal phalangeal joint (MPJ). The main function of the MPJ is proprioceptive, but it is also involved in propulsion. Furthermore, Travell and Simons note that a second metatarsal bone that is longer than the first metatarsal bone is a significant destabilizing factor causing eversion and pronation of the foot, and trigger point formation in the peroneus longus, the vastus medialis, and the gluteus medius muscles (10).

An important key to understanding the myofascial approach is the realization that pain referred from trigger points in proximal muscles can cause pain in distal muscles, in this case, in the heel and the arch of the foot. For example, Imamura et al. (11) accelerated the recovery of plantar fasciitis by treating trigger points in the leg muscles (gastrocnemius, soleus, and posterior tibialis muscles) (11) (see Figs. 14-13 and 15-3). Moreover, the treatment of heel and arch pain can be further enhanced by addressing the intrinsic muscles of the foot, including the flexor digitorum brevis, abductor digiti minimi, flexor hallucis brevis, abductor hallucis, and quadratus plantae muscles (Figs. 15-4–15-7). The intrinsic foot muscles stretch across the metatarsal phalangeal and midtarsal joints and are intimately involved in the function of the ankle and subtalar joints. Treatment of the trigger points in the intrinsic foot muscles and correction of the mechanics of gait as well as treatment of trigger points in the calf, knee, hip, and lower back muscles constitutes comprehensive management.

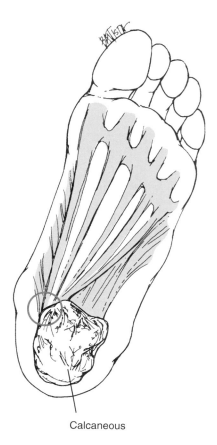

Calcaneous

FIGURE 15-2. Anatomic representation of the insertion of the plantar fascia at the medial tuberosity of the calcaneus (circled).

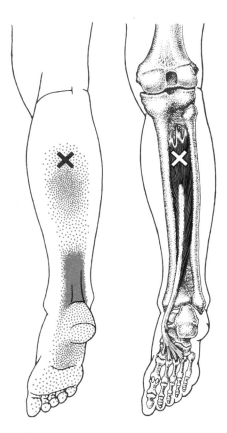

FIGURE 15-3. Posterior tibial trigger points and referred pain pattern. Reprinted with permission from Travell JG, Simons DG: Myofascial Pain and Dysfunction: The Trigger Point Manual, vol 2: The Lower Extremities. Baltimore: Lippincott Williams & Wilkins, 1993 (fig. 23.1), p. 461.

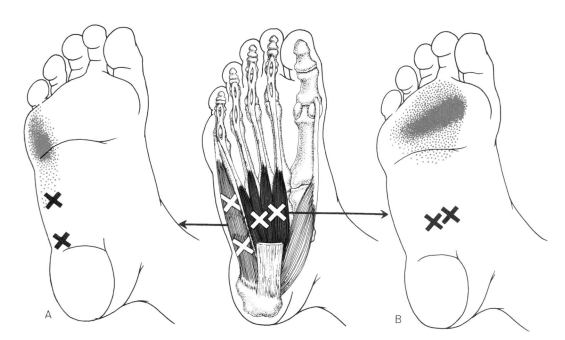

FIGURE 15-4. Abductor digiti minimi and flexor digitorum brevis trigger points and referral patterns. Reprinted with permission from Travell JG, Simons DG: Myofascial Pain and Dysfunction: The Trigger Point Manual, vol 2: The Lower Extremities. Baltimore: Lippincott Williams & Wilkins, 1993 (fig. 26.3), p. 505.

394

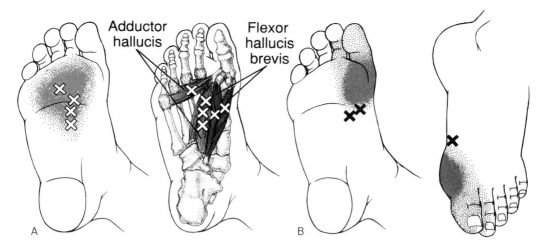

FIGURE 15-5. **Adductor hallucis and flexor hallucis brevis trigger points and referred pain patterns.**
Reprinted with permission from Travell JG, Simons DG: Myofascial Pain and Dysfunction: The Trigger Point Manual, vol 2: The Lower Extremities. Baltimore: Lippincott Williams & Wilkins, 1993 (fig. 27.2), p. 524.

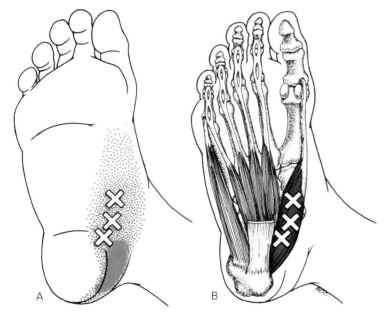

FIGURE 15-6. **Abductor hallucis trigger points and referred pain pattern.** Reprinted with permission from Travell JG, Simons DG: Myofascial Pain and Dysfunction: The Trigger Point Manual, vol 2: The Lower Extremities. Baltimore: Lippincott Williams & Wilkins, 1993 (fig. 26.2), p. 504.

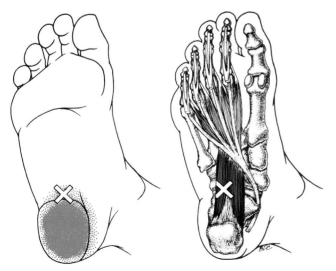

FIGURE 15-7. **Quadratus plantae trigger points and referred pain pattern.** Reprinted with permission from Travell JG, Simons DG: Myofascial Pain and Dysfunction: The Trigger Point Manual, vol 2: The Lower Extremities. Baltimore: Lippincott Williams & Wilkins, 1993 (fig. 27.1), p. 523.

CASE 15-1

Patient History

Mr. R.B., aged 45 years, complained of a painful left heel of gradually increasing severity for the past 3 months, with no history of trauma. He owned a fish store and spent 14-hour workdays standing on hard tile floors. He wore hard rubber boots or construction shoes while at work.

His medical history included obesity and hypertension. He was treated with a beta blocker for his hypertension.

Symptoms

Mr. R.B. complained of a throbbing ache in his left heel and arch that worsened when he first stood on getting out of bed, or on arising after long periods of sitting or resting. It took approximately 5 minutes to "walk-out" the pain. Pain decreased after walking but increased at the end of the day. He noticed no changes in the appearance of the left foot when he was in pain. Although he was self-medicating with nonprescription NSAIDs, he experienced no relief. He also bought over-the-counter innersoles, but experienced no relief using them.

Examination Findings

He was morbidly obese. The neurologic and vascular function of the lower extremity was intact. His shoes were significantly worn on the medial aspect of the heel, and under the first metatarsal phalangeal joint. He had mild **genu valgum** (knock-knees), **genu recurvatum** and early heel lift-off, with bilateral foot eversion. There was no swelling, redness, or sign of infection. There was callus along the medial aspects of the heel and great toe interphalangeal joints bilaterally. Hamstring, gastrocnemius, and soleus muscles were tight bilaterally. Dorsiflexion of the foot with the knee fully extended was limited. Severe tenderness was elicited by palpation of the medial longitudinal arch and at the medial calcaneal tuberosity, indicating trigger point involvement of the abductor hallucis muscle.

X-rays showed that he had inferior calcaneal spurs (heel spurs) bilaterally.

Diagnoses

Diagnoses included heel spur syndrome, myofascial pain syndrome of the abductor hallucis muscle with tenderness of the proximal plantar fascia, ankle equinus, genu recurvatum and genu valgum.

Treatment

Trigger point injections (local anesthetics) were performed at the point of maximum tenderness within the muscle belly of the abductor hallucis muscle. On the same visit, Campbell's rest strapping with **Low-dye** was applied. Orthopaedic felt, 1/8-inch, was applied within the strapping to the longitudinal arch to correct the gait. Half-inch felt heel lifts also were provided to be worn in his work shoes. These measures were taken to prevent foot movements that would reactivate the pain. The strapping was to be worn for at least 4 to 5 days, up to 1 week. He was instructed to purchase a well-fitting wedged athletic shoe with a removable innersole, a firm heel counter, a wide toe box, and a 3/4- to 1-inch heel height.

Follow-up

After wearing the strapping and the athletic shoe for 1 week, he reported a 50% decrease in symptoms. Plaster casts were made of his feet, non–weight-bearing, the feet placed in a neutral position, for full-length custom-made foot orthoses (Technique 15-1). Trigger point injections were again performed into the abductor hallucis muscle. Strapping of the foot was maintained. This treatment was repeated 1 week later, providing relief until the orthoses were ready. He experienced full resolution of his symptoms 4 weeks after starting treatment. Recovery may have been delayed because he had no time for physical therapy, manual trigger point release, or a self-stretching program. Nevertheless, the patient recovered well and has not required further care.

CASE 15-1 Continued

TECHNIQUE 15-1

Casting for Orthotics

The best results are achieved when casting for orthotics, by having the patient prone with the knees placed on a frontal plane. Using a water-soluble marker, the locations of the cut-out padding on the plantar surface of the foot are outlined. A dotted line is then drawn bisecting the Achilles tendon and then extending down, bisecting the calcaneus (A). When the plaster is applied, the thumb is placed on the fifth MPJ and the foot is gently dorsiflexed and the forefoot adducted to a position in which the dotted line on the Achilles and the center of the calcaneus is straightened rather than at an angle (B). Neutral position of the calcaneus relative to the calf is thus attained, rather than having the foot in either supination or pronation. This position is held until the plaster is dry. The casts are then sent to the lab with instructions to incorporate the cutouts into the orthotic.

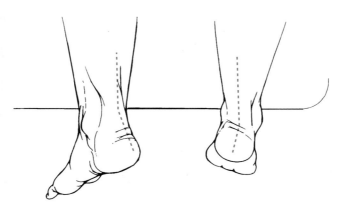

(A) Casting for orthotics. The foot is placed in a neutral position for casting. A line is drawn bisecting the Achilles tendon and calcaneus.

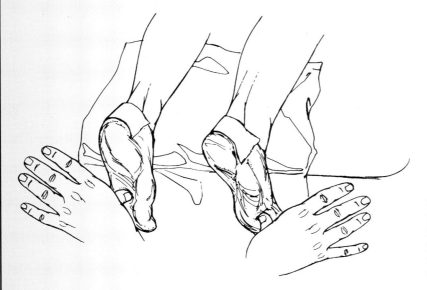

(B) Casting for orthotics. Pressure is placed on the lateral portion of the forefoot to gently dorsiflex and adduct the foot and straighten the line that was drawn. This pressure is held while the casting material sets.

CASE 15-2

Patient History

Ms. L.O., a 55-year-old horse trainer, was thrown from a horse 1 year before evaluation, suffering shoulder and neck injuries for which she was treated. At approximately the same time, when her activities were restricted as she was being treated for neck and shoulder injuries, she developed severe pain in her right heel. Several months later, she started to have pain in the left heel as well, but less severe.

Symptoms

Her heel pain occurred on arising in the morning, or after being seated for a period.

Examination Findings

She was a well-nourished white woman, 5'5" tall, weighing 125 pounds. Her gait was abnormal because of accommodation to bilateral painful heels. Pain was elicited on palpation of the right foot at the medial aspect of the heel a little more than 2 inches from the plantar aspect, at the plantar fascia (with the greatest pain at the origin of the plantar fascia at the calcaneal tuberosity) and at the insertion of the posterior tibial tendon at the first cuneiform-navicular joint. Palpation of the left foot elicited pain at the medial aspect of the heel in the area of the abductor hallucis, and at the plantar fascia. There was tenderness in the fibulocalcaneal areas bilaterally as well as at the dorsolateral aspects of the first metatarsal phalangeal joints bilaterally.

Pain in the right medial heel was quite intense and lasted a few seconds after pressure was released. Range of motion of the knees, ankles, subtalar, midtarsal, and MPJs was within normal limits, and the movement was without crepitus. The right medial heel was warm.

The first metatarsal phalangeal joint was dropped and malaligned along the metatarsal arch with the other MPJs, when non–weight-bearing. She had moderate **pes cavus.** Maximum dorsiflexion of the foot at the ankle, with the knees fully extended, was greatly diminished.

Diagnoses

Diagnoses included Baxter's neuritis of the right foot, bilateral plantar fasciitis, and bilateral functional hallucis limitus.

Treatment

Nerve block of the right calcaneal branch of the posterior tibial nerve was done with solution of 40 mg triamcinolone, 1,000 μg cyanocobalamin, and 2% lidocaine (no epinephrine), in a total volume of 5 mL (Technique 15-2). The left foot was not injected.

The feet were immobilized by using a modified Campbell's rest strap and Low-dye strapping with the addition of a 1/4-inch adhesive foam heel lift. In addition, the forefoot weight bearing was altered by adding a 1/8-inch metatarsal padding with a cut-out at the first metatarsal phalangeal joint. The forefoot padding followed the parabola of the second, third, and fourth MPJs and did not include the fifth MPJ. The whole was then reinforced with additional (overlapping by 1/2 inch), 1-inch micropore tape, starting from heel going forward to just distal to the MPJs.

She was instructed on moderate stretching exercises. The stretches included gastrocnemius and soleus stretches, which are described later.

The patient was told to take one dose of an over-the-counter NSAID and one acetaminophen two to three times daily. She left the office without pain, saying that she was able to walk with no pain for the first time in a year. She returned 1 week later and was restrapped after the application of ultrasound. One week later, still asymptomatic, she was casted for orthoses that were given to her 2 weeks later.

Follow-up

She has continued the stretching exercises and remained generally pain-free, unless there is a change in the barometric pressure.

CASE 15-2   Continued

TECHNIQUE 15-2

Injection Procedures Adapted for the Foot

The most painful part of the injection procedure is the penetration of the skin. The beveled hypodermic needle has a cutting edge. A thinner needle is easier to insert. A 25-gauge needle is routinely used. After cleansing, the skin is pulled taut over the area to be injected, such that the normal dermal topography is smoothed. Then, with the bevel of the needle facing upward, the skin is approached at a 30° to 40° angle. With a short stabbing motion, the skin is penetrated. Injecting the bottom of the foot should be avoided as much as possible, because such a procedure is extremely painful and generally is unnecessary. Injection is almost always done through the dorsum of the foot. If a particular area cannot be accessed directly in this fashion, then a weal of anesthesia can be raised near the intended injection site on the plantar surface of the foot, and an injection is performed through the weal, thus reducing plantar injection pain.

A nerve block for Baxter's neuritis is performed in a similar manner:

1. Using a 1.5-inch 25-gauge needle, a small weal of medication is placed subcutaneously to anesthetize the skin.

2. A small amount of the 5 mL liquid is released approximately every 1/4 to 3/8 inch as the needle is advanced. As the muscles relax, it becomes easier to inject along the course of the nerve.

Comment: The gradual nature of the injection procedure, and the distribution of the medication during the procedure, are tolerated much better than injecting more quickly and deeply and then injecting a large bolus of liquid in tissues around the nerve, where there is already local edema.

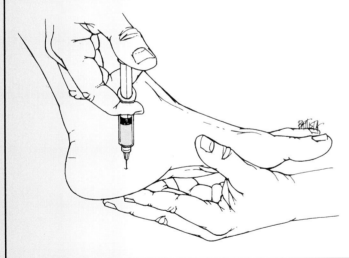

Injection procedure for abductor hallucis. The injection site is on the medial portion of the foot, but the needle is directed to the structures to be treated in the plantar region of the foot, in this case near the medial calcaneal tubercle.

An Overview of the Treatment of Heel and Arch Pain

The clinician must understand the normal mechanics of gait to treat heel pain and plantar fasciitis effectively. The patient's history serves to indicate the factor(s) that brought on the heel pain. The examination shows the abnormal foot mechanics that perpetuate the irritation of the structures involved in the pain.

The importance of a thorough medical history cannot be overstated. A careful exploration of the chief complaint should lead the clinician to tentative diagnoses even before the examination and x-rays are performed. A patient who has seen multiple specialists and primary care providers presents a particular challenge. The patient's description of her medical history and symptoms may be colored by the opinions of the practitioners she has previously seen.

The clinician should take care not to overlook information of great importance when obtaining the history (Box 15-1). Can the patient connect the onset of pain to a particular time or to specific activities? The type of shoe the patient wears is extremely important. For example, an elderly patient with foot pain may wear a sturdy, comfortable, extra-depth shoe with a shock-absorbing sole when going to the store or doctor's office. However, most of the day may be spent wearing flimsy slippers or walking barefoot at home. The patient who wears expensive shoes may not be pleased to learn that they provide little support or cushioning. A woman may complain of pain, because she wears a size 7 shoe when she really needs a size 8. Her foot may have changed size or shape over the years, developing **hammer toes** or **hallux abducto valgus.**

Knowledge of the occupational stresses on the patient's feet is often essential to crafting a workable treatment plan. The foot stresses for the postal worker or waiter are much different from those of the secretary or cab driver.

Normal Foot Mechanics During Gait

Gait encompasses essentially three phases: heel strike, stance, and toe-off. The heel should strike the ground in a supinated position of approximately 15°. Then, as the body moves forward, the weight is directed through the lateral heel to the fifth metatarsal base. The foot then moves into its pronatory phase, with the weight-bearing transferred from the lateral to the medial side of the foot through the midtarsal bones: from the fifth metatarsal tubercle to the cuboid, navicular, 3, 2, 1 cuneiforms, and then into the metatarsal bones. This constitutes the stance phase.

The toe-off phase involves a shift from pronation to supination as propulsion is achieved. Disorders result if the shift from pronation to supination fails to occur, because inordinate and pathologic stresses occur along the medial col-

---

> **BOX 15-1**
>
> ### History Taking for Foot and Arch Pain
>
> **A. Shoe Gear: Work, Home, Sporting/Recreational Activities**
>
> - Recent change in type of shoe gear
> - Patient's perception of good-quality shoes
> - Patient's perception of fit of shoe gear
>
> **B. Occupational Concerns**
>
> - Office/desk work
> - Long periods of standing or walking
> - Type of flooring: carpet, tile, cement, dirt
>
> **C. Environmental Concerns**
>
> - Wet, damp, cold, hot
> - Suburb, city
> - Ladders, clutch (standard shift)
>
> **D. Quality of Pain**
>
> - Burning, pins and needles, deep ache, sharp stabbing, dull ache
>
> **E. Occurrence of Pain**
>
> - Acute or gradual; trauma repeated over time
> - Constant or intermittent
> - Post-static dyskinesia
> - Pain at rest (burn off, night cramps)
> - Pain with weight-bearing
> - What increases or relieves pain

---

umn of the foot. The foot must accommodate to the pathologic forces, which can cause weakening of the talonavicular joints and subtalar joints. The entire limb has to be abducted without the redirection of stress from pronation to supination, As a result, pathologic weight-bearing is placed on the medial aspect of the heel, with resultant shearing forces at the origin of the structures emanating from the medial tubercle of the calcaneus. The fascia and the tendons of the intrinsic muscles will start to pull away from their calcaneal origin. This force is similar to an avulsion fracture, but gradual, in a cumulative microtrauma time frame.

The stretching and weakening of the medial plantar structures causes vascular, neurologic, and musculoskeletal injuries, including the posterior tibial tendon and nerve. The superficial branch of the lateral plantar branch of the posterior tibial nerve that innervates the flexor digiti minimi has been termed **Baxter's nerve** (Fig. 15-8). Baxter's nerve passes from medial to lateral deep to the origin of the plantar fascia. This branch of the nerve becomes inflamed and can become entrapped, requiring decompression.

The pathologic pronatory force occurs because of the impact of the short posterior muscle groups. The gastrocnemius and soleus muscles stretch as the body weight passes over the foot. When this muscle complex reaches its normative reflex length, it contracts and effects heel lift. This occurs when the body has moved over the foot to the midtarsal and midmetatarsal area of the foot, at stance phase. Anatomy and function are herein linked. The gastrocnemius muscle originates on the femur above the knee and inserts with the soleus muscle on the calcaneus, so that it crosses both the knee and the ankle joints. The plantar fascia arises from the calcaneus and inserts into the forefoot, spanning the subtalar joint and

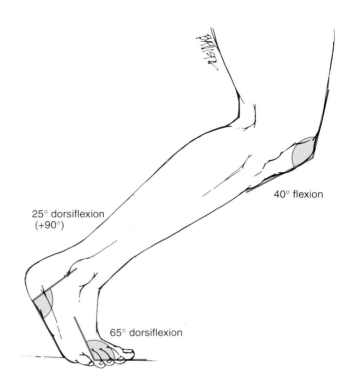

FIGURE 15-9. Range of motion at the knee, ankle, and first metatarsal–phalangeal joint required for normal gait. Forty degrees of flexion is required at the knee, and 25° of dorsiflexion (beyond 90° involved in normal stance) at the ankle, as well as 65° of dorsiflexion at the forefoot, are necessary for normal gait.

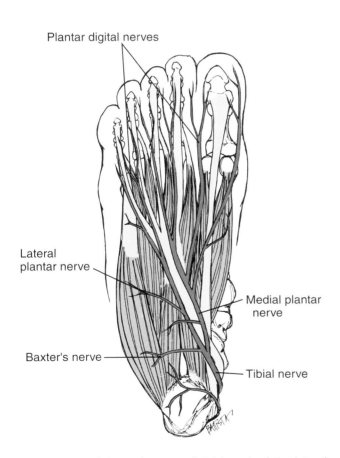

FIGURE 15-8. Calcaneal or superficial branch of the lateral plantar branch of the posterior tibial nerve: Baxter's nerve. Reprinted with permission from Hendrickson T. Massage for Orthopedic Conditions. Baltimore: Lippincott Williams & Wilkins, 2003 (fig. 9-3), p. 332.

midtarsal areas. As the Achilles tendon is activated, force is transmitted through the plantar fascia and associated structures to the first metatarsal–phalangeal joint. Sixty-five degrees of dorsiflexion of the first MPJ is required for normal function with the foot in a horizontal plane. Forty degrees of flexion is required at the knee for normal gait. Twenty-five degrees of additional dorsiflexion at the ankle also must be available to have normal mobility during walking, beyond the 90° angle between the foot and the shin that already exists when standing on a flat surface (Fig. 15-9). The foot becomes locked if the posterior muscle group contracts before the foot is in the stance phase, as the subtalar joint is ready to transmit the weight from the leg into the midtarsal joints and then to the first MPJ. When the foot is locked in this manner, the first MPJ cannot dorsiflex as in normal toe-off during forward gait. At this point, the foot, and hence the entire limb, must abduct and evert abnormally to accommodate the restriction of motion at the first metatarsal–phalangeal joint, thereby increasing the risk of developing myofascial trigger points, arthritis, tendinitis, and neuritis of the leg, knee, hip, spine, shoulder, and neck regions. When the lower limb is abnormally abducted and everted, the first MPJ bears weight on its medial instead of its plantar aspect. Medial weight-bearing on this joint is destabilizing and often causes bunions and hammer toes. In addition, the subtalar joint and the midtarsal joints tend to collapse and create flat feet. The posterior tibialis tendon can become tethered around the tibial malleolus and may cause posterior tibialis tenosynovitis and possible tendon rupture. The medial aspect of the knee can become compressed, stretching the lateral structures of the knee to damage and tear the menisci. The pelvis tilts because of a rotation shift of the iliac bone. There is increased pressure at the posterior aspect of the hip through excessive engagement of the femur and the acetabulum that can lead to erosion of the hip joint cartilage. Lumbar lordosis is accentuated, with accompanying disc compression. Kyphosis is accentuated; the shoulders are displaced forward, resulting in forward head posture, increased cervical lordosis, and increased cervical muscular strain. This abnormal accommodation pattern occurs more frequently in women than men, because of the wider female pelvis.

Treatment of the locked foot involves delaying heel lift until later in gait. Elevating the heel has the same effect as lengthening the posterior muscle group. By delaying its contraction and heel lift, the first MPJ is allowed to dorsiflex at the appropriate time. With the heel raised, the knee needs to bend less than 40° and the ankle less than 25°. Therefore, the first MPJ will need less than 65° of motion at toe-off.

Causes

Heel pain and arch pain result from accumulated stresses of improper foot mechanics. Generally, no specific inciting event or incident is found. However, sometimes the patient can identify a precipitating factor, such as walking barefoot on hard surfaces, a change in work activity with increased hours of standing, new shoes, weight gain, the use of a heavy clutch in city driving, the impact of jumping, or a sports injury.

Cautions

The clinician must consider a number of conditions that can produce heel and arch pain in the differential diagnosis during the diagnostic evaluation. There may be fractures of the calcaneus, the navicular, or the adjacent accessory navicular bone. An axial view of the calcaneus may be necessary to identify a sagittal fracture. Bone or soft tissue tumors are among the potential causes. Dupuytren's contracture can cause arch pain. Ankylosing spondylitis can refer pain to both heels. Infections that cause heel pain include gonorrheal septic arthritis and osteomyelitis. Osteomyelitis may produce heel pain, because the calcaneus is the most highly vascularized bone in the foot. Noninfectious arthritis, including rheumatoid arthritis, can cause heel pain as well. Kicking and impact sports can make the calcaneal bone hyperdense, a condition that is

painful itself. Peripheral vascular disease can cause ischemic foot pain felt in the arch area.

Myofascial Entrapments

Baxter's neuritis involves soft tissue entrapment of the calcaneal branch of the posterior tibial nerve. Usually heel pain abates on sitting or lying down, but in the case of Baxter's neuritis, a continued burning pain is present for minutes or hours after sitting or going into a non–weight-bearing position. The pattern of pain on initial weight-bearing is not as consistent as in plantar fasciitis. The point of most exquisite tenderness is not at the medial attachment of the plantar fascia and intrinsic muscles to the medial tubercle of the calcaneus, but rather is deeper and dorsal to the abductor hallucis, in the location of Baxter's nerve.

Often tenderness of the more proximal posterior tibial nerve may be present, which is palpable as a thin fibrous cord just posterior to the medial malleolus, when Baxter's neuritis is present. Neuritis of the posterior tibial neuritis can be assessed by eliciting pain through strumming the nerve with the finger or thumbnail (Fig. 15-10). Nerve irritation also can be assessed by putting the nerve on traction. A neurodynamic procedure for this is described by

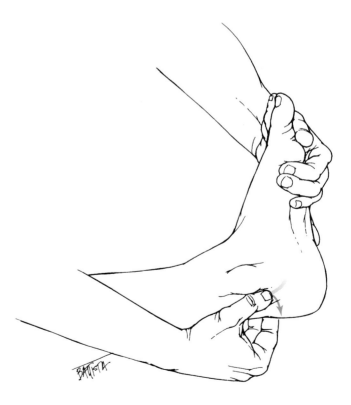

FIGURE 15-10. **The posterior tibial nerve can be palpated (snapped or strummed) posterior to the medial malleolus.** The degree of tenderness can be assessed and comparison can be made between the nerve tenderness at the right and left ankles.

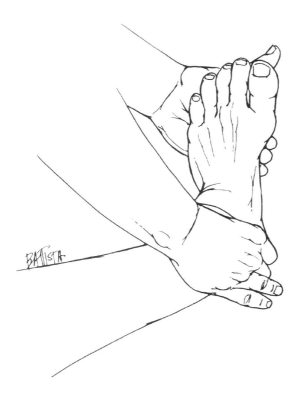

FIGURE 15-11. **Initial position for neurodynamic test of the posterior tibial nerve.** One hand is used to stabilize the talus so that movement takes place around this fulcrum. The other hand draws the medial foot and ankle into a position of dorsiflexion that places the posterior tibial nerve at maximal tension. The position required is with the outer foot dorsiflexed more than the inner foot. The next step is the introduction of straight-leg raising to assess whether the specific distal tension on the nerve alters the sensation compared with neutral dorsiflexion combined with straight-leg raising.

Butler and involves dorsiflexing the lateral aspect of the foot more than the medial, while holding the talus firmly in one hand as the pivot point, the patient lying supine (Fig. 15-11). When the slack has been taken up along the course of the posterior tibial nerve, then the leg is elevated as in the straight leg raising test. This generally will elicit significant discomfort when there is symptomatic nerve compression or neuritis. Discomfort is not present when the same procedure is performed with the foot dorsiflexed without medial foot tilt (12). (Note the sequence of movement. Performing the straight-leg raising first and then adding foot dorsiflexion is not a diagnostic test for peripheral nerve irritation or entrapment.) When both posterior tibial nerve and Baxter's nerve neuritis are present, treatment should address multiple sites of possible nerve entrapment.

Examination

Knowledge of muscle anatomy is essential to diagnose a restriction of joint motion caused by muscle dysfunction, and then to properly treat the appropriate muscle. Functional muscle anatomy is learned through the repeated examination of many patients. When confronted with a muscle identification that is in doubt, ask the patient to activate the muscle against resistance. Knowledge of the action of a particular muscle will lead to its anatomic identification when the patient performs the known function of that muscle.

The patient is examined while seated with the legs extended comfortably, and the posture of the foot is evaluated.

An arch is usually present in this position, even if the patient is flat-footed on weight-bearing. A very high arch as seen in **pes cavus** complicates foot biomechanics.

Movement patterns of the foot are evaluated by gently guiding the foot through normal movement and feeling for patterns of resistance. For example, the ankle is dorsiflexed and the talus is supported to avoid either pronation or supination. At the end of motion, it is possible to assess whether the great toe can extend sufficiently at the MPJ to allow for proper roll-through or toe-off. Normal medial subtalar roll is 20°, and lateral roll is 10°. Either muscle or joint dysfunction may be restrictive, but the result is the same in terms of abnormal gait patterns.

Mechanical stress is transmitted to numerous areas when the foot everts. This is seen as tenderness at the first MPJ, the lateral malleolus, the calcaneus joint, and the medial plantar aspect of the heel, including the medial tubercle of the calcaneus. Beaking (upward prominence) occurs at the first metatarsal–cuneiform joint. Improper foot mechanics also place stress on the knee, hip, and lower back, and in some cases contribute to problems up the spinal axis to the shoulder and neck, resulting in headache, neck, and shoulder pain.

The dorsalis pedis and posterior tibial pulses are palpated to determine whether peripheral vascular disease is present. One of the most common causes of heel and arch pain is functional limitation of the gastrocnemius and soleus muscle unit movement, affecting motion at the first MPJ. Although often separated into various segments, they function as a single unit in gait. The range of motion across each joint involved in gait is assessed. The knee joint is evaluated to see whether it can flex to at least 40°; the ankle is assessed to see whether it can dorsiflex at least 25°; and the first MPJ is checked to see whether it can dorsiflex at least 65° (see Fig. 15-9). If restriction is present at any of these joints, abnormal accommodation results, and excessive stresses on joint and soft tissue structures can be induced.

An easy way to assess overall shortening of the gastrocnemius–soleus muscle complex that affects the first MPJ is to have the patient stand with the foot everted 15°. In this position, the patient attempts to elevate the great toe. If the digit cannot be elevated from the horizontal plane, it should be assumed that the first MPJ will not function normally during gait.

The following are common causes of the limitation of motion of the gastrocnemius–soleus muscle unit just described:

- Pain at the dorsolateral aspect of the first MPJ

- Entrapment neuralgia of the deep peroneal nerve

- Plantar capsulitis of the second MPJ

- Tibial sesamoiditis

- Bursitis of the fifth MPJ

- Posterior tibial tenosynovitis

Observation of gait can uncover excessive supination, or the more common pronation. There may be early heel lift-off because of shortened posterior calf muscles.

The plantar surface of the foot is examined for a tight and tender band of fascia located under the medial portion of the foot that attaches to the heel. Underneath this taut fascia are the flexor hallucis brevis, the abductor hallucis, and the other intrinsic muscles of the foot. These muscles are assessed for tenderness and the presence of taut bands and trigger points. If the pain and tenderness are altered by palpation of these trigger points, then the patient probably suffers from a treatable myofascial disorder of the intrinsic muscles of the foot.

The gastrocnemius and soleus muscles are palpated for taut bands and trigger points. The posterior tibialis muscle and tendon are also palpated in the calf, ankle, and foot for trigger points and for tenderness of the tendon, which may be tender and swollen. When there is significant swelling in the tendon sheath, it can be visualized by magnetic resonance imaging (MRI).

Joint function also is evaluated for restriction and tenderness. Three somatic dysfunctions or subluxations appear to have the most effect on heel pain (Fig. 15-12). They are: 1) anterior positioning or restriction of the posterior glide of the talus; 2) dropping at the first cuneiform–navicular joint; 3) posterior positioning or restriction of the posterior-to-anterior joint play at the calcaneus.

Restriction of posterior glide at the talus often results from a sprain of the ankle, and it is most readily assessed by

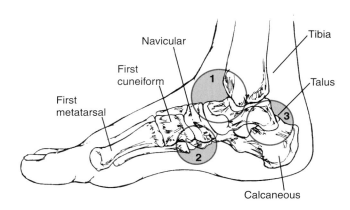

FIGURE 15-12. **Three common sites of joint restriction.** 1) Talus may be anterior (reduced posterior glide). 2) First cuneiform-navicular joint may drop rather than maintaining the curve of the arch. 3) The calcaneus may be posterior (reduced anterior glide).

palpating across the talus for resistance while dorsiflexing the foot at the ankle. Restriction of dorsiflexion of the foot limits the ability to achieve full stretch of the gastrocnemius–soleus muscle unit.

A plantar-displaced cuneiform–navicular joint can be palpated as a bony resistance underneath the medial border of the plantar fascia, just distal to the highest portion of the medial longitudinal arch. A tender prominence can be palpated in this location when this subluxation is present. Tenderness also will be present if there is tenosynovitis of the posterior tibialis tendon.

The calcaneus often becomes hypomobile in a posterior direction as a result of impact while jumping. The hypomobility increases the longitudinal tension on the plantar fascia and intrinsic muscles. The posterior displacement is most readily palpated with the ankle somewhat flexed but not at the end of the range of motion, because the full tension at the Achilles tendon will obscure the subtle changes in joint mobility.

Footwear is also examined, especially the well-worn shoe. Is the patient always in high heels? Is the shoe too rigid, with no give? Does the shoe lack support? Can it be twisted and bent easily? Has the heel counter broken down? Lateral wear to the heel is normal, but medial wear usually indicates a shortened gastrocnemius–soleus muscle unit that results in eversion and pronation of the foot very early in the gait cycle.

X-rays may show a calcaneal spur, and an MRI of the ankle can show abnormalities of the joint and of the tendons.

Treatment

Treatment is directed toward restoration and maintenance of normal foot biomechanics. To achieve this, the muscle must be treated to eliminate myofascial trigger points, and the muscle must be restored to its full length. Once this is accomplished, muscle strength and function is likely to be restored to normal, eliminating muscle-related restrictions of joint movement. Consequently, attention must be directed to muscle early in the treatment sequence. However, both nerve entrapments and joint mechanics must be treated. In practice, treatment often proceeds along the several lines of muscle, nerve, and joint therapy simultaneously.

Manual Myofascial Treatment

The manual therapist learns from the fact that injection or dry needling of calf and intrinsic foot muscle trigger points inactivates them and enhances restoration of normal muscle function and reduces pain, that manual techniques that achieve similar inactivation of trigger points can result in similar improvement in heel and arch pain.

Manual releases are often performed in two stages within the same treatment visit when there is a significant heel, arch, and calf tenderness. Initial releases tend to be gentle and modest and are performed along with increasing the range of motion of the affected joint, and then moist heat is applied. Afterward, a more rigorous regimen of myofascial release is administered, which is better tolerated because pretreatment tenderness is reduced.

Initial releases are performed with the patient in the prone position. To treat the trigger points in the intrinsic foot muscles, the knee is flexed, and pressure is lightly applied to them while the ankle and the toes are simultaneously dorsiflexed (Fig. 15-13). Treatment is extended proximally up the leg to the calf muscles. Dorsiflexion of the ankle is maintained while moderate pressure is placed on the trigger points in the soleus and posterior tibialis muscles (Fig. 15-14). The muscle stretch to increase range of motion can be kept static or nonmoving, but it often works better to perform

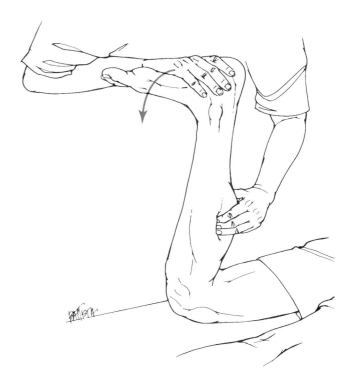

FIGURE 15-14. Myofascial release of trigger points in soleus and posterior tibialis muscles. The patient is prone with the knee flexed. Trigger point pressure release is performed on trigger points within these muscles while rocking the ankle into greater and lesser dorsiflexion to stretch the taut bands of muscle.

the stretch with a slow, rocking motion, while placing gentle pressure on the trigger points. The varying tension makes it easier to ease the fingers onto the taut trigger points. The limb movement seems to be more effective if it is active (performed by the patient) rather than passive (performed by the clinician to the patient). The knee is then straightened while a rocking motion is applied to the ankle. The gastrocnemius muscle is gently contacted and released as gentle pressure is applied to the trigger points (Fig. 15-15). If the trigger points are not releasing well, vapocoolant spray and stretch can be added to this sequence. Percussion technique, described in Chapter 4 (see Technique 4-1) is often useful as well, especially to achieve better release of the most knotted areas of muscle in the arch and calf. Contract-relax-release described in Chapter 11 also can be useful either at this point or later in the treatment sequence. Moist heat is then applied to the calf and arch for 10 minutes.

After the moist heat, a more rigorous release of the intrinsic foot muscle trigger points of the foot is performed with the patient prone, the knee bent 90°, and the foot easily accessible. Moderate tension is placed on the arch by dorsiflexing the ankle and toes, but the tension must not draw the plantar fascia so taut that it makes it difficult to palpate the deeper intrinsic muscles. The medial foot mus-

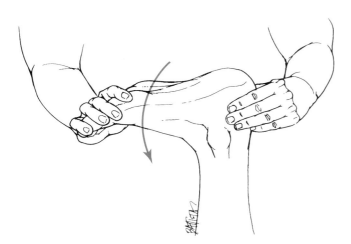

FIGURE 15-13. Myofascial release of trigger points in intrinsic muscles of the foot. The patient is prone with the knee flexed and the ankle dorsiflexed as the clinician stretches the foot muscles by dorsiflexing the forefoot and toes.

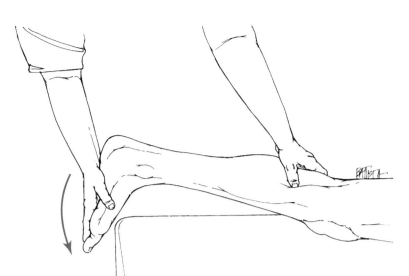

FIGURE 15-15. **Myofascial release of trigger points in the gastrocnemius muscle.** With the patient prone and the knee straight, trigger point pressure release is performed on the gastrocnemius trigger points while rocking the ankle into greater and lesser dorsiflexion, thus stretching the taut bands of muscle.

cles can be palpated medial to and under the medial border of the plantar fascia by inserting a finger under the medial border of the plantar fascia. The central and lateral muscles can be palpated through the plantar fascia. Each muscle can be selectively placed under tension to palpate the trigger points. The abductor digiti minimi muscle is brought to tension by extending (dorsiflexing) the little toe and drawing it slightly medial. The flexor digitorum brevis muscle is brought to tension by extending the middle toes. The flexor hallucis brevis and the abductor hallucis muscles are brought to tension by extending and adducting the big toe, respectively (Fig. 15-16). To treat the quadratus plantae, tension across the arch is reduced slightly to better palpate this deeper muscle. Digital pressure or the flat of the elbow can be used (Fig. 15-17). Percussion is an alternative means of inactivating the trigger points if they are not easily released by direct pressure. It is advantageous to treat the entire length of each of these muscles, even though the trigger points that refer pain to the heel may be quite localized in the muscle. There needs to be adequate compliance and elasticity across the arch, which requires that the entire taut band be relaxed. Taut muscles change the shape of the arch and render it difficult to properly fit orthotics. Myofascial release techniques reduce tenderness in the plantar fascia, and tension in the fascial tissues, because fascial tenderness can be referred from leg and intrinsic foot muscle trigger points. Myofascial release procedures are generally adequate to treat pain thought to arise from heel spurs or from the plantar fascia, even after other treatment procedures failed.

The patient is prone, and the knee is straightened to perform the deeper release work on the soleus, posterior tibialis, and gastrocnemius muscles. The ankle is taken through varying degrees of dorsiflexion while pressure is ap-

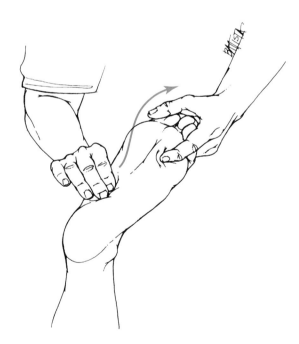

FIGURE 15-16. **Myofascial release of trigger points in flexor hallucis brevis and adductor hallucis.** The patient is prone with the knee flexed and the ankle dorsiflexed. The clinician presses on the intrinsic muscles under the medial border of the plantar fascia, while extending and adducting the big toe.

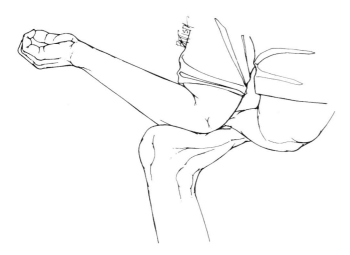

FIGURE 15-17. Myofascial release of trigger points in quadratus plantae. The patient is prone with the knee flexed and the ankle dorsiflexed. The clinician applies deep pressure with the flat of the elbow to the tender trigger points, while the forefoot is slightly dorsiflexed.

plied to the trigger points in the leg muscles. The proximal trigger point in the medial head of the gastrocnemius is often one of the most difficult trigger points to release; however, its referral pattern to the arch and heel makes it important to treat. Percussion can be used in addition to direct trigger point compression. The patient is asked to actively dorsiflex and release the ankle while pressure is applied to this trigger point.

If the trigger point is not releasing well, it is best to approach it from a different position. The supine position is assumed. The patient's foot is placed against the clinician's chest or abdomen and dorsiflexed to a varying degree to gently stretch the calf muscles, while trigger point compression is applied. To obtain a good release where the muscles converge on the Achilles tendon, apply digital pressure to the most anterior aspect of the muscles that can be palpated and apply traction posteriorly, away from the tibia and fibula (Fig. 15-18). The combination of an anterior and a posterior approach to the calf muscles, with the patient prone and then supine, often accomplishes better trigger point inactivation than would be possible with either approach alone. As these muscles are elongated, and the mechanics of calcaneal and talar function are addressed as needed, the range of motion at the ankle is often improved, and the stresses inherent in the gait cycle are dramatically reduced. This may take several visits to accomplish.

When symptomatic trigger points are present in the posterior tibial muscle, inactivating them helps to restore normal muscle length and reduce tendon strain. If the tendon has been strained, the foot may need to be immobilized for a time to allow the tendon to heal. Although some conventional treatment involves placing the foot in a non–

weight-bearing cast for 3 months, the ensuing restriction of motion can require physical therapy after the cast is removed to restore normal mobility.

A variation of the supine releases can be used to relieve pressure on the posterior tibialis nerve and its distal segment, Baxter's nerve. Myofascial releases 3 and 4 are described in Chapter 6 along with the rationale for this technique. The posterior tibial nerve lies between the posterior tibialis muscle and the soleus muscle, along with the posterior tibial artery and vein. It then passes posteriorly to the medial malleolus. The tender nerve is found slightly distal to the insertion of the intrinsic muscles and to the plantar fascia at the medial calcaneal tubercle. The nerve is higher in the arch than the tubercle. After the nerve is located, the intrinsic foot muscles across the arch are placed in a slightly shortened position, and then the muscles and nerve are elongated passively (MR3) or actively (MR4) while contact is maintained (Fig. 15-19). This is repeated three to four times. Then the tender nerve is then traced more proximally, and this same release procedure is performed every 1/2-inch or so along the course of the nerve (Fig. 15-20).

Often a burning pain is felt as the nerve is palpated. The calf muscles are relaxed and then the muscles and the nerve are passively or actively stretched three to four times with the clinician maintaining contact at each stop along the course of the nerve. Occasionally, nerve compression starts as high as the piriformis muscle. That needs to be addressed as well. Some lingering burning may be present along the course of the nerve for several hours after this treatment.

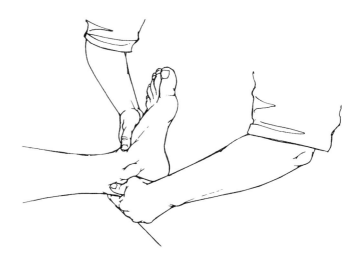

FIGURE 15-18. Supine myofascial release of trigger points in the soleus, gastrocnemius, and posterior tibialis. The patient's foot is against the clinician's chest or abdomen. The clinician applies trigger point pressure release and also can perform localized tissue traction along the entire length of the muscles. In the Achilles tendon area, the clinician applies trigger point pressure release from anterior-to-posterior on the front portion of the musculotendinous juncture.

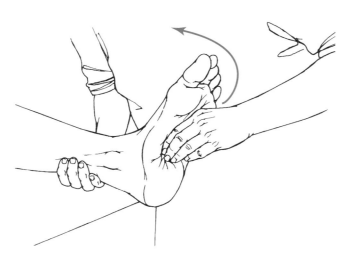

FIGURE 15-19. Myofascial release techniques 3 (passive stretch) and 4 (active stretch) are performed to mobilize the distal portion of the posterior tibial nerve: Baxter's nerve. The clinician's active contact is in the arch, more dorsal and higher in the arch than the calcaneal tubercle. Initially the foot is relaxed, and then it is dorsiflexed and pronated to stretch the tissues entrapping the nerve. The stretch during contact is repeated three or four times.

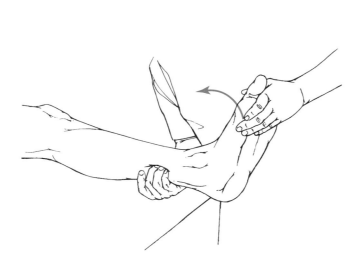

FIGURE 15-20. Myofascial releases 3 and 4 to mobilize the posterior tibial nerve in the calf. The clinician contacts the points along a line in the medial calf that are tender and often burning on contact. Initially the foot and ankle are relaxed. Contact is maintained while the nerve is stretched by dorsiflexing at the ankle and pronating the foot, passively or actively. This is repeated three or four times for each contact on the medial calf. Multiple points of contact are treated, by advancing the contact up the medial calf a few centimeters at a time, until the whole extent of the nerve in the calf has been treated.

However, patients often experience dramatic relief of what had been very chronic pain.

Other Aspects of Treatment

Treatment also includes correcting the biomechanical fault and addressing the environment within which the foot functions. Shoe gear is corrected, and treatment is prescribed so as to prevent the foot from assuming a range of motion that causes or aggravates the foot or ankle pain. Reassessment is performed on subsequent visits. Padding or strapping is used to correct the biomechanical abnormalities and relieve strain.

Two common types of strapping are Campbell's rest strap with Low-dye (Figs. 15-21 and 15-22) and Kushner's rest strap (Fig. 15-23). In some cases, more immobilization is required, and an Unna boot is used (Fig. 15-24). A 1/8-inch piece of felt is often placed under the heel of the strapping or in the shoe to attenuate the forces to the heel. Trig-

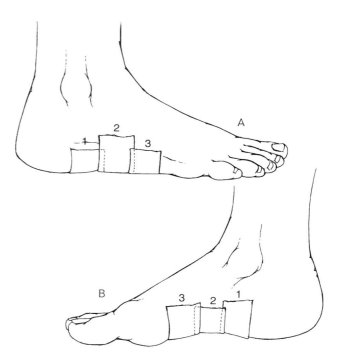

FIGURE 15-21. Campbell's rest strap. This strapping is used to reduce stress on the plantar aspect of the foot. Three of four strips of 1½-inch or 2-inch adhesive strips are used first. The first strip is applied from lateral (A) to medial (B), across the plantar aspect of the foot, starting just below the lateral malleolus, and ending at the top of the navicular, just below the medial malleolus. The next strip is placed distal and parallel to the first and overlaps it by one-third. The third strip and a fourth, if necessary, are placed in a similar fashion, overlapping by one-third, until the plantar aspect of the foot is covered, ending just proximal to the metatarsal heads. Two strips, each of 1-inch tape, are then placed as anchors across the medial and lateral ends of the previous taping.

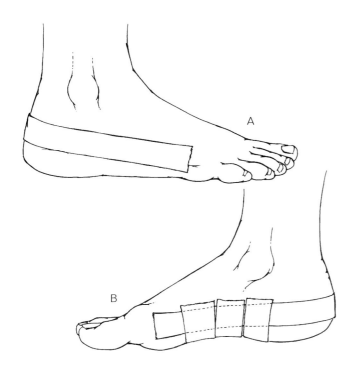

FIGURE 15-22. **Low-dye strapping.** This strapping is used to decrease the strain of pronation. **A.** First a 1-inch strip of adhesive tape is used to apply a heel lock. The tape is first placed at the side of the fifth metatarsal head, and then placed horizontally along the outer side of the foot and is secured around the heel. Before securing the tape to the medial side, the forefoot is adducted slightly and the tape ends at the medial side of the first metatarsal head. This helps to draw the first phalanx and metatarsal toward the midline. **B.** Campbell's Rest Strap, including the horizontal anchors, is applied over the heel lock.

ger point injections can be made into the trigger points identified by physical examination. Other modalities that are useful include continuous-wave ultrasound with zinc oxide cream. This helps to release the tender trigger points. Therapeutic ultrasound should not be performed after trigger point injections, because the patient cannot feel when the ultrasound is turned too high. Ultrasound is also contraindicated if there are screws or pins in the foot. Extracorporeal shock wave therapy also may be helpful. Whirlpool bathing of both feet can be performed for 10 minutes. Contrast baths of 5 minutes of ice alternating with 10 minutes of heat for several repetitions is also very helpful. Some patients appear to benefit from a course of NSAID or acetaminophen. A nerve block can be performed when necessary, when there has been entrapment of Baxter's nerve.

Orthotics often are prescribed for long-term improvement of gait, but it is important to have the foot in a pain-free state before casting for the orthotics. A functional hallucis rigidus must be addressed when present. When manual techniques for increasing range of motion, including myofascial release and manipulation or mobilization of joint restrictions, do not result in sufficient increased range of joint motion to restore normal gait, footwear should have some heel rather than being flat. As described earlier, elevating the heel has the same effect as lengthening the posterior muscle group. Athletic shoes can be selected that have a wedge structure at the heel. The amount of heel required is determined by the degree of movement restriction.

Patient Exercises and Home Care

Home exercises include stretches of the gastrocnemius and soleus muscles (see Fig. 14-16). Check to make sure that the foot is pointing straight forward when the gastrocnemius stretch is performed. Starting from this same position, to stretch the soleus muscle, the posterior knee is flexed and weight is dropped so that the patient goes into a partial squat, but the heel is kept in contact with the floor. In some cases, a plastic assistive device is used to enhance the stretching and enable the patient to target specific portions of the calf muscles (Fig. 15-25). Care must be taken not to overstretch the muscles when using such an assistive device for stretching the gastrocnemius and soleus muscles, especially when initiating the exercise. Another useful exercise is performed with a small weight strapped to the forefoot. The leg is extended and the patient moves as though writing the alphabet in the air, once per day. Calf muscle stretches are performed before and after any of these exercises.

Self-massage is performed as well. To feel the taut intrinsic muscles, one hand draws the muscles to tension by dorsiflexing the ball of the foot away from the heel, until the tender areas can be readily palpated and massaged. Massage of the trigger points in the muscles in the calf is often helpful as well. Self-massage before bedtime may help prevent muscle shortening when not weight-bearing, thereby reducing the pain on standing in the morning.

When the Baxter's nerve has been entrapped, exercises are prescribed to mobilize the entire posterior tibial nerve.

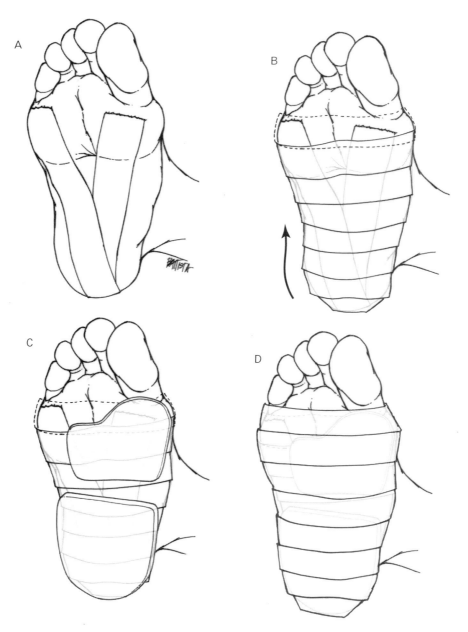

FIGURE 15-23. **Kushner's rest strap. A.** The bottom of the foot is coated with tincture of Benzoin. The patient is seated with the leg perpendicular to the torso, and the foot is brought to a 90° angle with the leg, but without tension. One-inch micropore tape is used to place two strips from the heel to the first and fifth MPJs. **B.** One-inch micropore tape is then applied to the plantar surface of the foot, extending approximately half the thickness of both the medial and lateral sides of the foot, starting at the heel and overlapping from proximal to distal. **C.** Add a 1/4-inch foam heel lift and a 1/8-inch felt modified dancer's pad as shown. The dancer's pad supports the first MPJ, but ends proximal to the second through fourth MPJs and does not extend laterally to the fifth metatarsal. **D.** Overlay the whole with a 1-inch micropore tape from proximal to distal. Finish with one strip of 1-inch micropore tape to reinforce the ends of the previous taping, as a horizontal strip extending along the medial side of the foot, starting at the first MPJ and wrapping around the side and back of the heel and extending along the outside of the foot to the fifth MPJ. Wear for 1 week.

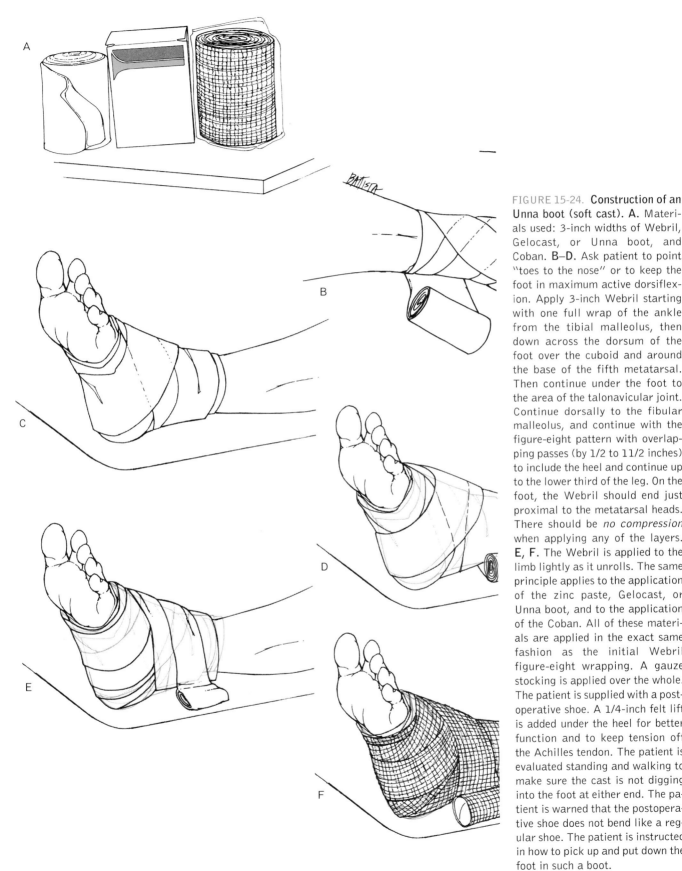

FIGURE 15-24. **Construction of an Unna boot (soft cast). A.** Materials used: 3-inch widths of Webril, Gelocast, or Unna boot, and Coban. **B–D.** Ask patient to point "toes to the nose" or to keep the foot in maximum active dorsiflexion. Apply 3-inch Webril starting with one full wrap of the ankle from the tibial malleolus, then down across the dorsum of the foot over the cuboid and around the base of the fifth metatarsal. Then continue under the foot to the area of the talonavicular joint. Continue dorsally to the fibular malleolus, and continue with the figure-eight pattern with overlapping passes (by 1/2 to 11/2 inches) to include the heel and continue up to the lower third of the leg. On the foot, the Webril should end just proximal to the metatarsal heads. There should be *no compression* when applying any of the layers. **E, F.** The Webril is applied to the limb lightly as it unrolls. The same principle applies to the application of the zinc paste, Gelocast, or Unna boot, and to the application of the Coban. All of these materials are applied in the exact same fashion as the initial Webril figure-eight wrapping. A gauze stocking is applied over the whole. The patient is supplied with a postoperative shoe. A 1/4-inch felt lift is added under the heel for better function and to keep tension off the Achilles tendon. The patient is evaluated standing and walking to make sure the cast is not digging into the foot at either end. The patient is warned that the postoperative shoe does not bend like a regular shoe. The patient is instructed in how to pick up and put down the foot in such a boot.

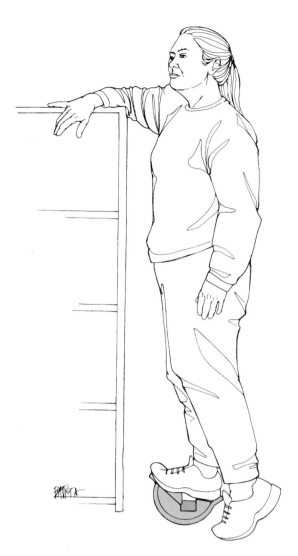

FIGURE 15-25. **Calf stretch with plastic assistive device.** Note that only partial weight is placed on the foot being stretched, and the shoe is on. The foot can be stretched in a neutral position, or the foot can be turned in slightly or turned out slightly to focus the stretch on the medial or lateral portions of the calf muscles. Care must be taken not to overstretch initially, until the tolerance of the tissues to stretch is ascertained.

A strap can be used to dorsiflex the foot, with the lateral side of the foot more dorsiflexed than the medial side, when seated or supine. When seated, the patient leans forward to stretch the entire sciatic/posterior tibial nerve tract. When supine, the patient can take the leg into a straight-leg raising position with the foot dorsiflexed as described. These maneuvers are taken only to the point of slight discomfort, and then the tension is released. The alternating stretch and release procedure is repeated for several minutes at least twice per day. If the patient experiences any increased pain afterwards, the exercise should be performed more gently. The tolerance of the nerve, muscles, and tendons to stretching generally increases gradually over time with repetition of this exercise, and nerve tenderness decreases concomitantly.

The patient also is instructed to wear a shoe at all times when out of bed and not bathing. A shoe with a wedge heel helps to control the gait. Activities that reproduce the stress that brought on the heel pain should be limited. Improvements in the person's work and home environment must be made, such as using a rubber mat on a hard floor surface, or driving a vehicle with a less stiff clutch.

CONCLUSION

A comprehensive approach to treatment of heel and arch pain, including correction of biomechanical factors, correction of the environment of the foot, and treatment of the muscle and tendon dysfunction, can result in rapid relief of pain and prompt restoration of function. The intrinsic muscles of the foot and the calf muscles that refer pain into the arch and heel are the focus of myofascial release techniques that resolve pain often attributed to heel spurs or plantar fasciitis. Furthermore, because the abnormal foot mechanics of a disordered gait affect other structures, including knees, hips, and lower back, addressing foot problems early is essential to dealing with factors that may have been perpetuating chronic or recurrent pain syndromes elsewhere in the body.

TREATMENT PROTOCOL

1. **Correct the biomechanical fault (such as functional hallux limitus and/or excessive pronation).**

2. **Treat the environment within which the foot functions.**

3. **Treat the involved muscles and tendons, including the intrinsic muscles of the foot, the gastrocnemius and soleus muscles, and the posterior tibialis muscle and tendon, and not just the plantar fascia.**

4. **Baxter's nerve also should be evaluated and treated when necessary.**

5. **Normal joint mobility is restored at the talus, the juncture of the navicular and cuneiform, and at the calcaneus.**

References

1. McCarthy D, Gorecki G. The anatomical basis of inferior calcaneal lesions—a cryomicrotomy study. J Am Podiatry Assoc 1979;69:527
2. Zacharie I. Surgical and Practical Observations of the Diseases of the Human Foot. London: Adams Brothers, 1860:47–82.
3. Steindler A, Smith AR. Spurs of the os calcis. Surg Gynecol Obstet 1933;66:663–665.
4. Baer WS. Painful heels. Bull Johns Hopkins Hosp 1905;264.
5. Contompasis JP. Surgical treatment of calcaneal spurs: a three year post-surgical study. J Am Podiatry Assoc 1974;16:264.
6. Lutter LD. Surgical decisions in athlete's subcalcaneal pain. Am J Sports Med 1986;14:481–485.
7. Bergman JN. History and mechanical control of heel spur pain. Clin Podiatr Med Surg 1990;7:243-259.
8. LeMelle DP, Kisilewicz P, Janis LR. Chronic plantar inflammation and fibrosis. Clin Podiatr Med Surg 1990;7:385–389.
9. Dreeben SM, Mann RA. Heel pain: sorting through the differential diagnosis. J Musculoskeletal Med 1992;9:21–37.
10. Travell JG, Simons DG. Myofascial Pain and Dysfunction, vol 2. Baltimore: Williams & Wilkins, 1992:370–396.
11. Imamura M, Fischer AA, Imamura ST, et al. Treatment of myofascial components in plantar fasciitis speeds up recovery: documentation by algometry. J Musculoskel Pain 1998;6:91–110.
12. Butler D. Mobilization of the Nervous System. Melbourne: Churchill Livingstone, 1991:127–146, 161–181.

Glossary

Activator: an impulse-generating tool for correcting joint subluxation and for introducing movement into restricted joints; considered a very-low-force modality

Adhesion: the uniting or sticking together of adjacent surfaces, used here to refer to connective tissues

Adjuvant: a substance used to enhance or potentiate the effect of another substance, generally used in relation to medications

Afferent: arising from the periphery and conducting toward the central, as in peripheral nerve input to the central nervous system

Afferentation: signal transmission from the periphery toward the center

Anterior drawer test: test for the integrity of the anterior and posterior cruciate ligaments and the anterior part of the medial and lateral tibio-meniscal ligaments. With the patient in the supine position and the knees flexed to 90°, the clinician sits on the toes of the patient. The clinician holds the proximal aspect of the tibia with both hands and places the index fingers on the medial and lateral hamstrings and the thumbs on the anterior joint line. The test involves the passive anterior translation of the tibia and is positive when excessive translation is noted.

Aphasia: the loss of learned speech, either loss of expression of thought or understanding, or both

Apley's compression test: test for the integrity of the posterior horns of the medial and lateral meniscus. With the patient in the prone position and the knee flexed to 90°, the clinician applies an axial downward force on the patient's heel with the tibia in either external or internal rotation. The test is positive if the patient complains of pain.

Arthrokinematics: pertaining to the function or movement between adjacent joint surfaces

Ballottement test: test for the presence of retropatellar effusion. With the patient in the supine position with the knee extended, the clinician gently pushes the patella into the femoral trochlear groove. The test is positive if the patella rebounds quickly.

Baxter's nerve: the calcaneal branch of the posterior tibial nerve

Baxter's neuritis: inflammation of Baxter's nerve caused by soft tissue entrapment; produces heel pain that does not subside quickly when not weight-bearing, in contrast to plantar fasciitis

Bechterew's test: seated leg extension of one leg at a time, to evaluate the effects of stretch on the sciatic nerve

Bruxism: clenching and grinding of the teeth, usually during sleep

Canine guidance: closure of teeth guided by the canine teeth

Carpal tunnel syndrome: compression of the median nerve, producing numbness, paresthesias, and sometimes pain, generally occurring during sleep, named for the site (or one of the sites) of compression where the median nerve and vascular structures pass with the flexor tendons of the thumb and fingers through a tunnel formed beneath the flexor retinaculum and over the carpal bones at the wrist or base of the hand

Cavitation: the popping sound produced when joints move or are moved quickly, a vacuum is produced in the joint space, and gases from the surrounding tissue are released into the vacuum

Centric occlusion: the position of the mandible that allows maximal intercuspation or closure of the teeth

Centric relation: the most stable position of the mandibular joint with unstrained condylar position in the mandibular fossa

Cervical lateral break: a lateral break performed on segments of the cervical spine

Class I occlusion: neutral occlusion

Class II division 1 occlusion: a deep malocclusion arising from the upper incisors overriding the lower incisors. The upper and lower lip cannot approximate, causing hyperactivity of the mentalis muscle.

Compression neuropathy: impairment of nerve function manifest by pain, weakness or sensory loss or paresthesias, resulting from compression forces on the nerve

Computed tomography: imaging technique produced by computer analysis of an x-ray array of imaging information that allows images to be made of body structures, including soft tissue structures and organs

Contract-relax-release: a gentle voluntary muscle contraction followed by relaxation and then passive muscle elongation (1)

Conduction block: a localized interference of the conduction of an impulse in a nerve, causing nerve dysfunction

Contract-relax-assist: a gentle voluntary muscle contraction followed by relaxation, and then by gentle contraction of the antagonist of the first muscle to facilitate elongation of the first muscle (1)

Contracture: static muscle contraction or shortening

Coryza: acute inflammation of the nasal passages

Crepitus: 1. noise or vibration produced when bone or irregular cartilage surfaces are rubbed against each other; example: a sound on movement of the temporomandibular joint; 2. noise or vibration produced when thickened soft tissues rub across each other; example: a sound that appears to arise in the interscapular region with movement of the shoulder

Cumulative trauma disorder (CTD): involves damage to muscles, tendons, joints, and nerves that arises from prolonged or repetitive exposure to forces such as vibration, repetitive motion, and sustained muscle contraction

Denervation: loss of motor or sensory innervation of a part of the body, such as muscle, skin, or internal organ

Diaphoresis: perspiration

Diastasis recti: a separation of the right and left sides of the rectus abdominis muscles at the linea alba, most often caused by pregnancy

Disordered hip complex: the pathomechanics or most frequent pattern of muscle and joint dysfunction seen in patients with hip or groin pain (described in Chapter 11)

Diverticulosis: the presence of a number of pouches or sacs in the wall of the colon

Double crush: the concept that a peripheral nerve can be entrapped or compressed at two sites

Dysmenorrhea: difficult or painful menstruation

Dyspareunia: painful sexual intercourse

Dystonia: a syndrome of sustained muscle contractions, frequently causing twisting and repetitive movements or abnormal postures

Eccentric contractions: a muscle contraction that occurs while a muscle is lengthening

Endometriosis: endometrial tissue that is outside of the uterus, within the pelvis or abdominal cavity

Flexor retinaculum (FR): a thick fibrous band that arches over the deep groove on the palmar surface of the carpal bones, forming the anterior surface of the fibro-osseous carpal tunnel through which the median nerve and associated vascular structures and the flexor tendons of the thumb and fingers pass. It is attached medially to the pisiform and the hamulus of the hamate and laterally to the tuberosity of the scaphoid and the medial part of the palmar surface and the ridge of the trapezium.

Fluctuation test: test for the presence of minor knee effusion. With the patient in the supine position and the knee flexed to 15°, the clinician cradles the proximal patella (over the suprapatellar bursa) with the thumb and index finger. The thumb and index finger of the other hand are placed anterior to the knee joint next to the patella. While repeatedly pushing down on the suprapatellar bursa, the clinician assesses the degree of synovial fluid that shifts under the thumb and index finger of the opposite hand. The test is positive if fluid shifting actually occurs.

Focal dystonia: a localized dystonia often affecting only specific actions or motions

Functional unit: a group of agonist and antagonist muscles that function together as a unit in opposition or in synergy to move or stabilize a body part [because they share common spinal reflex responses] (1)

Gnathologic: pertaining to the dynamics of forces developed by and on the structures of mastication during function

Hallux abducto valgus: permanent deformity involving deviation of the great toe toward the lateral side of the foot, generally accompanied by bunion formation

Hammer toes: permanent flexion deformity at the midphalangeal joint of one or more toes, generally involves a cocking-up of the proximal phalanx

Heel spur syndrome: used to describe pain at the site of muscle and plantar fascia attachment to the medial calcaneal tubercle, which is often the site of a heel spur (research indicates that pain can occur in this site without a heel spur, and that heel spurs at this site are not necessarily symptomatic; see plantar fasciitis)

Intercuspal position: indicating the relationship between the teeth of the upper and lower jaws

Interincisal distance: measurement of mandibular opening, measured between the upper and lower incisor teeth, with a normal range of 45 to 60 mm

Introitus: entrance into a hollow organ, as in the entrance to the vagina

Joint dysfunction: an alteration in normal joint play and mobility involving change in one or more of the normal joint functions. For most joints, these functions include flexion, extension, lateral flexion, and rotation.

Kemp's test: a seated test to evaluate nerve root compression or facet syndrome by passively laterally flexing the torso and thoracolumbar spine and then pressing down on the shoulder. If pain (usually sharp) results on the side of compression, the test is positive.

Lachman test: test for the integrity of the anterior cruciate ligament. With the patient in the supine position and the knee flexed to 20°–30°, the clinician stabilizes the distal thigh with one hand. The other hand is placed medially and posteriorly over the proximal tibia; this hand performs an anterior translation of the tibia. The test is positive when excessive translation is noted.

Lacrimation: the forming of tears

Lateral break: a form of spinal manipulative therapy involving lateral to medial impulse to address restriction in lateral to medial joint play

Lateral epicondylitis (LE): tennis elbow, a repetitive strain injury involving inflammation and/or fibrosis and pain at the extensor tendon attachment at the lateral epicondyle

Lateral pivot shift test: test for the integrity of the anterior cruciate ligament, the lateral capsule, and the arcuate complex. With the patient in the supine position and the hips and knees slightly flexed, the clinician holds the patient's foot with one hand and the proximal posterior fibula with the other hand. After bringing the tibia in approximately 20° of internal rotation, the clinician applies a valgus force through the knee and moves the knee into 20° to 40° of flexion. The test is positive when the knee "gives way."

Ligamentum flavum: a spinal ligament that connects the anteroinferior surface of one lamina with posterosuperior surface of the one below. It extends laterally to the articular capsule and is present in the cervical, thoracic, and lumbar spine.

Lithotomy position: supine with the buttocks on the end of the table, the knees flexed, and the feet generally in stirrups

Lower crossed syndrome: term used by Janda to denote a common dysfunction in the lower torso in which the abdominal and gluteal muscles are weaker than normal, whereas the back extensors (erector spinae) and hip flexors are tight and shortened

Magnetic resonance imaging (MRI): the technique of creating images of the body with non-ionizing energy. The patient is placed in a strong magnetic field that causes protons in water to align themselves with the magnetic field. A radiofrequency (RF) pulse changes the axis of alignment. Analysis of the changes produced by the RF pulse allows an image to be created

Masticatory myofascial pain (MMFP): a regional muscle pain disorder in the head or neck characterized by muscle tenderness in masticatory muscles and pain in the jaw, face, ear, teeth, head, or neck

McMurray test: test for the integrity of the medial and lateral meniscus. With the patient in the supine position, the clinician flexes the patient's hip and knee and either internally or externally rotates the tibia. While maintaining internal rotation, the clinician applies a varus force to the joint line of the knee and extends the knee. While maintaining external rotation, the clinician applies a valgus force to the joint line and extends the knee. Internal rotation and a varus force tests the integrity of the lateral meniscus; external rotation and a valgus force tests the integrity of the medial meniscus. The test is positive when the patient has pain during the test or a palpable or audible click occurs.

Menometrorrhagia: excessively prolonged or profuse menstruation

Meralgia paresthetica: burning pain and paresthesias in the distribution of the anterolateral cutaneous branch of the femoral nerve, arising from trauma to or entrapment of the nerve at the inguinal ligament (2)

Monoparesis: weakness of one limb

Myofascial release technique (MRT): term to describe a variety of techniques of release of tissue, used here to denote a series of techniques starting with static compression of trigger points (or tissue adhesions affecting nerves), progressing to compression of trigger points with passive muscle elongation or stretching, and progressing to compression of trigger points during active stretch of the shortened muscle. (For a fuller discussion, see Chapter 6.)

Myopathic: a disorder primarily involving muscle

Myotome: the muscles that receive innervation from one segmental spinal nerve

Nerve conduction velocity (NCV) study: a study to assess the speed with which a nerve impulse is conducted through a nerve

Nerve excursion: the ability of nerves to elongate and slide between adjacent tissues during normal movement

Neurolymphatic points: pressure massage reflex points in the Touch for Health system, used to activate muscle function, and thought of as stimulating lymphatic drainage

Neuropathic pain: pain that is primarily a disorder of the nerves

Nociceptive: capable of sensing and transmitting pain

Nonspecific back pain: a term used to denote back pain in which a specific pain-generating tissue has not been identified (indicates that the user of the term is probably not curious about the specific pain-generating structure or structures)

Oral para-functional habits: undesirable oral habits such as fingernail biting, pencil chewing, prolonged use of pacifiers

Organomegaly: abnormal enlargement of internal organs

Origin–insertion massage: a technique involving pressure on the origin and insertion of a muscle. When pressure is directed away from the center of the muscle and toward the bone, the technique is thought to inactivate the muscle, and when pressure is directed toward the center of the muscle, the pressure is thought to activate the muscle.

Paresthesias: abnormal sensations such as burning or tingling

Patellofemoral grinding test: test for the integrity of the joint surfaces of the patellofemoral joint. With the patient in the supine position and the knee flexed to approximately 20°, the clinician places the web space of one hand at the superior aspect of the patella. The patient is asked to contract the quadriceps muscle, while the clinician maintains a caudally applied force. The test is positive when the patient is apprehensive or when the test reproduces the patient's pain complaint.

Pelvic obliquity: a twisting or torsion of the pelvis, usually involving rotation of one or both ilia and restriction of normal sacroiliac joint play

Percussion technique: a repetitive rhythmic tapping with a reflex hammer used to inactivate trigger points

Peripheral entrapment neuropathy: nerve irritation or inflammation occurring in the peripheral rather than the central nervous system and resulting from compression between anatomic structures, most frequently involving one or several shortened muscles

Pes cavus: foot structure involving abnormal height of the medial longitudinal arch

Pilomotor activity: action of the sympathetically innervated smooth muscles that make body hair stand more erect

Plantar fasciitis: used to describe pain at the site of the medial calcaneal tubercle or adjacent tissues that is generally most pronounced on first arising to standing from a seated or lying down position (research indicates that the pain often may arise from myofascial trigger points rather than true tissue inflammation of the plantar fascia)

Post isometric relaxation (PIR): a stretching technique that employs isometric exertion of the muscle first and then takes advantage of the relaxation following contraction to lengthen the muscle

Post-static dyskinesia: term applied to heel pain, indicating that pain arises when the foot goes from a resting position to a weight-bearing position

Posterior drawer test: test for the integrity of the posterior cruciate ligament and the posterior capsule. With the patient in the supine position and the knees flexed to 90°, the clinician sits on the toes of the patient. The clinician holds the proximal aspect of the tibia with both hands and places the index fingers on the medial and lateral hamstrings and the thumbs on the anterior joint line. The test involves the passive posterior translation of the tibia and is positive when excessive translation is noted.

Posterior prematurities: a characteristic of occlusion in which the posterior teeth meet prematurely, before the rest of the teeth surfaces

Postural rest closure: the mandibular rest position in which the teeth are not in occlusion, and an interocclusal or freeway space is created

Prolotherapy: the injection of a local irritant, generally dextrose, into ligaments; intended to cause an inflammatory response and tissue fibrosis to strengthen a ligament that is thought to be lax or inadequately stabilizing a joint

Pronator teres syndrome (PTS): compression of the median nerve just distal to the elbow, an entrapment between the two heads of the pronator teres muscle. Symptoms are generally very similar to carpal tunnel syndrome because of the distal symptoms that often result from compression anywhere in a peripheral nerve; may be a contributing factor in cases of carpal tunnel syndrome.

Pseudo-dystonia: a dystonia-like syndrome that appears to derive from peripheral muscular imbalance and coordination caused by myofascial dysfunction rather than by a central nervous system disorder

Rotator interval: an area of the anterior shoulder joint capsule that some authors believe is weakened, predisposes the patient to instability, and should be obliterated during stabilization surgeries. It is defined as the space between the superior border of the subscapularis and the supraspinatus and includes the region of the following: the superior and middle glenohumeral, and the coracohumeral ligaments.

Sag test: test for the integrity of the posterior cruciate ligament and the posterior capsule. With the patient in the supine position with the hips and knees flexed to 90°, the clinician notes any "sagging" of the tibia posteriorly. The test is positive when the tibia indeed "sags" posteriorly.

Scapular dyskinesia: abnormal function and mobility of the scapula, generally involving alteration of scapulohumeral rhythm or the coordinated rotational movement of the scapula that accompanies abduction and adduction of the humerus

Sclerotome: tissues arising from the same fetal mesenchymal layer of cells (they migrate during fetal development and, by birth, are often no longer anatomically close to each other)

Scotomata (positive abnormal phenomena): a blind spot in the visual field or field of vision

Somatovisceral: arising from the soma or musculoskeletal structures but giving rise to changes in the viscera or organs, including referred pain from muscle trigger points to visceral organs

Sprain: injury involving disruption of ligamentous tissue

Stomatognathic: refers to the structures involved in speech and eating, including chewing and swallowing

Strain: injury involving disruption of muscle tissue

Subluxation: an abnormality of position or movement of spinal segments or other joints, also involving the accompanying changes in nerve conduction, muscle tension, circulation, and lymphatic drainage

Sudomotor activity: activity of the sympathetic nerves that stimulates the sweat glands to produce perspiration

Tachycardia: abnormally rapid heartbeat

Tachypnea: abnormally rapid respiration

Tennis elbow (TE): lateral epicondylitis, a repetitive strain injury involving inflammation and/or fibrosis and pain at the site of extensor muscle tendon attachment to the lateral epicondyle

Thoracic outlet syndrome: compression of elements of the brachial plexus in the neck or in the shoulder region. Symptoms include pain, sensory loss, and weakness in the arm and hand. The accompanying vascular structures such as the subclavian artery and vein also can be compressed, causing peripheral ischemic or embolic symptoms.

Transverse friction massage: technique used to dislodge tissue adhesions, fibrosis, or trigger points by vigorous rubbing across the direction of the muscle fibers, intended to produce minor injury and stimulate healing

Trigger point pressure release: application of slowly increasing non-painful [or readily tolerated] pressure over a trigger point until a barrier of tissue resistance is encountered. Contact is then maintained until the tissue barrier releases, and pressure is increased to reach a new barrier to eliminate the trigger point tension and tenderness. (1)

Vaginismus: painful spasm of the vaginal muscles preventing intercourse (or entry for examination purposes)

Valgus force: force applied to the lateral knee joint line in a lateral–medial direction

Valgus tests: test for the integrity of the medial capsule and tibial collateral ligament when performed in 30° of knee flexion; test for the integrity of the medial capsule, tibial collateral ligament, anterior and posterior ligaments, and posteromedial capsule when performed in full knee extension. With the patient in a supine position, the clinician abducts the leg and flexes the knee to approximately 30°. The clinician brings the tibia in a varus position and then abducts the tibia to check for excessive laxity in the medial joint space. The test is repeated with the knee in full extension. The test is positive when excessive laxity is observed with the knee in 30° of flexion or when any movement is observed with the knee in full extension.

Varus force: force applied to the medial knee joint line in a medial–lateral direction

Varus tests: test for the integrity of the lateral capsule and lateral collateral ligament when performed in 30° of knee flexion; test for the integrity of the lateral capsule, lateral collateral ligament, anterior and posterior ligaments, and posterolateral capsule when performed in full knee extension. With the patient in a supine position, the clinician abducts the leg and flexes the knee to approximately 30°. The clinician brings the tibia in a neutral or mid position (no abduction or adduction of the tibia) and then adducts the tibia to check for excessive laxity in the lateral joint space. The test is repeated with the knee in full extension. The test is positive when excessive laxity is observed with the knee in 30° of flexion or when any movement is observed with the knee in full extension.

Viscerosomatic: arising from the organs but referred to the soma or musculoskeletal structures

Vulvar vestibulitis: a subset of vulvodynia described as an intense burning pain when the vulvar tissues are touched; usually the tissues are not painful unless touched

Vulvodynia: an intense burning pain in the superficial tissues that are innervated by the pudendal nerve, includes external skin as well as burning and itching within the vagina

Whole nerve syndrome: concept that nerve entrapments often involve not one or two sites of entrapment, but a more general disturbance of nerve excursion with multiple tiny adhesions or larger sites of compression that produce a traction neuropathy

References

1. Simons DG, Travell JG, Simons LS. Travell & Simons' Myofascial Pain and Dysfunction: The Trigger Point Manual, vol 1: Upper Half of Body. 2nd Ed. Baltimore: Lippincott Williams & Wilkins, 1999:1–10.
2. Travell JG, Simons DG. Myofascial Pain and Dysfunction: The Trigger Point Manual, vol 2: The Lower Extremities. Baltimore: Lippincott Williams & Wilkins, 1993:226–235.

Index

Page numbers followed by an f denote figures; those followed by a t denote tables